AF593377

Occupational Medicine Practice Guidelines

EVALUATION AND MANAGEMENT OF COMMON HEALTH PROBLEMS AND FUNCTIONAL RECOVERY OF WORKERS

Second Edition

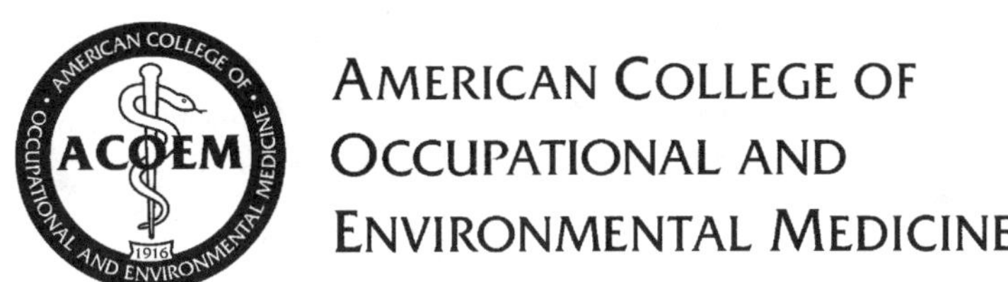

Edited by
Lee S. Glass, MD

Contributing Editors
Bernard R. Blais, MD, FACOEM, FAAO, FACS
Elizabeth Genovese, MD, MBA, FAADEP
Michael N. Goertz, MD, MPH, FACOEM
Jeffrey S. Harris, MD, MPH, MBA, FACOEM
Harold E. Hoffman, MD, CCFP, FACOEM, FRCPC
Julia E. Klees, MD, MPH, FACOEM
C. David Rowlett, MD, MS

OEM Press
Beverly Farms, Massachusetts

Second Edition

ISBN 1-883595-42-8

Library of Congress Cataloging in Publication Data

American College of Occupational and Environmental Medicine.
Occupational medicine practice guidelines : evaluation and management of common health problems and functional recovery in workers / the American College of Occupational and Environmental Medicine ; edited by Lee S. Glass. — 2nd ed.
p. ; cm.
Includes bibliographical references and index.
ISBN 1-883595-42-8
1. Medicine, Industrial—Standards. I. Glass, Lee S. II. Title.
[DNLM: 1. Occupational Diseases—diagnosis. 2. Occupational Diseases—therapy. 3. Occupational Health Services—standards. 4. Occupational Medicine—standards. WA 400 A513o 2003]
RC963.3.O245 2003
: 616.9′803—dc22 2003064962

Printed in the United States of America

OEM Press® is a registered trademark of OEM Health Information, Inc.

OEM Press
8 West Street
Beverly Farms, Massachusetts 01915
1-800-533-8046
1-978-921-7300
www.oempress.com

10 9 8 7 6 5 4 3 2

Disclaimer

The American College of Occupational and Environmental Medicine provides this segment of guidelines for practitioners and notes that decisions to adopt particular courses of actions must be made by trained practitioners on the basis of the available resources and the particular circumstances presented by the individual patient. Accordingly, the American College of Occupational and Environmental Medicine and OEM Health Information, Inc. disclaim responsibility for any injury or damage resulting from actions taken by practitioners after considering these guidelines.

Contents

I. Foundations of Occupational Medicine Practice

1. Prevention 1

2. General Approach to Initial Assessment and Documentation 21

3. Initial Approaches to Treatment 43

4. Work-Relatedness 55

5. Cornerstones of Disability Prevention and Management 75

6. Pain, Suffering, and the Restoration of Function 105

7. Independent Medical Examinations and Consultations 127

II. Presenting Complaints

8. Neck and Upper Back Complaints 165

10. Elbow Complaints 227

11. Forearm, Wrist, and Hand Complaints 253

12. Low Back Complaints 287

13. Knee Complaints 329

Tables

3. Initial Approaches to Treatment

5. Cornerstones of Disability Prevention and Management

7. Independent Medical Examinations and Consultations

8. Neck and Upper Back Complaints

9. Shoulder Complaints

10. Elbow Complaints

11. Forearm, Wrist, and Hand Complaints

12. Low Back Complaints

13. Knee Complaints

14. Ankle and Foot Complaints

15. Stress-related Conditions

16. Eye

Algorithms

8. Neck and Upper Back Complaints

9. Shoulder Complaints

10. Elbow Complaints

11. Forearm, Wrist, and Hand Complaints

12. Low Back Complaints

13. Knee Complaints

14. Ankle and Foot Complaints

16. Eye

Preface to the Second Edition

Like the first edition of the American College of Occupational and Environmental Medicine's *Occupational Medicine Practice Guidelines*, this second edition provides information and guidance on generally accepted elements of quality care in occupational and environmental medicine. Likewise, the goal of the second edition remains the same: to improve the efficiency with which the diagnostic process is conducted, the specificity of each diagnostic test performed, and the effectiveness of each treatment in relieving symptoms and achieving cure.

As the American College of Occupational and Environmental Medicine (ACOEM) prepared to begin the process of review and revision of the first edition material, medical societies representing virtually all specialties involved in occupational medicine were invited to appoint one or more of their members to assist ACOEM in updating the guidelines. Consequently, the guidelines in this volume represent the current, collective voice of health care professionals across the spectrum of specialists who treat work-related injuries and occupational diseases. The individual representatives of the various specialty societies and the independent reviewers involved in the process of updating this edition are listed in the Acknowledgments.

The audience for the first edition of these guidelines has included not only health care providers, but also insurance professionals, attorneys, and others involved in the administration of workers' compensation systems. To paraphrase Sir Winston Churchill (in his remarks about the British and Americans), our audience is comprised of a single people divided by a common language: For example, the term *causation* may turn a doctor's reflections to Koch's postulates, while the same word may trigger an attorney to think of a particular law or administrative regulation. In perhaps no other area of medicine is the ability of a patient to obtain needed medical care as closely tied to the ability of patients, physicians, insurance representatives, and others to communicate clearly as it is in occupational medicine. It is regrettable that mutual frustration, rather than mutual cooperation, is too often the norm in workers' compensation interactions. This edition of the *Guidelines* seeks to address such issues, in part by including an updated and expanded discussion of causation, standardizing the medical terminology, and addressing other matters of medicolegal significance.

This edition, like its predecessor, includes disability-duration data that reflect expert consensus opinion. New to this edition is disability-duration data that have been extracted from National Health Interview Survey (NHIS) data. NHIS databases are compiled by the Division for Health Interview Statistics for the National Center for Health Statistics, which in turn is part of the US Centers for Disease Control and Prevention (CDC). The databases represent the codified responses from structured interviews of individuals with a variety of medical conditions.

For purposes of further developing and improving the disability-duration recommendations in this edition, only data from interviews with individuals without workers' compensation claims has been included. The expert consensus disability-duration data from the first edition of the *Guidelines* has been updated and, for each condition, the disability-duration data reflecting the average median time the NHIS interviewees missed work in the past year, and the percentage of interviewees with the condition who missed no work as a result, has been added.

Because occupational eye injuries are unfortunately common and carry the potential for severe impairment, this edition of the *Guidelines* contains a completely rewritten and updated chapter on eye injuries. The clinician will find a comprehensive series of guidelines that provide practical recommendations for the prevention, evaluation, and treatment of these work-related conditions. Because it can be difficult for physicians seeing injured workers with occupational eye injuries and diseases to quickly obtain practical, straightforward information needed to treat them, ACOEM has created a problem-oriented chapter for this edition.

The Appendix, written by Elizabeth Genovese, MD, is new to this edition. It is a short, but thorough introduction to the topic of evidence-based medicine. Those of us who participated in updating the ACOEM *Guidelines* believe that quality, evidence-based medicine practice is a worthy goal for individual doctors as well as professional societies. We are confident that all who read the Appendix will garner a solid understanding of evidence-based medicine and the benefits it can bring to doctors, patients, our health care system, and society as a whole.

Lee S. Glass, MD
Chair, ACOEM Practice Guidelines Committee

Acknowledgments

The depth of services provided by each participant in the updating process was remarkable. Contributors reviewed at least one chapter each and reviewed the relevant medical literature that had been published since the creation of the original *Guidelines* in 1997. ACOEM gratefully acknowledges the medical library research services provided by Work Loss Data Institute, with which it contracted for that assistance. Following the chapter and literature review, participants provided written or verbal comments to ACOEM's Practice Guidelines Committee.

Verbal comments were in the form of participation in multi-specialty conference calls, during which the issues raised in each chapter were extensively discussed. Participation in such calls typically originated from all regions of the United States and Canada. Following these discussions, draft chapters were prepared and distributed by ACOEM to all chapter reviewers. Follow-up multi-specialty teleconference(s) were then held as appropriate, during which time the draft was again reviewed. Invariably, significant enhancements evolved as a result of the ensuing dialog that occurred during these teleconferences. In most cases, the teleconferences were conducted in four-hour time blocks, and all reviewers who participated in the extensive collective conversation that produced the guidelines in this volume did so without compensation.

ACOEM is deeply grateful and extends its sincere thanks for the commitment to the highest standards of professionalism that each reviewer has shown, and without which this edition would not have been possible.

Practice Guidelines Developers and Contributors

The second edition to the ACOEM *Occupational Medicine Practice Guidelines* were developed from the original by the ACOEM Practice Guidelines Committee under the direction of the Chair, Lee S. Glass, MD. Eight committee members acted as chapter leads for the various 16 chapters and appendix as follows:

1. **Prevention**
   Jeffrey S. Harris, MD, MPH, MBA, FACOEM
2. **General Approach to Initial Assessment and Documentation**
   Bernard R. Blais, MD, FACOEM, FAAO, FACS
3. **Initial Approaches to Treatment**
   Julia E. Klees, MD, MPH, FACOEM
4. **Work-Relatedness**
   Elizabeth Genovese, MD, MBA, FAADEP
5. **Cornerstones of Disability Prevention and Management**
   Michael N. Goertz, MD, MPH, FACOEM
6. **Pain, Suffering, and Restoration of Function**
   Lee S. Glass, MD
7. **Independent Medical Examinations and Consultations**
   Julia E. Klees, MD, MPH, FACOEM
8. **Neck and Upper Back Complaints**
   Michael N. Goertz, MD, MPH, FACOEM
9. **Shoulder Complaints**
   Harold E. Hoffman, MD, CCFP, FACOEM, FRCPC
10. **Elbow Complaints**
    Lee S. Glass, MD
11. **Forearm, Wrist, and Hand Complaints**
    C. David Rowlett, MD, MS
12. **Low Back Complaints**
    Elizabeth Genovese, MD, MBA, FAADEP
13. **Knee Complaints**
    Lee S. Glass, MD
14. **Ankle and Foot Complaints**
    Jeffrey S. Harris, MD, MPH, MBA, FACOEM
15. **Stress-related Conditions**
    Lee S. Glass, MD
16. **Eye**
    Bernard R. Blais, MD, FACOEM, FAAO, FACS

Appendix **Evidence-based Medicine: What does it mean? Why do we care?**
Elizabeth Genovese, MD, MBA, FAADEP

Other members of the committee who assisted in the preparation of the *Guidelines* were: Jennifer H. Christian, MD, MPH, FACPM; Philip I. Harber, MD, MPH, FACOEM, FCCP; John P. Holland, MD, MPH, FACOEM; Kathryn L. Mueller, MD, MPH, FACEP, FACOEM; Douglas J. Patron, MD, MSPH; Bernyce M. Peplowski, DO, MS; and Jack Richman, MD, CCFP, DOHS, FACOEM. Timothy J. Key, MD, MPH, FACOEM, as Responsible Officer and ACOEM President Elect, and Edward A. Emmett, MD, MS, FACOEM, Chair of the ACOEM Council on Occupational and Environmental

Medical Practice, contributed to the development of the guidelines as well. A special thanks is extended to ACOEM staff who oversaw the administration of this project: Marianne Dreger, Barry Eisenberg, Debra Paddack, Rebecca Schmarje, and Darleene Shah.

Affiliations of Practice Guidelines Committee Members

Bernard R. Blais, MD, FACOEM, FAAO, FACS, is Clinical Professor of Ophthalmology at Albany Medical College, Albany, New York, and President of Blais Consulting Ltd., Clifton Park, New York. He is Co-chair of the ACOEM Sensory Perception Committee and serves on the Council on Scientific Affairs. He is board certified in ophthalmology.

Jennifer H. Christian, MD, MPH, FACPM, is President and Chief Medical Officer of Webility Corporation in Wayland, Massachusetts. She is Chair of the ACOEM Work Fitness and Disability Section and the Committee on Return to Work, and serves on the Council on Occupational and Environmental Medical Practice and Council on Special Occupational Health Interests. She is board certified in occupational medicine.

Elizabeth Genovese, MD, MBA, FAADEP, is Medical Director for IMX Medical Management Systems of Bala Cynwyd, Pennsylvania, and Mercy WorkCare, and serves on the faculty of the University of Pennsylvania School of Medicine. She is Chair of the ACOEM Committee on Coding and Classification, a member of the Council on Occupational and Environmental Medical Practice, Course Director of the Musculoskeletal Examination and Treatment Course, and ACOEM representative to the CPT Advisory Panel. She is board certified in both occupational medicine and internal medicine.

Lee S. Glass, MD, is Associate Medical Director for the State of Washington, Department of Labor and Industries, in Olympia, Washington. He is a member of the ACOEM Council on Occupational and Environmental Medical Practice, current Chair of the Practice Guidelines Committee and editor of the second edition of the *ACOEM Occupational Medicine Practice Guidelines.*

Michael N. Goertz, MD, MPH, FACOEM, is the Medical Director for the Department of Occupational Medicine Park Nicollet Clinic in Minneapolis, Minnesota. He is board certified in occupational medicine.

Philip I. Harber, MD, MPH, FACOEM, FCCP, is Professor of Family Medicine, Vice Chair-Academic Affairs, and Chief, Division of Occupational and Environmental Medicine, at the University of California, Los Angeles. He is a member of the ACOEM Board of Directors and Chair of the Council on Scientific Affairs. He is board certified in occupational medicine, pulmonary medicine, and internal medicine.

Jeffrey S. Harris, MD, MPH, MBA, FACOEM, is Associate Clinical Professor, University of California at San Francisco, University of Utah, and Medical College of Wisconsin. He is President of J. Harris Associates, Inc. of Mill Valley, California and works for The Permanente Medical Group. He served as Chair of the ACOEM Practice Guidelines Committee from 1996-1998 and was editor of the first edition of the ACOEM *Occupational Medicine Practice Guidelines.* He holds IME and medical quality certifications and is board certified in occupational medicine, emergency medicine, and public health and general preventive medicine.

Harold E. Hoffman, MD, CCFP, FACOEM, FRCPC, is Adjunct Associate Clinical Professor, Department of Public Health Sciences, Faculty of Medicine and Dentistry, at the University of Alberta in Edmonton, Alberta, Canada. He serves as Director for ACOEM's Basic Curriculum in Occupational Medicine course. He is a Fellow of the Royal College of Physicians of Canada (occupational medicine).

John P. Holland, MD, MPH, FACOEM, is a Principle of Holland Associates, Inc., an occupational and environmental medicine and health services consulting firm in Seattle, Washington. He is an Assistant Clinical Professor in the Departments of Orthopedics and Environmental and

Occupational Health Sciences, University of Washington. He serves on the ACOEM Board of Directors as the current President (2003-2004) and was Chair of the Practice Guidelines Committee from 1998 to 2000. He is board certified in occupational medicine.

Julia E. Klees, MD, MPH, FACOEM, is Associate Corporate Medical Director of BASF Corporation of Mount Olive, New Jersey. She is board certified in both occupational medicine and internal medicine.

Kathryn L. Mueller, MD, MPH, FACOEM, FACEP, is Associate Professor in Preventive Medicine and Emergency Medicine at the University of Colorado Health Sciences Center, and Medical Director of the Colorado Division of Workers' Compensation. She serves as Associate Chair of the Practice Guidelines Committee and is a member of the ACOEM Board of Directors. She is board certified in occupational medicine.

Douglas J. Patron, MD, MSPH, is Medical Director for Concentra of Houston, Texas. He is board certified in both occupational medicine and internal medicine.

Bernyce M. Peplowski, DO, MS, is Regional Coordinator for Occupational Health Services for Southern California Permanente Medical Group in Baldwin Park, California. She is board certified in occupational medicine and has completed a fellowship in health professions education.

Jack Richman, MD, CCFP, DOHS, FACOEM, is Executive Vice President and Medical Director of Assessmed Inc. of Mississauga, Ontario, Canada. He is a member-at-large of the ACOEM Council on Occupational and Environmental Medical Practice. He holds a specialty certification in family practice and is certified by the Canadian Board of Occupational Medicine (CCBOM).

C. David Rowlett, MD, MS, is employed by the Medical Department of BWXT-Pantex of Amarillo, Texas. He holds masters degrees in both chemical engineering and preventive medicine. He is board certified in occupational medicine.

Specialty Society and Society Representative Listing

The American College of Occupational and Environmental Medicine (ACOEM) acknowledges the following organizations and their representatives who participated in the process to update the ACOEM *Occupational Medicine Practice Guidelines*, second edition. Their contributions are greatly appreciated.

Academy of Organizational and Occupational Psychiatry
Alexandria, Virginia
C. Donald Williams, MD, CGP
Yakima, Washington

American Academy of Disability Evaluating Physicians
Chicago, Illinois
Edwin Klimek, MD
Niagara Health System, Department of Medicine
St. Catharine's, Ontario, Canada

American Academy of Neurology
St. Paul, Minnesota
Edwin Klimek, MD
Niagara Health System, Department of Medicine,
St. Catharine's, Ontario, Canada

American Academy of Ophthalmology
San Francisco, California
M. Bowes Hamill, MD, FAAO
Baylor College of Medicine, Department of Ophthalmology
Cullen Eye Institute, Houston, Texas

American Academy of Physical Medicine and Rehabilitation
Chicago, Illinois
Jonathan S. Halperin, MD
Sharp Rees Stealy Medical Group
La Mesa, California

Michael Saffir, MD
Orthopaedic Specialty Group
Fairfield, Connecticut

Hillel M. Sommer, MD, FRCPC, FAAPMR
Associated Sports & Spine Physicians
Winnipeg, Manitoba, Canada

American Association for Hand Surgery, Chicago, Illinois
Kevin C. Chung, MD, MS, FACS
University of Michigan Medical Center
Ann Arbor, Michigan

M. Felix Freshwater, MD
Miami Institute of Hand and Microsurgery
Miami, Florida

Nash Naam, MD, FACS, FICS
St. Anthony's Memorial Hospital
Effingham, Illinois

American Association of Occupational Health Nurses, Inc.
Atlanta, Georgia
Mary Lou Wassel, MEd, RN, COHN-S/CM, ARM
Risk Consultants, Inc., Atlanta, Georgia

American Board of Independent Medical Examiners
Barrington, Illinois
Alan L. Colledge, MD
Labor Commission of Utah, Salt Lake City, Utah

American College of Emergency Physicians
Irving, Texas
Participation in the development of these guidelines does not imply endorsement by the ACEP
Raymond G. Hart, MD, MPH, FACEP
Center for Hand Injury Prevention and Research
Christine M. Kleinert Institute for Hand and Microsurgery, Louisville, Kentucky

William C. Dalsey, MD, MBA, FACEP
Kimball Medical Center, Lakewood, New Jersey

American College of Radiology
Reston, Virginia
David Rubin, MD
Mallinckrodt Institute of Radiology
St. Louis, Missouri

American Optometric Association
St. Louis, Missouri
Jeffrey L. Weaver, OD, MS, MBA, FAAO
American Optometric Association
St. Louis, Missouri

American Osteopathic Association
Chicago, Illinois
Tim Pinsky, DO, MPH, FACOEM, FAOCOPM, FAADEP
Best Med Consultants, Marlton, New Jersey

American Physical Therapy Association
Alexandria, Virginia
Jill Galper, PT, MEd
MossReHab, Philadelphia, Pennsylvania

American Podiatric Medical Association
Bethesda, Maryland
Pamela Colman, DPM
American Podiatric Medical Association
Bethesda, Maryland

David M. Schofield, DPM, FCFO
Elmira, New York

American Psychological Association
Washington, DC
Participation in the development of these guidelines does not imply endorsement by the APA
James R. Callan, PhD, FAPA
Pacific Science & Engineering Group
San Diego, California

Michael E. Geisser, PhD
University of Michigan Medical Center
Ann Arbor, Michigan

Dennis C. Harper, PhD, FAACP, FAPA, FAACPDM
Center for Disabilities and Development,
University of Iowa, Iowa City, Iowa

American Society of Anesthesiologists
Park Ridge, Illinois
David P. Martin, MD, PhD
Mayo Clinic, Department of Anesthesiology
Rochester, Minnesota

American Society of Plastic Surgeons
Arlington Heights, Illinois
Craig H. Johnson, MD
Mayo Clinic, Section of Plastic Surgery
Rochester, Minnesota

Association of Rheumatology Health Professionals
Atlanta, Georgia
Maura D. Iversen, ScD, MPH, PT
Division of Rheumatology, Immunology & Allergy, Boston, Massachusetts

Phillip McClure, PhD, PT
Arcadia University, Glenside, Pennsylvania

Carol A. Oatis, PhD, PT
Arcadia University, Department of Physical Therapy, Glenside, Pennsylvania

Ewa Roos, PT, PhD
Lund University Hospital, Department of Orthopedics, Lund, Sweden

Cheryl Riegger-Krugh, ScD, PT
University of Colorado Health Sciences Center
Denver, Colorado

Canadian Neurological Society
Calgary, Alberta, Canada
Participation in the development of these guidelines does not imply endorsement by the CNS
Edwin Klimek, MD
Niagara Health System, Department of Medicine
St. Catharine's, Ontario, Canada

Chiropractic Health Care Section of American Public Health Association
Washington, DC
Robert Mootz, DC, FICC, FABS
State of Washington Department of Labor and Industries, Olympia, Washington

Society for Vascular Surgery
Chicago, Illinois
Herbert I. Machleder, MD, FACS
University of California, UCLA Division of Vascular Surgery, Los Angeles, California

Independent Reviewers

Albert J. Osbahr, MD, FAAFP, FACOEM
Haywood Regional Medical Center
Clyde, North Carolina

Thomas J. Tredici, MD, FAAO
USAF School of Aerospace Medicine
Brooks Air Force Base, Texas

John M. Williams, Sr., MD, MPH, FAAO
Community Health Care Clinics
Wausau, Wisconsin

Edward G. Zurad, MD, FAAFP, MACOEM
Tyler Memorial Hospital
Tunkhannock, Pennsylvania

Editor's Note

This second edition of the ACOEM *Occupational Medicine Practice Guidelines* would be incomplete without special thanks to Jeffrey S. Harris, MD, MPH. Without Dr. Harris' leadership, the first edition of the *Guidelines* may never have been developed. It is upon the stable foundation of the earlier text that this edition rests.

Dr. Harris has continued his many contributions to the field of occupational medicine through his sustained, active participation in the development of this edition of the *Guidelines.* His many insights and cogently critical remarks have added greatly to the value of this work. We are deeply appreciative of Dr. Harris' on-going assistance.

I. *Foundations of Occupational Medicine Practice*

1 Prevention

General Principles

Prevention of work-related health complaints should be a top priority for occupational health professionals. Diagnosis and treatment of workers presenting with work-related health problems represent an opportunity to prevent recurrences in those workers (tertiary prevention), to mitigate the effects of current work-related hazards so as to reduce the duration of the problem (secondary prevention), and to prevent the same problems in coworkers and those in similar jobs (primary prevention).

Occupational health professionals can often identify opportunities for prevention. Understanding job and work requirements may suggest possibilities for primary prevention of work-related illness or injury through hazard identification. A workplace "walk through" is also useful to attain familiarity with job requirements and the work environment as one element of fitness-for-duty assessment. The discovery of significant work factors suggests that worksite intervention to prevent recurrences and hasten recovery may well be appropriate.

A cluster of cases in a work group suggests a probability of previously unidentified problems in work design or management. The presence of work-related discomfort, illness, or injury should trigger a search for causes (see Chapter 4, "Work-Relatedness") and plans for remediation. Different levels of certainty about the cause of the problem and differences in the severity of the adverse effects on health may justify different levels of response.

The practitioner's task in prevention is first to identify associated or causative workplace and personal factors. The practitioner should then suggest scientifically based selection and screening of personnel and engineering controls and task or job redesign, as well as treatment and disability management of the immediate health problem. Further preventive efforts may include personal protective equipment, administrative changes, education, and training at all levels of the company; close attention to the psychological needs of the employees; proper medical surveillance of the workplace; and the opportunity for contact with a health care provider if questions or complaints arise. Whether the job is a match with the capabilities of the individual worker should be investigated. There is enough variation in strength, flexibility, endurance, healing capacity, anatomy, and other factors among workers that individual investigation is warranted because statistical risks apply only generally to individuals (see "Person-Job Fit").

Evaluating the Evidence for Preventive Action: Causation and Association

DIAGNOSIS: KEY TO ANALYZING ASSOCIATION

The first element in seeking an association between a work-related health problem and a worksite factor is an accurate diagnosis. Epidemiologic studies generally correlate exposures with specific pathologic entities. Alternatively, some studies have correlated levels of symptoms, rather than diagnoses, with worksite exposures or tasks. These correlations are useful to help prevent health-related "complaints," but increased frequency or intensity of symptoms alone should not be equated with causation or potential prevention of specific pathologic entities (e.g., diagnoses), such as carpal tunnel syndrome or disk herniation, for example.

USE OF QUALITATIVE INFORMATION

Occupational health practitioners making recommendations for prevention of work-related complaints are still faced with a lack of quantitative associative information for many common problems. An individual worker's symptoms themselves may decrease productivity and cause discomfort. As such, clinicians are obligated by public health principles to mitigate the symptoms and to prevent a delay in recovery and recurrences in the individual as well as occurrences in others. Such actions often must be taken on a case-by-case basis using information about worker-job fit as well as preliminary or population data.

The current scientific literature about potentially work-related musculoskeletal disorders (WRMSDs), degenerative disorders such as degenerative joint or disk disease, and a number of other nonspecific symptoms and conditions (e.g., visual fatigue, commonly known as "eye strain," and associated headaches and neck and shoulder complaints, stress-related complaints, nonspecific chest pain, respiratory symptoms thought to be due to indoor air pollution, and others) is notable for a lack of studies that temporally and quantitatively define causal associations of work exposures. There are very few prospective studies; most are cross-sectional or case-control studies, which do not allow determination of temporal association. Other information is derived from physiology laboratory measurements rather than clinical observation in real work situations.

Further, almost all available studies either define exposure to work-related factors qualitatively or use job title as a proxy. In almost all cases there has been no quantification of specific ergonomic or other stressors to allow determination of a dose-response curve. If there were dose-response relationships, one might find thresholds at which WRMSDs and other work-related symptom complexes might or might not occur. Thus, at present, risk factors that have been found to be associated with or predictive of certain WRMSDs and other syndromes have not necessarily been found to be causal for these entities. Due to the absence of certainty regarding causality and the lack of quantitative exposure-response data, most recommendations for the prevention of WRMSDs will be qualitative. While practitioners must make good-faith efforts to prevent these complaints, these assumptions should not extend to opinions about causation for benefits or medicolegal purposes. The commonly seen statement "in the absence of other obvious causes, the problem is work related" is at odds with scientific logic and should not be used (see also Chapter 4).

COMPLEX CAUSATION

The occupational health practitioner also should be aware that many musculoskeletal, psychological, and other problems often are caused by several work- and non-work-related factors in varying combinations. Many potentially work-related complaints result from more than one factor. Some factors are work-related and others are personal. The work factors are necessary, but not sufficient in many cases. For example, not all workers exposed to certain numbers of repetitions and degrees of force during hand manipulations will develop tenosynovitis of the wrist and hand, but a few of them would develop the problem without significant ergonomic exposure at work or during performance of non-job-related daily activities or a hobby. In other cases, there may be a variety of possible causes for a disorder or complaint as well as personal and work factors that come into play. For example, pregnancy, hypothyroidism, or obesity may be associated with carpal tunnel syndrome in susceptible individuals. Population studies have identified such competing causes in a number of instances (see Chapter 4 for further details). Both work and personal factors may need to be addressed to prevent initial episodes, delayed recovery, or recurrences.

CHRONIC PAIN VERSUS WORK-RELATED PROBLEMS

Practitioners should be very careful to differentiate work-related problems from chronic pain (see Chapter 6). Musculoskeletal pain that develops with minimal exposure to defined work factors, that is related to positioning of equipment, and that involves several areas of the back or upper extremities may well be chronic pain that is not specifically related to job or task design. A history of such symptoms currently or in the past is helpful in making the distinction. These cases are often costly and involve a great deal of lost time and ineffective treatment.

PERSON-JOB FIT

Many "personal factors" are in reality a mismatch between the worker's abilities and job demands, or person-job fit. Ensuring proper person-job fit is important to prevent discomfort, loss of productivity, and physical injury to workers. (One conceptual view characterizes a person-job mismatch that leads to symptoms or the development of diffuse pain at work as work intolerance.) The general duty to provide a safe workplace mandates proper placement of workers while avoiding unjustifiable discrimination.

Workers may vary in their capacity to lift, exert force, perform fine motor tasks, etc. according to general or specific health status, age, conditioning, size, strength, and other factors. Physical functional abilities rise and fall over the worker's lifespan. Abilities also vary from worker to worker depending on conditioning, impairment, and innate capacity. The decline in cardiorespiratory and musculoskeletal functional capacity with age can be delayed or accelerated by physical conditioning (or lack thereof), overuse, illness (including chronic pain), and injury.

The visual system also undergoes predictable and anticipated changes during the lifespan of an individual. The natural hyperopia (far-sightedness) of an infant tends to lessen or to transition to myopia (near-sightedness) at approximately 20 years of age. All eyes have a progressive decrease in accommodation (focusing at near point).[1]

FITNESS-FOR-DUTY EVALUATION: ASSESSING PERSON-JOB FIT

Occupational physicians are often called on to determine this person-job match, sometimes termed "fitness for duty." To determine fitness for duty, it is often necessary to "medically" gauge the capacity of the individual compared with the objective physical requirements of the job based on the safety and performance needs of the employer and expressed as essential job functions. However, an objective statement from employers of the physical requirements of the job may not be available to physicians, so such assessment may be performed without complete workplace information. Further, as noted earlier, studies correlating physical testing with risk of complaints or injuries often are not validated or not available.

On a practical level, the fitness-for-duty evaluation of a worker must address a continuum of historical and physical findings from reports of occasional symptoms of musculoskeletal discomfort to a definitive diagnosis and active evidence of a significant musculoskeletal disorder that may functionally limit the individual. The challenge is to fairly and accurately evaluate the individual for fitness to perform the job, often not on the basis of quantifiable risk, but on professional opinion regarding what he or she can or cannot do. The worker's past history of pain or dysfunction in specific work settings can be quite useful in gauging the probable reaction to work factors, positioning, scheduling, the need for stretching and activity breaks, etc. For those whose work entails significant physical labor, a change in career or work duties may

[1] Infants have natural hyperopia of 2 to 30 diopters. At age 10, the amplitude of accommodation is 14 diopters, declining to 4 diopters at age 45 and 1 diopter at age 60. (It takes 3 diopters at the near point of accommodation to keep a target at 1 meter in focus.)

be necessary due to the decline in functional capacity with age or other factors. This also may be true of patients with current or past diffuse, rapid-onset, or chronic musculoskeletal pain.

Employers should carefully assess whether employees can tolerate a given job or work environment either at the time they are initially employed or on a routine basis subsequently, particularly when job requirements mandate a certain level of physical conditioning or, at the very least, the absence of undue sensitivities to physical, environmental, or mental stress. In circumstances where employees' physical or mental abilities are not compatible with job and worksite requirements due to baseline factors or due to aging or disease, it is not uncommon for them to experience physical or mental discomfort in the course of their employment.

Employers who consider worker-job fit may be able to prevent both injuries and symptomatic "work intolerance." In the case of age-related capacity, the first step is to identify particularly demanding jobs that are unlikely to remain suitable for employees until retirement. In identifying such jobs, one should be cognizant of high-grade evidence of increased incidence of symptoms or of injury with age, if it exists. (In many cases, it does not; see Chapter 4.) Speculation should be avoided. The next step is to discuss these issues explicitly within the company, with involved employees, and to anticipate the need for long-term succession plans to shift the duties of workers as they age.

PSYCHOSOCIAL FACTORS AND PERSON-JOB FIT

Employees who are invested in remaining at work will try to overcome obstacles resulting from work intolerance, perhaps by adapting or changing work practices to their abilities. Workers who are experiencing other forms of job-related dissatisfaction are less likely to seek to match their abilities to work demands.

Preventive Strategies and Tactics

Different strategies are needed to prevent first episodes of symptoms or activity limitations, to prevent recurrent episodes, to prevent or reduce lost workdays due to injury, to prevent chronic disability, and to reduce or prevent medical care utilization and its associated cost. Occupational health professionals should be clear about the goals of specific preventive efforts.

Primary Prevention

From a public health point of view, primary prevention is preferable to secondary and tertiary prevention. The primary prevention of work-related disorders depends on the reduction or elimination of exposure to factors causally associated with those disorders in individuals susceptible to such stressors. In the past, emphasis has been placed on risk factors that are physical in nature, such as force, repetition, posture, vibration, lighting, terminal design, and posture.

However, other factors, such as worker job satisfaction and relations with coworkers and supervisors, have been specifically noted to have a relatively strong relationship to musculoskeletal, visual, and other apparently ergonomic complaints.

The primary prevention of work-related complaints thus depends on reducing exposure to physical, personal, and psychosocial stressors. For example, engineering controls, including ergonomic workstation evaluation and modification, and job redesign to accommodate a reasonable proportion of the workforce may well be the most cost-effective measures in the long run. Personal protective equipment also can be an effective strategy for primary prevention. Primary preventive strategies based on maintaining activity and flexibility, such as exercise breaks for workers performing assembly tasks or a scheduled rotation of tasks, appear to be low in cost and generally effective based on physiologic principles. Strategies that improve work organization and management also should be addressed.

WORK DESIGN

Several general principles are important to prevent musculoskeletal disorders and visual fatigue or injury. These include protection from hazards via engineering controls (effective barriers to hazards), use of personal protective equipment, administrative controls, and adjustment of workstations, tasks, and tools to the individual worker's size and physiologic and work capacity.

Person-job fit is a basic principle that may markedly reduce occupational health concerns and the costs of lost productivity due to illness and injury as well as related medical costs. The same principles are used either to engineer jobs so that they fit many people or to adapt a job, task, or workstation to a specific person. These principles include:

- Decreasing force or load as well as repetitions through redesign, tool changes, or automation.
- Decreasing static exertions that result in excessive muscle fatigue.
- Providing reasonable and prudent exercise breaks, depending on the tasks involved. For example, stretch or light-exercise breaks may be reasonable every half hour or hour for static, repetitive, or sedentary jobs or tasks.
- Avoiding use of the hand as a tool, such as pounding on a tool or part.
- Providing lift-assist devices, particularly for those performing frequent, heavy lifts.
- Positioning work to avoid static, nonanatomic postures resulting in sustained muscle contraction.

Jobs and workstations should be designed so that they fit most workers' capacities. Workstations, equipment, or task components should be adjustable for workers of different stature, strength, and endurance to ensure a match between each worker and his or her tasks, thereby avoiding discomfort, loss of productivity, and injury. Management practices and psychosocial factors as they relate to person-job fit also should be assessed.

Ergonomic Tactics to Prevent Upper-Body Musculoskeletal Complaints and Disorders. In making recommendations for the design of tasks and workstations to prevent upper-body health concerns, the occupational health provider should be aware of the physical dimensions and range of motion needed to complete the tasks involved if they are well designed. The tools, machinery, or workstations should be flexible enough to accommodate any worker. Workers may be involved in the identification of physical job requirements and discomfort or overload situations by means of interviews, group sessions, and/ or questionnaires and scales.

Ergonomic research supports the following recommendations for the design of tasks that involve use of the neck, shoulders, and upper extremities in order to prevent musculoskeletal complaints and injuries:

- Jobs that require overhead reaching, work under load in that position, or hyperextending the neck should be modified to minimize these postures and movements in order to reduce shoulder and neck complaints as well as lack of visibility, especially in workers with presbyopia.
- Workstations should be designed to avoid repetitive twisting of the neck to refer to written materials.
- In a job where the operator is sedentary, he or she should be able to reach all materials and equipment without leaning, bending, or twisting at the waist. Twisting while bearing a load should be avoided whenever possible by proper placement of work materials. Reaching overhead and far to the sides, resulting in twisting motions of the torso, should be avoided. Proper placement of work materials within about a 90-degree arc, centered in front of the worker, minimizes reaching outside the "reach envelope." The forearm-only reach is preferable, although the full-arm reach is acceptable.
- Design of hand tools should be determined by hand anatomy and task design to:
  - Avoid ulnar or radial deviation or flexion or extension at the wrist.
  - Maximize grip strength by avoiding palmar flexion and other wrist deviations.
  - Provide as great a force-bearing area as possible in handles and grips.
  - Minimize the force and vibration transmitted to the hand and upper body.
  - Avoid repetitive finger action.
- To avoid neurovascular as well as tendon injury, the hand should not be used as a hammer.
- Vibration transferred to the hands, wrists, and remainder of the upper extremity should be reduced to the extent possible through the use

of vibration-damping wrappings and coatings, isolation suspension of vibrating machinery, or automation.

- Management support and participation in prevention programs, especially for repetitive-motion complaints, is often as important as mitigation of physical factors. Factors such as monotonous work, high perceived workload, low control or autonomy, and low levels of support should be addressed.

Ergonomic Tactics to Prevent Neck and Back Musculoskeletal Complaints and Disorders. Ergonomic research supports the following recommendations for the design of tasks that involve use of the neck and back in order to prevent musculoskeletal complaints and injuries:

- Twisting and bending while bearing a load should be avoided whenever possible by proper placement of work materials.
- Reaching outside the "preferred work area" should be avoided whenever possible by proper placement of work materials within approximately a 90-degree arc centered in front of the worker.
- Frequent bending and stooping, especially below knee level, should be avoided by:
  - Placement of the load.
  - Use of mechanical lifting devices.
- The following lifting recommendations are based on the National Institute for Occupational Safety and Health (NIOSH) *Applications Manual for the Revised NIOSH Lifting Equation* (revised 1991). Lifting should be:
  - Planned so as to conform to the following and to avoid slippery or cluttered areas:
    - Close to the body.
    - Between knee (preferably waist) and shoulder height.
    - Without bending or twisting the back.
    - With the chin tucked in, if lifting overhead.
    - With well-designed, secured handles (if handles are used).
    - Less than 50 percent of a worker's capacity (personal strength limits), as determined by preplacement testing.
    - Generally less than 25 to 35 pounds (11.3-15.8 kilograms), unassisted.
    - Less frequent than 20 lifts per minute, depending on lifting technique, physical conditioning, and personal factors.
    - Slow, with at least 3 seconds per lift.
- Pushing and pulling should be limited to forces of less than 50 pounds (22.5 kilograms) at the hands.
- Heavy carrying should be reduced to less than 33 percent of lean body weight by:
  - Dividing loads.
  - Use of mechanical transport devices.

- Using more than one worker to move heavy loads.
- Task assignment tailored to each worker and load size.

- The use of back belts as lumbar support should be avoided because they have been shown to have little or no benefit, thereby providing only a false sense of security.
- Unexpected movements should be avoided by:
  - Ensuring strong, easily gripped, thick handles with rounded edges.
  - Removal of slip, trip, and fall hazards.
  - Planning lifting maneuvers.
- Prolonged sitting and standing should be reduced by:
  - Providing rest and exercise breaks.
  - Task rotation or variation.
- Seating should generally be at a height of 16 to 20 inches (40-52 centimeters) with a lumbar support, adjustable reclining back (90-140 degrees), and a firm, flat, adjustable seat pan with a rounded edge no longer than 16 inches (40 centimeters) for prolonged sitting. Mobile workers may prefer a sit-stand option using a high stool with a seat 29 to 32 inches high (74-81 centimeters). Seating of the first type and sit-stand stools support back musculature and minimize intradiskal pressure. Foot rests and/or arm rests may be needed for some workers. All seating should be fully adjustable to accommodate workers of different heights and body habits.
- Job stress should be reduced and job satisfaction and task enjoyment should be increased by:
  - Varying repetitive or monotonous work.
  - Increasing workers' control over tasks.
  - Designing jobs so that workers see the output of their work.
  - Increasing workers' participation in decision making.
  - Matching authority and responsibility in jobs.
- Repetitive and monotonous work should be reduced whenever possible by:
  - Automatic feed devices.
  - Task, job, or worker rotation.
  - Breaks and exercises to maintain alertness.
- Whole-body vibration, such as that from motor vehicle and machinery operation, especially in the range of 4 to 8 cycles per second (but including 2 to 11 cycles per second), should be reduced as much as possible by:
  - Mechanical damping or balancing of machinery.
  - Damping cushions and padding.
  - Automating processes.
- The level of exertion should be limited to about 33 percent of a worker's aerobic capacity, as determined by preplacement testing. Anaerobic exercise may lead to fatigue-related errors and overload.
- Routine exercises specific to the back and neck have been shown to

be a preferred and effective utility in the prevention of neck and back strain and should be part of daily work for those at risk of developing musculoskeletal complaints.

Ergonomic Tactics to Prevent Visual Fatigue and Other Visual Disorders. "Visual fatigue" is a term used to describe phenomena related to intensive use of the eyes. It can include complaints of eye or periocular pain, itching or burning, tearing, oculomotor changes, focal problems, performance degradation, "aftercolors," and other phenomena. Ergonomic research supports the following:

- Placement of frequently used displays in the primary visual display area. The top of this area should be opposite the operator's eyes, with the eyes facing straight forward, extending down to a point where the operator is looking down at a 30-degree angle. Devices viewed as they are operated, such as buttons, keyboards, and controls, should be above and below this area, at the work surface, and above the plane of the operator's eyes.
- The optimal viewing distance for visual displays is about 20 inches (50 centimeters). Corrective lenses designed specifically for fine details, including display-screen work, can be used for workers with refractive error or presbyopia. Lenses of this type can be incorporated into multifocal eyeglasses as well.
- Proper illuminance is important. It should be evaluated for each task. It depends on the needs of the task, reflectance of surfaces in the area, and to some extent the age of the worker because older workers generally require brighter lighting with less glare for visual discrimination. In general, illuminance of 70 to 80 footcandles is needed for general office work, 100 to 150 footcandles for visually intensive tasks, and up to 500 to 1000 footcandles for very fine tasks. Specific task lighting is preferred, when needed, over excessive ambient area lighting.
- Lighting geometry should be configured to avoid glare. Glare should be reduced for display terminals by:
  - Placing visual display terminals out of direct line with windows.
  - Use of window films and coverings.
  - Use of dull, textured surfaces.
  - Reducing ambient lighting to below 500 lux (18-46 footcandles) and using supplemental lighting where needed.
  - Use of indirect lighting.
  - Parabolic louvers on fluorescent lights.
  - Shielding of auxiliary lighting.
  - Use of eye shades.
- Visual discomfort from glare and other sources cumulates during the workday, so task rotation may be a reasonable preventive measure if other measures are not possible or reasonable.

- Visual performance can be impaired by whole-body vibration in the range of 10 to 25 cycles per second. Such vibration, which may be generated by power saws, cranes, conveyors, and other machinery, should be damped or separated from the worker.

Periodic short periods of rest from fixed focal tasks for data-entry workers and other computer-related positions, such as a 5-minute period involving fixation of the eyes to infinity every 20 to 40 minutes, helps to reduce eye strain and discomfort while improving mood and performance.

PERSONAL RISK MODIFICATION

Strategies based on modification of individual risk factors (e.g., improving worker fitness, smoking cessation, weight loss) may be less certain, more difficult, and possibly less cost-effective. In particular, abdominal muscular strengthening to prevent low back pain is not supported by the existing evidence, whereas good aerobic condition is associated with a lower injury rate. Improving flexibility and strengthening of specific areas, such as the shoulder girdle, are recommended elsewhere (see Chapter 9, for example). An emphasis on aerobic conditioning may be appropriate to prevent musculoskeletal disorders. Aerobic fitness has other benefits as well, including improved productivity and job satisfaction.

Training in body mechanics and conditioning (sometimes referred to as "work hardening") also have been advocated to prevent musculoskeletal disorders and visual fatigue. While high-grade evidence supporting the efficacy of training in body mechanics is sparse, it is a logical step (perhaps primarily to prevent recurrences) and is supported by many experienced occupational health providers. Work hardening, in the form of conditioning at hire or reconditioning after absence from work for the specific demands of the job, is also a logical step from a physiologic standpoint because deconditioning has been implicated in both initial complaints and recurrences. However, because the evidence is inconclusive, these efforts may be more cost-effective if their focus is the prevention of recurrences rather than primary prevention.

PREPLACEMENT AND PERIODIC EXAMINATIONS

The preplacement/postoffer medical examination also may aid in reducing the risk for development of WRMSDs or other health conditions. The clinician must be clear about the purpose of the examination and its components. The examination should be designed by defining the type and level of risk to the worker and to others. In general, these examinations are most productive as selection screening in relation to the demands (time, load, repetitions), consequences of error, and person-job fit in areas of high injury with high job demands. The purpose of preplacement examinations should be narrowly job-related; their intention should not be to discover hidden diseases and treat them. Preplacement examinations may be used to establish a baseline, especially in workers who have sustained previous injuries or illnesses. It should be noted that these examinations typically are not regarded as establishing a doctor-patient relationship.

Job requirements should be in written form and should be framed in relation to quantified physical demands of the job, especially its essential functions. Quantified or statistics-based scales that rate or list physical demands, emotional demands, hours, working conditions, special equipment and tools used, faculties needed, and vocational qualifications can form the basis for evaluation of job requirements. A combination of descriptions by supervisors, site visits, and a group process used by teams of workers to define actual tasks (the Santa Barbara protocol), videotapes of the job as typically done, or structured questionnaires provides the necessary information for creating the most accurate job descriptions.

In evaluating the ability of a worker to do the job as described, the history is very important. If the candidate has had trouble with a similar job or demand in the past, this is a sensitive indicator for job evaluation or accommodation.

The clinician must be aware of the sensitivity and specificity of any tests used and their applicability to real job situations. Tests should have been evaluated in working populations and determined to reflect true job demands. At present, there is not good evidence that functional capacity evaluations are correlated with a lower frequency of health complaints or injuries. The preplacement examination process will determine whether the employee is capable of performing in a safe manner the tasks identified in the job-task analysis.

If a more comprehensive preplacement examination is done for health promotion or protection purposes, it may identify other risk factors and conditions such as obesity, thyroid disease, poor muscular conditioning, pregnancy, diabetes, and certain congenital anomalies. The employee should be counseled about factors associated with WRMSDs or other work-related health concerns and potential risks, particularly if he or she has any preexisting medical conditions. This process also allows the health care provider to communicate to the employer the need for appropriate restrictions, accommodations, or task redesign that would permit the employee to work safely.

PHYSICAL HAZARD CONTROL

If it is likely that physical work factors may contribute to subjective or objective health effects, the occupational health practitioner and the employer should consider methods of hazard control to mitigate the observed effects and improve productivity. Systematic job-task analysis will identify ergonomic and physical risk factors associated with various tasks. This identification should then lead to the implementation of appropriate control measures to reduce employee exposure to these risks. The following methods of physical and ergonomic hazard control are listed in order of preference:

Engineering controls. Engineering controls that reduce exposure levels are the preferred method of preventing the development of work-related musculoskeletal health effects. Engineering controls focus on job tasks or processes. Direct engineering changes in job operations may be made to minimize exposure of workers—for example, use of light curtains, barriers, or enclosed processes. To prevent job-related health effects due to ergonomic problems, the preferred means may be the development of special tools, jigs, or balances or the adjustment of workstations to fit each individual. A change in the work process itself can reduce exposure levels of various types significantly. Engineering change is best able to alter levels of necessary force; abnormal posturing, vibration, noise, and temperature; and exposures to chemical and physical hazards. The implementation of proper engineering controls may not preclude the need for administrative controls, employee training, or personal protective equipment, however. The implementation of engineering controls to reduce exposure levels is also the preferred method of controlling the development of work-related nonspecific eye complaints. However, personal protective equipment is often more practical.

Administrative controls. Administrative controls focus on the worker's capabilities and motivations and how the job task is done. These controls include job rotation, task separation, elimination of production incentives, reduction of overtime, optimal assignment of shift work, and the provision of appropriate break times. The implementation of such controls can reduce repetition rates and total repetitions, improve recovery time, and reduce the exposure to stressors. Administrative control also should be implemented to alter work-organization tasks that affect the psychological state of the employee. Psychosocial factors that have been associated with work-related complaints include job dissatisfaction, low enjoyment of tasks, poor relationships with supervisors or coworkers, excessive workload, low workload/monotony, ambiguity over career development, lack of employee control, social isolation, deskilling due to a single repeated job task, and simply individual differences leading to poor person-job fit. In some instances, psychosocial stressors have been found to be as important in contributing to work-related complaints as physical stressors.

Personal protective equipment. If engineering controls of physical, chemical, or biologic hazards are not feasible, appropriate and effective personal protective equipment (PPE) should be used. Hearing protection, impervious gloves, boots, respirators, and eye and face protectors are well-known examples of PPE. However, there are no forms of PPE that well-designed studies have proved effective in preventing WRMSDs.

MANAGEMENT EDUCATION

Education and information should be provided at all levels of a company. Upper management must understand the risk for WRMSDs, eye, hearing, and respiratory complaints and other health problems in the workforce; the financial and social cost associated with them; and the need for management's support of line supervisors to implement risk factor controls. Further training may be needed for environmental safety and health staff, plant engineers, human resources personnel, ergonomic teams, and the individual employees themselves. The Occupational Safety and Health Administration (OSHA) [29 CFR 1910.132] requires training on the workplace hazards and use of specific PPE to prevent injury for each of the tasks being performed.

EMPLOYEE EDUCATION AND INVOLVEMENT

Employees should have a baseline knowledge of the risk factors for work-related complaints, how to prevent them, and how to access medical care if a health concern develops. Employees also should understand their job responsibilities, job requirements, and duty to comply with health and safety standards developed by both regulatory agencies and the employer.

Employees should be encouraged to participate with management in identifying work factors associated with health concerns, and in suggesting methods to control exposure to them. Active participation may facilitate secondary and tertiary as well as primary prevention.

In making realistic recommendations, occupational health professionals also must balance the cost of preventive efforts (in time, effort, and money) against the expected benefit of designing broad-based or targeted programs. For example, some primary preventive efforts, such as back education or fitness programs, are often applied for all workers. However, back pain, while the most common complaint seen in occupational medicine, affects less than 2 percent of most workforces yearly, and about 10 percent of those workers account for more than 80 percent of the costs. In addition, because of the state of knowledge and individual variation in susceptibility and presence of non-work-related risk factors (see preceding discussion and Chapter 4), broad-based prevention efforts for some types of initial or recurrent health concerns may not be cost-effective. Effective targeting of preventive efforts may be difficult as well. A focus on secondarily preventing disability, which often leads to high-cost cases, may prove to be more cost-effective.

Secondary Prevention

Secondary prevention consists of detection and surveillance programs designed to identify early indicators of difficulty (e.g., symptoms, minor injuries, sprains, strains) and intervention to avoid reinjury and/or the worsening of conditions, including iatrogenic disability. Secondary prevention is aimed at reducing disability and hastening recovery once a health concern has become apparent. This is a more targeted approach, in that it has become apparent which workers will develop complaints, illnesses, or injuries. Since secondary prevention involves working in partnership with the worker, the cornerstones of this process are two-way communication, addressing myths and misconceptions, management of expectations, bilateral or trilateral planning, and management of the episode and the situation, as outlined in Chapter 3, "Initial Approaches to Treatment."

Modified or temporary duty is important to return workers to the worksite and prevents social isolation and deconditioning (see Chapter 5, "Cornerstones of Disability Prevention and Management"). Reconditioning and avoidance of static postures are important in musculoskeletal disorders both to hasten functional recovery and to prevent recurrences. Back schools are an example of an approach that combines these two areas with imparting of information and group support. Any problems with workstation or task design that contributed to the original problem should be corrected to avoid aggravating the condition.

SURVEILLANCE

Occupational health professionals may work with employers to develop and implement a surveillance system for the detection of work-related health complaints that may cause discomfort, develop into fixed pathology, or impair productivity. The components of an occupational surveillance program are the detection and enumeration of job-related morbidity and mortality, characterization of trends and identification of new patterns or clusters of disease, and monitoring of interventions to decrease frequency or severity. Health surveillance may identify a pattern of development of musculoskeletal, ocular, or other symptoms or of adverse health effects associated with some tasks that could not be predicted through task analysis. This is especially true when development of these conditions is associated with psychosocial more than physical factors.

Passive health surveillance may include retrospective review of OSHA logs, absenteeism records, or documents from workers' compensation insurers. Active health surveillance may include questionnaires or routine medical examinations or both. Well-designed medical surveillance may allow the employer to focus resources on those tasks that appear to be most predictive of development of musculoskeletal or other adverse health effects.

Tertiary Prevention

Tertiary prevention is vocational rehabilitation and functional restoration in a worker who has had a major alteration in work capacity or life whether due to a major biologic event (e.g., catastrophic injury, severe disease) or a constellation of factors (e.g., iatrogenic disability). Tertiary prevention in the work setting involves prevention of recurrences in a patient who has had a previous episode. The first action should be to evaluate the job or tasks and the person-job fit and then to modify the job, tasks, or workstation as necessary (see "Work Design"). Excessive loads, repetitions, abnormal postures, and other ergonomic problems should be addressed. If the individual cannot do the job as originally designed due to an impairment, reasonable accommodation should be attempted. If this is not possible, job placement elsewhere or retraining may be necessary.

As noted, reconditioning and avoidance of static position for long periods of time should help to prevent recurrences. Both aerobic conditioning and conditioning of specific muscle groups (e.g., forearm muscles or neck and shoulder musculature) should reduce the risk of future health problems.

References

BIOMECHANICS

Aaras A, Horgen G, Bjorset HH, Ro O, Walsoe H. Musculoskeletal, visual and psychosocial stress in VDU operators before and after multidisciplinary ergonomic interventions: a 6 year prospective study, part II. *Appl Ergon.* 2001;32(6):559-71.

Anderson CK, Chaffin DB. A biometric evaluation of five lifting techniques. *Appl Ergon.* 1986;17:2-8.

Anton D, Shibley LD, Fethke NB, Hess J, Cook TM, Rosecrance J. The effect of overhead drilling position on shoulder moment and electromyography. *Ergonomics.* 2001;44(5):489-501.

Chaffin DB, Andersson GBJ. *Occupational Biomechanics.* New York, NY: Wiley; 2002.

Herbert R, Gerr F, Dropkin J. Clinical evaluation and management of work-related carpal tunnel syndrome. *Am J Ind Med.* 2000;37(1):62-74.

Jokl P. The effect of the aging process on muscle and tendon injuries. In: Gordon SL, Gonzalez-Mestre X, Garrett WE Jr, eds. *Sports and Exercise in Midlife.* Rosemont, Ill: American Academy of Orthopaedic Surgeons; 1993:515-29.

Keyserling WM. Workplace risk factors and occupational musculoskeletal disorders, Part 1: A review of biomechanical and psychophysical research on risk factors associated with low-back pain. *AIHAJ.* 2000;61(1):39-50.

Leadbetter WB. Aging effects on the repair and healing of athletic injury. In: Gordon SL, Gonzalez-Mestre X, Garrett WE Jr, eds. *Sports and Exercise in Midlife.* Rosemont, Ill: American Academy of Orthopaedic Surgeons; 1993:177-233.

Li G, Haslegrave CM. Seated work postures for manual, visual and combined tasks. *Ergonomics.* 1999;49(8):1060-86.

Parnainpour M, Beijani FJ, Pavlidis L. Worker training: the fallacy of a single, correct lifting technique. *Ergonomics.* 1987;30:331-4.

Simoneau GG, Marklin RW. Effect of computer keyboard slope and height on wrist extension angle. *Hum Factors.* 2001;43(2):287-98.

PREVENTION

Armstrong TJ, Punnett L, Ketner P. Subjective worker assessments of hand tools used in automobile assembly. *Am Ind Hyg Assoc J.* 1989;50:639-45.

Baker EL, Melius JM, Millar JD. Surveillance of occupational illness and injury in the United States: current perspectives and future directions. *J Public Health Policy.* 1988;9:198-221.

Bigos SJ, Battié MC. Acute care to prevent back disability: ten years of progress. *Clin Orthop.* 1987;221:121-30.

Bigos SJ, Battié MC, Fisher LD, Hansson TH, Spengler DM, Nachemson AL. A prospective evaluation of commonly used pre-employment screening tools for acute industrial back pain. *Spine.* 1992;17:922-6.

Borenstein DG, Wiesel SW, Boden SD. *Low Back Pain: Medical Diagnosis and Comprehensive Management,* 2d ed. Philadelphia, Pa: Saunders; 1995.

Borg GA. Psychophysical bases of perceived exertion. *Med Sci Sports Exerc.* 1982; 14(5):377-81.

Burton WN, Chen CY, Conti DJ, Schultz AB, Edington DW. The value of the periodic executive health examination: experience at Bank One and summary of the literature. *J Occup Environ Med.* 2002:44(8):737-44.

Cady LD, Thomas PC, Karwasky RJ. Program for increasing health and physical fitness of fire fighters. *J Occup Med.* 1985;27:110-4.

Coe JV, Cuttle K, McClellan WC, Worden MJ. *Visual Display Units: A Review of Potential Health Problems Associated with Their Use.* Wellington, NZ: New Zealand Department of Health Regional Unit; 1980.

Collingwood TR. Fitness programs. In: O'Donnell MP, Harris JS, eds. *Health Promotion in the Work Place.* Albany, NY: Delmar; 1994:240-70.

Collins MJ, Brown B, Bowman KJ. *Visual Discomfort and VDTs.* Queensland, Australia: Centre for Eye Research, Department of Optometry, Queensland Institute of Technology; 1988.

Dababneh AJ, Swanson N, Shell RL. Impact of added rest breaks on the productivity and well-being of workers. *Ergonomics.* 2001;44(2):164-74.

Daltroy LH, Iversen MD, Larson MG, et al. A controlled trial of an educational program to prevent low back injuries. *N Engl J Med.* 1997;337(5):322-8.

Eastman Kodak Company, Human Factors Section, Health Safety and Human Factors Laboratory. *Ergonomic Design for People at Work.* Vol. 1. Belmont, Calif: Lifetime Learning Publications; 1983.

Eastman Kodak Company, Ergonomics Group, Health and Environment Laboratory. *Ergonomic Design for People at Work.* Vol. 2. New York, NY: Van Nostrand-Reinhold; 1986.

Elders LA, van der Beek AJ, Burdorf A. Return to work after sickness absence due to back disorders: a systematic review on intervention strategies. *Int Arch Occup Environ Health.* 2000;73(5):339-48.

Evanoff BA, Bohr PC, Wolf LD. Effects of a participatory ergonomics team among hospital orderlies. *Am J Ind Med.* 1999;35(4):358-65.

Halperin WE, Radcliffe J, Frazier TM, Wilson L, Becker SP, Shulte PA. Medical screening in the workplace: proposed principles. *J Occup Med.* 1986;28:547-52.

Harris JS, Fries J. The health benefits of health promotion. In: O'Donnell MP, Harris JS, eds. *Health Promotion in the Work Place.* Albany, NY: Delmar; 2001.

Herington T. Preplacement testing. In: LaDou J, ed. *Occupational Health and Safety.* 2d ed. Itasca, Ill: National Safety Council; 1994:229-36.

Himmelstein JS, Andersson GBJ. Low back pain: risk evaluation and preplacement screening. *Occup Med State Art Rev.* 1988;255-69.

Human Factors Society. *American National Standard for Human Factors Engineering of Video Display Terminal Workstations.* Santa Monica, Calif: HFS; 1987.

Illuminating Engineering Society. *IES Lighting Handbook.* New York, NY: IES; 1981.

Janowitz IL, White AA III. Preventing back injury. In: La Dou J, ed. *Occupational Health and Safety.* 2d ed. Itasca, Ill: National Safety Council; 1994:243-59.

Kaplansky BD, Wei FY, Reecer MV. Prevention strategies for occupational low back pain. *Occup Med.* 1998;3(1):33-45.

Keyserling WM, Armstrong TJ. Ergonomics. In: Last JM, Wallace RB, eds. *Maxcy-Rosenau-Last Public Health and Preventive Medicine.* 13th ed. Norwalk, Conn: Appleton & Lange; 1992:533-5.

Keyserling WM, Herrin GD, Chaffin DB. Isometric strength testing as a means of controlling medical incidents on strenuous jobs. *J Occup Med.* 1980;22:332-6.

Klaber Moffett JA, Chase SM, Portek I, Ennis JR. A controlled, prospective study to evaluate the effectiveness of a back school in the relief of chronic low back pain. *Spine.* 1986;11:120-2.

Kuijer PP, Visser B, Kemper HC. Job rotation as a factor in reducing physical workload at a refuse collecting department. *Ergonomics.* 1999;42(9):1167-78.

Kuorinka I, Jonsson B, Kilbom A, et al. Standardized Nordic questionnaire for the analysis of musculoskeletal symptoms. *Appl Ergon.* 1987;18:233-7.

Lankhorst GJ, Van deStadt RJ, Vogelaar TW, Vanderkorst JK, Prevo AJ. The effect of the Swedish back school in chronic idiopathic low back pain: a prospective controlled trial. *Scand J Rehab Med.* 1983;15(3):141-5.

Linton SJ. Occupational psychological factors increase the risk for back pain: A systematic review. *J Occup Rehabil.* 2001;11(1):53-66.

Linton SJ, Ryberg M. A cognitive-behavioral group intervention as prevention for persistent neck and back pain in a nonpatient population: a randomized, controlled trial. *Pain.* 2001;90(1-2):83-90.

Linton SJ, van Tulder MW. Preventive interventions for back and neck pain problems: what is the evidence? *Spine.* 2001;26(7):778-87.

Matte T, Baker E, Honchar P. The selection and definition of targeted work-related conditions for surveillance under SENSOR. *Am J Public Health.* 1989;79(suppl):21-5.

Mclean L, Tingley M, Scott RN, Rickards J. Computer terminal work and the benefit of microbreaks. *Appl Ergon.* 2001;32(3):225-37.

Mital A, Nicholson AS, Ayoub MM. *A Guide to Manual Materials Handling.* London: Taylor & Francis; 1993.

Ordin DL. Surveillance, monitoring and screening in occupational health. In: Last JM, Wallace RB, eds. *Maxcy-Rosenau-Last Public Health and Preventive Medicine*. 13th ed. Norwalk, Conn: Appleton & Lange; 1992: 551-8.

Saunders T, Driskell JE, Johnston JH, Salas E. The effect of stress inoculation training on anxiety and performance. *J Occup Health Psychol.* 1996;1(2): 170-86.

Schultz AB, Lu C, Barnett TE, et al. Influence of participation in a worksite health-promotion program on disability days. *J Occup Environ Med.* 2002;44(8):776-80.

Seradge H. Preventing carpal tunnel syndrome and cumulative trauma disorder: effect of carpal tunnel decompression exercises: an Oklahoma experience. *J Okla State Med Assoc.* 2000;93(4):150-3.

Seradge H. *AAOS Recommended Exercises to Prevent Carpal Tunnel Syndrome.* Rosemont, Ill: American Academy of Orthopaedic Surgeons; 1996.

Sheedy JE. Vision and work. In: LaDou J, ed. *Occupational Health and Safety.* 2nd ed. Itasca, Ill: National Safety Council; 1994:197-206.

Smilkestein G. The family APGAR: a proposal for a family function test and its use by physicians. *J Fam Prac.* 1978;6:1231-5.

Snook SH, Ciriello VM. The design of manual handling tasks: revised tables of maximum acceptable weights and forces. *Ergonomics.* 1991;34:1197-213.

Subcommittee on Medical Management, Committee Control of Cumulative Trauma Disorders, American National Standards Institute. Control of Cumulative Trauma Disorders. (Draft Standard Z365.) ANSI; 1995:7-710 and appendices.

Szabo RM. Carpal tunnel syndrome as a repetitive motion disorder. *Clin Orthop.* 1998;(351):78-89.

Thompson D, Rempel D. Industrial engineering and ergonomics. In: LaDou J, ed. *Occupational Health and Safety.* 2nd ed. Itasca, Ill: National Safety Council; 1994:163-86.

Tuchin PJ. Spinal care education as a preventative strategy for occupational health and safety: a new role for chiropractors. *Australas Chiropr Osteopath.* 1998;7(1):8-14.

US Preventive Services Task Force. Screening for Risk of Low Back Injury. In: *Guide to Clinical Preventive Services: Report of the U.S. Preventive Services Task Force.* Baltimore, Md: Williams & Wilkins; 1989:245-9.

van Poppel MN, Koes BW, van der Ploeg T, Smid T, Bouter LM. Lumbar supports and education for the prevention of low back pain in industry: a randomized controlled trial. *JAMA.* 1998;279:1789-94.

van Tulder MW, Jellema P, van Poppel MNM, Nachemson AL, Bouter LM. Lumbar supports for prevention and treatment of low back pain (Cochrane Review). In: *The Cochrane Library.* Issue 2; 2002. Oxford: Update Software.

Waddell G. A new model for the clinical treatment of low back pain. *Spine.* 1987;12:632-44.

Waris P, Kuorinka I, Kurppa K. Epidemiologic screening of occupational neck and upper limb disorders. *Scand J Work Environ Health.* 1979;5:25-38.

Yassi A, Cooper JE, Tate RB, et al. A randomized controlled trial to prevent patient lift and transfer injuries of health care workers. *Spine.* 2001;26(16):1739-46.

VISUAL (OCULAR) SCREENING

Brownell CP. Visual fact-finding discloses relationship of visual capacity and job performances. *Safety Eng.* 1947;93:24-6, 48-9.

Coe JV, Cuttle K, McClellan WC, Worden MJ. *Visual Display Units: A Review of Potential Health Problems Associated with Their Use.* Wellington, NZ: New Zealand Department of Health Regional Unit; 1980.

Cole BL, Breadon ID, Sharp K, et al. *Comparison of the Symptoms Reported by VDT Users and Non-VDT Users.* Bulletin No. 2. Melbourne, Australia: University of Melbourne; 1986.

Collins MJ, Brown B, Bowman KJ. *Visual Discomfort and VDTs.* Queensland, Australia: Centre for Eye Research, Department of Optometry, Queensland Institute of Technology; 1988.

Kuhn HS. *Eyes and Industry.* St. Louis, Mo: Mosby; 1950.

Kuhn HS. *Industrial Ophthalmology.* St. Louis, Mo: Mosby; 1944.

North RV. *Work and the Eye.* Oxford, England: Oxford University Press; 1993.

Novak JF. *Are the Eyes Right for the Job? Industrial and Traumatic Ophthalmology.* Symposium of the New Orleans Academy of Ophthalmology. St. Louis, Mo: Mosby; 1964.

Sheedy JE. Vision analysis. In: *Vision and Computer Displays.* 2nd ed. Walnut Creek, Calif: Vision Analysis; 1991.

TAAOO. Business Meeting, Committee of Industrial Ophthalmology, October 10, 1942; p. 143.

TAAOO. January/February 1943, A Panel Discussion on Industrial Ophthalmology Committee, p. 233.

Tiffin J. Visual skills and vision tests. In: *Industrial Psychology.* New York, NY: Prentice-Hall; 1943.

VISUAL JOB FIT

Duane A. Anomalies of the accommodation, clinically considered. *Arch Ophthalmol.* 1916;45:124.

Duane A. Accommodation. *Arch Ophthalmol.* 1931;5:1.

Herrnheiser JZ. Die refraktion sent wicklung des menschlichen Auges. *Zeitsch Heik.* 1892;13:342-377.

2 General Approach to Initial Assessment and Documentation

In assessing acute or subacute complaints, the occupational health practitioner should first exclude conditions that could threaten life or limb if not diagnosed and treated emergently or urgently. The recommended process is therefore to:

- Seek red flags[1] for potentially dangerous underlying conditions.
- In the absence of red flags, work-related complaints can be handled safely and effectively by occupational and primary care providers. The focus is on monitoring for complications, facilitating the healing process, and facilitating return to work in a modified or full-duty capacity. Evaluation and treatment generally can proceed in the acute phase without special studies because the findings from such studies seldom alter treatment. Yet, in some body systems (e.g., eye, bone, and head injuries), special studies may be mandatory.

The content of the evaluation may:

- Relate to the demands of the job in question.
- Relate specifically to the employee's medical condition (if there is a question that the medical condition may adversely affect the employee's ability to perform the essential job functions).
- Include understanding and documentation of the employee's disabling medical condition.
  - Consider using a functional capacity evaluation when necessary to translate medical impairment into functional limitations and determine work capability.
  - Consider the need for rehabilitation.

[1] The term red flag, as generally used by payors, is not applicable to this discussion. Payors generally use red flags to earmark a case that may become problematic from a claims management perspective. In these guidelines, red flag is a nonpejorative term that refers only to serious medical conditions. They are defined as a sign or symptom of a potentially serious condition indicating that further consultation, support, or specialized treatment may be necessary. The term yellow flag is used to indicate psychosocial or other barriers to recovery.

- Include consultation with the employee's treating physician when a difference of opinion arises regarding the employee's functional capacities, after obtaining the employee's written permission.

A focused medical history, work history, and physical examination generally are sufficient to assess the patient who complains of an apparently job-related disorder. The initial medical history and examination will include evaluation for serious underlying conditions, including sources of referred symptoms in other parts of the body. The initial assessment should characterize the frequency, intensity, and duration in this and other equivalent circumstances. In this assessment, certain patient responses and findings raise the suspicion of serious underlying medical conditions. These are referred to as red flags. Their absence rules out the need for special studies, immediate consultation, referral, or inpatient care during the first 4 weeks of care (not necessarily the first 4 weeks of the worker's condition), when spontaneous recovery is expected, as long as associated workplace factors are mitigated. In some cases a more complete medical history and physical examination may be indicated if the mechanism or nature of the complaint is unclear.

Diagnostic Labeling

The diagnoses applied by the physician or health care professional should be as precise as possible. For example, left lateral epicondylitis is preferable to work-related musculoskeletal disorder (WRMSD). Previously used terms such as cumulative-trauma disorder, repetitive-motion disorder, overuse syndrome, and so on should not be used. Some of the reasons such terms largely have been discarded include the following:

- Such diagnostic labels link a purported exposure with a nonspecific, multifactorial disease. This attribution is no more appropriate than labeling, for example, a "diabetic heart attack."
- These diseases may occur without any physical exposure.
- Repetition does not appear to be the most important physical risk factor; rather, force appears to be. Such terms also connote that repetition is the prime risk factor for intervention.
- The performance of unaccustomed activities appears to be a risk factor, but these labels imply that it is not.
- WRMSDs may occur with only one exertion rather than being due to something repeated.
- Nonspecific diagnostic labels do not help to communicate the body part injured. Thus safety personnel actions and prevention activities may be hindered.

Medical History

The categories presented in this section are meant to be guidelines only. An inquiry focused on the patient's past medical history may include surgery, hospitalizations, medications, allergies, and illnesses that require periodic attention and provide the professional with an opportunity for counseling when appropriate.

The examining physician should use some judgment about what should or should not be done. Most examinations will need to focus on the presenting complaint. From the items presented, the physician should select what needs to be done.

Besides detecting serious conditions, identifying and categorizing presenting symptoms, and collecting information about the mechanism of injury and apparent work-relatedness, the history establishes rapport between patient and clinician. Asking open-ended questions is a useful way to start the inquiry. The patient's description of the mechanism of injury or illness (so far as is known), his or her presenting symptoms, the duration of symptoms, exacerbating factors, and history of previous episodes will help to define the problem. This description also provides insight into the patient's concerns and expectations, as well as the work, socioeconomic, and psychosocial issues that may affect the patient's response to treatment, functional status, and return to work.

The medical history includes the patient's estimate of activity tolerance given his or her symptoms. Perceived activity intolerance contributes to the clinical assessment of the presenting problem, guides treatment and self-care, provides the basis for disability and case management, and establishes a baseline for resuming the activity and evaluating progress. The medical history also should determine whether the present injury or illness is correlated now or in the past with a certain vocational or avocational activity.

Presenting Symptoms and Related Information

IDENTIFICATION OF BODY PART(S) INVOLVED

The most important aspect of an evaluation of a painful condition is to first identify the body part(s) involved, followed by an inquiry regarding the specific location of the pain. The patient almost invariably will raise a hand/finger to signal the location of the problem, and in two questions, 90% or more of problems typically can be diagnosed (all subsequent testing tends to be "rule in" or "rule out"). For example, the patient says that he or she has elbow pain. The next question is where in the elbow do you have pain? The patient may raise his or her left hand and signal the lateral aspect of the right elbow, and immediately the doctor should know that the diagnosis is most likely right lateral epicondylitis.

The focused occupational history elicits the following information about presenting symptoms:

- Date and time of onset
- Nature of onset (very gradual, increasing, acute)
- Mechanism: how the patient thinks it happened
- For acute trauma—the *four Ws*:
    - *Where*: Location of the accident
    - *When*: Time and date
    - *Who*: Other individuals involved
    - *What*: A detailed description of accident circumstances, including force and load
- Nature of symptoms: location, character
    - Changes in symptoms since onset
        - Means of increasing or decreasing symptoms
        - Limitation of function at home, at work, or in other situations
    - Past history of and therapy for similar complaints
    - Results of previous tests, treatments, and procedures
    - Site of accident
    - Other physicians or practitioners seen for this or similar complaints

Sources of historical information may include patient, the first responder(s), or other personnel involved or associated with accident.

Review of Body Systems

The history could include questions about the following:

FOR VISUAL SYSTEM COMPLAINTS (see Chapter 16 for details):

- Changes in central vision
- Changes in peripheral vision
- Presence of color vision abnormalities
- Double vision
- Ocular pain
- Sensation of foreign body in the eye(s)
- Red eye
- Discharge

FOR THE MUSCULOSKELETAL SYSTEM

- Pain (location, character, and radiation; see appropriate body part chapters for details)
- Deformity or dislocation
- Open wounds and/or blood loss
- Specific limitation of motion or other function

- Dysesthesias or paresthesias (location, character, and radiation)
- Weakness
- Atrophy

When a patient complains of pain, assessment tools such as pain drawings and visual analogue pain rating scales may help to further document the patient's perceptions and progress.

PSYCHOLOGICAL/BEHAVIORAL HISTORY FOR STRESS-RELATED COMPLAINTS (See Chapter 15 for details)

- Emotional distress
- Predominately sad, anxious, angry, or indifferent mood
- Flashbacks or nightmares with similar situations to a traumatic event[2]
- Recurrent intrusive thoughts
- Heightened arousal
- Concentration problems
- Sleep disturbance
- Hypervigilance
- Disruption in social or occupational functioning (e.g., withdrawal from activities, decreased work productivity).
- Increased use of substances or substance abuse
- Perceived stressors or excessive demands:
    - Work
        - Number of jobs held and work or shift schedules
        - Physical work environment (e.g., heat, cold, noise, risk)
        - Social and organizational structure of workplace (e.g., pace of job demands, overload, support of coworkers, and attitude of supervisors)
        - Organizational role (e.g., conflict, clarity of responsibility, demands, and degree of fit between worker and job/organization)
    - Family
        - Demands placed on working parents, multiple roles
    - Financial situation

[2] In the case of accident-related injury or significant stress, symptoms of posttraumatic stress disorder may be seen and include persistent reexperience of the event in the form of flashbacks, nightmares, intense distress when exposed to situations that remind the patient of the accident, and/or recurrent, intrusive thoughts of the incident. In addition, such workers often will avoid situations or feelings associated with the trauma and may experience emotional unresponsiveness. Persistent symptoms of heightened arousal (e.g., sleep disturbance, irritability, and anger), concentration problems, and hypervigilance also are characteristic features. Exacerbation of these symptoms may occur relatively frequently and may be associated with higher levels of pain, disability, and psychological distress.

- Effect of hobbies and after-work activities
- Other stressful life events or daily hassles
- Stress-related physical complaints
    - Cardiovascular (e.g., hypertension)
    - Headaches
    - GI dysfunction (e.g., ulcers, irritable bowel syndrome)
    - Sleep disturbance
    - Somatization or tendency to convert stress into physical symptoms
    - Neuroticism
    - Lack of self-esteem
    - Personality traits associated with difficulties in socialization

FOR CARDIOVASCULAR DISEASE

A number of workplace conditions have been implicated as risk factors for cardiovascular disease (CVD), including:

- Long work hours
- Shift work
- Chemical conditions (e.g., carbon disulfide, nitrate esters, carbon monoxide, methylene chloride, solvents)
- Physical conditions (e.g., cold, heat, noise, passive smoking, sedentary work)
- Degree of perceived threat/necessary vigilance[3]

FOR PULMONARY DISEASE

A relatively detailed history of the patient's complaints and environmental or occupational exposures is essential. It should include the following:

- Job title (e.g., machine operator, maintenance mechanic)
- The product being made (e.g., beryllium-containing airplane parts)
- The service being rendered (e.g., ventilation system cleaning)
- Actual work practices
- Types and duration of exposures
- Is ventilation adequate?

[3] Evidence strongly suggests a causal association between job strain (a combination of high psychological demands and low job decision latitude or low job control) and hypertension and CVD. Low decision latitude is also a risk factor for CVD. As yet limited but convincing evidence exists for a role of another psychosocial factor, effort-reward imbalance (ERI), with similar observed effect sizes as job strain. In addition, threat-avoidant vigilant (TAV) work has been identified through studies of single occupations as a potentially helpful explanatory variable as to why groups such as professional drivers—whose work is characterized by high TAV—have the most consistent evidence of CVD.

- Is visible dust, mist, or smoke present? (If yes, the ventilation in the work area may be inadequate.)
- Is respiratory protective equipment used?
- Is a two-part system used to make a paint or coating material? (If yes, occupational asthma is possible.)
- Are chemical odors present, or do headaches occur at work? (Yes to either suggests the possibility of overexposure to solvent or other vapors.)
- Does the work process involve friction, grinding, heat, blasting, generation of fine particles, or enclosed spaces? (If yes, the exposures are likely to be high.)

- Sources for determining and measuring exposure
    - MSDSs list the ingredients of the product and profile their important health, safety, and chemical properties.
    - Measurements of environmental concentrations of the agent(s) to which the patient was exposed may be obtained if available.
    - An industrial hygiene survey of the workplace may be requested if more exposure information is needed to evaluate the potential linkage between a patient's respiratory illness and occupational exposure.
- Other
    - Condition(s) found in the patient's home
    - Hobbies
    - Social habits

FOR ABDOMINAL DISORDERS

A relatively detailed history of the patient's complaints and environmental or occupational exposure is recommended. Beyond this, a gastrointestinal review of systems (ROS) may be appropriate and may include symptoms of occupational liver disease evaluation.

Abdominal Hernia. A hernia, the protrusion of an organ(s) through the abdominal wall, may be caused by any factor that increases pressure in the abdomen, such as

- Lifting heavy objects
- Coughing or sneezing a lot
- Constipation and straining for a bowel movement
- Obesity
- Pregnancy
- In men, pushing too hard to urinate when an enlarged prostate is causing a blockage.

Temporal relationship to the onset of symptoms/occurrence of a hernia during a work activity can be evaluated. Symptoms associated with a groin hernia may include

- Pain or discomfort in lower abdominal or groin area
- A bulge that cannot be pushed back in, a potentially life-threatening problem because the bowel (or other organ) may be trapped or strangulated

FITNESS

Does the patient do any routine regular or periodic physical activities in order to maintain better aerobic and overall muscle tone?

Work History

It is critical for the occupational health practitioner to obtain an accurate and complete yet focused picture of the patient's work situation, essential job functions, hobbies, and home activities and the possible work-relatedness of the patient's health concern. This is important in order to obtain an accurate diagnosis, to prevent delayed recovery and recurrences, and to determine compensability or liability.

The clinician should inquire about the patient's specific job, including a description of the worksite, range of motion performed, frequency of activity, rest periods, and posture. Having the patient demonstrate the requirements of the job often is useful in spotting a posture or movement that might cause or aggravate a condition. The clinician also should inquire about preventive programs, management, and relations with supervisors and coworkers. A history of exposures to possible causative factors, in terms as quantitative and complete as possible, is central to diagnosing, treating, and preventing each work-related complaint.

Further, the clinician may inquire about the frequency and types of illnesses not considered traditional occupational ailments, such as migraine headaches, allergic disorders, infectious diseases, and depression. These ailments can subtly and dramatically affect work performance. For example, recent epidemiologic studies have shown a relatively high prevalence of unrecognized, untreated depression that significantly affects work.

Job History and Description

The clinician should ask about and clearly document the following:

- Job title, description, and design
  - Specific tasks and time devoted to each task
  - Job or task rotation and other administrative controls

    - Safety and job training
    - Nightshift or rotating shift
- Additional or part-time jobs
    - Specific tasks and time devoted to each
    - Job or task rotation and other administrative controls
    - Safety and job training
    - Night shift or rotating shift
- Historical background
    - Has the patient changed companies or job title because of any health problem over the last 5 years?
    - If so, has the patient permanently changed the kinds of things he or she does at work because of the problem?

Exposure and Protection

- Exposure to trauma or other physical hazards, such as electricity, electromagnetic radiation, noise, vibration, chemicals, and/or biologic hazards on all jobs
- Exposures and protection at home, in hobbies, or at additional or part-time jobs
- History of such exposure in the past
    - What part of your health problem most affects you when you work?
    - Do you think something at work could have caused the problem?
    - Do you think something at work may make the problem worse, even if it did not cause it?
- Adequacy of protection from hazards (engineering, personal, job or task rotation, exercise breaks, conditioning)
    - Using personal protective equipment when exposed
    - Chemical sampling, ergonomic evaluations, and other relevant job evaluation
- At times, a medical problem can make work difficult. If you could change something at work to make it easier for people with medical conditions such as yours, what would it be?

FOR POTENTIAL CHEMICAL EXPOSURE

- *The name of chemical* [Description or Material Safety Data Sheet (MSDS)[4] information]

[4] Under federal law (29 CFR 1910.1200, Hazard Communication), MSDSs are to be furnished by the employer to the worker or his or her health care provider on request. Unfortunately, the quality of the information on MSDSs varies greatly because the information is supplied by the manufacturer of the product, and there is no effective mechanism in place to ensure that it is accurate.

- *The type of chemical* (alkali, acid, solvent)
- *The type of exposure* (liquids, solids, fumes)
- *The dose of exposure*
- The pH of the material
- The concentration of the material
- The solubility of the material
- The contact time (time from exposure until decontamination)
- Emergency medical care provided by the first responder(s)
- Product manufacturer

Chemical data may be available from Material Safety Data Sheets, the Internet, standard texts, or the Regional Poison Control Center.

FOR MUSCULOSKELETAL DISORDERS

- Intensity of exertion (How much force was used?)
- Frequency of exertion (How often did these exertions occur?)
- Duration of exertion (How long has the person performed this job? How long has the task been performed by the worker?)
- Static work (Are activities performed in one position with the development of localized muscle fatigue?)
- Use of the hand as a hammer or tool (Does the worker pound the hand on a part or tool?)
- Vibration (Is there low-frequency vibrating tool exposure and for how long?)
- Posture (How high must the person reach, or how low must he or she bend?)
- Is there rotation on the job? (Is there substantial variability in the job, or does the person rotate to a substantially different job?)
- Are lifting devices available for heavy lifts?
- Cold temperatures (Are the temperatures cold enough that greater force may have to be expended to hold the product or tool?)

Effect of Present Illness or Injury

- Time missed from work due to the current problem or health concern
- Time missed from work due to all health concerns (current and past)
- Work hours and days
    - Any recent changes
    - Concerns about job stability, safety, supervision, coworkers
- Relation of symptoms to work hours and days; symptoms on weekends and vacations

- Similar symptoms in coworkers or family members
- Preplacement testing relative to this area or organ system and test results
- Periodic testing or surveillance relative to this area or organ system and test results
- First report of illness or injury filed for this complaint; filing of a workers' compensation claim
- Discussing with the patient his or her typical functional level would be helpful to effectively determine the effect of this present illness or injury on his or her baseline functionality. Questions such as: What activities, if any, did you engage in previously? What were your restrictions? What are your restrictions now?
- The combination of medical history; occupational, ergonomic, and psychosocial stressors; symptom severity; and the way patient copes with pain are important predictors of clinical outcome.

Role of Epidemiology in the Assessment of Work-Relatedness[5]

Results from epidemiologic studies can contribute to the evidence of causality relationship between workplace risk factors and musculoskeletal disorders (MSDs). The framework for evaluating evidence for causality includes strength of association, consistency, temporality, exposures, response relationship, and coherence of evidence.

Using this framework, the evidence for a relationship between workplace factors and the development of MSDs from epidemiologic studies is classified into one of the following categories:

Strong evidence of work-relatedness (+++). A causal relationship is shown to be very likely between intense or long duration exposure to the specific risk factor(s) and MSD when the epidemiologic criteria of causality are used. A positive relationship has been observed between exposure to the specific risk factor and MSD in studies in which chance, bias, and confounding factors could be ruled out with reasonable confidence in at least several studies.

Evidence of work-relatedness (++). Some convincing epidemiologic evidence shows a causal relationship when the epidemiologic criteria of causality for intense or long-duration exposure to the specific risk factor(s) and MSD are used. A positive relationship has been observed between exposure to the specific risk factor and MSD in studies in which chance, bias, and confounding factors are not the likely explanation.

[5] MSDs and workplace factors in the Centers for Disease Control and Prevention (CDC) publication, Revised NIOSH: A Critical Review of Epidemiological Disorders for Work-Related Musculoskeletal Disorders of the Neck, Upper Extremity, and Low Back, DHHS (NIOSH) Publication No. 97-141.

Insufficient evidence of work-relatedness (+/0). The available studies are of insufficient number, quality, consistency, or statistical power to permit a conclusion regarding the presence or absence of a causal association. Some studies suggest a relationship to specific risk factors, but chance, bias, or confounding may explain the association.

Evidence of no effect of work factors (−). Adequate studies consistently show that the specific workplace risk factor(s) is not related to development of MSD.

A substantial body of credible epidemiologic research provides strong evidence of a connection between MSDs and certain work-related physical factors when there are high levels of exposure and especially in combination with exposure to more than one physical factor (e.g., repetitive lifting of heavy objects in extreme or awkward postures).

The strength of the associations reported in the various studies for specific risk factors and adjustments for other factors varies from modest to strong. The largest increases in risk generally are observed in studies with a wide range of exposure conditions and careful observance or measurement of exposures.

Role of Individual Factors in the Assessment of Work-Relatedness

Individual factors also may influence the degree of risk from specific exposures. There is evidence that some individual risk factors influence the occurrence of MSDs (e.g., elevated body mass index and carpal tunnel syndrome or a history of past back pain and current episodes of low back pain). There is little evidence, however, that these individual factors interact synergistically with physical factors. All these disorders also can be caused by nonwork exposures. The majority of epidemiologic studies involve health outcomes that range in severity from mild (workers reporting these disorders continue to perform their routine duties) to more severe disorders (workers are absent from the workplace for varying periods of time). The milder disorders are more common. A limited number of studies investigate the natural history of these disorders and attempt to determine whether continued exposure to physical factors alter their prognosis.

The number of jobs in which workers routinely lift heavy objects, are exposed on a daily basis to whole-body vibration, routinely perform overhead work, work with their necks in chronic flexion position, or perform repetitive forceful tasks is unknown. While these exposures do not occur in most jobs, a large number of workers may indeed work under these conditions.

Within the highest-risk industries, however, it is likely that the range of risk is substantial, depending on the specific nature of the physical exposures experienced by workers in various occupations within that industry. The risk factors for various parts will vary but generally will consist of repetition, force, posture, and vibration. Posture, in disorders of upper extremity, is not considered to be a risk factor by the National Institute for Occupational Safety and Health (NIOSH). Both the strongest studies (based on their criteria) were statistically negative for circulation trauma syndrome. Based primarily on pain complaints, there was strong evidence of neck/neck-shoulder disorders. Regarding the back, lifting, forceful movements, awkward posture, heavy physical work, whole-body vibration, and static work postures head up the list of risk factors.

The epidemiologic literature identified a number of specific physical exposures strongly associated with specific MSDs when exposures are intense and prolonged and particularly when workers are exposed to several risk factors simultaneously.

Physical Examination

Guided by the medical history, the areas covered in the physical examination should be selected and may include:

- General observation of the patient
  - Posture, station, and overall fitness level
  - General demeanor, affect, facial expression, mood changes
  - Gait and weight bearing
- Vital signs
  - Blood pressure
  - Pulse
  - Height
  - Weight
- Focused regional examination
- Neurologic, ophthalmologic, or other specific screening
- More comprehensive examination areas with related or potentially referred symptoms, as indicated by the history or the physician's knowledge of the tentative diagnostic entity
- Evaluation of nonorganic symptoms and signs

The content of focused examinations is determined by the presenting complaint and the area(s) and organ system(s) affected. (See the appropriate body part chapters in this book for details based on the system or part of the body involved.)

Examining the musculoskeletal system and elements of other organ systems, particularly those involving tenderness, pain, range of motion, or effort, are subjective to some extent because the patient's response or interpretation is required for findings on the examination. Some patients with musculoskeletal and other complaints will have no objective findings.

Communicating the Results of the Initial Assessment: Evaluating Fitness for Duty and/or Return to Work

After completing the initial assessment, the patient's condition may require communicating with his or her employer about any prescribed medical restrictions. It is obviously important for physicians to attempt to provide clear, concise, and specific restrictions when possible. However, it is critical that physicians understand and recognize the limitations in their own ability to either predict an individual's functional capacity or define what is safe and/or reasonable for an individual to do. For example, physicians must recognize that lifting limitations assigned often are arbitrary. How something is lifted is often much more important than how much is lifted.[6]

There is limited science to provide clear, concise, and specific guidance in assignment of restrictions. Therefore, arbitrary and opinionated restrictions are all too frequently observed. Physicians need to understand that such arbitrary designations (e.g., unable to lift more than 1 pound) are taken by court systems as unbending and inflexible truths. Simple transcription of a patient's complaint into the medical record with subsequent assertion that these reports have special scientific or clinical weight is inappropriate. In many cases, when restrictions are assigned, they are used by vocational rehabilitation specialists and others and translated into the *Dictionary of Occupational Title* definitions. At the very least, physicians should be fully aware of the implications of their restrictions.

Beyond evaluating a patient's health status, it is necessary to address how that status may affect the patient's ability to perform the essential functions of his or her current job or reasonably anticipated modified duty. The examining physician should not disclose to the employer any specific findings, diagnoses, or information unrelated to the patient's occupation or work environment.

The following may be noted in communicating with the employer:

- Specific and objective limitations
- Specialized equipment requirements
- Permanent or temporary restrictions
- Day/work-hour limitations
- Time period for restrictions/scheduled follow-up

Reasons for communicating with employers include:

- Informing supervisors and managers about medically indicated permanent and temporary restrictions on the patient's work or duties.
- Informing first aid and safety personnel, when appropriate, whether the patient's health status might require emergency treatment or

[6] Parameters that affect lifting capacity particularly as related to spinal capacities are available in the CDC publication, *Applications Manual for the Revised NIOSH Lifting Equation*. DHHS (NIOSH) Publication No. 94-110.

whether any specific assistance is needed in case of fire or other evacuations.

- Helping to ensure safety for the returning employee and coworkers.

Recordkeeping

The information obtained at the time of the first contact with the patient will, in the United States, normally be part of the Occupational Safety and Health Administration (OSHA) Form 301 (Injury and Illness Report) and any other reports, such as workers' compensation reports, that may be required. Employers in the United States are required to record work-related injuries or illnesses that result in one of the following: death, days absent from work, restricted work or transfer to another job, medical treatment beyond first aid,[7] loss of consciousness, or diagnosis of a significant injury/illness by a physician or other licensed health care professional. Further, an adequately documented, legible report is essential for accurate billing and legal purposes.[8]

Records generally contain the following:

- Full name and address data
- Date of birth
- Date of hire
- Gender
- Date and time the injury/illness occurred
- Nature of the injury/illness (part of the body affected)
- How did it happen?

[7] According to OSHA, 29 CFR 1904(b)(5)(ii), "first aid" means the following: (a) using a nonprescription medication at nonprescription strength (for medications available in both prescription and nonprescription forms, a recommendation by a physician or other licensed health care professional to use a nonprescription medication at prescription strength is considered medical treatment for record keeping purposes); (b) administering tetanus immunizations (other immunizations, such as hepatitis B vaccine or rabies vaccine, is considered medical treatment); (c) cleaning, flushing, or soaking wounds on the surface of the skin; (d) using wound coverings such as bandages, Band-Aids, gauze pads, etc. or using butterfly bandages or Steri-Strips (other wound-closing devices such as sutures, staples, etc. are considered medical treatment); (e) using hot or cold therapy; (f) using any nonrigid means of support, such as elastic bandages, wraps, nonrigid back belts, etc. (devices with rigid stays or other systems designed to immobilize parts of the body are considered medical treatment for record keeping purposes); (g) using temporary immobilization devices while transporting an accident victim (e.g., splints, slings, neck collars, back boards, etc.); (h) drilling of a fingernail or toenail to relieve pressure or draining fluid from a blister; (i) using eye patches; (j) removing foreign bodies from the eye using only irrigation or a cotton swab; (k) removing splinters or foreign material from areas other than the eye by irrigation, tweezers, cotton swabs, or other simple means; (l) using finger guards; (m) using massages (physical therapy or chiropractic treatment are considered medical treatment for record keeping purposes); or (n) drinking fluids for relief of heat stress.

[8] Incomplete or illegible recording for billing purposes can lead to inaccurate coding, billing, insufficient reimbursement, and loss of reimbursement.

- What was the employee doing just before the incident occurred?
- What object or substance directly harmed the employee?
- Where was treatment given? At the worksite?
- If treatment was administered away from the worksite, where was it given?
- Who was in charge of treatment?
- Was the employee hospitalized as an inpatient? Who was the attending practitioner? What was his or her subspecialty?
- If the employee died, when and where did the death occur? Who pronounced the employee dead?

Privacy of Records

The confidentiality of medical information and records is protected and required by statutes, regulations, and codes of medical ethics, which govern their maintenance, retention, and release. Medical information concerns the medical status of individual patients, including historical, physical, and laboratory findings. Medical records are the physical or data-storage form of medical information gathered from or applying to patients and should be considered protected health information. Examples of information reflected in medical records include:

- Oral information, including telephone communication, noted by a physician or other allied health professional.
- Reports of medical examinations, progress notes, laboratory results, consultations, assessments, and recommendations.
- Electronically or optically stored or transmitted information.
- Photographs taken for medical purposes.
- Radiologic studies.
- Billing data or records.

Medical records should be secured, with access limited to physicians, their qualified designees, and others who have a legal right to access. An authorization for release of medical information, signed by the patient and meeting the applicable legal requirements, must be executed before medical records are released. When medical information or records are transmitted, only that information pertinent to the issue at hand should be sent unless otherwise authorized.

Medical confidentiality may be waived by operation of law and by authorization of the patient or the patient's legal representative. The former commonly occurs in legal proceedings in which the patient places his or her physical condition at issue. For example, in some states, the filing of a workers' compensation claim is deemed to allow the insurer access to all medical records that relate to a condition relevant to the claim, regardless of whether the injured worker authorizes such release. The latter is the more common manner by which physicians obtain authorization to release medical information.

Only pertinent information and records should be released. Absent patient consent or specific legal authority, physician recommendations communicated to an employer concerning a patient's medical clearance, performance, and/or safety in the workplace should not include medical diagnoses.

Providers should familiarize themselves with the laws of their states that relate to the disclosure of confidential medical information. In the United States, complex issues involving the supremacy of federal law in a particular circumstance may arise depending on the wording of certain state statutes. It is beyond the scope of this publication to explore such issues. It is a sound practice for providers, whenever possible, to require that they be provided with current, properly worded releases that specify the records to be released and the recipients who are to receive them. Once in possession of such documentation, providers should take care not to release information that is beyond the scope of the authorization that has been received.

References

MEDICAL HISTORY: PRESENTING SYMPTOMS

Barsky AJ, Goodson JD, Lane RS, et al. The amplification of somatic symptoms. *Psychosom Med.* 1988;50:510-9.

Blais BR. Occupational ophthalmology. In: Tasman W, Jaeger EA, eds. *Duane's Clinical Ophthalmology.* Philadelphia, Pa: Lippincott Williams & Wilkins; 2002:5:37.

Sullivan MJ, Katon WJ. Somatization: the path between distress and somatic symptoms. *APS J.* 1993;2:141-9.

OSHA Federal Law, 29 CFR 1910.1200. Hazard Communication.

REVIEW OF BODY SYSTEMS

Andersson GBJ, Fine LJ, Silverstein BA. Musculoskeletal disorders. In: Levy BS, Wegman DH, eds. *Occupational Health: Recognizing and Preventing Work-Related Disease.* Boston, Mass: Little, Brown and Company; 1995.

Balmes JR. Occupational respiratory diseases. *Prim Care.* 2000;27(4):1009-38.

Belkic K, Schnall P, Ugljesic M. Cardiovascular evaluation of the worker and workplace: a practical guide for clinicians. *Occup Med.* 2000;15(1):213-22, iv.

Dworkin SF, Von Korff M, LeResche L. Multiple pains and psychiatric disturbance: an epidemiologic investigation. *Arch Gen Psychiatry.* 1990;47:239-44.

Frank AL. The occupational and environmental history and examination. In: Rom WN, ed. *Environmental and Occupational Medicine.* Boston, Mass: Little, Brown and Company; 1992.

Wiley SD. Deception and detection in psychiatric diagnosis. *Psychiatr Clin North Am.* 1998;21(4):869-93.

EXPOSURE AND PROTECTION

OSHA Federal Law, CFR 1910.132. Personal Protective Equipment.

CORRELATION WITH PRESENT ILLNESS OR INJURY

Boedeker W. Associations between workload and diseases rarely occurring in sickness absence data. *J Occup Environ Med.* 2001;43(12):1081-8.

Feuerstein M, Huang GD, Haufler AJ, Miller JK. Development of a screen for predicting clinical outcomes in patients with work-related upper extremity disorders. *J Occup Environ Med.* 2000;42(7):749-61.

Katon WJ, Lin E, Von Korff M, et al. Somatization: a spectrum of severity. *Am J Psychiatry.* 1990;148:34-40.

Moore JS, Garg A. A comparison of different approaches for ergonomic job evaluation for predicting risk of upper extremity disorders. IEA 94. *Occup Health Saf* 2.

ROLE OF EPIDEMIOLOGY IN THE ASSESSMENT OF WORK-RELATEDNESS

Silverstein BA. The prevalence of upper extremity cumulative trauma disorders in industry. Doctoral dissertation, University of Michigan; 1985.

Silverstein BA, Fine LJ, Armstrong TJ. Hand-wrist cumulative trauma disorders in industry. *Br J Ind Med.* 1986;43(11):779-84.

Silverstein BA, Fine LF, Armstrong RJ. Occupational factors and the carpal tunnel syndrome. *Am J Ind Med.* 1987;11:343-58.

PHYSICAL EXAMINATION

Bridges K, Goldberg D, Evans B, et al. Determinants of somatization in primary care. *Psychol Med.* 1991;21:473-83.

Herrington T. Preplacement testing. In: LaDou J, ed. *Occupational Health and Safety.* 2nd ed. Chicago: National Safety Council; 1995.

Herrington TN, Morse LH. *Occupational Injuries: Evaluation, Management, and Prevention.* St. Louis, Mo: Mosby-Year Book; 1995.

COMMUNICATION OF RESULTS OF THE INITIAL ASSESSMENT AND EVALUATION OF FITNESS FOR DUTY AND/OR RETURN TO WORK

Boswell RT, McCunney RJ. Musculoskeletal disorders. In: McCunney RJ, ed. *A Practical Approach to Occupational and Environmental Medicine.* 3rd ed. Philadelphia, Pa: Lippincott, Williams & Wilkins, 2003.

Brigham CR, Ensalada LH, Talmadge JB, eds. Evaluation of Impairments. *Clin Occup Environ Med.* 2001;6(4).

Clark WL. Disability evaluation. In: LaDou J, ed. *Occupational Medicine.* Norwalk, Conn: Appleton & Lange; 1990.

Demeter SL, Andersson GBJ, Smith GM. *Disability Evaluation.,* 2d ed. St. Louis, Mo: Mosby; 2003.

Foye PM, Stitik TP, Marquardt CA, Cianca JC, Prather H. Industrial medicine and acute musculoskeletal rehabilitation: 5. Effective medical management of industrial injuries: from causality to case closure. *Arch Phys Med Rehabil.* 2002;83(3 Suppl 1):S19-24, S33-9.

Islam SS, Velilla AM, Doyle EJ, Ducatman AM. Gender differences in work-related injury/illness: analysis of workers compensation claims. *Am J Ind Med.* 2001;39(1):84-91.

Margoshes B. Disability management and occupational health. *Occup Med.* 1998;13(4):693-703, iii.

McCunney RJ. Health and productivity: a role for occupational health professionals. *J Occup Environ Med.* 2001;43(1):30-5.

Miller TR. *Evaluating Orthopedic Disability: A Commonsense Approach.* Oradell, NJ: Medical Economics Books; 1987.

Randolph DC, Ranavaya MI, eds. Risk and disability evaluation in the work place. *Occup Med.* 2000;15(4):review.

Viederman M. Active engagement in the consultation process(1). *Gen Hosp Psychiatry.* 2002;24(2):93-100.

Wyman DO. Evaluating patients for return to work. *Am Fam Physician.* 1999;59(4):844-8.

RECORDKEEPING

Courtney TK, Webster BS. Disabling occupational morbidity in the United States: an alternative way of seeing the Bureau of Labor Statistics' data. *J Occup Environ Med.* 1999;41(1):60-9.

Occupational injury and illness recording and reporting requirements. Occupational Safety and Health Administration (OSHA), US Department of Labor: Final rule. *Fed Reg.* 2001;66(13):5916-6135.

OSHA Federal Law, CFR 1910.151. Medical and First Aid.

GENERAL

Atcheson SG, Brunner RL, Greenwald EJ, Rivera VG, Cox JC, Bigos SJ. Paying doctors more: use of musculoskeletal specialists and increased physician pay to decrease workers' compensation costs. *J Occup Environ Med.* 2001;43(8):672-9.

Blais BR. Occupational ophthalmology. In: McCunney R, ed. *A Practical Approach to Occupational and Environmental Medicine.* 3rd ed. Philadelphia, Pa: Lippincott Williams & Wilkins; 2003:477-509.

Frank AL. Approach to the patient with an occupational or environmental illness. *Primary Care: Clin Office Pract.* 2000;27(4):877-94.

Harber P, Mullin M, Merz B, Tarazi M. Frequency of occupational health concerns in general clinics. *J Occup Environ Med.* 2001;43(11):939-945.

Imbus HR. Clinical aspects of occupational medicine. In: Zenz C, Dickerson OB, Horvath EP, eds. *Occupational Medicine.* St. Louis, Mo: Mosby-Year Book; 1994.

Rundall TG. Health planning and evaluation. In: Last JM, Wallace RB, eds. *Public Health and Preventive Medicine.* Norwalk, Conn: Appleton & Lange; 1992.

Additional Resources

RETURN-TO-WORK DURATION GUIDELINES

Bruckman RZ, Rasmussen H. *Healthcare Management Guidelines,* Vol. 7: *Workers' Compensation.* Seattle, Wash: Milliman & Robertson; 1996.

Denniston PL, Ranavaya MI, eds. *Official Disability Guidelines 2003,* 8th ed. Corpus Christi, Texas: Work Loss Data Institute; 2002.

Reed P, ed. *The Medical Disability Advisor: Workplace Guidelines for Disability Duration.* 4th ed. Boulder, Colo: Reed Group; 2001.

IMPAIRMENT GUIDELINES

Cocchiarella L, Andersson GBJ, eds. *Guides to the Evaluation of Permanent Impairment.,* 5th ed. Chicago, Ill: American Medical Association Press; 2001.

Appendix 2A: HIPAA Privacy Guidance

The Secretary of the Health and Human Services (HHS) has assigned oversight of HIPAA (45 CFR Parts 160 and 164 created December 28, 2000, amended August 14, 2002) privacy compliance to the Office of Civil Rights (OCR). A practice may want to bookmark OCR's Web site (www.hhs.gov/ocr/hipaa/assist.html) to review or download the document, "Frequently Asked Questions About the HIPAA Privacy Rule." This document will be updated as OCR responds to questions posted on its Web site or develops additional guidance on privacy issues.

Guidance on HIPAA issues is based on information contained in "Small Practice Implementation Guide," version 2.0 (www.wedi.org/snip/public/articles/200211012.0final.pdf, © 2002 The Workgroup on Electronic Data Interchange).

The standards for Privacy of Individually Identifiable Health Information, 45 Code of Federal Regulations (CFR), Parts 160 and 164, set forth the mandatory requirements on privacy of records, summarized as follows:

(A) *Standard.*

A covered entity may not use or disclose protected health information, except as permitted or required by Part 164 or by subpart C of Part 160.

(1) Permitted uses and disclosures. A covered entity is permitted to use or disclose protected health information as follows:

- (i) To the individual;
- (ii) For treatment, payment, or health care operations as permitted by and in compliance with Part 164
- (iii) Incident to a use or disclosure otherwise permitted or required by this subpart, provided that the covered entity has complied with the applicable requirements with respect to such otherwise permitted or required use or disclosure.

(2) Required disclosures. A covered entity is required to disclose protected health information:

- (i) To an individual, when requested
- (ii) When required by the Secretary Health and Human Services under subpart C of part 160 of this subchapter to investigate or determine the covered entity's compliance with this subpart.

(B) *Standard: minimum necessary.*

(1) Minimum necessary applies. When using or disclosing protected health information or when requesting protected health information from another covered entity, a covered entity must make reasonable efforts to limit protected health information to the minimum necessary to accomplish the intended purpose of the use, disclosure, or request.

- *Assurances from business associates to safeguard confidential information that your practice shares with them.* A business associate is defined as a person or organization that is not a member of your staff but performs a function that uses confidential information from your practice. A good example of a business associate might be a health care clearinghouse that submits the practice's claims. Plumbers, electricians, office equipment repair people, and mail carriers are not considered business associates unless the practice has contracted with them to handle or shred medical records. Practices will need written contracts or similar agreements with business associates that list the permitted and required uses and disclosures of confidential information. Practices may look at the sample contract language on the U.S. Department of Health and Human Services (HHS) Office of Civil Rights Web site listed in "Sample Business Associate Contract Provisions."
- *Procedural and physical safeguards to protect and ensure the security of confidential information.* What are the practice's procedures for patients' and other visitors' access to the office beyond the waiting room? How are the records maintained and secured? What measures do you take to ensure the security of the confidential information when it is housed on your computer system or transmitted by modem or fax? If a fire, flood, or computer breakdown occurs, what is your contingency

plan to recover and secure the records? You will have to document the answers to these questions in writing and include the documentation in the privacy manual.

- *Access and audit control.* Each practice must establish and document levels of staff access to patient records. During this process it is important to ensure that the staff understands what the practice considers to be unauthorized use, disclosure, modification, and destruction of confidential patient information. In electronic medical records systems, a mechanism must be in place for identifying and tracking who has accessed or attempted to access confidential information. The privacy manual must specify who may access the log and how the log will be reviewed to identify potential weaknesses or actual breaches of security. Because of the required privacy provisions, it seems possible that all electronic health systems will soon have auditing capability. At the present time, however, there is no comparable requirement for paper medical records.
- *Training.* All members of your staff must receive sufficient training so that they can implement properly your practice's policies and procedures for handling confidential information. Training could be done individually or in a staff meeting to discuss how the practice will handle privacy concerns or by having the staff review the practice's notice of privacy policies. During training, the practice's privacy officer can emphasize that the practice is open to staff observations of lapses in compliance with privacy procedures and that staff members can feel comfortable approaching the privacy officer about their observations.
- *What if confidential information is disclosed?* A practice is obligated to make a reasonable effort to mitigate any harm that might result from using or disclosing confidential information in violation of its policies and procedures. A practice also must impose sanctions against staff members or business associates who do not comply with its policies and procedures. At a minimum, sanctions could mean retraining on privacy policies and perhaps noting the violation in an employee's record. If the disclosure is serious or flagrant enough, dismissing the staff member or canceling a contract with a business associate may be necessary.

When developing, organizing, and refining the practice's policy manual, remember that its contents must include procedures to address each item listed in the "Notice of Privacy Practices."

3 *Initial Approaches to Treatment*

Patient Information, Discussion, and Involvement

In the absence of red flags, the occupational health practitioner should discuss with the ill or injured worker clear, objective information about:

- The natural history of the acute complaint and the particular diagnosis.
- The generally favorable outlook for recovery (assuming that the condition is acute).
- The timeline for recovery, including goals and expectations of function.
- Testing and treatment options, with an explanation of the sensitivity, specificity, yield, risks, and benefits in lay terms or with print or audiovisual aids.
- Safe return to work as a primary expectation and that patients who return early to full or modified work typically have better long-term outcomes.

If the initial assessment does not detect any serious conditions, the physician can assure the patient that a dangerous problem does not exist and that a rapid recovery from the acute complaint can be expected. The need for discussion and information varies among patients and at various stages of care. Labeling nonspecific conditions should be avoided. While an acute condition must be identified for compensation under most workers' compensation statutes, labeling a regional pain syndrome as an injury creates a mind-set in the patient that there is specific anatomic damage when in fact such conditions are idiopathic and self-resolving in the absence of inactivity or iatrogenesis.

Determining whether a patient suffers from a pathologic condition may not always be straightforward. Some workers may believe that symptoms resulting from a lack of fit with job activities reflect physical injury or an occupational disease. When they present for evaluation, they may describe their problem as characterized by the gradual development of symptoms (primarily pain) over time or the development of symptoms after a minor physiologic stress. Often they may have multiple symptoms with nonspecific physical findings. Some health care providers may perform multiple tests and procedures to attempt to determine the source of these employees' complaints. In the absence of reproducible objective findings that are known to be work-related in population studies, an incomplete or inaccurate approach to the patient assessment may set the stage for the prolongation of medical care, delayed recovery, and later the range of behaviors that develop in order to prove that the symptoms reflect an injury or occupational disease that precludes a return to the work environment.

When patients are actively involved in decision making, it is possible to decrease inappropriate testing and treatment and hasten recovery. The therapeutic alliance between the occupational health practitioner and the patient is critical to prompt recovery. The need for patient discussion and information varies among patients (some patients need more detailed information and discussion) and at various stages of care. Conveying all information to the patient can foster informed decision making. The clinician should discuss the uses and yields of tests, both appropriate and inappropriate, as well as the content, effects, mechanics, and effectiveness of proposed treatment methods.

Labeling nonspecific conditions (regional pain syndromes) should be avoided because labeling creates a mind-set that specific anatomic damage exists. Such conditions are usually self-resolving if inactivity and iatrogenesis are avoided.

Instruction in self-care methods is critical for ongoing self-management. For patients with specific, more common conditions, the use and explanation of overall norms and medians for length of disability may be helpful in including the patient in the decision-making process. The physician can consult a few disability-duration references for more information regarding length of disability.[1] Understanding and awareness are the precursors for action.

An apprehensive patient requires more detailed information and discussion. History should be obtained regarding the patient's attempt to control symptoms and the effectiveness of those methods. However, a number of points should be covered with all patients, including diagnosis and treatment, controlling symptoms, restoring function, return to work, preventing recurrences, and appropriate tests and treatments:

- Musculoskeletal symptoms can be managed with a combination of heat or cold therapy, short-term pharmacotherapy (oral medication), a short period of inactivity, specific recommendations regarding employment and recreational activities, and judicious mobilization and resumption of activity, even before the patient is pain-free.[2]
- Most patients will recover function to reasonable levels and have a decrease in both pain and limitation of activity within days to weeks; if recovery takes longer, the patient should communicate with the physician.
- For the conditions discussed in these guidelines, few useful or cost-

[1] See "Other References" at end of this chapter.

[2] See specific body part chapters later in this book for additional information.

effective tests exist for the average patient or problem in the first few days or weeks.

- Inactivity and/or immobilization should be limited because they result in deconditioning and bone loss after relatively short periods of time.
- Communication of physical therapy assessment and progress can be used as a means of monitoring, ensuring compliance, and getting the patient back to work.
- Return to work has a variety of benefits for ill or injured workers as they recover (see Chapter 5, "Cornerstones of Disability Prevention and Management").

There are risks and benefits for recommended and popular, but sometimes unproven or non-cost-effective, test and treatment options, including various imaging procedures, physical modalities, medications, and surgery; the clinician should present the patient with specific treatment options and discuss the following items:

- Sensitivity, specificity, and yield for tests
- Actions, side effects, complications, and costs of medications
- Quantitative risks and benefits for procedures
- Differences between proven and unproven tests and treatments

The clinician also should discuss with the patient and employer potential practical strategies for modifying worksite situations, including ergonomic risk factors, load and pacing, supervision, interpersonal factors, and task design. Finally, a patient's concern about his or her role, financial matters, employment security, and family can increase stress and delay recovery. These concerns also should be part of the exchange between the clinician and patient.

The clinician may present this at the patient's own pace (with allowance for repetition), using interactive media such as CD-ROMs or videotapes, if these are available. Using an anatomic model also can be helpful when video resources are not available. Midlevel practitioners can reinforce and discuss the information as needed. In some cases, small groups can be used for discussion and support, for example, at the worksite or in group practices, especially for patients with recurrent problems. Giving patients generic or specific summary information to take home for reference can be quite valuable in increasing their knowledge of and active involvement in recovery. Surveys of patient satisfaction can be useful to evaluate the effectiveness of education and discussion, as well as the provision of testing and treatment. Lastly, office environment, friendliness and knowledge of staff, and minimal waiting periods and patient trust can lead to greater patient satisfaction and faster, more efficient recovery.

Variance from Expectations

If the patient is not recovering as he or she expects, the patient and clinician should seek reasons for the delay and address them appropriately. Patients who do not improve within a few days (i.e., those with eye complaints) or weeks (i.e., those with musculoskeletal complaints) may need more extensive information and discussion about their problems, as well as reassurance that special studies may be considered if consistent with the working diagnosis and if recovery continues to be slow. Patients with neurologic or structural disorders may have a longer expected recovery time than patients with nonspecific symptoms and thus may need more discussion, information, and reassurance.

Communication between the clinician, patient, and patient's employer will ensure that the patient/employee and employer understand why the functional recovery is progressing more slowly than expected and what is being done to aid the process. If kept involved and informed in the process, the employer may be more likely to provide modified work possibilities for the recovering worker. Although verbal contact is best, physicians should minimize communication gaps with a simple form or written explanation for employers and the worker.

Managing Expectations

Managing patient and employer expectations is part of total care management. Imparting general information to the patient is useful, but it must be personalized. The clinician should have an open discussion with the patient to understand what the health condition means to the patient and the patient's knowledge, beliefs, and expectations about the effects of the condition and functional recovery. In addition, the physician should deal with commonly held misconceptions about many complaints, such as back pain and wrist pain, by conveying information about causation, prevention, and accurate diagnosis. Patients may believe that they must be inactive to avoid further damage, that they have serious structural problems or instabilities, that they will be permanently disabled, or that they will require surgery. They may have other, more personal concerns, which may be based on the experiences of friends or relatives, whether medically justified or not. Because they may not voice their concerns directly, providing such information may have a significant benefit. Managing expectations in this way often can hasten recovery. Besides providing the patient with a realistic set of expectations, the clinician also must manage the expectations of the employer, insurance carrier, and perhaps a union or a lawyer. Written and verbal contact is the best way to keep these parties educated, informed, and aligned.

PATIENT COMFORT

Physical comfort, often a major concern of patients, can and should be achieved in several ways:

- Reducing anxiety by sharing concerns, providing information about the patient's condition, and frankly discussing the expected course of recovery and the risks and benefits of medications

- Physical methods (self- and provider-provided)
- Rest, immobilization, and activity
- Medication, tests, and surgery

Oral Pharmaceuticals

Oral pharmaceuticals are a first-line palliative method. Nonprescription analgesics provide sufficient pain relief for most patients with acute work-related symptoms. If treatment response is inadequate (i.e., symptoms and activity limitations continue), physicians should add prescribed pharmaceuticals or physical methods. Consideration of comorbid conditions, side effects, cost, and efficacy of medication versus physical methods and provider and patient preferences should guide the physician's choice of recommendations. The physician should discuss the efficacy of medication for the particular condition, its side effects, and any other relevant information with the patient to ensure proper use and, again, to manage expectations.

ACETAMINOPHEN AND NONSTEROIDAL ANTI-INFLAMMATORY DRUGS

The safest effective medication for acute musculoskeletal and eye problems appears to be acetaminophen. Nonsteroidal anti-inflammatory drugs (NSAIDs), including aspirin and ibuprofen, also are effective, although they can cause gastrointestinal irritation or ulceration or, less commonly, renal or allergic problems. Studies have shown that when NSAIDs are used for more than a few weeks, they can retard or impair bone, muscle, and connective tissue healing and perhaps cause hypertension. Therefore, they should be used only acutely. Phenylbutazone is not recommended due to the risk of bone marrow suppression. Initial treatment of symptoms should be limited to nonprescription analgesics. Acetaminophen may be used safely in combination with NSAIDs or other pharmacologic or physical methods.

MUSCLE RELAXANTS

Muscle relaxants seem no more effective than NSAIDs for treating patients with musculoskeletal problems, and using them in combination with NSAIDs has no demonstrated benefit, although they have been shown to be useful as antispasmodics. Side effects including drowsiness have been reported in up to 30% of patients taking muscle relaxants. Muscle relaxants act on the central nervous system and have no effect on peripheral musculature. They may hinder return to function by reducing the patient's motivation or ability to increase activity.

OPIOIDS

Opioids appear to be no more effective than safer analgesics for managing most musculoskeletal and eye symptoms; they should be used only if needed for severe pain and only for a short time. Opioids cause significant side effects, which the clinician should describe to the patient before prescribing them. Poor patient tolerance, constipation, drowsiness, clouded judgment, memory loss, and potential misuse or dependence have been reported in up to 35% of patients. Patients should be informed of these potential side effects.

Injections

Injections of corticosteroids or local anesthetics or both should be reserved for patients who do not improve with more conservative therapies. Steroids can weaken tissues and predispose to reinjury. Local anesthetics can mask symptoms and inhibit long-term solutions to the patient's problem. Both corticosteroids and local anesthetics have risks associated with intramuscular or intraarticular administration, including infection and unintended damage to neurovascular structures. Injections of opioids are never indicated except for conditions involving acute, severe trauma.

Rest, Immobilization, and Activity

Restriction of activity or immobilization should be employed only for short periods of time because both result in deconditioning and bone loss in a matter of days. Bone or muscle lost in this way cannot be restored without undertaking a reconditioning program. In addition, aching, stiffness, and pain will occur if muscles and joints are not used. As pain decreases, mobilization of painful areas can proceed carefully. Depending on the condition in question, aerobic and specific activities may improve comfort both acutely and as recovery progresses. In the case of eye complaints, refer to Chapter 16.

Physical Methods

During the acute to subacute phases for a period of 2 weeks or less, physicians can use passive modalities such as application of heat and cold for temporary amelioration of symptoms and to facilitate mobilization and graded exercise. They are most effective when the patient uses them at home several times a day. Although not for long-term use, transcutaneous galvanic and electrical stimulation can keep symptoms at bay temporarily, diminishing pain long enough so that patients begin to mobilize. Little evidence exists for the effectiveness of other passive modalities.

The value of physical therapy increases when a physician gives the therapist a specific diagnosis of the lesion causing the patient's symptoms. With a prescription that clearly states treatment goals, a physician can use communication with the therapist to monitor such variables as motivation and compliance. Therapists can be very effective as a member of the treatment team, can amplify the physician's directions to the patient, and can provide substantial encouragement regarding return to work.

Manipulative therapy on appropriately selected patients may be effective in aiding recovery, as opposed to providing merely short-term comfort, only in patients with low back pain for defined periods of time (less than 4 weeks' duration). There is some controversy regarding the use of spinal manipulation on patients with radiculopathy.

Physicians must be aware of presenting patient characteristics because some will respond better than others. Manipulative therapy works especially well on patients who are open-minded and optimistic, as well as on those who have had previous success with physical modalities. However, caution is warranted because some patients develop treatment dependence. Patients who may react negatively include those who have never had any prior experience with manipulation and are anxious or uneducated about manipulation and those who are extremely sensitive to touch. For these types of patients, even the physical therapist should be told to be careful during treatment. In most cases involving the anxious patient, extra time and medication from the physician and pain medication have the most success. Finally, limited-duty (restricted) work that allows the patient to remain engaged with the workplace and strong encouragement so that the patient feels "something is being done" may help this particular personality type more than any physical treatment. See Table 3-1 for a summary of recommendations on initial approaches to treatment.

Table 3-1. Summary of Recommendations on Initial Approaches to Treatment

	Recommended	Optional	Not Recommended
Patient discussion education, and involvement	Patient discussion[c] Patient involvement[b]	Patient education[c]	
Medication	Acetaminophen[c] NSAIDs[b]	Opioids, short course[c] Steroid injections[d]	Muscle relaxants[c] NSAIDs[c] Opioids > 2 weeks[c] Topical medications
Physical treatment methods	Early physical intervention	Self-application of heat or cold[d] Manipulation without radiculopathy[b] Manipulation, radiculopathy present[c]	Manipulation, prior to diagnosis of progressive or severe neurologic deficits[d] Traction[b] TENS[a]

[a]Strong research-based evidence (multiple relevant, high-quality scientific studies).
[b]Moderate research-based evidence (one relevant, high-quality scientific study or multiple adequate scientific studies).
[c]Limited research-based evidence (at least one adequate scientific study).
[d]Panel interpretation of information not meeting inclusion criteria for research-based evidence.
Source: Adapted from Bigos, 1994.

Other Methods and Modalities

Specific treatment methods are evaluated and discussed in Chapters 8 through 16.

References

GENERAL

Bigos SJ, Bowyer O, Braen G, et al. *Acute Low Back Problems in Adults.* Clinical Practice Guideline No. 14. Rockville, MD: U.S. Department of Health and Human Services, Public Health Service, Agency for Health Care Policy and Research, AHCPR Pub. No. 95-0642; 1994.

Krause N, Frank JW, Dasinger LK, Sullivan TJ, Sinclair SJ. Determinants of duration of disability and return-to-work after work-related injury and illness: challenges for future research. *Am J Ind Med.* 2001;40(4):464-84.

PATIENT INFORMATION, DISCUSSION, AND INVOLVEMENT

Barry MJ, Fowler FJ Jr, Mulley AG Jr, Henderson JV Jr, Wennberg JE. Patient reactions to a program designed to facilitate patient participation in treatment decisions for benign prostatic hyperplasia. *Med Care.* 1995;33(8):771-82.

Bandura A. Self-Efficacy Mechanism in Physiological Activation and Health-Promoting Behavior. Presented at the National Health Management Conference, San Francisco, September 1991.

Belzer EJ. Improving patient communication in no time. *Fam Pract Manag.* 1999;6(5):23-8.

Bigos SJ, Battie MC. Acute care to prevent back disability: ten years of progress. *Clin Orthop.* 1987;221:121-30.

Braddock CH III, Edwards KA, Hasenberg NM, Laidley TL, Levinson W. Informed decision making in outpatient practice: time to get back to basics. *JAMA.* 1999;282(24):2313-20.

Brines J, Salazar MK, Graham KY, Pergola T, Connon C. Injured workers' perceptions of case management services: a descriptive study. *AAOHN J.* 1999;47(8):355-64.

Brody DS, Miller SM, Lerman CE, et al. Patient perceptions of involvement in medical care: relationship to illness attitudes and outcomes. *J Gen Intern Med.* 1989;4:506-11.

Bush T, Cherkin D, Barlow W. The impact of physician attitudes on patient satisfaction with care for low back pain. *Arch Fam Med.* 1993;2:301.

Cohen JE, Goel V, Frank JW, et al. Group education interventions for people with low back pain: an overview of the literature. *Spine.* 1994;19:214-22.

Deyo RA, Diehl AK. Patient satisfaction with medical care for low back pain. *Spine.* 1986;11:28-30.

Deyo RA, Diehl AK, Rosenthal M. Reducing x-ray utilization: can patient expectations be altered? *Clin Res.* 1986;34:269A.

Deyo RA, Cherkin DC, Weinstein J, Howe J, Ciol M, Mulley AG Jr. Involving patients in clinical decisions: impact of an interactive video program on use of back surgery. *Med Care.* 2000;38(9):959-69.

Edwards A, Elwyn G, Mulley A. Explaining risks: turning numerical data into meaningful pictures. *Br Med J.* 2002;324(7341):827-30.

Eisenthal S, Koopman C, Lazare A. Process analysis of two dimensions of the negotiated approach in relation to satisfaction in the initial interview. *J Nerv Mental Dis.* 1983;171:49-54.

Fowler FJ Jr, Wennberg JE, Timothy RP, Barry MJ, Mulley AG Jr, Hanley D. Symptom status and quality of life following prostatectomy. *JAMA.* 1988;259(20):3018-22.

Gardner HH, Shneiderman CA. Ensuring value by supporting consumer decision making. In: Harris JS, Belk HD, Wood LW, eds. *Managing Employee Health Care Costs: Assuring Quality and Value.* Beverly, Mass: OEM Press; 1992.

Gerr F, Mani L. Work-related low back pain. *Primary Care: Clin Office Pract.* 2000;27(4):865-76.

Greenfield S, Kaplan S, Ware JE. Expanding patient involvement in care: effects on patient outcomes. *Ann Intern Med.* 1985;102:520-8.

Kemper DW, Lorig K, Mettler M. The effectiveness of medical self care interventions: a focus on self-initiated response to symptoms. *Patient Educ Couns.* 1993;21:29-39.

Lorig K, Kraines RG, Brown BW, et al. A workplace health education program that reduces outpatient visits. *Med Care.* 1985;23:1044-54.

Lorig K, Mazonson PD, Holman HR. Evidence suggesting that health education for self management in patients with chronic arthritis has sustained health benefits while reducing health care costs. *Arthritis Rheum.* 1993;36:439-46.

Mani L, Gerr F. Work-related upper extremity musculoskeletal disorders. *Clin Office Pract.* 2000;27(4):845-64.

Mayer TG. Rehabilitation: what do we do with the chronic patient? *Neurol Clin.* 1999;17(1):131-47.

McGrail MP Jr, Lohman W, Gorman R. Disability prevention principles in the primary care office. *Am Fam Phys.* 2001;63(4):679-84.

McNeil BJ, Weichselbaum R, Parker SG. Fallacy of the five-year survival in lung cancer. *N Engl J Med.* 1978;299:1397-401.

McNeil BJ, Weichselbaum R, Parker SG. Speech and survival: tradeoffs between quality and quantity of life in laryngeal cancer. *N Engl J Med.* 1981;305:982-7.

Mertz MG. What does Walt Disney know about patient satisfaction? *Fam Pract Manag.* 1999;6(10):33-5.

Mullen PD, Green LW, Persing RG. Clinical trials of patient education for chronic conditions: A comparative analysis of intervention types. *Prev Med.* 1985;14:753-81.

Mulley AG Jr. Supporting the patient's role in decision making. In: Harris

JS, Belk HD, Wood LW, eds. *Managing Employee Health Care Costs: Assuring Quality and Value.* Beverly, Mass: OEM Press; 1992.

Nelson EC, Larsen C. Patients' good and bad surprises: how do they relate to overall patient satisfaction? *Quality Rev Bull.* 1993;19(3):89-94.

Phillips, William R. Building the future of health care on the foundations of family practice. *Fam Pract Manag.* 2000;7(1):41-3.

Radosevich DM, McGrail MP Jr, Lohman WH, Gorman R, Parker D, Calasanz M. Relationship of disability prevention to patient health status and satisfaction with primary care provider. *J Occup Environ Med.* 2001;43(8):706-12.

Roter D. The enduring and evolving nature of the patient-physician relationship. *Patient Educ Counsel.* 2000;39(1):5-15.

Spunt BS, Deyo RA, Taylor VM, Leek KM, Goldberg HI, Mulley AG. An interactive videodisc program for low back pain patients. *Health Educ Res.* 1996;11(4):535-41.

Taylor WP, Stern WR, Kubiszyn TW. Predicting patients' perceptions of response to treatment for low back pain. *Spine.* 1984;9:313-6.

Teichman PG. Documentation tips for reducing malpractice risk. *Fam Pract Manag.* 2000;7(3):29-33.

Vickery DM, Medical self care. In: O'Donnell MP, Harris JS, eds. *Health Promotion in the Work Place.* 2d ed. Albany, NY: Delmar; 1994.

Vickery DM, et al. Effect of a self-care education program on medical visits. *JAMA.* 1983;250:2952-6.

Vickery DM, Golaszewski TJ, Wright EC, et al. The effect of self-care interventions on the use of medical services within a Medicare population. *Med Care.* 1988;26:580-8.

Wallston KA. Theoretically based strategies for health behavior change. In: O'Donnell MP, Harris JS, eds. *Health Promotion in the Work Place.* 2nd ed. Albany, NY: Delmar; 1994.

Weingarten S. Translating practice guidelines into patient care: Guidelines at the bedside. *Chest.* 2000;118(2 Suppl):4S-7S.

Weisel SW, Boden SD, Feffer HL. A quality-based protocol for management of musculoskeletal injuries: a ten-year perspective outcome study. *Clin Orthop.* 1994;301:164-76.

Wennberg JE, Fowler FJ. A test of consumer contributions to small area variations in health care delivery. *J Maine Med Assoc.* 1977;68:275-9.

White B. Measuring patient satisfaction: how to do it and why to bother. *Fam Pract Manag.* 1999;6(1):40-4.

Williamson P, Breitman BD, Katon W. Beliefs that foster physician avoidance of psychosocial aspects of health care. *J Fam Pract.* 1981;13:999-1003.

Wilson SR, Scamagas P, German DF, et al. A controlled trial of two forms of self-management education for adults with asthma. *Am J Med.* 1993;94:564-76.

MEDICATION

Agency for Health Care Policy and Research. *Acute Pain Management: Operative or Medical Procedures and Trauma.* Clinical Practice Guideline. Rockville, Md: USGPO; 1992.

Bigos SJ, Bowyer O, Braen G, et al. *Acute Low Back Problems in Adults.* Clinical Practice Guideline No. 14. Rockville, MD: U.S. Department of Health and Human Services, Public Health Service, Agency for Health Care Policy and Research, AHCPR Pub No. 95-0642; 1994.

Brooks PM, Day RO. Nonsteroidal antiinflammatory drugs: differences and similarities. *N Engl J Med.* 1991;324:1716-25.

Chawla PS, Kochar MS. Effect of pain and nonsteroidal analgesics on blood pressure. *WMJ.* 1999;98(6):22-5, 29.

Cooper SA, Engel J, Ladove M, et al. An evaluation of oxycodone and acetaminophen in the treatment of postoperative dental pain. *Clin Pharmacol Ther.* 1979;25:219.

Filho JL. Multicenter study of piroxicam in the treatment of acute musculoskeletal diseases involving 3011 patients. *Eur J Rheumatol Inflamm.* 1983;6: 119-25.

Fowler PD, Aspirin, paracetamol and non-steroidal anti-inflammatory drugs: a comparative review of side effects. *Med Toxicol.* 1987;2:338-66.

Gall EP, Capterton EM, McComb JE, et al. Clinical comparison of ibuprofen, fenoprofen calcium, naproxen and tolmetin sodium in rheumatoid arthritis. *J Rheumatol.* 1982;9:402-7.

Hamill-Ruth RJ, Marohn ML. Evaluation of pain in the critically ill patient. *Crit Care Clin.* 1999;15(1):35-54, v-vi.

Heishman SJ, Stitzer ML, Bigelow GE, et al. Acute opioid physical dependence in humans: effect of varying the morphine-naloxone interval. *J Pharmacol Exp Ther.* 1978;250:485-91.

Hickey RFJ. Chronic low back pain: A comparison of diflunisal with paracetamol. *N Z Med J.* 1982;95:312-4.

Hopkinson JH III, Bartlett FH Jr, Steffens AO, et al. Acetaminophen versus propoxyphene hydrochloride for relief of pain in episiotomy patients. *J Clin Pharmacol.* 1973;13:251-63.

Jaranek GC, Kimmey MB, Saunders DR, Willson RA, Shanahan W, Silverstein PE. Misoprostol reduces gastroduodenal injury from one week of aspirin: an endoscopic study. *Gastroenterology.* 1989;96:656-61.

Lanza F, Peace K, Gustitus L, et al. A blinded endoscopic comparative study of misoprostol versus sucralfate and placebo in the prevention of aspirin-induced gastric and duodenal ulcerations. *Am J Gastroenterol.* 1988;8:143-6.

Mahmud MA, Webster BS, Courtney TK, Matz S, Tacci JA, Christiani DC. Clinical management and the duration of disability for work-related low back pain. *J Occup Environ Med.* 2000;42(12):1178-87.

Moreland LW, St Clair EW. The use of analgesics in the management of pain in rheumatic diseases. *Rheum Dis Clin North Am.* 1999;25(1):153-91, vii.

Muncie HL Jr, King DE, DeForge B. Treatment of mild to moderate pain of acute soft tissue injury: diflunisal vs. acetaminophen with codeine. *J Fam Pract.* 1986;23:125-7.

Patel AT, Ogle AA. Diagnosis and management of acute low back pain. *Am Fam Phys.* 2000;61(6):1779-86, 1789-90.

Schorn D. Tenoxicam in soft-tissue rheumatism. *S Afr Med J.* 1986;69: 301-3.

Scott DL, Roden S, Marshall T, et al. Variations in responses to non-steroidal anti-inflammatory drugs. *Br J Clin Pharmacol.* 1982;14:691-4.

Stevenson, DD. Approach to the patient with a history of adverse reactions to aspirin or NSAIDs: diagnosis and treatment. *Allergy Asthma Proc.* 2000; 21(1):25-31.

Tacci JA, Webster BS, Hashemi L, Christiani DC. Clinical practices in the management of new-onset, uncomplicated, low back workers' compensation disability claims. *J Occup Environ Med.* 1999;41(5):397-404.

Thorling J, Linden B, Berg R, et al. A double-blind comparison of naproxen gel and placebo in the treatment of soft-tissue injuries. *Curr Med Res Opin.* 1990;12:242-8.

Wallenstein SL, Houde RW. Clinical comparison of analgetic effectiveness of *N*-acetyl-*p*-aminophenol, salicylamide and aspirin. *Fed Proc.* 1954;13: 414-7.

PHYSICAL MODALITIES

Deyo RA. Conservative therapy for low back pain: distinguishing useful from useless therapy. *JAMA.* 1983;250:1057-62.

Deyo RA, Walsh NE, Martin DC, et al. A controlled trial of transcutaneous electrical nerve stimulation (TENS) and exercise for chronic low back pain. *N Engl J Med.* 1990;322:1627-35.

Linz DH, Shepherd CD, Ford LF, Ringley LL, Klekamp J, Duncan JM. Effectiveness of occupational medicine center-based physical therapy. *J Occup Environ Med.* 2002;44(1):48-53.

Shekelle PG, Adams AH, Chassin MR, Hurwitz EL, Brook RH. Spinal manipulation for low-back pain. *Ann Intern Med.* 1992;117(7):590-8.

Zigenfus GC, Yin J, Giang GM, Fogarty WT. Effectiveness of early physical therapy in the treatment of acute low back musculoskeletal disorders. *J Occup Environ Med.* 2000;42(1):35-9.

Other References

Bruckman RZ, Rasmussen H. *Healthcare Management Guidelines,* Vol. 7: *Workers' Compensation.* Seattle, Wash: Milliman & Robertson; 1996.

Denniston PL, Ranavaya MI, ed. *Official Disability Guidelines 2002.* 7th ed. Corpus Christi, Texas: Work Loss Data Institute; 2001.

Reed, P, ed. *The Medical Disability Advisor: Workplace Guidelines for Disability Duration.* 4th ed. Boulder, CO: Reed Group; 2001.

4 Work-Relatedness

Occupational physicians and other clinicians often are asked for an opinion as to whether or not a problem is work related. It is incumbent upon the clinician to make certain that any opinion given reflects careful analysis of all available clinical findings and high-grade scientific evidence. Determining whether a symptom, illness, or injury is due to work is important to the individual patient and to other workers exposed to similar conditions. From a health standpoint, specific measures may be needed to prevent recurrences in this individual and to prevent similar problems in others. A determination that a symptom, injury, or illness was caused by work can lead to immediate preventive assessments or protective efforts (see Chapter 1, "Prevention"). Economically, assessing causation may affect payment for lost time, medical care, rehabilitation, and permanent loss of earning capacity. It is important to note that states may have different legal standards for work-relatedness, and occupational health professionals need to be aware of the statutory and case-law definitions that are applicable to the case in which an opinion is being expressed. However, legal distinctions do not alter the science involved in establishing an association (or lack thereof) between work and health.

Medical causation and legal causation are different concepts, and it is important that the occupational medicine physician understand the differences. Medical causation is physical or biological in nature. For example, a physician may conclude, based on sound scientific evidence, that a substance in a workplace is likely to be the cause of a patient's pulmonary adenocarcinoma. Legal causation, on the other hand, generally has two components: cause in fact and proximate cause. Cause in fact exists when the occurrence of an event brings about a result. As an example, prior close contact with a patient with meningitis may be deemed the cause in fact of a patient's meningococcemia. Proximate cause relates to concepts such as the predictability or remoteness of an event. As a society we have concluded that there must be some cut-off point beyond which, even if the causal relationship dots can be connected, no liability will attach. When the result of concern is beyond that point, a court might find that there is cause in fact, but that proximate cause has not been demonstrated. For example, suppose a physician prescribes a patient a medication, which is consumed later at home by the patient's child, who dies as a result. A court may find that prescribing the medication was the cause in fact, but not the proximate cause, of the child's death. Legal cause exists only when both cause in fact and proximate cause have been proven. What constitutes legal cause may vary from state to state, and may differ between states and the federal government. Unless otherwise stated, references to causation in this practice guideline are synonymous to "medical" causation or "cause in fact."

Legislatures may create presumptions that in turn establish rights and liabilities, even in the absence of medical causation. For example, a state might establish an irrefutable presumption that lung cancers are work related if they occur in emergency workers. An emergency worker who actually has no harmful exposures develops pulmonary adenocarcinoma; as a result, the patient's occupation may be deemed by courts, but not physicians, to be the cause of his or her lung cancer. Legislatively created presumptions also may have the opposite effect. For example, a law might state that for workers' compensation purposes, no occupational exposure shall be deemed the cause of a lung cancer in those patients who have a ten-pack-per-year or greater smoking history; as a result, a heavy smoker with chronic exposure to a known workplace carcinogen will not be able to establish legal liability on the part of the employer for the cancer. Presumptions differ markedly from state to state. In the example just given, the exposed worker may have no difficulty prevailing in a different state—say, the state in which the manufacturer of the carcinogen is headquartered. Workers' compensation law often includes presumptions, often of great importance. For example, the presumption that an attending physician's opinion carries greater weight than that of a consulting physician may result in accepting the attending physician's opinion and rejecting the consultant's opinion. This might be true even when the attending physician had no success after years of treating the injured worker's condition, and the consultant is a respected academician of stellar repute and integrity.

Definitions of Causation and Related Terms

While assessing causation can be relatively straightforward, as it is commonly in direct trauma, determining whether a complaint is related to work often requires careful analysis and weighing all associated or apparently causal factors operative over time. Physicians and others who analyze causation need to use clear, unambiguous terminology to describe their findings and analysis. When asked for an opinion on causation, physicians also need to do so only on the basis of scientific evidence. The commonly seen statement "in the absence of other obvious causes, the problem is work related" should not be used. Such language is not reflective of the scientific basis upon which such opinions should rest, and does provide adequate support for conclusions that must be made regarding financial and legal responsibility.

Of equal importance is the need for those analyzing causation to assess whether or not a worker's symptoms are truly representative of an injury *per se*, or simply reflective of a normal musculoskeletal response following the performance of an activity to which the worker was unaccustomed. In general, if there is no clear mechanism of injury and the physical examination is negative, it is preferable to provide analysis, reassurance, and recommendations regarding prevention rather than give a vague tissue diagnosis suggesting an "injury."

It is usually best to classify them accordingly rather than attribute them to an "injury" in the absence of evidence that an injury actually occurred. In such instances, it is often helpful to involve the patient in the analytic process and in his or her causation analysis.

Single, Multiple, or Competing Causation

The physician may determine and state whether a workplace factor is the only cause, one among several contributing causes, or one of several possible causes, each of which could independently produce the disorder. A direct cause can generally be attributed if both the immediate trauma and the effect are clearly observable. Direct trauma can result from the interaction of several forms of energy with the patient's body. If a clear, direct relationship exists between an illness or injury and a source of energy, such as a moving or falling object (kinetic energy), a fall (potential energy), a chemical burn (chemical energy), or an electric shock or radiation (electromagnetic energy), a sole, direct cause is said to exist.

Health problems may develop as the result of a combination of factors, only some of which may be work related. For example, a given patient's hearing loss may occur as a result of aging as well as occupational noise exposure (although the two often can be distinguished). In addition, occupational and nonoccupational exposures may have a combined effect. For example, carpal tunnel syndrome cases that occur in the context of physical exposures, rather than those that arise due to personal risk factors such as diabetes mellitus or rheumatoid arthritis, may develop following exposures arising from both hobbies and work-related activities. Personal factors also can be part of the "web of causation." For example, tall individuals have a greater probability of developing back pain in certain settings, and there is some evidence that anatomic factors in the wrist may contribute to tendinitis or carpal tunnel syndrome. In these circumstances, physicians are obliged to assess whether causality is truly multifactorial or reflects just one of several competing factors.

Competing causation differs from combined causation in that either a workplace factor or a nonoccupational factor, but not both, can be responsible independently for the adverse health effect. For example, because pregnancy, diabetes, myxedema, tobacco, and stereotypical high-force motions have been independently associated with carpal tunnel syndrome, a patient with diabetes who does very little stereotypical work will most likely develop carpal tunnel syndrome due to the diabetes, not the nature of his or her work. In both combined and competing causation, it may be useful to attain a thorough understanding of the patient's exact work activities, including the degree to which the condition under investigation is found in coworkers. This permits physicians to understand both the operant biomechanical forces and assess whether their effects were seen in others besides the patient, even though at a lesser level (suggesting combined causation), or limited predominantly to the patient (suggesting competing causation with the nonoccupational factor of greater significance than occupational factors).

Likelihood and Certainty

For medical purposes, different definitions of causation are used, depending on the purpose of the assessment of work-relatedness. In the clinical setting, relatively specific case definitions are used to define occurrence (as described further in these guidelines for individual conditions). In clinical occupational practice, action based on the assessment of causal association and on the seriousness of the health effect may be commensurate with the degree of certainty about causation, based on the available information on temporal, physiologic, and physical links between the exposure and the effect. Use logic rather than opinion to link the population and research evidence with clinical findings and exposure data (also see Chapter 7, "Independent Medical Examinations and Consultations"). Otherwise, preventive efforts are unlikely to be effective. From a public health standpoint, a reasonable likelihood of causation should lead to preventive actions. Again, physicians can weigh the cost and benefit of the intervention against the degree of certainty as to causation. For example, an ergonomic evaluation of the worksite could be triggered by workers' complaints of discomfort, while removing a worker from a job would require more study and associative certainty.

The physician's expressed opinion of likelihood should not be affected by the administrative or legal context. The available evidence often does not support an absolute link between the exposure and the effect, so the clinician's opinion about causation cannot be absolute. Rather, it may address the likelihood of causation. The degree of certainty expressed by the clinician should be supported primarily by the available evidence and it should be a product of logic and informed judgment. Words or phrases such as "more likely than not" (equal to or greater than 51%) or "conclusive" (95%) are legal rather than medical terms and need to be used as defined and intended.

Complaints presented for causality analysis might represent recurrences, exacerbations, or aggravations of preexisting conditions. The distinction between a recurrence, exacerbation, and an aggravation of a condition also is important medically and legally.

A recurrence of an ongoing condition arises from the same etiology as the preexisting condition, which may be a prior work injury. Recurrence generally involves the reappearance of signs or symptoms attributable to a prior injury with minimal or no provocation (i.e., in the absence of a clearly definable injury or precipitating factor). An example would be anatomically appropriate radicular pain that develops after minimal effort in a patient with a previously documented work-related disk herniation.

An aggravation of a preexisting condition is a new event, which permanently worsens an existing condition. Aggravations can include those situations in which a process was without symptoms until the precipitating event occurred. Some workers' compensation systems recognize "temporary" aggravations.

Exacerbation is the transient worsening of a prior condition by an injury or illness, with the expectation that the situation will eventually return to baseline. The term "exacerbation" is used in this volume, rather than "temporary aggravation."

Acute trauma can be superimposed on prior work-related or non-work-related conditions. If an underlying condition is aggravated or exacerbated at work, it is important to document the impairment, pain, and activity limitation due to the aggravating or exacerbating factors. Restoring prior activity levels is a principal goal of treatment. When and if that goal is reached, the exacerbation will be said to have ceased. Because an aggravation of a prior condition has, by definition, led to a permanent alteration in the patient's underlying condition, the work injury cannot be described as cured; regardless of whether a full return to work occurs, there is potential for future recurrence of symptoms. Should symptoms recur, it may—depending upon the workers' compensation laws involved—be necessary to determine whether their recurrence is due to the aggravating incident or the preexisting condition.

Types of Causation Analysis

A provisional causation analysis generally is conducted soon after the first clinical encounter. Although the occupational health professional is advised to ascertain exposure and answer all the questions listed above, information may still be incomplete. However, a provisional opinion as to causation may be necessary to initiate appropriate preventive measures and to determine whether workers' compensation or other benefits will be provided, even if a concrete diagnosis has not yet been made.

The definitive case analysis often is conducted after reaching a conclusive diagnosis and/or obtaining considerably more information about the individual case, work conditions, and prior medical history. Reviewing other pertinent medical information and scientific literature often is necessary.

An epidemiologic causation analysis, based on patterns observed in groups of workers, may be important in some instances. However, it might be required if the complaint is relatively common or nonspecific or is not uniquely associated with work exposures, in which case the frequency of the complaints among coworkers provides a point of reference. It may be needed if a question arises as to whether a group of workers has an injury or illness pattern causally related to work. In situations such as these, the employer, insurer, or both will generally request and follow the analysis.

Methods for Determining Work-Relatedness

There are different approaches to the determination of work-relatedness that have been published. One of those published by the National Institute for Occupational Safety and Health (NIOSH) consists of a six-step process:

- *Evidence of Disease.* What is the disease? What certainty is there that the diagnosis is correct? What evidence supports or fails to support that diagnosis?
- *Epidemiology.* What is the epidemiological evidence for that condition? Is there support for a relationship with work?
- *Evidence of Exposure.* What evidence, particularly objective, is there that the level of exposure is of the frequency, intensity, and duration of exposure to rise to the level that would support a work-relatedness determination?
- *Consideration of Other Relevant Factors.* What other factors are present in this case? For example, is the worker with carpal tunnel syndrome (CTS) pregnant or obese?
- *Validity of Testimony.* Is there information that suggests that the information above is inaccurate, for example, from a collateral source?
- *Conclusions.* This step is a synthesis of the above five steps.

Evaluating the Evidence

For epidemiologic surveillance, a highly sensitive (e.g., broadly phrased) but relatively nonspecific case definition frequently is employed. This increases the rate of screening yield for study but may produce a number of false-positives as well. If surveillance results suggest an effect, more formal research can be done to carefully evaluate the apparent association. The epidemiologic research-study definition of causal association is much more rigid, traditionally implying 95% certainty that the purported causal relationship is not statistically spurious. Quality scientific literature about musculoskeletal disorders (MSDs) that defines causal associations with work exposures is notably lacking, making it difficult to predict whether those risk factors that have been found to be associated with, or predictive of, certain MSDs and other syndromes are necessarily causal for these entities.

Criteria for the Evaluation of Epidemiologic Evidence

Criteria to assess the evidence for the work-relatedness of various health effects have been accepted by the epidemiologic and public health communities. When considering recommendations for preventive measures, occupational health practitioners can use these criteria to evaluate the possible effects of exposures for individuals and groups.

The first four of the following criteria are generally considered the most important:

- Temporal association between the exposure or work factor and the health concern (i.e., the exposure must precede the disease)
- Strength of the association (e.g., how large is the relative risk or odds ratio that compare the exposed with the unexposed workers?)
- Dose-response (also known as biological gradient) showing increased risk estimates across at least three levels of exposure)
- Consistency of the association among epidemiological studies
- Predictive performance of the association in predicting future health problems
- Experimental evidence from animal models
- Analogy (e.g., evidence of effects from a chemical with analogous structure)
- Specificity of the association in showing that the exposure causes one problem rather than a large group of unrelated problems
- Plausibility of the purported exposure-disease relationship
- Reversibility (e.g., that the tissue abnormalities resolve with cessation of exposure)
- Coherence of the association with existing physiologic data, trends in exposure levels over time, and other knowledge

Clinicians need to be very specific about the frequency, intensity, and duration of purported ergonomic factors that might be associated with a specific case of any of these entities. A considered judgment about the causal association by the clinician may directly facilitate the effectiveness of treatment and prevention.

For some conditions, systematic reviews exist. Those reviews are helpful in evaluating the quality of the available epidemiologic studies.

Basics of Causation Analysis

Unless the causal factor's effect on the patient is immediate and visible, imputing causation to a work factor (whether it be an acute event or exposure, organizational or psychological condition, or chronic or recurrent exposure) requires that the evidence supporting an association between a medical condition and a given physical, biologic, or chemical exposure allow physicians to conclude that the condition would not have occurred otherwise or would have occurred in a lesser form. The coexistence of the exposure and the effect is necessary but not sufficient. In the occupational setting, temporary or permanent impairment is a particularly salient health effect. (Disability, which can result from impairment, results from the interaction between the impairment and available work functions the worker/patient can safely and effectively perform [see Chapter 5].) Other than acute trauma, for an exposure to be causally associated with a health effect, the clinician must be able to define the effect, thoroughly understand the mechanism of injury linking the exposure to symptoms, and be aware of and apply the available epidemiologic evidence for causal association of the entity in question in general.

Causality Initial Assessment—Mechanism

While the provisional assessment often is conducted with limited facts, it must be conducted carefully because it affects subsequent care, compensability, and Occupational Safety and Health Administration (OSHA) recording. Information needed to reach a definitive analysis may be available at the time of the first visit, but obtaining additional information may be necessary. The minimum initial assessment of causality, for preventive purposes, can be based on the time course and a well-grounded suspicion that there is a causal factor. However, the degree of uncertainty should be communicated clearly to the patient and the employer. With regard to causality, the objectives of the initial assessment are to:

- Determine whether a specific clinical disorder is present—make a diagnosis
- Evaluate potential causative workplace exposure factors
- Assess whether other causal factors are likely

The initial contact with the patient often is the best time to acquire time-sensitive or unbiased information from him or her. The patient's memory of acute events is most accurate immediately following those events. Information needed for the definitive analysis of causation often comes from other sources or is found in medical or work records.

History (Initial and Interval)

A careful medical history, essential in establishing the work-relatedness of a complaint, emphasizes the organ system that is the focus of the presenting complaint or thought to be the target of the exposure. Elicit a description of activity limitations and pain levels both before and after a work injury or aggravation. This information can provide insight into possible nonworkplace causes as well as the premorbid level of function. It also is beneficial to obtain a psychiatric history in situations where the patient presents with psychiatric or stress-related complaints.

One link between exposures and health effects is their temporal relationship. The clinician may determine the time course of events, carefully documenting the time of potential exposures or trauma and of symptom onset. While the onset of subacute or chronic conditions may be gradual, the patient can generally provide time estimates. Also of relevance is whether or not symptoms decrease overnight or during weekends, holidays, or other times the patient is not "exposed," in the absence of a defined physical deficit, such as a fracture, where one would ordinarily expect to see some degree of symptom resolution once exposure to the injurious factor has ceased. It should be noted that determining temporal causality might be difficult with certain psychiatric problems such as posttraumatic stress disorder because the onset of symptoms may be delayed temporally for quite some time relative to the trauma causing them.

Workplace exposures also need to be quantified as much as possible in the history. The patient can describe his or her typical workday and any unusual events preceding the onset of complaints. Unusual events might include changes in workload, in physical or chemical processes, the absence or breakdown of engineering controls, or personal protective equipment.

A history of trauma requires a quantified account of relevant work- and non-work-related activities during the time that symptoms were progressing. Psychiatric or stress-related complaints require assessing worksite exposure to acute stresses, such as workplace violence, and more subtle conditions, such as mismatched workload, skills and abilities, role ambiguity, and lack of control and autonomy. These conditions may be local to the specific job, or they may be more general to the process, worksite, or employer. Interpersonal relationships with supervisors and coworkers may be documented as well.

The inquiry includes relevant personal habits (especially substance use, including tobacco, alcohol, and others with adverse health effects), coexisting disease states, and family history. The patient also can be asked about similar occupational or nonoccupational problems and their resolution in the past. Carefully address nonwork activities, particularly regarding the patient's participation in recreational activities or hobbies that could precipitate similar symptoms because they may be relevant in either causing initial symptoms or hindering their resolution.

In short, when taking the worker's history, the goal should always be to obtain answers to the following questions:

- Was there a temporal relationship between the exposure and the alleged effect? (Did the work exposure occur before the health effect?) If so, was the time that elapsed between the exposure and its putative effect consistent with what ordinarily is found, given the nature of the exposure (temporal contiguity)?
- Was the amount (duration, dose, strength) of the exposure sufficient to cause an effect in most workers? If not, was the amount of the exposure sufficient to cause an effect in this particular worker (i.e., does the worker have any special sensitivities)?
- Does the association with work fit logically with previous biologic or statistical evidence as to how the symptom or disorder could develop (termed the coherence of the association)?

Other specifics of the case must also be considered:

- Could other causes (personal, comorbid, or nonoccupational) possibly account for the symptom, illness, or injury in question?
- Could the exposure have been mitigated by engineering controls, personal protective equipment, immunization, or other means?
- Is the health effect causing functional impairment? Is it causing work exclusion (e.g., some infectious diseases)?

Workplace Environment Assessment

Although in many instances causation can be definitely concluded or excluded based purely upon the patient's history, a more detailed history of exposure is necessary at times to guide the definitive assessment and meet OSHA and other regulatory requirements. This is seen especially in those cases in which the injury is not readily apparent and is attributed to low-level chronic factors rather than an acute, easily definable, event. In situations such as these, patients may be required to provide information about workplace ergonomic exposures by describing in detail his or her typical job duties and maximal effort needed to perform the job, with specific descriptions and comparisons being more useful than general descriptions such as "heavy." The clinician might inquire about the total force used, local concentration of force (a forcefully applied grasp on a sharp tool handle edge), the frequency of specific motions or tasks, awkward postures, psychological and managerial issues, job satisfaction, and other factors, such as cold and vibration.

Information obtained directly from the patient ideally is supplemented with information from the worksite. Descriptions of events from coworkers and supervisors may prove useful in corroborating or refuting a patient's history. Summaries of health effects from material safety data sheets (MSDSs) may prove useful in guiding the clinical inquiry and subsequent literature searches. Actually measuring exposure, particularly chemical exposure, often is necessary to assess causation. While qualitative measurements to determine whether or not a chemical, physical, or biological hazard is present are a good first step, quantitative measurements over time are needed to determine the level, duration, and temporal pattern of exposure. Use the appropriate measure for chemical, physical, and biologic agents (time-weighted averages versus peak exposures). If possible, measurements should be concurrent with the time course of the problem, rather than using current measurements to impute previous exposure. If current measurements must be used, some assurance that conditions have not changed would be useful in order to have some degree of confidence that the relationship is plausible. A worksite visit by the occupational physician may be useful. Measurements by an ergonomist or an industrial hygienist, depending on the issue, may be needed to quantify exposure.

Area or personal monitoring data are more useful to prove and quantify exposure and, when relevant, can be obtained at a time or times when they would be expected to most closely replicate worksite conditions at the time of exposure.

Any further information that is available for exposure assessment, such as job records, videotapes of job tasks, and monitoring data, can be reviewed at this stage. A definitive assessment would require objective, quantified evidence of exposure to proven causative factors at levels known to have the adverse health effects in question.

Record Review

Definitive causation analysis often requires considerably more information than is available at the time provisional assessments are made. A detailed and thorough medical history must be obtained or reviewed, and relevant prior or coexisting complaints, illnesses, or injuries should be noted. The source of information for the history may be the patient, concurrent medical records from other physicians, past records, preplacement testing, or periodic medical surveillance data. In unusual cases, hospital or pharmacy records may prove useful. Treat all information confidentially and release it only if required and only with the patient's consent.

Literature Review

In some cases, additional information from the scientific literature also may be needed. Reviews of epidemiologic or toxicologic literature may be required to clarify the existing evidence linking exposure to health effects. Epidemiologic surveys may be needed to clarify the prevalence of complaints or health effects.

A careful review of the published scientific literature may reveal a pattern of association between the apparent exposures and the patient's health effect. In most instances, epidemiologic studies will be based on workers in similar jobs or industries. The study populations may be compared to the circumstances of the patient in question, including exposure duration, dose, and so on. In reviewing the scientific literature, one should, in general, ask the following questions:

- What is the quality of the available literature? Are supportive studies descriptive or analytic in nature? What was the study design used (e.g., prospective cohort or cross-sectional)? Were various potential sources of bias (recall bias, healthy worker effects, volunteer bias, selection bias, and similar problems) analyzed and accounted for?
- What is the specific quantification of the exposure-effect relationship? Is there statistical significance? Were potential confounders addressed (matched, excluded, stratified, or statistically adjusted)? Are case definitions consistent among studies? Can a change in symptoms or disease

be predicted by a change in the intensity, duration, body burden, or dose of the chemical, physical, psychological, or biologic factor?

It is important to conduct a balanced review of the literature rather than relying on single studies that support a particular point of view. If the epidemiologic studies are inadequate, it may be necessary to refer to toxicologic studies in animals. In assessing the relevance of animal studies to the patient's situation, the physician can consider the comparability of the specific agent, dose, route of exposure, and so on. Interspecies variations (e.g., enzyme system differences) need to be taken into account. Similar effects in several species carry more weight than a positive finding in a single nonprimate species.

Epidemiologic Surveys

In the absence of support in the scientific literature for a causal relationship between disease process and a given event, series of events, or injury, the presence of multiple, similarly defined cases in the same worksite raises the probability of work-relatedness, but also may indicate clustering due to behavioral factors (e.g., mass hysteria syndromes, which may be associated with nonspecific complaints such as nausea, headache, and offending odors). Nonetheless, case clusters cannot be ignored without further investigation. If several cases are seen, the occupational health professional can determine the attack rate (number of cases/number of employees at risk). If clusters are found, more formal surveys of the entire exposed population and comparison groups should prove useful. Occasionally, the health effect is so unusual (e.g., angiosarcoma of the liver or bischloromethyl ether-related small cell lung cancer) that calculating the attack rate is not necessary.

Summary

Determining work-relatedness is important to assure delivery of appropriate workers' compensation benefits and to prevent exacerbations and recurrences of the condition. Preventive efforts also are needed to be sure that other workers do not experience similar problems.

An initial assessment of work-relatedness usually can be done at the first clinical encounter with the patient. Work-relatedness is generally easy for acute traumatic injuries, but more difficult for subjective complaints, cumulative injuries, and occupational disease. The initial assessment must, therefore, be considered preliminary. More detailed analysis, including information from the patient, other providers, medical records, exposure records, the literature, and the worksite may be needed for a detailed assessment.

At the level of the individual worker, assessing work-relatedness can lead to preventive measures, including engineering controls, personal protective equipment, administrative or process changes, or training. If work causes or contributes to illness and the exposure cannot be controlled, reassigning the worker may be necessary. At the employee group level, prevention efforts can protect workers in similar jobs from hazards and therefore prevent other cases of occupational illness or injury.

Causation by work is the key determinant of workers' compensation; such determination of causation should be carefully reasoned and consistent with available evidence. Determining early in the clinical course that a problem is not work related may avoid claim denial at a later date and help a significantly impaired worker receive compensation and reimbursement for health services from an appropriate source.

References

CAUSALITY

Berry K. Root cause analysis in response to a "near miss." *J Health Care Qual.* 2000;22(2):16-8.

Chaffin DB, Andersson GBJ. *Occupational Biomechanics.* New York, NY: Wiley; 1991.

Cullinan P. Epidemiological assessment of health effects from chemical incidents. *Occup Environ Med.* 2002;59:568-72.

Demeter SL. A patient seeking disability. *Am Fam Physician.* 2001;63(1):161-2, 164.

Demeter SL, Andersson GBJ. *Disability Evaluation.* Chicago, Ill: AMA Press; 2003.

Evans A. Causation and disease: a chronological journey. *Am J Epidemiol.* 1978;108(4):249-58.

Forst LS. A state trauma registry as a tool for occupational injury surveillance. *J Occup Environ Med.* 1999;41(6):514-20.

Garabrant DH. Epidemiologic principles in the evaluation of suspected neurotoxic disorders. *Neurol Clin.* 2000;18(3):631-48.

Goldsmith DF. Importance of causation for interpreting occupational epidemiology research: a case study of quartz and cancer. *Occup Med.* 1996;11(3): 433-49.

Guidotti TL, Rose SG. *Science on the Witness Stand, Evaluating Scientific Evidence in Law, Adjudication, and Policy.* Beverly Farms, Mass: OEM Press; 2001.

Harber P. *Medical Causation Analysis: Suggested Guidelines.* San Francisco, Calif: Industrial Medical Council; 1994.

Harber P, Schusterman D. Medical causation analysis heuristics. *J Occup Environ Med.* 1996;38(6):577-86.

Hill AB. The environment and disease: association or causation? *Proc R Soc Med.* 1965;58:295.

Jokl P. The effect of the aging process on muscle and tendon injuries. In: Gordon SL, Gonzalez-Mestre X, Garrett WE Jr, eds. *Sports and Exercise in Midlife.* Rosemont, Ill: American Academy of Orthopaedic Surgeons; 1993:515-29.

Leadbetter WB. Aging effects on the repair and healing of athletic injury. In: Gordon SL, Gonzalez-Mestre X, Garrett WE Jr, eds. *Sports and Exercise in Midlife.* Rosemont, Ill: American Academy of Orthopaedic Surgeons; 1993:177-233.

Michael B Jr, Daubert K. Doctors and differential diagnosis: treating medical causation testimony as evidence. *Defense Counsel J.* 1999;66(4):525.

Moore J. Biomechanical models for the pathogenesis of specific distal upper extremity disorders. *Am J Ind Med.* 2002;41(5):353-69.

Moye LA. *Epidemiologic Tenets of Causality.* University of Texas School of Public Health Web site, December 2002. www.sph.uth.tmc.edu:8053/Biometry/LMoye/StatAnalysis%202001/PH1820%202001/lectenet.htm

Muir DC. Cause of occupational disease. *Occup Environ Med.* 1995;52(5):289-93.

Samuels SW. Philosophic perspectives: community, communications, and occupational disease causation. *Int J Health Serv.* 1998;28(1):153-64.

Susser M. What is a cause and how do we know one? A grammar for practical epidemiology. *Am J Epidemiol.* 1991;133:635-48.

Talmage J. Basic Science 101. Power Point Presentation. January 2, 2003.

Weed DL. On the logic of causal inference. *Am J Epidemiol.* 1986;123:265-79.

Williams JK. Understanding evidence-based medicine: a primer. *Amer J Obstetrics Gynecology.* 2001;185(2).

EPIDEMIOLOGY

Andersson GBJ. Epidemiological aspects of low back pain in industry. *Spine.* 1981;6:53-60.

Andersson GBJ. Epidemiology of occupational neck and shoulder disorders. In: Gordon SL, Blair SJ, Fine LJ, eds. *Repetitive Motion Disorders of the Upper Extremity.* Rosemont, Ill: American Academy of Orthopaedic Surgery; 1995:31-42.

Andersson GBJ, Fine LJ, Silverstein BA. Musculoskeletal disorders. In: Levy BS, Wegman DH, eds. *Occupational Health: Recognizing and Preventing Work-Related Disease.*, 3rd ed. Boston, Mass: Little, Brown and Company; 1995:455-87.

Atroshi I, Gummesson C, Johnsson R, et al. Prevalence of carpal tunnel syndrome in a general population. *JAMA.* 1999;282(2):153-8.

Barnhart S, Demers P, Miller M, et al. Carpal tunnel syndrome among ski manufacturing workers. *Scand J Work Environ Health.* 1991;17:46-52.

Battie MC, Videman T, Gill K, Moneta GB, et al. 1999 Volvo Award in clinical sciences. Smoking and lumbar intervertebral disc degeneration: an MRI study of identical twins. *Spine.* 1991;16(9):1015-21.

Bekkelund SI, Pierre-Jerome C, Torbergsen T, Ingebrigtsen T. Impact of occupational variables in carpal tunnel syndrome. *Acta Neurol Scand.* 2001;103(3):193-7.

Bergquist-Ullman M, Larsen U. Acute low back pain in industry. *Acta Orthop Scand.* 1977;170:1-117.

Biering-Sorenson F. A prospective study of low back pain in a general population. *Scand J Rehabil Med.* 1983;15:71-96.

Biering-Sorenson F. A one-year prospective study of low back trouble in a general population: the prognostic value of low back history and physical measurements. *Dan Med Bull.* 1984;31:362-75.

Biering-Sorenson F. Physical measurements as risk indicators for low back trouble over a one-year period. *Spine.* 1984;9:106-19.

Bigos SJ, Spengler DM, Martin N, et al. Back injuries in industry: a retrospective study. II. Injury-related factors. *Spine.* 1986;11:246-51.

Bigos SJ, Spengler DM, Martin N, et al. Back injuries in industry: a retrospective study. III. Employee related factors. *Spine.* 1986;11:251-6.

Bigos SJ, Battie MC, Fisher LD. Methodology for reevaluating predictive factors for the report of back injury. *Spine.* 1991;16:669-70.

Bigos SJ, Battie MC, Fisher LD, et al. A prospective study of work perceptions and psychosocial factors affecting the report of back injury. *Spine.* 1991;16:1-6.

Bigos SJ, Battie MC. Risk factors for industrial back problems. *Semin Spine Surg.* 1992;4:2-11.

Boedeker W. Associations between workload and diseases rarely occurring in sickness absence data. *J Occup Environ Med.* 2001;43(12):1081-8.

Bovenzi M, Hulshof CT. An updated review of epidemiologic studies on the relationship between exposure to whole-body vibration and low back pain (1986-1997). *Int Arch Occup Environ Health.* 1999;72(6):351-65.

Chaffin DB, Park KS. A longitudinal study of low back pain as associated with occupational weight lifting factors. *Am Ind Hyg Assoc J.* 1973;32:513-25.

Chiang H-C, Ko Y-C, Chen S-S, et al. Prevalence of shoulder and upper-limb disorders among workers in the fish-processing industry. *Scand J Work Environ Health.* 1993;19:126-31.

Chiang H, Chen S, Yu H, et al. The occurrence of carpal tunnel syndrome in frozen food factory employees. *Kaohsiung J Med Sci.* 1990;6:73-80.

Davis L, Wellman H, Punnett L. Surveillance of work-related carpal tunnel syndrome in Massachusetts, 1992-1997: a report from the Massachusetts Sentinel Event Notification System for Occupational Risks (SENSOR). *Am J Ind Med.* 2001;39(1):58-71.

Deyo RA, Bass JE. Lifestyle and low back pain: the influence of smoking and obesity. *Spine.* 1989;501-6.

Dillane JB, Fry K, Kalton G. Acute back syndrome: a study from general practice. *Br Med J.* 1966;2:82-4.

Dillon C, Petersen M, Tanaka S. Self-reported hand and wrist arthritis and occupation: data from the U.S. National Health Interview Survey-Occupational Health Supplement. *Am J Ind Med.* 2002;42(4):318-27.

Dryson EW, Walls CB. The distribution of occupations in two populations with upper limb pain. *Int J Occup Environ Health.* 2001;7(3):201-5.

English C, Maclaren W, Court-Brown C, et al. Relations between upper limb soft tissue disorders and repetitive movements at work. *Am J Ind Med.* 1995;27:75-90.

Fraser TM. *Human Stress, Work and Job Satisfaction: A Critical Approach.* Occupational Health and Safety Series No. 50. Geneva, Switzerland: International Labour Office; 1983.

Frymoyer JW, Pope MH, Clements JH, Wilder DG, MacPherson B, Ashikaga T. Risk factors in low back pain. *J Bone Joint Surg.* 1983;65A: 213-8.

Frymoyer JW. Back pain and sciatica. *N Engl J Med.* 1988;318:291-300.

Garg A. Basis for guide: epidemiologic approach. In: Waters TR, Putz-Anderson V, eds. *Scientific Support Documentation for the Revised 1991 NIOSH Lifting Equation: Technical Contract Reports.* Springfield, Va: U.S. Department of Commerce, National Technical Information Service; 1991.

Garland FC, Doyle EJ Jr, Balazs LL, Levine R, Pugh WM, Gorham RD. Carpal tunnel syndrome and occupation in U.S. Navy enlisted personnel. *Arch Environ Health.* 1996;51(5):395-407.

Gerr F, Marcus M, Ensor C, et al. A prospective study of computer users: I. Study design and incidence of musculoskeletal symptoms and disorders. *Am J Ind Med.* 2002;41:221-35.

Gerr F, Marcus M, Ortiz D. Methodological limitations in the study of video display terminal use and upper extremity musculoskeletal disorders. *Am J Ind Med.* 1996;29(6):649-56.

Gordon SL, Blair SJ, Fine LJ, eds. *Repetitive Motion Disorders of the Upper Extremity.* Rosemont, Ill: American Academy of Orthopaedic Surgery; 1994.

Gorsche R, Preston W, Renger R, et al. Prevalence and incidence of stenosing flexor tenosynovitis (trigger finger) in a meat-packing plant. *J Occup Environ Med.* 1998;40(6):556-60.

Grieco A, Molteni G, De Vito G, Sias N. Epidemiology of musculoskeletal disorders due to biomechanical overload. *Ergonomics.* 1998;41(9):1253-60.

Hagberg M, Morgenstern H, Kelsh M. Impact of occupations and job tasks on the prevalence of carpal tunnel syndrome. *Scand J Work Environ Health.* 1992;18(6):337-45.

Hakim A, Cherkas L, Zayat S, et al. The genetic contribution to carpal tunnel syndrome in women: a twin study. *Arthritis Rheum.* 2002;47(3):275-9.

Hanrahan LP, Higgins D, Anderson H, Smith M. Wisconsin occupational carpal tunnel syndrome surveillance: the incidence of surgically treated cases. *WMJ.* 1993;92(12):685-9.

Harrington J, Carter J, Birrell L, Gompertz D. Surveillance case definitions for work related upper limb pain syndromes. *Occup Environ Med.* 1998; 55(4):264-71.

Heliovaara M, Makela M, Knekt P, et al. Determinants of sciatica and low back pain. *Spine.* 1991;16:608-14.

Hildebrandt VH, Bongers PM, Dul J, van Dijk FJ, Kemper HC. The relationship between leisure time, physical activities and musculoskeletal symptoms and disability in worker populations. *Int Arch Occup Environ Health.* 2000;73(8):507-18.

Hill AB. The environment and disease: association or causation? *Proc R Soc Med.* 1965;58:295.

Hoogendoorn WE, van Poppel MN, Bongers PM, Koes BW, Bouter LM. Systematic review of psychosocial factors at work and private life as risk factors for back pain. *Spine.* 2000;25(16):2114-25.

Kelsey JL, Githens PB, O'Connor T, et al. Acute prolapsed lumbar intervertebral disc: an epidemiologic study with special reference to driving automobiles and cigarette smoking. *Spine.* 1984;9:608-13.

Kelsey JL, Githens PB, White AA III, et al. An epidemiologic study of lifting and twisting on the job and risk for acute, prolapsed lumbar disc. *J Orthop Res.* 1984;2:61-6.

Kelsey JL, Hardy RJ. Driving motor vehicles as a risk factor for acute herniated lumbar intervertebral disc. *Am J Epidemiol.* 1988;102:63-73.

Kelsey JL, Hochberg MC. Musculoskeletal disorders. In: Last JM, Wallace RB, eds. *Maxcy-Rosenau-Last Public Health and Preventive Medicine.* 13th ed. Norwalk, Conn: Appleton & Lange; 1992:913-26.

Keyserling WM, Armstrong TJ. Ergonomics: musculoskeletal disorders. In: Last JM, Wallace RB, eds. *Maxcy-Rosenau-Last Public Health and Preventive Medicine.* 13th ed. Norwalk, Conn: Appleton & Lange; 1992:533-45.

Keyserling WM. Workplace risk factors and occupational musculoskeletal disorders, Part 1: A review of biomechanical and psychophysical research on risk factors associated with low-back pain. *AIHA J.* 2000;61(1):39-50.

Kihlberg S, Hagberg M. Hand-arm symptoms related to impact and nonimpact hand-held power tools. *Int Arch Occup Environ Health.* 1997;69(4):282-8.

Kuorinka I, Hagberg M, Silverstein B, et al., eds. *Work Related Musculoskeletal Disorders: A Reference Book for Prevention.* New York, NY: Taylor & Francis; 1995.

Kusnetz S, Hutchison MK, eds. *A Guide to the Workrelatedness of Disease (rev.).* US DHEW, CDC, NIOSH. Pub No. PB298-561;1979.

Latko W, Armstrong T, Franzblau A, et al. Cross-sectional study of the relationship between repetitive work and the prevalence of upper limb musculoskeletal disorders. *Am J Ind Med.* 1999;36:248-59.

Levi L. *Stress in Industry: Causes, Effects and Prevention.* Occupational Health and Safety Series No. 51. Geneva, Switzerland: International Labour Office; 1984.

Lewis M, Hay EM, Paterson SM, Croft P. Effects of manual work on recovery from lateral epicondylitis. *Scand J Work Environ Health.* 2002;28(2):109-16.

Linton SJ. Occupational psychological factors increase the risk for back pain: a systematic review. *J Occup Rehabil.* 2001;11(1):53-66.

Lloyd DCEF, Troup JDG. Recurrent back pain and its prediction. *J Soc Occup Med.* 1983;3:66-74.

Lundstrom R, Nilsson T, Burstrom L, et al. Exposure-response relationship between hand-arm vibration and vibrotactile perception sensitivity. *Am J Ind Med.* 1999;35:456-64.

Macfarlane G, Hunt I, Silman A. Role of mechanical and psychosocial factors in the onset of forearm pain: prospective population based study. *BMJ.* 2000;321(7262):676-9.

Magora A. Investigation of the relationship between low back pain and occupation. *Ind Med Surg.* 1972;41:5-9.

Marras WS. Occupational low back disorder causation and control. *Ergonomics.* 2000;43(7):880-902.

Matias AC, Salvendy G, Kuczek T. Predictive models of carpal tunnel syndrome causation among VDT operators. *Ergonomics.* 1998;41(2):213-26.

McCormack RR Jr, Inman RD, Wells A, et al. Prevalence of tendinitis and related disorders in a manufacturing work force. *J Rheumatol.* 1990;17: 958-64.

Molteni G, De Vito G, Sias N, Grieco A. Epidemiology of musculoskeletal disorders caused by biomechanical overload. *Med Lav.* 1996; 87(6):469-81.

Moore J, Garg A. Upper extremity disorders in a pork processing plant: relationships between job risk factors and morbidity. *Am Ind Hyg Assoc J.* 1994;55(8):703-15.

Murata K, Araki S, Okajima F, et al. Subclinical impairment in the median nerve across the carpal tunnel among female VDT operators. *Int Arch Occup Environ Health.* 1996;68(2):75-9.

Nachemson AL. The natural course of low back pain. In: White AA, Gordon SL, eds. *American Academy of Orthopedic Surgeons Symposium on Idiopathic Low Back Pain.* St. Louis, Mo: Mosby; 1982.

Nakazawa T, Okubo Y, Suwazono Y, et al. Association between duration of daily VDT use and subjective symptoms. *Am J Ind Med.* 2002;42:421-6.

Pedersen LK, Jensen LK. Relationship between occupation and elbow pain, epicondylitis. *Ugeskr Laeger.* 1999;161(34):4751-5.

Pope MH, Andersson GBJ. *Occupational Low Back Pain.* St. Louis, Mo: Mosby-Year Book; 1991.

Rempel DM, Harrison RJ, Bernhardt S. Work related cumulative trauma disorders of the upper extremity. *JAMA.* 1992;267:838-42.

Rempel DM, Punnett L. Epidemiology of the wrist and hand. In: Pope MH, Nordin M, eds. *Work Related Musculoskeletal Disorders.* St. Louis, Mo: Mosby; 1996.

Robinson E. Cases of telegraphists' cramp. *BMJ.* 1882;November 4:880.

Rossignol M, Stock S, Patry L, et al. Carpal tunnel syndrome: what is attributable to work? The Montreal study. *Occup Environ Med.* 1997;54:519-23.

Sauter SL, Swanson NG. The relationship between workplace psychosocial factors and musculoskeletal disorders in office work: suggested mechanisms and evidence. In: Gordon SL, Blair SJ, Fine LJ, eds. *Repetitive Motion Disorders of the Upper Extremity.* Rosemont, Ill: American Academy of Orthopaedic Surgery; 1995:65-76.

Silverstein B, Welp E, Nelson N, Kalat J. Claims incidence of work-related disorders of the upper extremities: Washington state, 1987 through 1995. *Am J Public Health.* 1998;88(12):1827-33.

Silverstein M, Silverstein B, Franklin G. Evidence for work related musculoskeletal disorders: a scientific counterargument. *J Occup Environ Med.* 1996;38(5):477-84.

Spengler DM, Bigos SJ, Martin NA, et al. Back injuries in industry: a retrospective study. I: overview and cost analysis. *Spine.* 1986;11:133-42.

Stevens JC, Beard CM, O'Fallon WM, Kurland LT. Conditions associated with carpal tunnel syndrome. *Mayo Clin Proc.* 1992;67(6):541-8.

Stevens J, Witt J, Smith B, et al. The frequency of carpal tunnel syndrome in computer users at a medical facility. *Neurology.* 2001;56(11):1568-70.

Svensson HO, Andersson GBJ. Low-back pain in 40-47 year old men: work history and work environment factors. *Spine.* 1983;8:272-6.

Tanaka S, Petersen M, Cameron L. Prevalence and risk factors of tendinitis and related disorders of the distal upper extremity among US workers: comparison to carpal tunnel syndrome. *Am J Ind Med.* 2001;39:328-35.

Theorell T, Harms-Ringdahl K, Ahlberg-Hulten G, et al. Psychosocial job factors and symptoms from the locomotor system: a multicausal analysis. *Scand J Rehabil Med.* 1991;23:165-73.

Tornqvist EW, Kilbom A, Vingard E, et al. MUSIC-Norrtalje Study Group. The influence on seeking care because of neck and shoulder disorders from work-related exposures. *Epidemiol.* 2001;12(5):537-45.

Troup JDG, Chapman AE. *Manual Handling and Lifting: An Information and Literature Review with Special Reference to the Back.* London: Her Majesty's Stationery Office; 1985.

Troup JDG, Martin JD, Lloyd DCEF. Back pain in industry: a prospective study. *Spine.* 1981;6:61-9.

Vasseljen O, Westgaard R. A case-control study of trapezius muscle activity in office and manual workers with shoulder and neck pain and symptom-free controls. *Int Arch Occup Environ Health.* 1995;67:11-8.

Venning PJ, Walter SD, Stitt LW. Personal and job-related factors as determinants of incidence of back injuries among nursing personnel. *J Occup Med.* 1987;29:820-5.

Viikari-Juntura E. The role of physical stressors in the development of hand/wrist and elbow disorders. In: Gordon SL, Blair SJ, Fine LJ, eds. *Repetitive Motion Disorders of the Upper Extremity.* Rosemont, Ill: American Academy of Orthopaedic Surgery; 1995:7-30.

Viikari-Juntura E, Silverstein B. Role of physical load factors in carpal tunnel syndrome. *Scand J Work Environ Health.* 1999;25(3):163-85.

Weber H. Lumbar disc herniation: a controlled, prospective study with 10 years of observation. *Spine.* 1983;8:131-40.

Werner RA, Franzblau A, Albers JW, Armstrong TJ. Median mononeuropathy among active workers: are there differences between symptomatic and asymptomatic workers? *Am J Ind Med.* 1998;33(4):374-78.

Werner RA, Gell N, Franzblau A, Armstrong TJ. Prolonged median sensory latency as a predictor of future carpal tunnel syndrome. *Muscle Nerve.* 2001;24(11):1462-7.

Wickstrom G. Effect of work on degenerative back disease: a review. *Scand J Work Environ Health*. 1978;4:1-12.

Wieslander G, Norback D, Gothe C-J, et al. Carpal tunnel syndrome (CTS) and exposure to vibration, repetitive wrist movements, and heavy manual work: a case-referent study. *Br J Ind Med*. 1989;46:43-7.

5 *Cornerstones of Disability Prevention and Management*

This chapter emphasizes the importance of keeping life as normal as possible for ill and injured workers, keeping them at work, or safely returning them to appropriate work as soon as possible. In addition, the chapter examines tools and techniques which have proven effective in assisting workers to remain engaged in society at all levels. It also examines the role of each of the participants in the stay-at-work/return-to-work (SAW/RTW) process (the employee, provider, insurer, and employer).

Most workers who report a work-related health concern can return to regular-, temporary-, or modified-duty immediately or within a short time. Occupational physicians and other health professionals who treat work-related injuries and illness can make an important contribution to the appropriate management of work-related symptoms, illnesses, or injuries by managing disability and time lost from work as well as medical care.

Prompt return to work in a capacity suitable for the worker's current capabilities and needs for rest, treatment, and social support prevents deconditioning and disabling inactivity, reinforces self-esteem, reduces disability, and improves the therapeutic outcome in most individual cases and on an aggregate basis. Ill or injured workers can be temporarily placed in different jobs from their usual jobs (temporary-duty), or their usual jobs can be temporarily modified to accommodate their limitations and remaining abilities (modified or temporary transitional work). Accommodation, with progressively fewer restrictions as healing occurs, generally has a greater chance of success; the highest success rates are achieved when workers return to a modification of their pre-injury job. Disability management conveys respect for injured or ill employees and provides social support that hastens recovery.

Consequences of Disability to the Individual

The consequences of disability to the individual are profound and multidimensional in scope, yet many workers and their families are unaware of the harm that may result from unnecessary absence from work.

Most adults derive a good deal of their self-image from their work role. The inability to do one's job removes a pillar of his or her self-esteem and sense of well-being, and leads to a profound change in identity. Inactivity leads rather quickly to muscle and joint aches, pain, and stiffness that may become a vicious cycle of inactivity and worsening musculoskeletal complaints. Within a matter of days, muscle mass, tendon strength, and bone mass begin to decline. Reversing these changes often takes much longer than the inactivity that caused them, particularly in older patients. Even limited activity, which often is easier to accomplish at the worksite, can prevent or mitigate these changes. For this and other reasons, patients with no absences from work have the best chance of recovery. Preferential consideration should be given to plans that involve (in descending order) light or modified work, flexible schedules, and reduced hours. Injured workers often experience a decrease in health due to the injury and pain medications. In many cases, depression occurs due to a sharp decrease in an injured worker's quality of life, including a loss of independence.

While absent from work, some ill or injured workers may no longer receive salary increases, medical benefits, bonuses, overtime or holiday pay. In addition, they may incur many added expenses, depending on the injury. They may need to hire help to mow the lawn, shovel the driveway, maintain the home, repair vehicles, or do other tasks they could do prior to their injury or illness. Savings, if any, may dwindle, and debt may increase as they strive to accommodate their disability. Furthermore, they may incur other losses, such as the inability to obtain disability insurance when purchasing a home, renewing a mortgage, or buying a car.

The consequences of disability can affect an entire family, across generations, and often change and reverse traditional societal roles. Individuals may be unable to fulfill their normal roles as spouse or parent, and other members of the family may be forced to assume new duties. The new role may be a barrier to functional recovery.

Consequences of Disability to the Employer

The cost of disability to employers is substantial. Recent available statistics based on data from the Centers for Disease Control National Center for Health Statistics (NCHS), extracted from the National Health Interview Survey (NHIS) and the Healthcare Cost and Utilization Project (HCUP) for the year 2000, indicates that total lost-time cost is $458,150 per year per 100 workers. This cost includes indirect disability costs of $366,520 (including replacement, rehiring, retraining, overtime, downtime, and lost productivity) and direct costs (actual weekly wages paid) of $91,630. Add to that annual medical costs of $268,539, and the resulting total cost of disability per 100 employees per year is $726,689.

Functional Recovery and Return to Work

In order for an injured worker to stay at or return successfully to work, he or she must be physically able to perform some necessary job duties. This does not necessarily mean that the worker has fully recovered from the injury, or is pain-free; it means that the worker has sufficient capacity to safely perform some job duties. Known as functional recovery, this concept defines the point at which the worker has regained specific physical functions necessary for re-employment.

While return to modified- or temporary-duty work is an important first step in the functional improvement of workers with health concerns, it must be managed carefully. The factors contributing to absences from work are complex. Some factors are medically related; others are personal or related to family, job, worksite, or the economy.

Certain factors have been shown to promote an ill or injured worker's functional recovery, including:

- Encouragement and support from the worker's employer, coworkers, doctor, family, and friends.
- Injured workers' perceptions that their jobs (whether the usual job or the modified-duty job) are commensurate with their qualifications and that they can perform the job duties adequately.
- Access to quality medical care after the injury. This includes a positive relationship between the worker and his or her doctor, in which the doctor provides adequate information about proposed treatments and recovery expectations and discusses the worker's job duties and ways to avoid aggravation or re-injury. Additional components of quality care include resuming aerobic activity as soon as possible to avoid deconditioning, and exhausting reasonable care methods prior to electing surgery (unless surgery is clinically indicated).
- Injured workers' positive expectations and experiences with medical care and work-related injuries. This includes previous positive experiences the workers have had with quality medical care and/or managing work-related injuries. These experiences may be their own or shared by coworkers, family, and friends. These previous experiences often shape expectations about the success of proposed medical treatments or modified-duty proposals.

Early Steps to Reduce Time Away from Work

Understanding the consequences of disability to the employer, the ill or injured worker, his or her family, and our society should provide motivation enough to proactively develop a plan for early return-to-work.

Many peer-reviewed studies show that proactive return-to-work programs, including modified- or light-duty options for injured workers, reduce overall employer costs directly through savings on workers' compensation insurance premiums and indirectly through minimized costs associated with recruiting, hiring, and training for replacement employees.

Studies also indicate that employer-sponsored return-to-work programs tend to promote safer work environments by modifying job duties or equipment in order to reduce the likelihood of exacerbating an existing injury or preventing re-injury. By demonstrating a desire to integrate injured workers back into the workplace, employers reinforce their commitment to the safety and well-being of employees while fostering a sense of workplace security and cooperation.

Perhaps most importantly, studies indicate that without an effective return-to-work program, medical care alone is relatively ineffective in reducing lost time. Participation and communication among all participants is crucial to the success of proactive efforts to achieve an early return to work. Each has a role in the process and should understand the importance of promptly assuming responsibility for that role. Whether the program is formalized or merely an unwritten commitment to the approach, the responsibilities are the same.

A. Employer's Role

A successful return-to-work program must have multiple levels of responsibility that include the employer, safety professionals, supervisors, and the injured worker. To be most effective, the return-to-work process starts before any injury has occurred. This process includes educating management and workers and is best supported by a nonhostile work environment in which a positive supervisor/management response follows an injury or onset of symptoms. In situations involving unsophisticated, passive or actively hostile employers in which the worker may perceive dangerous working conditions or a negative interpersonal climate, there is little incentive for a worker to return if alternatives, such as extended workers' compensation benefits or sick leave are available.

The optimal system allows early return to modified work and communication with the employee, provider, and insurance carrier. Ideally, the employer will have job descriptions readily available for provider review and be willing to participate in job/schedule modification as necessary. A lost-time injury can often be avoided if the employer, physician, and insurer communicate and collaborate to get the employee's life back to normal. Typically, the medical care associated with these model programs is conservative and guided by evidence-based treatment guidelines. The employer's (or insurer's) willingness and ability to eliminate obstacles, and arrange an appropriate on-the-job recovery, based on the provider's work prescription, will determine the date when the employee actually gets back to work. Additionally, employers consistently monitor and evaluate the progress of return-to-work programs in order to identify opportunities for improvement.

B. Clinician's Role

Under the optimal system, a clinician acts as the primary case manager. The clinician provides appropriate medical evaluation and treatment and adheres to a conservative evidence-based treatment approach that limits excessive physical medicine usage and referral. Ideally, the clinician has previously visited the job site and knows the functional demands of the position. If this is not possible, a review of the job description is appropriate.

Clinicians must step beyond their usual medical treatment approach and actively communicate with other members of the return-to-work program including employers and/or payers. It is paramount that the clinician understands the importance of communication with the worker on return to full function as early as possible in a participatory management approach.

Several key points should be kept in mind when dealing with the ill or injured worker:

- Early events are key. Occupational health practitioners' involvement early in a case can be some of the most valuable work they do. During those critical first few days, they set the tone.
- Occupational health practitioners can ask about disruption of normal activities as well as work. They also can check to see that patients released to work have actually returned to work.
- Clinicians can assume patients will work during the medical work-up and treatment. Treatment plans can always include staying at or returning to work (with modifications as necessary to keep the patient safe and as comfortable as possible), unless bed or home confinement is specifically medically indicated.
- Clinicians can provide extra support to make sure anxious or reluctant patients return to full function as soon as possible in order to avoid inadvertently rewarding avoidance behavior or phobic-like reactions. Even when the medical condition is not expected to change appreciably from week to week, frequent follow-up visits are often warranted for monitoring in order to provide structure and reassurance.
- It is important to stay alert to the issue of elapsed time away from work: Over four weeks should be considered in the danger zone. By one month, many patients begin to develop a disability mindset.

Ascertain whether specific obstacles are preventing the patient from returning to work and ask: What is the specific reason the patient is not working? Nonmedical or administrative details often delay return to work and cannot be rectified unless first identified.

Nonmedical issues, once identified, need to be referred or, if possible, managed by the provider. These issues can be handled in the same way as a regular medical specialist referral. In other words, physicians need to find their comfort point and refer the situations that are beyond it. This may require developing a network of resources to call when nonmedical issues prolong disability. The clinician should judiciously select and refer to specialists who will support functional recovery as well as provide expert medical recommendations. Close communication is necessary and should emphasize the occupational health clinician's role as the primary case manager.

FORMULATING AND COMMUNICATING A WORK PRESCRIPTION TO THE EMPLOYER/INSURER

When treating work illness or injuries, providing guidance regarding the worker's ability to stay at work or return to work, estimating work capacities, and describing medical restrictions and limitations are among the most important assessments occupational health practitioners can make. It is appropriate to view this activity as formulating a medical prescription for functional activity with a particular focus on work. Providers should strive to provide unbiased, objective, and dispassionate advice. Their reasoning should follow a logical sequence such as that described here:

Step 1. Determine if absence from work is medically required. If not, then the patient can be cleared to do medically appropriate work during recovery. The next steps will determine the specifications for that appropriate work. Typically, absence is medically required when:

- Attendance is required at a place of care (hospital, doctor's office, physical therapy).
- Recovery (or quarantine) requires confinement to bed or home.
- Being in the workplace or traveling to work is medically contraindicated (poses a specific hazard to the public, coworkers, or to the worker personally, i.e., risks damage to tissues or delays healing).

Step 2. Look for any obvious mismatch between the patient's medical condition and the demands of the regular job (or any proposed modified-duty job). For example, what part of the patient's body needs to be protected? What kinds of activities or functions should the patient avoid? Are special protection, reduced demands on capability or endurance, or a special accommodation needed? If so, for how long?

In order to assess the situation accurately, clinicians may need to augment their clinical judgment with further input from the employer. Office staff can request this data, which might include job descriptions including tasks, data on physical demands and chemical exposures of the job, and information regarding whether accommodations can be made allowing an employee to function in his or her original job category despite physical limitations.

Step 3. Describe any medical restrictions (i.e., what the patient *should not* be allowed to do, or what the employer *should* do). Distinct from work capacities and limitations, these are specific medical concerns or protective circumstances that are required in order to protect and keep the patient safe while working. An example is a prohibition against working at heights for a patient with a balance problem or seizure disorder. Determining restrictions *is* a medical issue. The physician's medical knowledge and some knowledge of potential hazards at work and at home are required. These restrictions should not be modified by either the patient or the employer without the physician's consent, even if the patient is fully capable of performing the task.

Step 4. Describe the functional limitations (i.e., what the patient *cannot* or *is* unable to do). Limitations represent the difference between the patient's current physical stamina, agility, strength, and cognitive ability and potential job requirements. If specific job demands are known, it will be possible to describe more precisely the fit between the patient's current capability and actual job requirements.

Determining limitations is *not* really a medical issue; clinicians are simply being asked to provide an independent assessment of what the patient is currently able and unable to do. In many cases, physicians can listen to the patient's history, ask questions about activities, and then extrapolate, based on knowledge of the patient and experience with other patients with similar conditions. It may be necessary to obtain a more precise delineation of patient capabilities than is available from routine physical examination. Under some circumstances, this can best be done by ordering a functional capacity evaluation of the patient.

Whatever the basis of work capacities or restrictions, it is necessary for physicians to state their sources of information. In particular, avoid relying solely on the patient or the employer for input; instead, seek objective information or third-party corroboration, especially when controversy exists.

This is particularly true when a patient may be asked to do work that may exceed his or her limitations and lead to further injury or create a hazard. In addition to considering functional testing, these circumstances may necessitate arranging for a conference with the patient, his or her supervisor, and/or the insurer to eliminate any possible misunderstandings. If the employer refuses or is unable to abide by the physician's work prescription, the physician should be available to discuss and explain the basis of limitations and the implication of not following them. The physician is not an arbitrator, but may help identify resources to resolve any disagreement.

Medically discretionary disability is time away from work at the discretion of a patient or employer that is

- Associated with a diagnosable medical condition that may have created some functional impairment but left other functional abilities still intact.

- Most commonly due to a patient's or employer's decision not to make the extra effort required to find a way for the patient to stay at work during illness or recovery.

Occupational health practitioners need to remember that while impairment is defined as an anatomic change or a reduction in physiologic or psychological function (World Health Organization, 1979), impairment may or may not result in disability. Employers who provide accommodations based on essential job function matched to worker abilities can prevent an impairment from causing disability. Unfortunately, employers often choose not to provide accommodations for a worker who is medically able to do some productive work and increase the likelihood of disability.

Many employers feel ill-prepared to make accommodations even though they are willing to do so (e.g., they may have a lack of knowledge about adaptive equipment or creative solutions). Occupational health professionals can assist by suggesting practical and simple accommodations: including workstation adjustment (including task alignment); load; seating; support; unbundling heavy collections of objects; and/or periodic assistance by coworkers for infrequent but demanding tasks and rest breaks. Occupational health professionals can refer employers to guides for accommodation under the Americans with Disabilities Act (ADA) as a model for this process. Remember that disabilities covered by the ADA are permanent, while those discussed here are generally temporary.

Step 5. Identify any nonmedical obstacles that appear to be primary or secondary barriers to return to work. Medically unnecessary disability occurs whenever a person stays away from work because of nonmedical issues such as:

- The misperception that a diagnosis alone (without demonstrable functional impairment) justifies work absence.
- Other problems that masquerade as medical issues, e.g., job dissatisfaction, anger, fear, or other psychosocial factors.
- Poor information flow or inadequate communications.
- Administrative or procedural delay.

Ideally, the provider is aware of risk factors for needless disability or delayed recovery from the first visit. Depending on the presentation, the clinician may address the risk factors early on or monitor them closely and recruit other resources, as necessary, to address them.

Step 6. Provide three intervals as part of the "prognosis," on an ongoing basis, so others can plan accordingly.

a. When the patient will next need to be seen?

b. How long will it take for a next-step improvement in functional capacity?

c. How much time should it take until the medical condition is fully resolved? To monitor progress, a provider may use return-to-work guidelines. All members of the team should be aware of the pros and cons of using such guidelines.

Step 7. Let others determine the actual return to work date (i.e., the extent and speed with which the clinician's recommendations regarding work capacities and restrictions are translated into actual employment decisions). Remember, while the provider's role is to assess work capacities and restrictions, the employer's responsibility is to determine how and when they are accommodated.

C. Employee's/Patient's Role

To achieve functional recovery, patients must assume certain responsibilities. It is important that patients stay active or increase activity to minimize disuse, atrophy, aches, and musculoskeletal pain, and to raise endorphin levels. They must adhere to exercise and medication regimens, keep appointments, and take responsibility for their moods and emotional states. They must work within their medical restrictions, and refuse unreasonable requests by coworkers and supervisors to function over their limitations in a way that could endanger their health or safety.

D. Payer's Role

Payers must act expeditiously in evaluating responsibility for a claim. If the claim is accepted worker payments must be timely in accordance with applicable statutes. Claims should be monitored for indicators of delayed recovery and, if necessary, trigger early case management to support providers in their efforts. They should play a nonadversarial role and work with the employer to define their approach.

Barriers to Recovery and Yellow Flags Requiring Intervention

Most patients smoothly and promptly recover their ability to function after an occupational health problem, usually within a matter of days to weeks. The few who do not recover quickly account for the majority of cost, lost workdays, and frustration for employers, practitioners, families, and the community. Thus, primary prevention, early detection, and secondary prevention of delayed recovery are key parts of the occupational health practitioner's role.

Statistics from several uncontrolled studies of employed populations indicate that workers absent for more than six months due to a work-related complaint have approximately a 50% probability of returning to work, those absent more than one year have a 25% probability, and those absent more than two years have virtually no chance of returning to work.

A delay in recovery from an acute work-related condition might be due to psychosocial or employment factors of various types or to a medical problem that was not identified on initial examination (missed diagnosis or comorbid condition). Failure-to-recover function as expected (as predicated in these guidelines), should prompt an inquiry into previously unknown or disregarded factors that could contribute to slower-than-expected improvement in activity tolerance and work ability.

WORKSITE FACTORS

Besides risk factors associated with ill or injured workers, job-related barriers also can delay timely return to work. These barriers include:

- Lack of employer-sponsored modified-duty options for injured workers. Smaller employers, workplaces with restrictive human resource policies, and employers with highly specialized job requirements are less likely to make modified-duty positions available for injured workers.
- Job duties that require significant physical modifications (e.g., permanent changes in work schedule or additional travel requirements), ergonomic adjustments, or qualifications (e.g., education requirements) in order for the worker to perform. This may disproportionately affect certain industries such as construction or agriculture where physical job modifications are often difficult.
- Unstable or negative work environment. Inconsistent or vague employer personnel policies, low job satisfaction, perceived unfairness with performance evaluations, supervisor/employee communication problems, and perceived lack of job security may inhibit an injured worker's willingness to return to work in a timely fashion.
- Union agreements that may influence return to work. Some unions actively help members obtain modified work, while others are limited in their ability to do so.
- The presence or absence of second-injury laws, which structurally may provide incentives or disincentives to return to work.

PATIENT FACTORS

Table 5-1 lists risks for delayed recovery that have been identified in cohort or cross-sectional studies, which are viewed as being statistically related to delayed return-to-function. Previous episodes of work absence due to delay in functional recovery, seriousness of injury, physical demands, chemical expo-

Table 5-1. Risk Factors for Delayed Functional Recovery

Factors
Demographic factor
Age
Historical factors
Previous injuries
Recent prolonged absence from work
Absence from work
Multiple absences from work
Being a victim of past abuse
Social factors
Family history of disability
Change in family role
Family support
Union membership
Personal health
Chemical dependency
Depression
Emotional distress
Employment-related factors
Job satisfaction
Task enjoyment
Adversarial job relationship
Job demands
Alternative work available (absence of modified work)
Perception of work-relatedness
Union agreements
Presence or absence of second injury funds
Injury-related factors
Severity of (self-rated) symptoms and/or health status
Expectations of work capacity
Severity of signs
Delayed presentation
Chronic pain symptoms
Multiple diagnoses
Diagnosis of low back pain or carpal tunnel syndrome
Prior negative treatment experiences
Excessive/inappropriate physical medicine treatment
Economic and legal factors
Income
Education
Compensability
Legal representation
Litigation pending

sures, and socioeconomic variables, such as educational ease of changing the job, are the most strongly correlated with delayed return to work. A worker's level of education and income are strongly correlated; many believe that income is the driving variable. Some investigators believe that age as a risk for delayed return-to work may be related to lengthening of the time required for musculoskeletal healing with aging, while others believe it may be a covariant or confounding factor. (Aging also increases access to retirement benefits, reducing the economic incentive to return to work.) Probably both theories are correct to some extent in deconditioned individuals. (Odds ratios or *P* values are not listed; however, readers can refer to the studies cited in the references at the end of this chapter.) A variety of factors have been shown to delay an injured worker's functional recovery. Clearly, not all workers encounter these factors, and the presence of a risk factor does not guarantee a delay, but it does increase the statistical probability that a delay will occur. When one or more of these factors are present, however, managing them proactively increases the probability of successful re-employment.

These risk factors for delayed functional recovery include:

- The existence of multiple diagnoses for a work-related injury, which may include a severe injury involving multiple body parts, an injury that is exacerbated and later develops into a different medical condition, or a misdiagnosis.
- Low back injuries and diagnoses of carpal tunnel syndrome. Studies have shown that these two medical conditions consistently have longer treatment and disability durations in workers' compensation compared with similar types of injuries in other parts of the body. In general medicine, these conditions do not have the same treatment/disability duration trends.
- Previous negative experiences with medical care and work-related illness or injuries.
- The existence of chronic pain or other medical complications (e.g., chronic regional pain syndrome, among others).
- Ill or injured workers' perceptions regarding their current health status and proposed medical treatment, the severity of their medical symptoms and pain, their fear of aggravation or reinjury, their perception that unrelated medical conditions are work related, and their fear of losing workers' compensation benefits (or of difficulty in restarting benefits) if modified-duty attempts are not successful.
- Preexisting and coexisting medical or psychological conditions that may affect physical recovery (e.g., diabetes, musculoskeletal disorders, smoking, alcoholism, depression, and anxiety, among others).
- Excessive or clinically inappropriate use of physical medicine treatments (e.g., manipulations or therapeutic exercises, among others) or surgery.
- Involvement in workers' compensation disputes or litigation.

- Demographic characteristics such as female workers, older workers, and workers with lower income and education levels.

Clinicians may note that the above-mentioned indicators should raise the index of suspicion, but must be viewed in the context of the patient's whole life and in terms of how his or her mood and coping skills are affected. However, in cases in which psychosocial factors play a role (i.e., patients with pain who also have emotional or behavioral problems), it is sometimes difficult to determine whether the psychosocial problem predated and contributed to delayed recovery or vice versa (i.e., delayed recovery contributed to the psychosocial problem). In addition, there have not been cohort or cross-sectional studies that have shown a strong statistical correlation between delayed recovery and variables such as depression, or other mood or behavioral changes.

It should be noted that patients with specific (as opposed to nonspecific) diagnoses (e.g., sciatica rather than regional low back pain), and those with a history of prior injury, psychological impairment, or psychosocial risk factors, statistically have a longer recovery period. However, clinicians need to be aware of individual variation; with good case management, some workers with previous injury or other risk factors for delayed recovery can return to work in a relatively short time.

BEHAVIORAL WARNING SIGNS OR RISK FACTORS FOR DELAYED RECOVERY

Some of the above-mentioned barriers to return to work are considered yellow flags because they could be eliminated with prompt and proper intervention, often by a behavioral health professional. These barriers should be recognized and handled as soon as possible. They may include substance abuse, family disorders, work conflict (especially with supervisors), and psychological problems (e.g., depression). Other possible obstacles to returning to work are the patient's lack of motivation, illness behavior (symptom exaggeration), inappropriate or ineffective treatment, a desire to use rehabilitation to change a job the worker dislikes, or the patient's having received legal advice to accept a lump sum payment instead of rehabilitation. The behavioral health professional might inquire about the reasons the patient believes he or she is not able to return to work and cooperatively develop strategies to overcome the perceived barriers. There also should be discussion of how the patient has been functioning, what is going on in his or her life, and what plans the patient has for the future. If personal or psychosocial factors are contributing to delayed recovery, psychological, psychiatric, or other behavioral health intervention is more appropriate than continuing medication, physical therapy, or surgery; continuing such treatment in the face of treatment failure simply creates the expectation of disability.

SYSTEM-INDUCED FUNCTIONAL DISABILITY

A new yellow flag of particular concern has been identified as iatrogenic disability. However, this is a misnomer because the term iatrogenic implies that the problem stems from a patient's medical care, when, in fact, it is an unintended and undesirable result of an injured or ill person's contact with a disability benefits system as a whole. Ill or injured people with this type of disability have developed a strong, unshakable belief that they are sicker and less able to function than they really are, leading many to describe their disability as functional in nature.

Functional disability is not the same as malingering. Using the term malingerer indicates that the individual is conscious of his or her behavior and is specifically feigning illness or injury for secondary gain. A malingerer may limp out of the exam room only to stride briskly to his or her car and engage in strenuous activity later that day. Patients with functional disability truly believe they are too ill to work. Initially, they may know they are using a relatively minor medical problem as an excuse not to do something they should (referred to as partial malingering); but over time, many patients become so invested in their need to prove they are sick that their illness behaviors become a disease in and of themselves. Some may also achieve primary gain from discovering that they get more attention than they could otherwise if they are ill and cannot perform their usual activities, including work activities. Thus, primary and secondary gain factors feed upon each other to the point where the differentiation between the two is blurred, and the patient has entered a functional disability state.

When health care providers and other members of the health care team, which should include the employer and insurer, are alert to the aforementioned issues, patients who are developing signs of delayed recovery can be "intercepted" before they have fully developed a functional disability syndrome and the accompanying cascade of unfortunate life events.

Because the components of disability systems are so fragmented—insurance, medical, administrative, vocational, legal, and employer representatives all playing a part and each having its own agenda—it's not unusual that no single component is accountable for assuring the best outcome for the injured or ill patient. Instead, each component simply tries to fulfill its own obligations.

It is difficult to feel very powerful in such a complex system. This is especially true for the ill or injured worker, people who suddenly must deal both with an injury or illness and an unfamiliar, complicated process in an unfamiliar bureaucratic system. Workers are basically left to fend for themselves at a time when their illness or injury makes them vulnerable. A resulting sense of abandonment may be the root cause of most functional disability cases. Ill or injured workers often interact with professionals, who reinforce the process by acting as if an illness or injury is causing time off work, even though the time off is actually due to other causes, including slow communication, paperwork delays, the lack of a piece of adaptive equipment, a policy against light duty, poor management, or weak motivation. When injured or ill people hear their employer, claims examiner, case manager, or doctor talk in that manner, they may start to believe that there is a medical reason for their time off work. They may develop a habit of thinking: *As long as I have this condition, I won't be able to work; or alternatively, I should not be released to work.* If reinforced by environmental, societal, or psychological factors, these ideas can trigger the process that leads to system-induced functional disability.

Managing Delayed Recovery

Clinical Reassessment

The clinician can always think about differential diagnoses, whether they are of an occupational or nonoccupational nature. This does not have to be a long process. By stepping back and reevaluating the patient and the entire clinical picture, symptoms or physical findings may be identified that have developed since the injury and that may not be consistent with the original diagnosis. A detailed history and physical examination should be conducted. Special studies, as discussed more thoroughly in Chapters 8 through 16, may be used to determine the presence of conditions that might be helped by surgical or medical therapy more intensive or specialized than that described in these guidelines. However, the occupational health professional managing the case must be sure that the studies are indicated and are specific and sensitive for the related condition. Testing can be done to confirm clinical data. In addition, effective therapy should be available for any condition that the clinician attempts to identify.

Many patients will have normal results of studies or findings consistent with age. Because an evaluation is usually successful in detecting the rare case of serious pathology, but in most cases will not find a specific cause for musculoskeletal pain, the patient may need reassurance. Prestudy counseling to reinforce this point is usually very helpful. In some instances, the delay in appropriate return to work stems from the need for adequate communication of exposure information rather than inadequate communication of physical demands. However, when special studies fail to define the exact cause of symptoms, no patient should receive the impression that the clinician thinks "nothing is wrong" or that the problem could be "in his or her head." Assure the patient that a clinical workup is usually highly successful in detecting serious conditions, but does not reveal the precise cause of many common musculoskeletal, visual, psychophysiologic, or pain symptoms.

A. Reassessing Function and Functional Recovery

The first step in managing delayed recovery is to document the patient's current state of functional ability (including activities of daily living) and the recovery trajectory to date as a time line. As a starting point for the assessment, obtain a complete history from the patient and other objective observers, including the employer or onsite occupational health professional, with regard to abilities and effectiveness at work. Goals for functional recovery can then be framed with reference to this baseline.

A number of functional assessment tools are available, including functional capacity exams and videotapes. Most assess general functioning, but modifications to test work-related functioning are under development or can be created by the clinician. Examples include the SF-36, as modified for musculoskeletal disorders by task forces of the American Academy of Orthopedic Surgeons and assessment tools discussed in Chapter 7, "Consultations and Independent Medical Examinations." Some are more subjective and strive to identify psychological factors. One needs to look at the resources available in the area.

B. Case Management in Delayed Recovery

Patients who do not recover as expected usually have several interrelated causes of delayed functional recovery. Cases of delayed functional recovery require close management rather than simple care. The occupational health clinician can act as the manager of the case or can enlist the help of a skilled case manager, who is typically an occupational health nurse or a social worker.

The patient and the employer should be full parties to the development of a plan to achieve functional recovery. The patient must assess his or her own capabilities and reasons for delayed functional recovery and create or agree to a realistic stepwise plan for improvement. He or she must also agree to stop doctor-shopping and work with the coordinator of care. Ideally, the employer will agree to job modification and progressive return to duty or to retraining the patient for another job if necessary.

It is important to list and proactively manage each risk for delayed recovery before the recovery trajectory extends beyond the expected duration. Chemical dependency, work problems, family disorders, and vocational issues all require separate but integrated action plans. Some of these may be system problems or behavioral disorders requiring specialized approaches that are beyond the scope of these guidelines. However, the clinician should be aware of, and avoid, enabling behaviors and practices.

Contingencies, supports, and work limits are useful in working with patients who have difficulty increasing their level of function. Time off work can be contingent on participation in treatment or with the plan. Medication and physical therapy should be time contingent, not "as needed." Regularly scheduled time-limited appointments are usually best to limit patients' emotional demands and foster their independence. Patients should be monitored for compliance with appointments. Group interventions are often useful to provide support and help with problem solving. They are often more successful than individual interactions and allow more time to be devoted in the aggregate.

C. Approach to the Patient

In working with the ill or injured patient, the occupational health practitioner can show a nonjudgmental, respectful attitude and accept the patient's concerns as valid. However, many patients whose functional recovery is taking longer than expected are angry, despairing, or depressed (see Chapter 6, "Pain, Suffering, and Restoration of Function"). The practitioner can deflect these feelings rather than become emotionally involved or take sides in disputes with other health care providers, insurers, or employers. It also is counterproductive for the practitioner to be defensive about past treatment that did not succeed. The practitioner must avoid being intimidated by the patient into ordering unjustifiable studies, referrals, or treatment.

It is important to explore signs of passivity in the patient, which may herald depression. Passivity also may be a sign that the patient needs redirection to resume active control of his or her life in order to recover function. The occupational health practitioner can encourage dialogue with the patient about his or her fears, sense of loss, work-related status, and hopes for the future. At any impasse in the discussion, the practitioner can clarify his or her intent to be helpful.

Although the preceding section discussed the patient's responsibilities in cases of delayed recovery, particular emphasis also may need to be placed on providing additional support, such as helping the patient develop coping skills, having the patient's family intervene, and helping with career plans. Further compliance with appointments and the consequences of noncompliance also can be emphasized.

Functional recovery is often delayed because the cumulative effect of work and other issues has overwhelmed the patient's ability to cope. A number of techniques are available to teach coping skills, depending on the patient's specific needs and skill deficits. Many patients benefit from training in communications skills and assertiveness. With this training, patients are better able to deal with family- or employment-related issues that may be interfering with their functional recovery or return to work. Time management and prioritization also are important skills. Hardiness training has been used in some instances to change negative or self-defeating mindsets and thus hasten recovery. If low self-esteem is an issue, psychological counseling may be useful. Fear avoidance can sometimes interfere with a patient's ability to cope (see Chapter 6). Other techniques can also be used to enhance coping skills. Referral to a behavioral health professional trained in these areas may be a very important investment in the patient's overall outcome.

To optimize the chances of success, the patient's family or support system must be enlisted in the recovery effort. The practitioner can explain that the patient must take care of him or herself and assume the responsibilities outlined above. Co-dependent or enabling behavior will markedly impede the recovery effort. However, shifting responsibilities such as childcare, laundry, and housekeeping to the worker may impede recovery.

Vocational and career interventions may be needed to facilitate return to productive work. As noted above, low income and limited education, as well as heavy occupations, are associated with delayed recovery. It is likely that these three variables are proxies for restricted career choices, monotonous jobs, and low levels of task control, leading to low levels of job enjoyment. Therefore, it is helpful to discuss career aspirations with the patient very early in the course of the episode. Patients can be asked to write their own career plan and investigate options for transfer, retraining, and so on, so that they take charge of the vocational planning process. This often helps patients realize that some of their expectations were unrealistic and to change their direction and goals.

Referrals

Referral may be appropriate if the practitioner is uncomfortable with the line of inquiry outlined above, with treating a particular cause of delayed recovery (such as substance abuse), or has difficulty obtaining information or agreement to a treatment plan. Depending on the issue involved, it often is helpful to "position" a behavioral health evaluation as a return-to-work evaluation. The goal of such an evaluation is, in fact, functional recovery and return to work. Collaboration with the employer and insurer is necessary to design an action plan to address multiple issues, which may include arranging for an external case manager. The physician can function in this role, but it may require some discussion to insure compensation for assuming this added responsibility.

Functional Restoration

If an early return to work has been achieved and the return-to-work process is working well, the likelihood of debilitation should be limited. If, however, there is a delay in return to work or a prolonged period of inactivity, a program of functional restoration can be considered. Such a program could include components of aerobic conditioning as well as strength and flexibility assessment where necessary. It is also worth noting that preinjury and postinjury or illness strength and endurance may be limited and might be less than the job requires. If this is the case, the likelihood of reinjury or prolonged problems may increase. Though it may not be part of the process for treating an acute injury, the provider and employer may have to address these issues either through focusing on modifying the job to suit the patient's abilities or considering alternative placement.

References

GENERAL

Abenhaim L, Suissa S. Importance and economic burden of occupational back pain: a study of 2,500 cases representative of Quebec. *J Occup Med.* 1987;29:670-4.

Ahlgren C, Hammarstrom A. Has increased focus on vocational rehabilitation led to an increase in young employees' return to work after work-related disorders? *Scand J Pub Health.* 1999;27(3):220-7.

Bigos SJ, McKee JE, Holland JP, Holland CL, Hildebrandt J. Back pain, the uncomfortable truth-assurance and activity problem. *Schmerz.* 2001; 15(6):430-4.

Blair SJ, Fine LJ, eds. *Repetitive Motion Disorders of the Upper Extremity.* Rosemont, Ill: American Academy of Orthopaedic Surgeons 1995:65-76.

Bruening LA, Beaulieu D. The return-to-work phase for the patient with cumulative trauma. In: Hunter JM, Schneider LH, Mackin EJ, et al. *Rehabilitation of the Hand: Surgery and Therapy.* St. Louis, Mo: Mosby; 1990:1192-6.

Butler RJ, Johnson WG, Baldwin ML. Managing work disability: why first return to work is not a measure of success. *Ind Labor Rel Rev.* 1995;48: 452-69.

Carmean G, et al. *The Santa Barbara Project. Vols 1, 2.* Santa Barbara: County of Santa Barbara; 1984.

Clarke JA, Cole DC, Ferrier SE. *Work-Ready 1: Report of Qualitative Component from Ontario.* Toronto, Ontario: Institute for Work and Health; 1999.

Colledge AL, Johnson HI. S.P.I.C.E.—a model for reducing the incidence and costs of occupationally entitled claims. *Occup Med.* 2000;15(4):695-722, iii.

Colledge AL, Johns RE Jr, Thomas MH. Functional ability assessment: guidelines for the workplace. *J Occup Environ Med.* 1999;41(3):172-80.

Cornes P. The vocational rehabilitation index: a guide to accident victims' requirements for return to work assistance. *Int J Disabil Studies.* 1990;12: 32-6.

Crook J, Moldofsky H. The probability of recovery and return to work from work disability as a function of time. *Qual Life Res.* 1994; Suppl 1:S97-109.

Denniston PL, ed. *Official Disability Guidelines. 8th ed.* Corpus Christi, Texas: Work-Loss Data Institute, 2003.

DiBenedetto DV. Demonstrating the cost effectiveness of an expert occupational and environmental health nurse: application of AAOHN's success tools. *AAOHN J.* 2001;49(12):547-56.

Dworkin RH, Handlin DS, Richlin DM, et al. Unraveling the effects of compensation, litigation and employment on treatment response in chronic pain. *Pain.* 1985;49-59.

Elders LA, van der Beek AJ, Burdorf A. Return to work after sickness absence due to back disorders—a systematic review on intervention strategies. *Int Arch Occup Environ Health.* 2000;73(5):339-48.

Fass A, Van Erik JTM, Chavannes AW, Gubbels JW. A randomized trial of exercise therapy in patients with acute low back pain: efficacy on sickness absence. *Spine.* 1995;20:941-7.

Field TF, Norton LP. *ADA Resource Manual for Rehabilitation Consultants.* Atlanta, Ga: Elliott and Fitzpatrick; 1992.

Frank JW, Kerr MS, Brooker AS, et al. Disability resulting from occupational low back pain. Part I: What do we know about primary prevention? A review of the scientific evidence on prevention before disability begins. *Spine.* 1996;21:2908-17.

Frank J, Sinclair S, Hogg-Johnson S, et al. Preventing work-related disability from work-related low back pain. New evidence gives new hope—if we can just get all the players onside. *CMAJ*. 1998;158(12):1625-31.

Frymoyer JW, Cats-Baril WL. An overview of the incidence and costs of low back pain. *Orthop Clin NA*. 1991;22:263-71.

Gaines WG Jr, Hegmann KT. Effectiveness of Waddell's nonorganic signs in predicting a delayed return to regular work in patients experiencing acute occupational low back pain. *Spine*. 1999;24(4):396-400; discussion 401.

Gard G, Sandberg AC. Motivating factors for return to work. *Physiother Res Int*. 1998;3(2):100-8.

Gatchel RJ, Polatin PB, Kinney RK. Predicting outcome of chronic back pain using clinical predictors of psychopathology: a prospective analysis. *Health Psychol*. 1995;14(5):415-20.

Green-McKenzie J, Parkerson J, Bernacki E. Comparison of workers' compensation costs for two cohorts of injured workers before and after the introduction of managed care. *J Occup Environ Med*. 1998;40(6):568-72.

Harris JS, Mueller KL, Low P, et al. Beliefs about and use of occupational medicine practice guidelines by case managers and insurance adjusters. *J Occup Environ Med*. 2000;42(4):370-6.

Hartigan C, Miller L, Liewher SC. Rehabilitation of acute and subacute low back and neck pain in the work-injured patient. *Orthop Clin North Am*. 1996;27(4):841-60.

Hendler N. Return-to-work barriers: how to overcome them. *J Workers Comp*. 1995;5(Summer):9-20.

Hilde G, Hagen KB, Jamtvedt G, Winnem M. Advice to stay active as a single treatment for low back pain and sciatica. *Cochrane Database Syst Rev*. 2002;(2):CD003632.

House JS, Landis KR, Umbertson D. Social relationships and health. *Science*. 1988;241:540-5.

Indahl A, Haldorsen EH, Holm S, Reikeras O, Ursin H. Five year follow-up study of a controlled clinical trial using light mobilization and an informative approach to low back pain. *Spine*. 1998;23(23):2625-30.

Indahl A, Velund L, Reikeraas O. Good prognosis for low back pain when left untampered. A randomized clinical trial. *Spine*. 1995;20(4):473-7.

Johnson WG, Butler RJ, Baldwin M. First spells of work absence among Ontario workers. In: Thomason T, Chaykowski RP, eds. *Research in Canadian Workers Compensation*. Kingston, Ontario: IRC Press; 1995:72-84.

Jokl P. The effect of the aging process on muscle and tendon injuries. In: Gordon SL, Gonzalez-Mestre X, Garrett WE Jr, eds. *Sports and Exercise in Midlife*. Rosemont, Ill: American Academy of Orthopaedic Surgeons; 1993:515-29.

Katz JN, Keller RB, Fossel AH, et al. Predictors of return to work following carpal tunnel release. *Am J Ind Med*. 1997;31(1):85-91.

Keller RB, Atlas SJ, Soule DN, Singer DE, Deyo RA. Relationship between rates and outcomes of operative treatment for lumbar disc herniation and spinal stenosis. *J Bone Joint Surg Am*. 1999;81:752-62.

Kuorinka I, Forcier L, eds. *Work Related Musculoskeletal Disorders (WMSDs): A Reference Book for Prevention.* London: Taylor and Francis; 1995.

Lehmann TR, Spratt KF, Lehmann KK. Predicting long-term disability in low back injured workers presenting to a spine consultant. *Spine.* 1993;18: 1103-11.

Lutz GK, Butzlaff ME, Atlas SJ, Keller RB, Singer DE, Deyo RA. The relationship between outcomes and expectations in surgery for sciatica. *J Gen Intern Med.* 1999;14:740-4.

McIntosh G, Frank J, Hogg-Johnson S, Bombardier C, Hall H. Prognostic factors for time receiving workers' compensation benefits in a cohort of patients with low back pain. *Spine.* 2000;25(2):147-57.

Melamed S, Ben-Avi I, Luz J, Green MS. Objective and subjective work monotony: effects on job satisfaction, psychological distress, and absenteeism in blue-collar workers. *J Appl Psychol.* 1995;80:29-42.

Nachemson A. Work for all: those with back pain as well. *Clin Orthop.* 1983; 179:77-85.

Niedhammer I, Bugel I, Goldberg M, Leclerc A, Gueguen A. Psychosocial factors and sickness absence in the Gazel cohort: a prospective study. *Occup Environ Med.* 1998;55:735-41.

North FM, Syme SL, Feeney A, Shipley M, Marmot M. Psychosocial work environment and sickness absence among British civil servants: the Whitehall II study. *Am J Pub Health.* 1996;86:332-40.

Physician Education Project in Workplace Health. *Injury/Illness and Return to Work/Function.* Toronto, Canada: Workplace Safety and Insurance Board; 2000.

Pransky G, Benjamin K, Himmelstein J, et al. Work-related upper-extremity disorders: prospective evaluation of clinical and functional outcomes. *J Occup Environ Med.* 1999;41(10):884-92.

Prezzia C. The use of evidence-based duration guidelines. *J Workers Comp.* 2001;10(4):43-53.

Rael EG, Stanfeld SA, Shipley M, Head J, Feeney A, Marmot M. Sickness absence in the Whitehall II study: the role of social support and material problems. *J Epid Comm Health.* 1995;49:474-81.

Ranavaya MI. Evidence based disability duration guidelines. *Disability Med.* 2002;2(3):75-8.

Rasmussen H, Minifie RL, Bruckman RZ, et al. *Workers' Compensation Medical Management System.* Seattle, Wash: Milliman and Robertson; 1996.

Reed, PO III, ed. *The Medical Disability Advisor.* 2nd ed. Horsham, Pa: LRP Publications; 1994.

Sauter SL, Swanson NG. An ecological model of musculoskeletal disorders in office work. In: Moon SD, Sauter SL, eds. *Beyond Biomechanics: Psychosocial Aspects of Musculoskeletal Disorders in Office Work.* London: Taylor and Francis; 1996.

Thompson D, Rempel D. Industrial engineering and ergonomics. In: LaDou J, ed. *Occupational Health and Safety.* 2nd ed. Itasca, Ill: National Safety Council; 1994:163-86.

Theorell T, Harms-Ringdahl K, Ahlberg-Hulten G, et al. Psychosocial job factors and symptoms from the locomotor system: a multicausal analysis. *Scand J Rehabil Med.* 1991;23:165-73.

Vallfors B. Acute, subacute and chronic low back pain: clinical symptoms, absenteeism and working environment. *Scand J Rehabil Med.* 1985; 11(suppl):1-98.

Wesel SW, Feffer HL, Rothman RH. Industrial low back pain—a prospective evaluation of a standardized diagnostic and treatment protocol. *Spine.* 1984;9:199-203.

World Health Organization. *International Classification of Impairments, Disabilities and Handicaps.* Geneva: World Health Organization; 1980.

EPIDEMIOLOGY

Andersson GBJ. Low back pain in industry: epidemiologic aspects. *Scand J Rehabil Med.* 1979;11:163-8.

Andersson GBJ, Svensson HO, Oden A. The intensity of work recovery in low back pain. *Spine.* 1983;8:880-4.

Barnes D, Smith D, Gatchel RJ, et al. Psychosocioeconomic predictors of treatment success/failure in chronic low back pain patients. *Spine.* 1989; 14:427-30.

Bergquist-Ullman M, Larsson U. Acute low back pain in industry: a controlled prospective study with reference to therapy and confounding factors. *Acta Orthop Scand Suppl.* 1977;170:1-117.

Bigos SJ, Spengler DM, Martin NA, Zeh J, Fisher L, Nachemson A. Back injuries in industry: a retrospective study. III: employee related factors. *Spine.* 1986;11:252-6.

Bigos SJ, Battie MC, Fisher LD, et al. A prospective study of work perceptions and psychosocial factors affecting the report of back injury. *Spine.* 1991;16: 1-6.

Butler RJ, Johnson WG, Baldwin ML. Managing work disability: why first return to work is not a measure of success. *Ind Labor Rel Rev.* 1995;48: 452-69.

Butler RJ, Worrall JD. Gamma duration models with heterogenicity. *Rev Econ Stat.* 1991;73:161-6.

Butler RJ, Worrall JD. Work injury compensation and the duration of nonwork spells. *Econ J.* 1985;95:714-24.

Cats-Baril WL, Frymoyer JW. Identifying patients at risk of becoming disabled because of low back pain: the Vermont Rehabilitation Engineering Center predictive model. *Spine.* 1991;16:605-7.

Chaffin DB. Back disorders and nonneutral trunk postures of automobile assembly workers. *Scand J Work Environ Health.* 1991;17:337-64.

Cheadle A, Franklin G, Wolfhagen C, et al. Factors influencing the duration of work-related disability: a population based study of Washington workers' compensation. *Am J Public Health.* 1994;84:190-5.

Cornes P. The vocational rehabilitation index: a guide to accident victims' requirements for return to work assistance. *Int J Disabil Studies.* 1990;12: 32-6.

Depression Guideline Panel. *Depression in Primary Care: Volume 1, Detection and Diagnosis.* Clinical Practice Guideline No. 5. Rockville, Md: U.S. Department of Health and Human Services, Public Health Service, Agency for Health Care Policy and Research, AHCPR Pub No. 93-0550; 1993.

Deyo RA, Diehl AK. Predicting disability in patients with low back pain. *Clin Res.* 1986;34:814A.

Deyo RA, Diehl AK. Psychosocial predictors of disability in patients with low back pain. *J Rheumatol.* 1988;15:1557-64.

Deyo RA, Tsui-Wu Y-J. Functional disability due to low back pain. *Arthritis Rheum.* 1987;30:1247-53.

Dworkin RH, Handlin DS, Richlin DM, et al. Unraveling the effects of compensation, litigation and employment on treatment response in chronic pain. *Pain.* 1985;23(1):49-59.

Frymoyer JW, Cats-Baril W. Predictors of low back pain disability. *Clin Orthop Rel Res.* 1987;221:89-98.

Frymoyer JW, Pope MH, Clements JH, et al. Risk factors in low back pain. *J Bone Joint Surg.* 1983;65A:213-8.

Frymoyer JW, Rosen JC, Clements J, et al. Psychologic factors in low back disability. *Clin Orthop.* 1985;195:178-84.

Gallagher RM, Rauh V, Haugh LD, et al. Determinants of return-to-work among low back pain patients. *Pain.* 1989;39:53-69.

Goertz M. Prognostic indicators for acute low back pain. *Spine.* 1990;15:1307-10.

Greenough CG, Fraser RD. The effect of compensation on recovery from low back injury. *Spine.* 1989;14:947-55.

Haddad GH. Analysis of 2932 workers' compensation back injury cases: the impact of costs to the system. *Spine.* 1987;12:765-9.

Johnson WG. Work disincentives of benefits payments. In: Worrall JD, ed. *Safety and the Work Force: Incentives and Disincentives in Workers' Compensation Insurance.* Ithaca, NY: ILR Press; 1983:138-53.

Johnson WG, Baldwin M. Returns to work by Ontario workers with permanent partial disabilities. Report to the Workers' Compensation Board of Ontario; 1993.

Johnson WG, Baldwin ML, Burton JF Jr. Why is the treatment of work-related injuries so costly? New evidence from California Inquiry. 1996; 33(1):53-65.

Johnson WG, Butler RJ, Baldwin M. First spells of work absence among Ontario workers. In: Thomason T, Chaykowski RP, eds. *Research in Canadian Workers' Compensation.* Kingston, Ontario: IRC Press; 1995:72-84.

Johnson WG, Ondrich J. The duration of post-injury absence from work. *Rev Econ Stat.* 1990;72:578-86.

Kamerow DB, Pincus HA, MacDonald DI. Alcohol abuse, other drug abuse, and mental disorders in medical practice: prevalence, costs, recognition and treatment. *JAMA.* 1986;255:2054-7.

Kobasa S, Maddi S, Kahn S. Hardiness and health: a prospective study. *J Pers Soc Psychol.* 1982;42:168-77.

Lehmann TR, Spratt KF, Lehmann KK. Predicting long-term disability in low back injured workers presenting to a spine consultant. *Spine.* 1993;18: 1103-12.

Leigh JP. An empirical analysis of self-reported, work limiting disability. *Med Care.* 1985;310-9.

Loisel P, Abenhaim P, Durand JM, et al. A population-based, randomized clinical trial on back pain management. *Spine.* 1997;22(24):2911-8.

Maeland JG, Havik OE. Psychological predictors for return to work after a myocardial infarction. *J Psychosom Res.* 1987;471-81.

MacKenzie EJ, Shapiro S, Smith RT, et al. Factors influencing return to work following hospitalization for traumatic injury. *Am J Public Health.* 1987;77:329-34.

Nagi S. Disability concepts revisited. In: Pope AM, Tarlov AR, eds. *Disability in America: Towards a National Agenda for Prevention.* Washington, DC: National Academy Press; 1991.

Pederson PA. Prognostic indicators in low back pain. *J R Coll Gen Pract.* 1981;209-16.

Pulvertaft RG. Psychological aspects of hand injuries. *Hand.* 1975;7:93-103.

Rossignol M, Suissa S, Abenhaim I. Working disability due to occupational back pain: three-year follow up of 2,300 compensated workers in Quebec. *J Occ Med.* 1988;30:502-5.

Rossignol M, Abenhaim L, Seguin P, et al. Coordination of primary health care for back pain. A randomized controlled trial. *Spine.* 2000;25(2):251-8.

Rost K, Burnam MA, Sith GR. Development of screeners for depressive disorder and substance disorder history. *Med Care.* 1993;31:189-200.

Ruser JW. Workers' compensation and occupational illnesses and injuries. *J Labor Econ.* 1987;325-50.

Sander RA, Meyers JE. The relationship of disability to compensation status in railroad injuries. *Spine.* 1986;11:141-3.

Scheer SJ, Radack KL, O'Brien DR Jr. Randomized controlled trials in industrial low back pain relating to return to work. Part 1. Acute interventions. *Arch Phys Med Rehabil.* 1995;76(10):966-73.

Scheer SJ, Radack KL, O'Brien DR Jr. Randomized controlled trials in industrial low back pain relating to return to work. Part 2. Discogenic low back pain. *Arch Phys Med Rehabil.* 1996;77(11):1189-97.

Scheer SJ, Watanabe TK, Radack KL. Randomized controlled trials in industrial low back pain. Part 3. Subacute/chronic pain interventions. *Arch Phys Med Rehabil.* 1997;78(4):414-23.

Sinclair SJ, Hogg-Johnson SA, Mondloch MV, Shields SA. The effectiveness of an early intervention for workers with soft tissue injuries: the Early Claimant Cohort Study. *Spine.* 1997;22:2919-31.

Smith SR, O'Rourke DF. Return to work after a first myocardial infarction: a test of multiple hypotheses. *JAMA.* 1988;259:1673-7.

Stansfeld SA, Fuhrer R, Head J, Ferrie J, Shipley M. Work and psychiatric disorder in the Whitehall II study. *J Psychosom Res.* 1997;43:73-81.

Stutts JT, Kasdan ML. Disability: a new psychosocial perspective. *J Occup Med.* 1993;825-7.

Tate RB, Yassi A, Cooper J. Predictors of time loss after back injury in nurses. *Spine.* 1999;24(18):1930-5.

Taylor VM, Deyo RA, Ciol M, et al. Patient-oriented outcomes from low back surgery: a community-based study. *Spine.* 2000;25:2445-52.

Theorell T, Harms-Ringdahl K, Ahlberg-Hulten G, et al. Psychosocial job factors and symptoms from the locomotor system: a multicausal analysis. *Scand J Rehab Med.* 1991;23:165-73.

Troup JDG, Martin JD, Lloyd DCEF. Back pain in industry: a prospective study. *Spine.* 1981;6:61-9.

Troup JDG, Foreman TK, Baxter CE, et al. The perception of back pain and the role of psychophysical tests of lifting capacity. *Spine.* 1987;12:645-57.

Tulkin S. Emotional and Behavioral Components of Disability: Focus on Chemical Dependency and Developing an Action Plan. Presented at the 6th Kaiser Permanente Interregional Conference on Primary Care and Musculoskeletal Medicine, Kauai, Hawaii; April 1996.

Tulkin S. Clinical Skills and Attitudes Needed to Recognize and Respond to Somatization. Presented at the 6th Kaiser Permanente Interregional Conference on Primary Care and Musculoskeletal Medicine, Kauai, Hawaii; April 1996.

Vallfors B. Acute, subacute and chronic low back pain: clinical symptoms, absenteeism and working environment. *Scand J Rehabil Med.* 1985; 11(Suppl):1-98.

van Tulder MW, Koes BW, Bouter LM. Conservative treatment of acute and chronic nonspecific low back pain. A systematic review of randomized controlled trials of the most common interventions. *Spine.* 1997;22(18): 2128-56.

Vasudevan SV. Clinical perspectives on the relationship between pain and disability. *Neurol Clin.* 1989;7:429-39.

Volinn E, Van Koevering D, Loeser JD. Back sprain in industry: the role of socioeconomic factors in chronicity. *Spine.* 1991;16:542-8.

Waddell G, Feder G, Lewis M. Systematic reviews of bed rest and advice to stay active for acute low back pain. *Br J Gen Pract.* 1997;47(423):647-52.

Wells KB, Stewart A, Hays RD, et al. The functioning and well being of depressed patients: results from the medical outcomes study. *JAMA.* 1989; 262:914-9.

MANAGEMENT

Abenhaim L, Rossignol M, Valat JP, et al. The role of activity in the therapeutic management of back pain. Report of the International Paris Task Force on Back Pain. *Spine.* 2000;25(4 Suppl):1S-33S.

Abenhaim L, Rossignol M, Gobielle D, Bonvalot Y, Fines P, Scot S. The prognostic consequences in the making of the initial medical diagnosis of work-related back injuries. *Spine.* 1995;20:791-5.

Baldwin ML, Johnson WG, Butler RJ. The error of using returns-to-work to measure the outcomes of health care. *Am J Ind Med.* 1996;29:632-41.

Bandura A. Self-efficacy mechanism in psychological activation and health-promoting behavior. In: Madden J, ed. *Neurobiology of Learning, Emotion and Affect.* New York, NY: Raven Press; 1991.

Battie M. Minimizing the impact of back pain: work place strategies. *Semin Spine Surg.* 1992;4:20-8.

Bernacki EJ, Guidera JA, Schaefer JA, Tsai S. A facilitated early return to work program at a large urban medical center. *J Occup Environ Med.* 2000;42(12):1172-7.

Bernacki EJ, Guidera JA. The effect of managed care on surgical rates among individuals filing for workers' compensation. *J Occup Environ Med.* 1998; 40(7):623-31.

Bernacki EJ, Tsai SP. Managed care for workers' compensation: three years of experience in an "employee choice" state. *J Occup Environ Med.* 1996;38(11):1091-7.

Bigos S, Bowyer O, Braen G, et al. *Acute Low Back Problems in Adults: Clinical Practice Guideline No. 14.* AHCPR Publication 95-0642. Rockville, Md: AHCPR, PHS, USDHHS; 1994.

Boseman J. Disability management. Application of a nurse based model in a large corporation. *AAOHN J.* 2001;49(4):176-86.

Brain GF, Conlon MF. The case management approach to work-related injuries. *Orthop Clin North Am.* 1996;27(4):831-40.

Brines J, Salazar MK, Graham KY, Pergola T, Connon C. Injured workers' perceptions of case management services. A descriptive study. *AAOHN J.* 1999;47(8):355-64.

Brines J, Salazar MK, Graham KY, Pergola T. Return to work experience of injured workers in a case management program. *AAOHN J.* 1999;47(8): 365-72.

Brody DS, Thompson TL II, Larson DB, et al. Strategies for counseling depressed patients by primary care physicians. *J Gen Intern Med.* 1994;9: 569-75.

Brooker A-S, Smith JM, Cole DC, Hogg-Johnson SA. *Workplace Arrangements to Return Injured Workers to Work: Evidence from a Prospective Cohort of Workers with Soft Tissue Injuries.* Toronto, Ontario: Institute for Work and Health; 1998.

Brooker A-S, Frank JW, Tarasuk VS. Effective disability management and return to work practices. In Sullivan T, ed. *Injury and the New World of Work.* Vancouver, BC: University of British Columbia Press; 2000.

Buchsbaum DG, Buchannan RG, Centor RM, et al. Screening for alcohol abuse using CAGE scores and likelihood ratios. *Ann Intern Med.* 1991; 115:774-7.

Burton WN, Conti DJ. Disability management: corporate medical department management of employee health and productivity. *J Occup Environ Med.* 2000;42(10):1006-12.

Butler RJ, Johnson WG, Baldwin ML. Managing work disability: why first return to work is not a measure of success. *Ind Labor Rel Rev.* 1995;48: 452-69.

Caudill M, Schnable R, Zuttermeister P, Benson H, Friedman R. Decreased clinic use by chronic pain patients: response to behavioral medicine interventions. *Clin J Pain.* 1991;7:305-10.

Christian, J. "Talking About Ability to Work": a continuing medical education course for physicians. Webility Corporation, 2003. Wayland, Ma. (Acknowledgement: Some of the material in sections of this chapter has been adapted and reprinted with permission from Webility Corporation.)

Council of Musculoskeletal Specialty Societies. *Disabilities of the Arm, Shoulder and Hand Outcomes Data Collection Package.* Rosemont, Ill: American Academy of Orthopaedic Surgeons; 1996.

Council of Musculoskeletal Specialty Societies. *Disabilities of the Spine Outcomes Data Collection Package.* Rosemont, Ill: American Academy of Orthopaedic Surgeons; 1996.

Council of Musculoskeletal Specialty Societies. *Disabilities of the Lower Limb Outcomes Data Collection Package.* Rosemont, Ill: American Academy of Orthopaedic Surgeons; 1996.

Depression Guideline Panel. *Depression in Primary Care: Volume 2, Treatment of Major Depression.* Clinical Practice Guideline No. 5. Rockville, Md: US Department of Health and Human Services, Public Health Service, Agency for Health Care Policy and Research, AHCPR Pub. No. 93-0551; 1993.

Devine EC. Effects of psychoeducational care for adult surgical patients: a meta-analysis of 191 studies. *Pat Ed Couns.* 1992;19:129-42.

Feuerstein M, Burrell LM, Miller VI, Lincoln A, Huang GD, Berger R. Clinical management of carpal tunnel syndrome: a 12-year review of outcomes. *Am J Ind Med.* 1999;35(3):232-45.

Feurstein M. A multidisciplinary approach to the prevention, evaluation, and management of work disability. *J Occup Rehab.* 1991;1:5-12.

Friedman R, Sobel D, Myer P, et al. Behavioral medicine, clinical health psychology and cost offset. *Health Psychol.* 1995;14:509-18.

Gillette RD. Behavioral factors in the management of back pain. *Am Fam Physician.* 1996;53:1313-8.

Green-McKenzie J, Rainer S, Behrman A, Emmett E. The effect of a health care management initiative on reducing workers' compensation costs. *J Occup Environ Med.* 2002;44(12):1100-5.

Hasenbring M, Marienfeld G, Kuhlendahl D, et al. Risk factors of chronicity in lumbar disc patients: a prospective investigation of biologic, psychologic, and social predictors of therapy outcome. *Spine.* 1994;19:2759-65.

Helman CJC, Budd M, Borysenko J, et al. A study of the effectiveness of two group behavioral medicine interventions for patients with psychosomatic complaints. *Behav Med.* 1990;16:165-73.

Kalina CM. Strategies in disability management. Corporate disability management programs implemented at the work site. *Ann N Y Acad Sci.* 1999; 888:343-55.

Kalina CM. Linking resources to process in disability management. Successful program. *AAOHN J.* 1998;46(8):385-90.

Kaplan S, Greenfield S, Ware JE. Assessing the effects of physician-patient interactions on the outcomes of chronic disease. *Med Care.* 1989;27:S110-27.

Karjalainen K, Malmivaara A, van Tulder M, Roine R, Jauhiainen M, Hurri H, Koes B. Multidisciplinary rehabilitation for fibromyalgia and musculoskeletal pain in working age adults. *Cochrane Database Syst Rev.* 2000;(2): CD001984.

Klaber-Moffett JA, Chase SM, Portek BS, et al. A controlled, prospective study to evaluate the effectiveness of a back school in the relief of chronic low back pain. *Spine.* 1986;11:120-2.

Klapow JC, Slater MA, Patterson TL, et al. An empirical evaluation of multidimensional clinical outcome in chronic low back pain patients. *Pain.* 1993;55:107-18.

Lanes TC, Gauron EF, Spratt KF, et al. Long-term follow up of patients with chronic back pain treated in a multidisciplinary rehabilitation program. *Spine.* 1995;20:801-6.

Lincoln AE, Feuerstein M, Shaw WS, Miller VI. Impact of case manager training on worksite accommodations in workers' compensation claimants with upper extremity disorders. *J Occup Environ Med.* 2002;44(3):237-45.

Loisel P, Durand P, Abenhaim I, et al. Management of occupational back pain: the Sherbrooke model. Results of a pilot and feasibility study. *Occ Environ Med.* 1994;51:597-602.

Lorig K, Holman H, Sobel D, et al. *Living a Healthy Life with Chronic Conditions.* Palo Alto, Calif: Bull Publishing; 1994.

Mahmud MA, Webster BS, Courtney TK, Matz S, Tacci JA, Christiani DC. Clinical management and the duration of disability for work-related low back pain. *J Occup Envir Med.* 2000;42(12):1178-87.

Malmivaara A, Hakkinen U, Aro T, et al. The treatment of acute low back pain: bed rest, exercises, or ordinary activity. *N Engl J Med.* 1995;332(6):351-5.

Marras WS, Lavender SA, Leurgans SE, et al. The role of dynamic three-dimensional trunk motion in occupationally related low back disorders: the effects of workplace factors, trunk position, and trunk characteristics on risk of injury. *Spine.* 1993;18:617-28.

Marshall M, Gray A, Lockwood A, Green R. Case management for people with severe mental disorders. *Cochrane Database Syst Rev.* 2000;(2): CD000050.

McGill CM. Industrial back problems: a control program. *J Occup Med.* 1968;10:174-8.

McGrail MP Jr, Tsai SP, Bernacki EJ. A comprehensive initiative to manage the incidence and cost of occupational injury and illness. Report of an outcomes analysis. *J Occup Environ Med.* 1995;37(11):1263-8.

Mobley EM, Linz DH, Shukla R, Breslin RE, Deng C. Disability case management: an impact assessment in an automotive manufacturing organization. *J Occup Environ Med.* 2000;42(6):597-602.

Mumford E, Schlessinger HJ, Glass G, et al. A new look at evidence about reduced cost of medical utilization following mental health treatment. *Am J Psychiatry.* 1984;141:1145-58.

Paulsen JS, Altmaier EM. The effects of perceived versus enacted social support on the discriminative cue function of spouses for pain behaviors. *Pain.* 1995;60:103-10.

Shaw WS, Feuerstein M, Lincoln AE, Miller VI, Wood PM. Case management services for work related upper extremity disorders. Integrating workplace accommodation and problem solving. *AAOHN J.* 2001;49(8):378-89.

Shrey DE. Disability management in industry: the new paradigm in injured worker rehabilitation. *Disabil Rehabil.* 1996;18(8):408-14.

Sobel D. Rethinking medicine: improving health outcomes with cost-effective psychosocial interventions. *Psychosom Med.* 1995;57:234-44.

Straaton KV, Maisiak R, Wrigley JM, Fine PR. Musculoskeletal disability, employment, and rehabilitation. *J Rheumatol.* 1995;22(3):505-13.

Stutzman LJ. Medical Management—How do they manage that? Evidence-based return-to-work guidelines. CWCE Magazine. August 2001:36.

Tacci JA, Webster BS, Hashemi L, Christiani DC. Clinical practices in the management of new onset, uncomplicated, low back workers' compensation disability claims. *J Occup Envir Med.* 1999;41(5):397-404.

Talo S, Puukka P, Rytokoski U. Can treatment outcome of chronic low back pain be predicted? Psychological disease consequences clarifying the issue. *Clin J Pain.* 1994;10:107-21.

Tota-Faucette ME, Gil KM, Williams DA, et al. Predictors of response to pain management treatment: the role of family environment and changes in cognitive processes. *Clin J Pain.* 1993;9:115-23.

Trief PM, Carnrike CL Jr, Drudge O. Chronic pain and depression: is social support relevant? *Psychol Rep.* 1995;76:227-36.

Wassel ML, Wachs JE. Improving return to work outcomes. *AAOHN J.* 2002;50(6):275-85.

Wickizer TM, Franklin G, Plaeger-Brockway R, Mootz RD. Improving the quality of workers' compensation health care delivery: the Washington State Occupational Health Services Project. *Milbank Q.* 2001;79(1):5-33.

Workplace Safety and Insurance Board. *Injury/Illness and Return to Work/Function: A Practical Guide for Physicians.* Toronto, Ontario: WSIB; 2000. www.wsib/on.ca/wsib/wsibsite.nsf/Public/HealthPhysiciansGuideRTW.

Wright ME. Long-term sickness absence in an NHS teaching hospital. *Occup Med.* 1997;47:401-6.

Zigenfus GC, Yin J, Giang GM, Fogarty WT. Effectiveness of early physical therapy in the treatment of acute low back musculoskeletal disorders. *J Occup Environ Med.* 2000;42(1):35-9.

6 Pain, Suffering, and the Restoration of Function

Pain is a symptom rather than a disease. It can be a valuable, albeit unpleasant, guide to diagnosing and resolving illness or injury. It also can be a troubling problem that interferes with function at work and at home. Pain perception occurs in the context of each person's life situation, affecting work, interpersonal, and social functioning, as well as the ability or willingness to be active; inactivity can in turn aggravate pain.

It is important for the physician to assess pain in relation to objective findings, to understand each worker's reaction to pain, and to manage pain as work-related health problems progress over time. Early recognition and effective management of pain that is out of proportion to physical damage is a critical skill in preventing excessive dysfunction, suffering, and cost. Many of the longest, most frustrating, and most expensive workers' compensation cases involve complaints of persistent pain.

Understanding pain today takes physicians beyond the classic medical model. Though incompletely understood, the perception and response to pain may have a significant genetic component. Used in all medical training, the classic model is based on correlating specific tissue pathology with distinctive symptoms. In this model, acute injury causes pain as the result of tissue damage. As such, it can be a guide to the location and severity of work-related injury. The situation becomes more difficult to assess and treat when there is no specific injury or after the acute lesion should have healed. Pain symptoms in those situations have often become dissociated from physical injury.

Until recently, physicians considered pain without evidence of tissue damage to be primarily a psychological disorder. During the last ten to twenty years, research has revealed that central nervous system factors may account for pain sensations despite the absence of tissue damage or after healing has taken place.

Pain, whether acute or chronic, is the most prevalent health condition in the U.S. workforce and the most costly in terms of lost productive work time. Pain from common conditions such as headaches and backache costs U.S. employers about $80 billion a year in lost productivity. The bulk of the loss, about $64 billion, is largely invisible to employers because it occurs when workers are on the job but in too much pain to perform up to job standards, not when they take sick days.

Pain in today's workplace presents a challenge to the occupational physician. Although mistreating or undertreating pain is of concern, an even greater risk for the physician is overtreating the chronic pain patient, especially with opioids and other medication. Overtreatment often results in irreparable harm to the patient's socioeconomic status, home life, personal relationships, and quality of life in general. However, because opioids are "easy" and represent a path of little resistance, they may prevent the patient, the physician, or both from vesting in a difficult and uncomfortable rehabilitation course. A physician's choice to palliate and not rehabilitate is a profound clinical, ethical, and medico-economic decision not be taken lightly or be based on unfounded dogma. A patient's complaints of pain should be acknowledged. Patient and clinician should remain focused on the ultimate goal of rehabilitation leading to optimal functional recovery, decreased healthcare utilization, and maximal self-actualization. Early identification and appropriate management of the patient exhibiting signs of delayed recovery (see Chapter 5) may decrease the likelihood that he or she will go on to develop chronic pain.

This chapter focuses primarily on chronic pain. Acute pain is addressed within specific body part chapters, and readers should refer to the appropriate chapters for more detailed recommendations on managing body-part specific pain due to injury or trauma. Evidence that factors other than the nature of the injury are primary determinants of disability clearly suggests that treating pain, even acute pain, should emphasize functional restoration rather than relief of pain because the latter may reinforce psychological, environmental, and psychosocial factors that predispose progression to chronic pain states.

Pain that is disproportionate to the physical findings raises many questions: When does acute pain become chronic? Is the diagnosis incorrect? Is there a second diagnosis? What else is going on in the patient's life, either at home or at work, which may be aggravating his or her feelings of pain? How can nonphysiological pain be articulated to a system that is based on labels and coding? How can that concept of pain be put into a medicolegal context when dealing with workers' compensation issues? Does the current treatment improve function? What role should patients play in promoting optimal function in everyday living and enabling meaningful family, workplace, and social relationships?

The following discussion sheds light on these questions and suggests an interdisciplinary model to address the multiple components of the patient's pain experience.

Pain Perception

Pain cannot be measured objectively. Its central nervous system and psychological dimensions go beyond the sensory examination. Pain is a complex phenomenon that has been described as an experience rather than a sensation. The experience, and the way each patient manifests it, is the product of cultural factors; previous personal, family, and social experiences with injury and pain; the patient's general stress and anxiety level; family and social roles and support; expectations for recovery, income, and financial support; and character structure and coping methods. The clinician should inquire about these issues in a neutral and supportive way to understand each patient's pain presentation and the relationship of that presentation to the objective findings for that patient as well as the natural history of the probable pathologic entity underlying the presenting complaint.

The Seattle model hypothesizes several levels or dimensions to pain. The first level is at the cellular-chemical level and includes tissue damage, inflammation, and nociception (the afferent transmission of impulses from small, thin fibers located throughout the body in peripheral nerves, which register trauma to nearby tissue). The second level is the nervous system transmission and perception (burning, aching, needles, etc.). The third level is the response-reaction including fear, anger, and frustration with a possible affective component such as depression or suffering. The fourth level is the psycho-socio-behavioral dimension with components such as somatization, learned illness behaviors, secondary gain, malingering, and personality disorders. To understand and manage pain the physician must be aware of these dimensions and the role that each plays in how pain is perceived, recognizing that some components may be present and others noncontributory, depending on the patient. Pain is subjective, and clinicians have no objective way of determining how much pain a patient is experiencing.

Successful pain management hinges on appreciating the dynamics of each patient's case and on proactively managing factors that might delay return to work or restoration of function. The immediate focus should be on functional improvement rather than on abolishing pain. Physicians also should be aware that while complete cessation of pain may not be a realistic goal for some patients, self-care, functional restoration, and successful reintegration into the workforce can be attainable goals even though the complete elimination of pain may not be possible.

Acute Versus Chronic Pain

Although the focus of this chapter is the management of chronic pain, a brief discussion of acute versus chronic pain may be useful as the basis for managing delayed recovery and preventing chronic pain in patients with an acute complaint.

Acute musculoskeletal pain is often a signal of real or impending tissue damage. Acute pain may generate sympathetic responses such as anxiety, tachycardia, and elevated blood pressure as well as somatic and neuroendocrine responses. Acute pain generally fluctuates in intensity and with exacerbating events. It generally disappears with healing. However, it is also a psychological experience that is interpreted in the context of the patient's experiences, environment, and cultural background. Thus, no two patients experience pain in exactly the same way. In the patient with acute pain, removing the physical cause of the pain eliminates the psychological reactions as well as the noxious nociceptive input.

The distinction between acute and chronic pain is somewhat arbitrary. Chronicity may be reached from one to six months postinjury. The International Association for the Study of Pain has stated that three months is the definitional time frame, while the American Psychiatric Association uses a six-month limit. The most clinically useful definition might be that "chronic pain persists beyond the usual course of healing of an acute disease or beyond a reasonable time for an injury to heal."

The central nervous system may be altered by chronic pain. Changes may occur that make people more sensitive to incoming impulses, which amplify the pain. This is thought to occur at the level of the spinal cord and brain. Chronic pain is typically accompanied by few autonomic responses. Patients with chronic pain are often preoccupied with somatic symptoms, sleep, appetite and libido disturbances, and disruption in interpersonal relationships.

In patients with chronic pain, psychological reactions to the pain become the major contributors to impaired functioning. These include anxiety, helplessness, escape/avoidance behaviors, depression, and increased pain behaviors. The perpetuation of pain thus has emotional, behavioral, and physiologic components. Before pain becomes chronic, there is an important therapeutic window for preventing chronic, centrally mediated pain. During this period, patients present with some or all of the chronic pain characteristics, but their pain is still related to tissue damage. It is well localized, rather than poorly localized, and is not yet compounded by the motivational, affective, cognitive, and behavioral overlay that is often a frustrating aspect of chronic pain. Dysfunctional movements and patterns such as antalgic gait, abnormal postures, or guarding may contribute to the chronicity of pain. If these movement patterns are normalized, symptoms may be reduced and function increased. Normalization may be achieved through a combination of physical methods and workstation or task redesign (see Chapter 1, "Foundations of Occupational Medicine Practice").

The key, then, is to promptly recognize this transitional period (when the patient begins to deviate from the expected recovery trajectory for his or her complaint, illness, or injury) and to institute pain management techniques or make a timely referral if these techniques are not part of the physician's personal armamentarium. Typically, the chronic pain patient cannot be treated by the interventions that are appropriate for acute pain.

Barriers to Optimizing the Management of Pain

Physicians should endeavor to maintain a supportive, nonjudgmental approach to the patient with chronic pain.

Patients who embellish a medical or work history, exaggerate pain drawings, or respond to physical examination in a way that is inconsistent with known physiology can be particularly challenging. Patients may exhibit inconsistencies such as a greater range of motion when distracted than when asked to perform that specific part of the exam. Verbal or nonverbal communication of distress or suffering, such as amplified grimacing, distorted gait or posture, exaggerated reaction to passive or active motion, and moaning or rubbing the affected area, may make it difficult to determine the extent of physical pathology or physiologic dysfunction or may otherwise cloud medical issues.

Physicians may find themselves becoming angry with such patients. Anger is not constructive in this context, nor is interpreting inconsistencies, pain behaviors, or passivity as malingering, manipulation, or purely as a personality issue. Such reactions or labeling do not benefit the patient or the physician. It is more useful to view such behavior as the patient's attempt to enlist the physician as an advocate, or as a plea for help. The patient could view him- or herself as trapped in a job whose activity requirements do not match his or her age, physical condition, or health. In many cases, compensation insurance payment or legal actions could be at issue. Many patients simply do not view themselves as capable of assisting in their own recovery, either because of a skill deficit or a belief that someone else is responsible for their health.

Patients with recurring musculoskeletal problems, inconsistencies, and amplifications may have been reinforced by clinicians' responses to their complaints during previous medical interactions. It is important to objectively identify any psychosocial factors, work-related issues, or legal matters involved. These should be dealt with in a positive, overt, cooperative manner to facilitate recovery and minimize the chance of physical debilitation and chronic or long-term disability.

The treatment of chronic pain requires specialized knowledge, substantial time, and access to multidisciplinary care. Judicious involvement of other professionals, including psychologists, exercise and physical therapists, and other healthcare professionals who can offer extra physical or mental therapy while the physician continues to orchestrate the whole therapeutic process can be helpful. Close communication between all participating professionals is mandatory.

Types of Patients and Specific Pain Syndromes

Pain disorder is diagnosed when pain is the predominant focus of the patient's complaint, and causes significant distress and impairment in social, occupational, or other important areas of functioning. Psychological factors must play a significant role. Pain disorders associated with a general medical condition are identified with the codes for the condition or anatomic area. Pain symptoms also may be manifestations of other mental disorders, e.g., depressive, anxiety, psychotic, or personality disorders. Other pain-related disorders include conversion disorder, somatization disorder, and factitious disorder.

The Minnesota Multiphasic Personality Inventory (MMPI) results, coping style, and locus of control concepts all may be predictive of chronic pain development and treatment outcome. The way in which the physician manages the patient with evidence of delayed recovery can materially affect the degree to which progression to a chronic pain syndrome will occur. Once the patient is exhibiting evidence of chronic pain, a systematic, thorough approach to patient evaluation will provide information that can assist in managing it.

A. The History in Delayed Recovery Associated with Chronic Pain

In cases of delayed recovery associated with chronic pain, the physician should ask the patient to describe the pain and its location, the intensity or severity, aggravating and relieving factors, the patient's cognitive response to pain, and his or her goals for pain control. The primary treating physician, ancillary health care personnel, and consultants should approach pain complaints as an integral element of each history and physical examination. Pain should be compared to an appropriately focused physical examination and not be evaluated by interview and pain scales alone. Each physician should:

- Determine specifically how pain is limiting physical, work, and social activity
  - What factors increase pain symptoms at work? At home?
  - How is the worker specifically limited at work? At home?
- Assess the injured worker's reaction to injury and expression of symptoms at the first and subsequent visits
  - Is there abnormal guarding of the area in question?
  - Is the worker upset or concerned out of proportion to the signs of injury or illness?
  - What is the expression of and meaning of pain to the worker in his or her cultural context?
  - What therapeutically relevant information do pain-assessment tools and scales (which should be used judiciously) provide?
- Assess the worker's coping and problem-solving skills at home and at work
  - Does the worker feel in control of most situations?
  - Can the worker obtain needed support and objectives?
  - Does the worker experience pain or other symptoms in response to stressful situations or ideas?
- Understand the context of the work-related health complaint
  - How is life at home?
  - Are there problems at work?
  - Is the worker encountering problems with the ergonomics of the job or workstation?
    - Describe work times, movement and breaks for sedentary jobs
    - Describe tasks, workstation structure, load, repetitions, etc. compared to the worker's height, habitus, etc.
- Ask about the worker's preinjury physical condition and briefly assess it on examination

- What was the worker's aerobic capacity, strength, body mass, and general flexibility?
- Determine the preinjury amount and frequency of use of pain-mitigating or psychoactive substances
  - Over-the-counter pain medications
  - Prescription pain medications
  - Alcohol
  - Tobacco
  - Other psychoactive drugs
- Identify any factors that would affect the worker's pain threshold and increase or decrease expressions of pain (see also Chapter 5, "Cornerstones of Disability Prevention and Management") including:
  - Who is responsible for the worker's health (health locus of control)?
  - Who is responsible for the health problem?
  - Is the employer concerned?
  - Has the worker's home role changed as a result of pain?
- Discuss any prior or similar health problems and the worker's functional recovery
  - Was recovery delayed?
  - Was pain a significant element in delayed recovery?
  - How was it managed?
  - Was functional recovery complete?
- Treat pain from physical injury quickly and appropriately by agreement with the injured worker
- Provide positive support but be realistic about functional recovery
  - Explain the relevant anatomy and possible pain sources (or lack thereof)
  - Explain ways to manage pain and dysfunction and their relative effectiveness
    - Immobilization
    - Resumption of activity
    - Medication
    - Physical modalities
- Prescribe rapid but careful resumption of function
  - Active mobilization of injured areas
  - Progressively increasing transitional work
- Recognize and describe symptoms that are greater than objective findings at every visit
- Assess the effects of treatment
  - Are symptoms decreasing appropriately over time?
  - Are the symptoms unresponsive to nonsteroidal anti-inflammatory drugs (NSAIDs) or opiate analogs such as hydrocodone?
  - Are the symptoms unresponsive to centrally acting muscle relaxants?
  - Are symptoms unresponsive to injections of generally proven efficacy?

- Follow the injured worker's functional recovery trajectory closely
- Consider referral

Physicians should consider referral for further evaluation and perhaps cooperative treatment if:

- Specific clinical findings suggest undetected clinical pathology.
- Pain distribution is nonanatomic or described in a bizarre or atypical manner.
  - Some examples include glove- or stocking-like pain or paresthesias, shock-like pain, pain that radiates up and down the neck and back, burning pain, and pain that is present constantly regardless of position, medication use, or physical treatments.
- Medication use does not decrease as expected, or increases.
- Appropriate active physical therapy does not appear to be improving function as expected.
- Complaints of pain or dysfunction start to involve other areas of the body, including instances in which the patient:
  - Ceases to discuss returning to work in a specific time frame but rather in relation to a "cure."
  - Fails to benefit from any, or all, rational therapeutic interventions.
  - Experiences increased pain, or at the very least, pain does not decrease, over time.
  - Is unwilling to discuss his or her family situation or expresses comfort with role reversal at home.
  - States that the illness or injury has caused all of his or her problems.
  - Directs excessive anger at the employer or coworkers, the physician, or an insurer and/or demonstrates an attitude of revenge or wanting to prove that he or she is sick.
  - Is less interested in the home therapy program or even in recovery of function.

Judicious referral also is warranted to corroborate the absence of physical pathology, which can be the basis of assurances to the patient that increased participation in usual activities will not be detrimental to his or her overall physical status.

B. Psychosocial and Behavioral Components of Pain

Pain may:

- Trigger anxiety, fear, crisis reactions, and stress
- Impact spirituality, meaningfulness, and hope
- Effect perceptions of control and self-efficacy

- Cause depression, a wish to die, suicidal risks
- Impact habits, roles, occupational performance, and future quality of life

One of the most significant outcomes of research into the psychosocial factors and pain are fear-avoidance models. The theoretical model is based on the premise that pain-related fear (beliefs that pain is a sign of damage or harm to the body, and activities that might cause pain should be avoided) is increasingly being recognized as an important contributor to disability and adjustment among persons with chronic pain.

Pain-related fear is believed to contribute to pain and disability in several ways. First, avoidance of pain is natural, given that it is aversive. However, persons who are high in pain-related fear tend to avoid a greater number of situations that they believe may cause pain. Research also suggests that these persons tend to overestimate the amount of pain experienced during functional activity, leading to greater activity avoidance. In this fashion, pain-related fear and associated avoidance of activity are believed to contribute to disability independent of pain itself. Pain-related fear and avoidance have also been proposed to lead to greater physical deconditioning, which in turn heightens disability. In addition, pain-related fear has been shown to be related to musculoskeletal abnormalities such as muscle guarding while bending, which in turn may directly contribute to the pain experience.

Several studies support the notion that pain-related fear is significantly related to greater perceived disability, even when controlling for biomedical factors, demographic variables, and self-reported pain.

Exposing patients to activities they fear as a way to reduce their pain-related fear can be a powerful intervention for chronic pain. A decline in pain-related fear may reduce pain vigilance, resulting in a decline in reported pain intensity.

Studies suggest that reduction in pain-related fear may be partially responsible for improvement in functional restoration treatment because the duration of many treatment programs is too short to attribute improvement to the physiological effects of exercise.

C. Physician Guidelines for Dealing with Potentially Chronic or Chronic Injuries

In general, intervention for treating pain should be time-limited and goal-oriented. Persons returning to work in six months or less after injury tend to have the best outcomes. Persons who have been out of work for a year or more tend to have poor return-to-work outcomes. Early detection of potential chronicity also may be an important step in defining early treatment approaches to treating pain or disability because early intervention may increase successful return to work. Clinicians may use several published tools to examine the potential of developing a chronic pain problem (see "Pain Assessment Models and Tools," at the end of this chapter). Properly interpreted, such tools may help identify persons who need more than just interventional pain care and are unlikely to respond to simple pain-treatment approaches.

Research suggests that multidisciplinary care is beneficial for most persons with chronic pain, and likely should be considered the treatment of choice for persons who are at risk for, or who have, chronic pain and disability. Flor et al. (1992) conducted a meta-analytic review of multidisciplinary pain treatment for chronic back pain, which concluded that chronic pain patients treated in multidisciplinary programs were functioning better than 75% of control patients who either received no treatment or who were treated by conventional unimodal approaches.

Multidisciplinary treatment was found to be superior to conventional physical therapy alone, had benefits that persisted over time, and was beneficial in improving return to work and decreasing use of health care. While the components and approaches of multidisciplinary care often differ, the hallmarks of such programs include:

- Thorough, multidisciplinary assessment of the patient
- The establishment of a time-limited treatment plan with clear functional goals
- Frequent assessment of the patient's progress toward meeting such goals
- Modification of the treatment plan as appropriate, based on the patient's progress

Typically, such programs involve ongoing medical care or supervision, exercise or specific physical therapy intervention, psychosocial intervention, and occupational therapy or other services related to daily functioning and/or vocational rehabilitation. Specific multidisciplinary approaches, such as functional restoration, report return-to-work rates of more than 80% following treatment, with a high percentage of these persons still working after one year. Because not all chronic pain patients may need intensive multidisciplinary interventions, some programs offer comprehensive multidisciplinary evaluations resulting in specific treatment recommendations for the patient.

Principles of Pain Management

As noted previously, the physician should acknowledge the patient's pain. Pain should be considered an experience, not a sensation, an injury, or a disease. Exaggerated pain behaviors may indicate that the patient's psychological state is modifying pain expression.

The physician should indicate acceptance of the patient's expression of pain within the patient's own context. Trivializing or minimizing expressions of pain typically cause pain behaviors to increase rather than decrease because the patient attempts to convince the physician that the symptoms are serious. Pain expression is often a cry for help. Open, neutral, dispassionate communication best serves both patient and physician in these cases.

The physician should discuss the physical and psychological mechanisms of pain at each patient encounter using the questions described previously. The physician should view the psychological dimensions of pain as just as real as the physical dimensions to avoid stigmatizing the patient with the psychological aspect of pain. The physician should explore the meaning and significance of pain to each patient as a foundation for the therapeutic plan.

Physicians should discuss expectations for recovery at the initial encounter with the patient. Recovery expectations have a significant effect on the duration, intensity, and problems associated with pain. Time necessary for recovery, durations of probable need for medication, and reassurances that renewals probably will not be needed result in more rapid and complete return to function.

Preventing and Managing Chronic Pain

Acute pain should be relieved promptly and effectively to prevent development of abnormal, self-perpetuating pain reflexes. The goals of pain management are to normalize sympathetic arousal and change pain perception. Pharmacologic agents may be used in doses that are adequate to relieve symptoms, but that do not exceed the patient's needs. Drugs or immobilization that prevents appropriate physical activity can hamper recovery. Prolonged use of narcotic medications may cause both physiologic and psychological addiction and may reduce the body's supply of endorphins, causing depression and delayed recovery.

Mobilization, even in the face of some residual pain or stiffness, should be encouraged, and it should be increased as the healing process progresses. A recent study by Indahl et al. (1995) illustrates the point that activity prescription among persons with low back pain can be beneficial. The authors randomly assigned persons with an eight-week history of back pain to a group that received conservative medical treatment, or to a group to which light, normal activity, including bending, was prescribed. Persons in the latter group experienced a significantly greater rate of return to work.

If a patient fails to functionally improve as expected with treatment, the patient's condition should be reassessed in order to identify incorrect or missed diagnoses. Further treatment should be appropriate for the diagnosed condition(s), and should not be performed simply because of continued reports of pain.

The clinician should be alert to the incipient development of chronic pain syndrome and should secure a psychological assessment if necessary. Referral for pain management also may be indicated.

Pain medications are typically not useful in the subacute and chronic phases and have been shown to be the most important factor impeding recovery of function in patients referred to pain clinics. This may reflect failure of providers to set up the expectation of improved function as a perquisite for prescribing them.

The long-term use of sustained-release opioid medications may be considered in the treatment of chronic musculoskeletal pain, if:

- The patient has signed an appropriate pain contract.
- Functional expectations have been agreed to by the clinician and the patient.
- Pain medications will be provided by one physician only.
- The patient agrees to use only those medications recommended or agreed to by the clinician.

Functional status must be reassessed at every visit, and changes in opioid prescribing should be consistent with observed functional status.

Enhancing Coping Skills

Pain that persists or does not completely resolve may challenge a patient's coping skills. By identifying coping skills acquired prior to the pain experience, the clinician or a psychologist to whom the clinician has referred the patient can establish a base for the patient to build on to resume a normal role in society. Many clinicians who treat patients with transitional and chronic pain believe that the pain experience, particularly if compounded by other life events or circumstances, can overwhelm the patient's ability to cope with personal and work life, leading to a focus on pain symptoms and deterioration in his or her family life and work. The appropriate treatment may be reinforcement of coping skills rather than attempts to suppress a self-perpetuating pain cycle with medication or surgery.

End Points and Outcomes

Many patients can work with some degree of pain, while others appear disabled out of proportion to physical findings. Therefore, the pain management plan should focus on coping and adaptation in order to restore function. Pain often decreases as other areas of life are normalized. The desired end point in pain management is return to function rather than complete or immediate cessation of pain. Patients may be reassured that with increasingly normal physical function, pain will become increasingly more manageable.

Summary

Physicians should acknowledge the patient's experience of pain. Pain can be independent of the degree of physical pathology. The pain experience is modified by coping mechanisms; cultural and personal expectations; the patient's current psychological state; tissue damage and repair; and the influences, expectations, and responses of health care providers. It is critical for physicians to convey acceptance of, and empathy with, information the patient shares.

Anomalous or exaggerated expressions of pain indicate that medical and psychological evaluations may be warranted.

Pain management focuses on functional restoration. Because return to function is essential to a return to health, occupational health professionals are concerned with return to function. It is very important to identify, at as early a point as possible, the development of chronic pain patterns and responses. Maintaining function will minimize the stiffness, aches, and atrophy that result from being sedentary. Typically, when function improves, so does perceived pain.

References

NATURAL HISTORY

Indahl A, Velund L, Reikeraas O. Good prognosis for low back pain when left untampered: a randomized clinical trial. *Spine.* 1995;20(4):473-7.

RISK FACTORS

Andersen JH, Kaergaard A, Frost P, et al. Physical, psychosocial, and individual risk factors for neck/shoulder pain with pressure tenderness in the muscles among workers performing monotonous, repetitive work. *Spine.* 2002; 27(6):660-7.

Fransen M, Woodward M, Norton R, Coggan C, Dawe M, Sheridan N. Risk factors associated with the transition from acute to chronic occupational back pain. *Spine.* 2002;27(1):92-8.

PREVENTION

Kendall NA. Psychological approaches to the prevention of chronic pain: the low back paradigm. *Baillieres Best Prac Res Clin Rheumatol.* 1999;13(3): 545-54.

Linton SJ. Early identification and intervention in the prevention of musculoskeletal pain. *Amer J Independent Med.* 2002 May.

Philips HC. Avoidance behavior and its role in sustaining chronic pain. *Behav Res Ther.* 1987;25:273-9.

GENERAL

Agency for Healthcare Research and Quality. Washington, DC. *Management of cancer pain.* www.ahrq.gov/clinic/canpainsum.htm (March 1, 2001).

Agency for Health Care Policy and Research. *Acute Pain Management: Operative or Medical Procedures and Trauma. Clinical Practice Guidelines.* Rockville, Md: 1992.

American Academy of Pain Medicine. *The Necessity for Early Evaluation of the Chronic Pain Patient.* www.painmed.org/productpub/statements/earlyevalstmt.html. (February 6, 2001).

Bonica JJ. Definitions and taxonomy of pain, anatomic and physiologic basis of nocioception and pain, and feneral considerations of chronic pain. In: Bonica JJ, ed. *The Management of Pain.* Philadelphia, Pa: Lea & Febiger; 1990.

Institute of Medicine, Committee on Pain, Disability and Chronic Illness Behavior. Osterweis M, Kleinman A, Mechanic D, eds. *Pain and Disability: Clinical Behavioral and Public Policy Perspectives.* Washington, DC: National Academy Press; 1987.

International Association for the Study of Pain, Committee on Taxonomy. Pain terms: a list with definitions and notes on usage. *Pain.* 1979;6:249-52.

Melzack R. Neurophysiological foundations of pain. In: Sternbach R, ed. *The Psychology of Pain.* New York, NY: Raven Press; 1986.

Melzack R, Wall PD. Pain mechanisms: a new theory. *Science.* 1965;150:971-9.

Osterweis M, Kleinman A, Mechanic D, eds. *Pain and Disability — Clinical, Behavioral, and Public Policy Perspectives.* Committee on Pain, Disability and Chronic Illness Behavior, National Academy of Sciences. Washington, DC: National Academy Press; 1987.

Raj PP, ed. *Practical Management of Pain,* 2nd ed. St. Louis, Mo: Mosby-Year Book; 1992.

Ranavaya M, Talmage J. AMA guides to the evaluation of permanent impairment: What's New in the 5th edition? *Disability Medicine.* 2001;1(1).

Salga PL, Bennett RM, Irving GA, McCarberg W, McKeever CD, Pastor RZ, Todd KH. *The Pain Management Challenge.* Medical Crossfire CME Certified Publication Special Edition. Vol 3, No7, June 2002.

Vasudevan SV. The relationship between pain and disability: an overview of the problem. *J Disabil.* 1991;2:44.

CHRONIC PAIN

Aronoff, GM. Chronic pain and the disability epidemic. *Clin J Pain.* 1991;7:330-8.

Bennett RM. *Understanding Chronic Pain and Fibromyalgia: A Review of Recent Discoveries.* National Fibromyalgia Association. http://fmaware.org/doctor/bennettpain.htm.

Caudill M, Schnable R, Zuttermeister P, Benson H, Friedman R. Decreased clinic use by chronic pain patients: response to behavioral medicine interventions, *J Clin Pain.* 1991;7:305-10.

Cook AJ; Chastain DC. The classification of patients with chronic pain: age and sex differences. *Pain Research Manage.* 2001;6(3):142-51.

Cox GB, Chapman CR, Black RG. The MMPI and chronic pain: the diagnosis of chronic pain. *J Behav Med.* 1978;1(4):437-43.

Headley BJ. Chronic pain management. In: O'Sullivan SB. *Physical Rehabilitation: Assessment and Treatment.* Philadelphia, Pa: F.A. Davis; 1994:577-602.

Ryley jf, Ahern DK, Follick MJ. Chronic pain and functional impairment. *Arch Phys Med Rehabil.* 1988;69:579-82.

State of Colorado Department of Labor and Employment, Division of Workers' Compensation. *Chronic Pain Disorder (Evaluation and Management) Medical Treatment Guidelines.* March 15, 1998.

REFLEX SYMPATHETIC DYSTROPHY

Grabow TS, Raja SN. Complex regional pain symdrome I (reflex sympathetic dystrophy). *Anesthesiology.* 2002;96(5).

Gulevich SJ, Conwell TD, Lane J, et al. Stress infrared telethermoghaphy is useful in the diagnosis of complex regional pain syndrome, type i (formerly reflex sympathetic dystrophy). *Clin J Pain.* 1997;13:50-9.

Jadad AR, Carroll D, Glynn CJ, McQuay HJ. Intravenous regional sympathetic blockade for pain relief in reflex sympathetic dystrophy: a systematic review and a randomized, double-blind crossover study. *J Pain Symptom Manage.* 1995;10:13-20.

Kirkpatrick AF, ed. *Clinical Practice Guidelines for the Diagnosis, Treatment, and Management of Reflex Sympathetic Dystrophy Syndrome (Complex Regional Pain Syndrome).* Milford, Conn: The Reflex Sympathetic Dystrophy Association of America; 2000. www.rsds.org/cpgeng.htm.

Perez R, Kwakkel G, Zuurmond W, et al. Treatment of reflex sympathetic dystrophy (CRPS Type 1): a research synthesis of 21 randomized clinical trials. *J Pain Symptom Manage.* 2001:21:511-26.

Ramamurthy S, Hoffman J. Guanethidine Study Group. Intravenous regional guanethidine in the treatment of reflex sympathetic dystrophy/causalgia: a randomized, double-blind study. *Anesth Analg.* 1995;81:718-23.

State of Colorado Department of Labor and Employment, Division of Workers' Compensation. *Reflex Sympathetic Dystrophy/Complex Regional Pain Syndrome Medical Treatment Guidelines.* March 3, 1998.

PAIN ASSESSMENT

Bergner M, et al. The sickness impact profile: development and final revision of a health status measure. *Med Care.* 1981;19:787-805.

Brena SF, Spektor S. Systematic assessment of impairment and residual functional capacity in pain-impaired patients. *J Back Musculoskel Rehabil.* 1993;3:6.

Deyo RA. Measuring the functional status of patients with low back pain. *Arch Phys Med Rehabil.* 1988;69:1044-53.

Fairbank JL, Davies JB, Couper J, et al. The Ouswestry low back pain disability questionnaire. *Phys Ther.* 1980;66:271-3.

Field GB, Parry J. Pain control: some aspects of day-to-day management. *Eur J Cancer Care (Engl).* 1994;2:79-86.

Fordyce WE, Lansky D, Calsyn DA, et al. Pain measurement and pain behavior. *Pain.* 1984;18:53-9.

Haig AJ, Geisser ME, Theisen M, Michel B, Yamakawa K. *The spine team assessment: physical and psychosocial performance of 429 adults with chronic low back pain disability.* Presented at the annual meeting of the American Academy of Physical Medicine and Rehabilitation, San Francisco, Ca. November 2-5, 2000.

Harden R, Bruehl S, Gass S, et al. Signs and symptoms of the myofascial pain syndrome: a national survey of pain management providers. *Clin J Pain.* 2000;16:64-72.

Hendler N, Vierstein M, Gucer P, Long D. A preoperative screening test for chronic back pain patients. *Psychosomatics.* 1979;20:801.

Kerns RD, Turk DC, Rudy TE. The West Haven-Yale Multidimensional Pain Inventory (WHYMPI). *Pain.* 1985;23:345.

Main CJ, Williams A C de C. ABC of psychological medicine: Musculoskeletal pain. *BMJ.* 2002;325(7363):534-7.

Mayer TG, Gatchel RJ, Mayer H. A prospective two year study of functional restoration in industrial low back injury: an objective assessment procedure. *JAMA.* 1987;258:1763-7.

McNeil TW, Sinkora G, Leavitt F. Psychological classification of low-back pain patients: a prognostic tool. *Spine.* 1986;11(9):955-9.

Melzack R. The McGill Pain Questionnaire: major properties and scoring methods. *Pain.* 1975;1:277-99.

Millard RW. The Functional Assessment Screening Questionnaire: application for evaluating pain-related disability. *Arch Phys Med Rehabil.* 1989;70:303-7.

Pope MH, et al. *Occupational Low Back Pain: Assessment, Treatment and Prevention.* St. Louis, Mo: Mosby-Year Book; 1991.

Ransford AO, Carson DC, Mooney V. The pain drawing as an aid to the psychologic evaluation of patients with low-back pain. *Spine.* 1976;1:127.

Roland M, Morris R. A study of the natural history of back pain: part I: development of a reliable and sensitive measure of disability in low-back pain. *Spine.* 1983;8:141-4.

Sipkoff M, *Tools Help Assess Pain Objectively.* QI Physician.com; December 2000.

Turk DC. Evaluation of pain and disability. *J Disability.* 1991;2:24.

Turk DC, Melzack R, eds. *Handbook of Pain Assessment.* New York, NY: Guilford Press; 1992.

Turk DC, Okifuji A. Assessment of patients' reporting of pain: an integrated perspective. *Lancet.* 1999;53:1784-8.

van Tulder M, Koes B, Bouter L. Conservative treatment of acute and chronic nonspecific low back pain: a systematic review of randomized controlled trials of the most common interventions. *Spine.* 1997; 22(18):2128-56.

van Tulder MW, Esmail R, Bombardier C, Koes BW. Back schools for non-specific low back pain (Cochrane Review). In: *The Cochrane Library.* Issue 2; 2002. Oxford: Update Software.

Vasudevan SV. Impairment, disability and functional capacity assessment. In: Turk DC, Melzack R, eds. *Handbook of Pain Assessment.* New York, NY: Guilford Press; 1992.

Waddell G, McCulloch JA, Kummell E, et al. Nonorganic physical signs in low back pain. *Spine.* 1980;5:117-25.

Waddell G, Somerville D, Henderson I, Newton M. Objective clinical evaluation of physical impairment in chronic low back pain. *Spine.* 1992;17:617-28.

Ware JE, Sherbourne CD. The MOS 36-Item Short Form Health Survey (SF-36). *Med Care.* 1992;30:473-83.

PSYCHOSOCIAL EVALUATION

Agency for Health Care Policy and Research. *Depression in Primary Care: Detection, Diagnosis and Treatment.* Clinical Practice Guideline. Rockville, Md; 1993.

Asmundson GJG, Norton GR, Allerdings MD. Fear and avoidance in dysfunctional chronic back pain patients. *Pain.* 1997;69:321-36.

Asmundson GJ, Norton PJ, Norton GR. Beyond pain: the role of fear and avoidance in chronicity. *Clin Psychol Rev.* 1999;19(1):97-119. Review.

Bacon NM, Bacon SF, Atkinson JH, et al. Somatization symptoms in chronic low back pain patients. *Psychosom Med.* 1994;56(2):118-27.

Chapman CR, Turner JA. *Psychological and Psychosocial Aspects of Acute Pain.* Philadelphia, Pa: Lea & Febiger; 1990.

Chapman SL, Pemberton JS. Prediction of treatment outcome from clinically derived MMPI clusters in rehabilitation for chronic low back pain. *Clin J Pain.* 1994;10:267-76.

Crombez G, Vervaet L, Baeyens F, Lysens R, Eelen P. Do pain expectancies cause pain in chronic low back patients? A clinical investigation. *Behav Res Ther.* 1996;34:919-25.

Crombez G, Vlaeyen JWS, Heuts PHTG, Lysens R. Pain-related fear is more disabling than pain itself: evidence on the role of pain-related fear in chronic back pain disability. *Pain.* 1999;80:329-39.

Derogatis LR, Rickels K, Rock AF. The SCL-90 and the MMPI: a step in the validation of a new self-report scale. *Br J Psych.* 1976;128:280-9.

Ensalada LH. The importance of illness behavior in disability management. *Occup Med.* 2000;15(4):739-54, iv. Review.

Feuerstein M, Berkowitz SM, Haufler AJ, Lopez MS, Huang GD. Working with low back pain: workplace and individual psychosocial determinants of limited duty and lost time. *Amer J Independent Med.* 2001;40(6):627-38.

Flor H, Turk DC. Chronic back pain and rheumatoid arthritis: predicting pain and disability from cognitive variables. *J Behav Med.* 1988;11:251-65.

Geisser ME, Haig AJ, Theisen ME. Activity avoidance and function in persons with chronic back pain. *J Occup Rehabil.* 2000;10:215-27.

Gatchel RJ, Gardea MA. Psychosocial issues: their importance in predicting disability, response to treatment, and search for compensation. *Neurol Clin.* 1999;17(1):149-66.

Gatchel R, Polatin P, Kinney R. Predicting outcome of chronic back pain using clinical predictors of psychopathology: a prospective analysis. *Health Psychol.* 1995:14(5);415-20.

Groves JE. Taking care of the hateful patient. *N Engl J Med.* 1978;298:883-7.

Hadler NM. Fibromyalgia, chronic fatigue, and other iatrogenic diagnostic algorithms. Do some labels escalate illness in vulnerable patients? *Postgrad Med.* 1997;102(2):161-2, 165-6, 171-2.

Hill HE, Belleville RE, Wikler A. Studies on anxiety associated with anticipation of pain. *Arch Neurol Psychiatry.* 1955;73:602-8.

Hoogendoorn WE, Bongers PM, De Vet HC, Ariens GA, Van Mechelen W, Bouter LM. High physical work load and low job satisfaction increase the risk of sickness absence due to low back pain: results of a prospective cohort study. *Occup Environ Med.* 2002;59(5):323-8.

Jensen MP, Turner JA, Romano JM, Lawler BK. Relationship of pain-specific beliefs to chronic pain adjustment. *Pain.* 1994b;57:301-9.

Keefe FJ, Kashikar-Zuck S, Robinson E, et al. Pain coping strategies that predict patients' and spouses' ratings of patients' self-efficacy. *Pain.* 1997; 73:191-9.

Kori SH, Miller RP, Todd DD. Kinesiophobia: a new view of chronic pain behavior. *Pain Manage.* 1990;3:35-43.

LaChapelle DL, Hadjistavropoulos HD, McCreary DR, Asmundson GJ. Contributions of pain-related adjustment and perceptions of control to coping strategy use among cervical sprain patients. *Eur J Pain.* 2001;5(4):405-13.

Lethem J, Slade PD, Troup JDG, Bentley G. Outline of a fear-avoidance model of exaggerated pain perceptions. *Behav Res Ther.* 1983;21:401-8.

Love AW, Peck CL. The MMPI and psychological factors in chronic low back pain: a review. *Pain.* 1987;28(1):1-12. Review.

Lynch NT, Vasudevan SV. *Persistent Problematic Pain: Psychosocial Assessment and Intervention.* Boston, Mass: Kluwer, 1988.

McCracken LM, Gross RT. The role of pain-related anxiety reduction in the outcome of multidisciplinary treatment for chronic low back pain: preliminary results. *J Occup Rehabil.* 1998;8:179-89.

McCracken LM, Gross RT, Sorg PJ, Edmands TA. Prediction of pain in patients with chronic low back pain: effects of inaccurate prediction and pain-related anxiety. *Behav Res Ther.* 1993;31:647-2.

McCracken LM, Spertus IL, Janeck AS, Sinclair D, Wetzel FT. Behavioral dimensions of adjustment in persons with chronic pain: pain-related anxiety and acceptance. *Pain.* 1999;80:283-9.

Rogers R. *Clinical Assessment of Malingering and Deception.* New York, NY: Guilford Press; 1988.

Sternbach RA, Timmermans G. Personality changes associated with the reduction of pain. *Pain.* 1975;1:177-81.

Tait RC. Psychological factors in the assessment of disability among patients with chronic pain. *J Back Musculoskel Rehabil.* 1993;3:20.

Trief PM,Yuan HA. Use of the MMPI in a chronic pain rehabilitation program. *J Clin Psychol.* 1983;39(1):46-53.

Turk DC, Rudy TD. Persistent pain and the injured worker: integrating biomedical, psychosocial and behavioral factors in assessment. *J Occup Rehabil.* 1991;1(2):159-79.

van Lankveld W, Naring G, van't Pad Bosch P, et al. The negative effect of decreasing the level of activity in coping with pain in rheumatoid arthritis: an increase in psychological distress and disease impact. *J Behav Med.* 2000;23(4):377-91.

Turk DC, Rudy TD, Kubinski JA, Zaki HS, Greco CM. Dysfunctional patients with temporomandibular disorders: evaluating the efficacy of a tailored treatment protocol. *J Consult Clin Psychol.* 1996;64:139-46.

Vlaeyen JWS, de Jong J, Geilen M, Heuts PHTG, van Breulelen G. The treatment of fear of movement/(re)injury in chronic low back pain: further evidence on the effectiveness of exposure in vivo. *Clin J Pain.* 2002;18: 251-61.

Vlaeyen JWS, Kole-Snidjers AMJ, Rotteveel AM, Rvesink R, Heuts PHTG. The role of fear of movement/(re)injury in pain disability. *J Occup Rehabil.* 1995;5:235-52.

Vlaeyen JWS, Seelen HAM, Peters M, et al. Fear of movement/(re)injury and muscular reactivity in chronic low back pain patients: an experimental investigation. *Pain.* 1999;82:297-304.

Waddell G, Main CJ. Assessment of severity in low back disorders. *Spine.* 1984;9:204-8.

Waddell G, Morris EW, DiPaola M, et al. Chronic low-back pain, psychologic distress and illness behavior. *Spine.* 1984;9(2):209-13.

Waddell G, Newton M, Henderson I, Somerville D, Main C. A Fear-Avoidance Beliefs Questionnaire (FABQ) and the role of fear-avoidance beliefs in chronic low back pain and disability. *Pain.* 1993;52:157-68.

Watson PJ, Booker CK, Main CJ. Evidence for the role of psychological factors in abnormal paraspinal activity in patients with chronic low back pain. *J Musculoskeletal Pain.* 1997;5:41-56.

PHYSICAL METHODS

International Association for the Study of Pain. *Outline Curriculum on Pain for Schools of Occupational Therapy and Physcial Therapy, 1994.* www .iasp-pain.orglot-pt toc.html.

van Tulder MW, Malmivaara A, Esmail R, Koes BW. Exercise therapy for low back pain (Cochrane Review). In: *The Cochrane Library.* Issue 2; 2002. Oxford: Update Software.

INJECTIONS

Cheshire WP, Abashian SW, Mann JD. Botulinum toxin in the treatment of myofascial pain syndrome. *Pain.* 1994;59:65-9.

Foster L, Clapp L, Erickson M, Jabbari B. Botulinum toxin A and chronic low back pain. A randomized, double blind study. *Neurol.* 2001;56:1290-3.

Lew MF, Adornato BT, Duane DD, et al. Botulinum toxin type B: a double-blind, placebo-controlled, safety and efficacy study in cervical dystonia. *Neurol.* 1997;49:701-7.

Nelemans PJ, Bie RA de, Vet HCW de, Sturmans F. Injection therapy for subacute and chronic benign low back pain (Cochrane Review). In: *The Cochrane Library.* Issue 2; 2002. Oxford: Update Software.

Wheeler AH, Goolkasian P, Gretz SS. A randomized, double-blind, prospective pilot study of botulinum toxin injection for refractory, unilateral, cervico-thoracic, paraspinal, myofascial pain syndrome. *Spine.* 1998;23:1662-7.

OTHER MEDICATIONS

Academy of Pain Medicine. Use of opioids for the treatment of chronic pain. www.painmed.org/productpub/statements/opioidstmt.html. (February 6, 2001).

Berndt S, Maier C, Schutz HW. Polymedication and medication compliance in patients with chronic non-malignant pain. *Pain.* 1993;52:331-9.

Ciccone DS, Just N, Bandilla MA et al. Psychological correlates of opioid use in patients with chronic nonmalignant pain: a preliminary test of the downhill spiral hypothesis. *J Pain Symptom Manage.* 2000;20:180-92.

Federation of State Medical Boards of the U.S. Inc. Model Guidelines for the Use of Controlled Substances for the Treatment of Pain. 1998. www.medsch.wisc.edu/painpolicy/domestic/model.htm (November 27, 2000).

Harden RN. Chronic opioid therapy: another reappraisal. *American Pain Soc Bul.* Jan-Feb 2002. www.ampainsoc.org/pub/bulletin/jan02/poli1.htm.

Katz N. MorphiDex (MS:DM) double-blind, multiple-dose studies in chronic pain patients. *J Pain Symptom Manage.* 2000;19(1):S37-41.

McLean W, Boucher E, Brennan M. et al. Is there an indication for the use of barbituate-containing analgesic agents in the treatment of pain. Guidelines for their safe use and withdrawl management. *Can J Clin Pharm.* 2000;(7)4:191-7.

Moulin DE, Iezze A, Amireh R, Sharpe WK, Boyd D, Merskey H. Randomised trial of oral morphine for chronic noncancer pain. *Lancet.* 1996;347:143-7.

Phillip M, Fickinger M. Psychotropic drugs in the management of chronic pain syndromes. *Pharmacopsychiatry.* 1993;26:221-34.

Rousmaniere PF. Pain medication in workers' compensation. *Risk Insurance Mag.* April 2002.

Rowbotham M, Harden N, Stacey B, Bernstein P, Magnus-Miller L. Gabapentin for the treatment of postherpetic neuralgia. A randomized controlled trial. *JAMA.* 1998;280:1837-42.

Stein C. The control of pain in peripheral tissue by opioids. *N Engl J Med.* 1995;332:1685-90.

Turner JA, Denny MC. Do antidepressant medications relieve chronic low back pain? *J Fam Pract.* 1993;37:545-53.

EDUCATIONAL/MULTIDISCIPLINARY METHODS

Burton AK, Waddell G, Tillotson KM, Summerton N. Information and advice to patients with back pain can have a positive effect. A randomized controlled trial of a novel educational booklet in primary care. *Spine.* 1999;24(23):2484-91.

Cutler RB, Fishbain DA, Rosomoff HL, et al. Does nonsurgical pain center treatment of chronic pain return patients to work? A review and meta-analysis of the literature. *Spine.* 1994;19:643-52.

Flor H, Fydrich T, Turk DC. Efficacy of multidisciplinary pain treatment centers: a meta-analytic review. *Pain.* 1992;49:221-30.

Guzman J, Esmail R, Karjalainen K. et al. Multidisciplinary rehabilitation for chronic low back pain: systematic review. *BMJ.* 2001;322:1511-16.

Haldorsen EMH, Grasdal AL, Skouen JS, Risa AE, Kronholm K, Ursin H. Is there a right treatment for a particular patient group? Comparison of ordinary treatment, light multidisciplinary treatment, and extensive multidisciplinary treatment for long-term sick-listed employees with musculoskeletal pain. *Pain.* 2002;95:49-63.

Hazard RG, Fenwick JW, Kalish SM, Redmond J, Reeves V, Reid S, Frymoyer JW. Functional restoration with behavioral support: a one year prospective study of patients with chronic low back pain. *Spine.* 1989;14:157-61.

Jensen MP, Turner JA, Romano JM. Correlates of improvement in multidisciplinary treatment of chronic pain. *J Consult Clin Psychol.* 1994a;62:172-9.

Karjalainen K, Malmivaara A, van Tulder M, et al. Multidisciplinary biopsychosocial rehabilitation of subacute low back pain in working-age adults: a systematic review within the framework of the Cochrane Collaboration Back Review Group. *Spine.* 2001;26(3):262-9.

Mayer TG. Rehabilitation: what do we do with the chronic patient? *Neurol Clin.* 1999;17(1):131-47.

Mayer TG, Gatchel RJ. *Functional Restoration for Spinal Disorders: The Sports Medicine Approach.* Philadelphia, Pa: Lea & Febiger; 1988.

Mayer TG, Mooney, Gatchel RJ. *Contemporary Conservative Care for Painful Spinal Disorders.* Philadelphia, Pa: Lea & Febiger; 1991.

Turk DC, Okifuji A, Sinclair JD, Starz, TW. Differential responses by psychosocial subgroups of fibromyalgia syndrome patients to an interdisciplinary treatment. *Arth Care Res.* 1998;11:397-404.

COMPLEMENTARY AND ALTERNATIVE MEDICINE

Barrows KA, Jacobs BP. Mind-body medicine. An introduction and review of the literature. *Med Clin North Am.* 2002;86(1):11-31.

van Tulder MW, Cherkin DC, Berman B, Lao L, Koes BW. Acupuncture for low back pain (Cochrane Review). In: *The Cochrane Library.* Issue 2; 2002. Oxford: Update Software.

Appendix 6A. Pain Assessment Models and Tools

The Joint Commission on Accreditation of Health Care Organizations recently released guidelines urging health care facilities to assess pain in all patients (when pain is present). Further, The American Pain Society has called on physicians to recognize pain as "the fifth vital sign" and assess pain along with pulse, blood pressure, temperature, and respiration.

The role of the occupational health physician is to understand the effects of the pain experience on the patient and his or her ability to function, so that work and social function can be restored. To do this, pain assessment tools may be used by the occupational physician or a pain specialist upon referral.

Several basic concepts, expressions, and definitions used within the area of pain assessment are important to understand, including the following:

Acute Pain Model. Using a traditional framework to view the pain experience, this model suggests that if a patient has pain, visible signs of discomfort (behavioral or physiological) will be present. Research has shown this model to be of limited value. It is known, for example, that individuals adapt rapidly to the effects of pain and that the absence of behavioral or physiological signs of pain does not necessarily mean the absence of pain.

Adaptation to Pain. Adaptation is a phenomenon in which the body seeks homeostasis and returns to a former physiological state despite severe pain. It includes the suppression of behaviors, such as crying and moaning, despite severe pain.

Admission Assessment. For this assessment, a patient's biophysical data is gathered upon entry to a particular facility.

Brief Pain Inventory (BPI). This inventory is used for patients with a complicated chronic pain problem. The BPI is a comprehensive pain assessment tool that may be used with a patient whose pain has not been satisfactorily controlled.

Faces Rating Scale. There are several published *faces scales* that are administered visually and use facial expressions to suggest various pain intensities (i.e., Wong Baker, Bieri). The Faces Rating Scale is used primarily with young children, but also may be useful when treating adults who have difficulty using the numbers of a *visual analog scale* (VAS), a common pain assessment tool.

Flowsheets. These worksheets are used to document progress toward achieving and maintaining pain management goals. Physicians use flow sheets to record time, pain ratings, facts about analgesic administration, and side effects. The information on a pain management flowsheet can be incorporated into other forms to avoid duplicate charting.

Graphic Rating Scale (GRS). The GRS builds on the VAS by adding words or numbers between the extreme ends of the scale. If words are added, such as "no pain," "mild," "moderate," and "severe," it is called a *verbal graphic rating scale.* If numbers are added, such as zero through ten, it becomes a *numerical graphic rating scale.*

Numerical Rating Scale (NRS). This scale is administered verbally or visually from zero to ten or zero to five and uses words and numbers along a vertical or horizontal line. Zero equals "no pain" and five or ten equals the "worst possible pain."

Simple Descriptor Scale (SDS). This scale uses a list of words describing different levels of pain intensity. A simple and clinically useful example is "no pain," "mild," "moderate," or "severe" pain.

Visual Analog Scale (VAS). The VAS uses a horizontal 10-centimeter line with words at the extremes, such as "no pain" and "pain as bad as it could be." The patient makes a mark along the line to represent pain intensity. A number is obtained by measuring the millimeters from the end to the point the patient has indicated.

7 Independent Medical Examinations and Consultations

The occupational health practitioner may refer to other specialists if a diagnosis is uncertain or extremely complex, when psychosocial factors are present, or when the plan or course of care may benefit from additional expertise. An independent medical assessment also may be useful in avoiding potential conflict(s) of interest when analyzing causation or when prognosis, degree of impairment, or work capacity requires clarification. When a physician is responsible for performing an isolated assessment of an examinee's health or disability for an employer, business, or insurer, a limited examinee-physician relationship should be considered to exist. A referral may be for:

- **Consultation:** To aid in the diagnosis, prognosis, therapeutic management, determination of medical stability, and permanent residual loss and/or the examinee's fitness for return to work. A consultant is usually asked to act in an advisory capacity, but may sometimes take full responsibility for investigation and/or treatment of an examinee or patient.
- **Independent Medical Examination (IME):** To provide medicolegal documentation of fact, analysis, and well-reasoned opinion, sometimes including analysis of causality. An IME differs from consultation in that there is no doctor-patient relationship established and medical care is not provided. It may be a means of medical clarification or adjudication in which the physician draws conclusions regarding diagnosis, clinical status, causation, work-relatedness, testing and treatment efficacy and requirements, physical capacities, impairment, and prognosis based on available information. The evaluations must be independent, impartial, and without bias. The client often may be the employer, insurer, state authority, or attorney.

Accepted Purposes of Independent Medical Examinations (IMEs)

Independent medical examinations have at least four accepted purposes. To be most effective, IMEs must be complete, focused, rigorously and clearly reasoned, impartial, and supply the information needed by the person who requested them. Independent medical examinations are discussed below primarily in the context of workers' compensation. However, not only workers' compensation systems rely upon IMEs; they are, at times, equally valuable for assessing non-work-related illnesses and injuries, and the work issues surrounding them.

First, IMEs are intended to provide specific, relevant, and impartial information to guide adjudication of a workers' compensation or other claim when required information has not been made available by other means, or when the existing information is believed to be inaccurate. Claims adjusters may use IMEs to provide guidance about entitlement issues such as the work-relatedness of a medical condition, the need for further medical or income benefits, and the nature and extent of permanent impairments.

Second, IMEs may be used to guide management of medical care, disability, and rehabilitation when the claims adjuster is concerned that the care may be inadequate, inappropriate, or that return to work is unreasonably delayed. Case managers and rehabilitation specialists may need clarification of the diagnosis, appropriateness of treatment, or need for work modifications or absence. IMEs also may be used to elicit hitherto unknown facts in a situation or to uncover the reasons for delayed functional recovery. While IMEs are not the preferred method for obtaining basic medical information, they can be an invaluable aid when a claims adjuster has questions and needs expert corroboration or guidance. This is particularly true when the health problem is unusual or the nature or need for the proposed treatment is controversial.

Third, IMEs may be used to provide technical data and written opinions in order to comply with requirements of the claims adjudications process, or to move even an uncontested claim to a next step. Statutes, regulations, organizational policies, or tradition often consider a signed doctor's report as a precondition to moving to the next step. Examples include work releases, closing exams, maximal medical improvement (MMI) findings, impairment ratings, and so forth. Independent medical examinations may provide these data if they are not provided by the treating physician.

Fourth, IMEs can be a source of expert medical opinions on issues of diagnosis, causality, treatment, or impairment for defense or claimants' attorneys and workers' compensation commissioners or judges. Attorneys, adjusters, and judges generally are seeking information to clarify a disputed point. In some jurisdictions, the IME report itself is not admissible evidence; the testimony of the examiner is considered the evidence, whereas the report is hearsay unless both parties agree to the contrary, or the administrative law judge accepts the report in evidence.

During the course of a workers' compensation claim, IMEs may be appropriately used to evaluate testing and treatment appropriateness or disability management. The best practice in protracted treatment is to obtain an IME promptly after the recommended care in evidence-based guidelines has been exceeded. Many payers obtain IMEs if there is prolonged or apparently ineffective treatment. The best practice in using IMEs to manage delayed recovery is contingent on the availability of information and the time in which it is available.

At case closure, IMEs are appropriate to obtain an opinion of MMI, an assessment of impairment rating, or prediction of future medical needs if the information is not available from the attending physician, is felt to be biased or inaccurate, or is needed to resolve a dispute. If the claimant appears to be at MMI, but the attending physician does not agree, an IME may be appropriate. Most states require an impairment assessment or rating at the conclusion of the claim if the attending physician states that the claimant has not recovered to his or her preinjury status. For workers' compensation, there is a treating physician presumption (official or unofficial) in most states, making the attending physician the preferred initial source of information. This presumption may be changed by the recent U.S. Supreme Court decision, *Black & Decker Disability Plan v. Nord.*

Legal and Regulatory Requirements for Independent Medical Examinations (IMEs)

Each state has legal and regulatory provisions governing the collection and use of medical information, the circumstances under which IMEs may be obtained, and the qualifications and selection process for examiners. Most states allow the workers' compensation board to order a physical examination of a claimant by a physician of its choice, and allow insurers or employers to order a physical examination of a claimant by a physician of their choice.

Some states allow IMEs at the discretion of the employer/insurer or "as needed." The majority of states allow IMEs to resolve disputes, especially regarding treatment, nature of injury, and disability. Some states use IMEs mostly for permanent partial disability ratings. Some states require a hearing before the Board can order an IME. Simply accreting more opinions on one side or the other, or creating a "tie-breaker," is not viewed as the best use of an IME, but the "dueling docs" phenomenon is the reason for many IMEs.

In summary, IMEs are used to provide information and opinions for the understanding and guidance of causality analysis, diagnosis, medical testing and therapy, and functional recovery programs. To be most effective in meeting these needs, IMEs must be complete, focused, rigorously and clearly reasoned, impartial, and supply the information requested.

Qualifications of a Consultant or an Independent Medical Examiner

Physicians obtaining external opinion from consultations or IMEs should refer examinees to other physicians who are independent of the practitioner managing the case, other physicians involved with the case, the payer, and any attorneys who may be involved, e.g., in workers' compensation or environmental liability cases.

Consultants and IME physicians have the same obligations as physicians in other contexts: to evaluate objectively the examinee's health or disability.

They should not be influenced by the preferences of the examinee, employer, or insurance company when making a diagnosis.

Consultants and IME physicians should:

- Be licensed and in good standing in the jurisdiction where the examination occurs. Physicians should list licensure such as MD, DO, etc., after their signature so that payers know who performed the IME and the physician's licensure.
- Be board certified, defined as successful completion of an American Board of Medical Specialties (ABMS) prescribed residency in an Accreditation Council for Graduate Medical Education (ACGME) accredited institution and subsequent certification by the applicable board in the area of inquiry or possible exposure. Comparable certification should be demonstrated for physicians in other countries.
- Demonstrate evidence of ongoing continuing medical education accredited by Accreditation Council for Continuing Medical Education (ACCME) and good standing with the professional specialty board or association.
- Return primary care to the practitioner managing the case following the examination and assessment.

In addition to the above, independent medical examiners should:

- Demonstrate experience in the performance of IMEs.
- Be able to rate impairment and differentiate impairment from disability.[1]
- Declare any financial or other interest they may have in the findings or outcome of the examination.
- Disclose any important health information or abnormalities discovered during the course of the examination.
- Be independent contractors providing medical examinations within the realm of their specialty, in contrast to industry-employed physicians (IEPs), whom businesses or insurance companies employ to conduct medical examinations.
- Be objective in performing and reporting IMEs as well as actively ascertaining potential conflicts of interest. Potential bias relevant to any evaluation should be documented to show that such bias exists.

[1]The official WHO (World Health Organization) definition of *Impairment* is "any loss or abnormality of psychological, physiological or anatomical structure or function." WHO's definition for *Disability* is: "any restriction or lack of ability to perform an activity in a manner or within the range considered normal for a human being." The term *disability* reflects the consequences of impairment in terms of functional performance and activity by the individual.

Examiner Skills and Abilities

Examiners should be trained and knowledgeable about the body systems and health problems that the examinee appears to have. The examiner should know how to elicit and interpret key symptoms and signs. For example, if the worker complains of low back pain, the examiner should be knowledgeable about the anatomy and physiology of both the musculoskeletal and nervous systems, and diagnosis of disorders of the low back.

If causation is an issue, the examiner should be able to assess work and home exposure to ergonomic factors, chemicals, and other sources of work-related health problems. He or she should also have a thorough knowledge of the high-grade scientific evidence linking exposures and adverse health effects if asked to assess health issues other than direct trauma.

Communication, and interpersonal and language skills are crucial elements of the independent medical examination skill set. Because the results of an IME may affect the ability to obtain financially desired or needed benefits, it can be a threatening experience to the examinee. Further, not all examinees are excellent historians without careful questioning and interpretation. One of the main complaints about independent medical examiners is failure to listen or to cover points that are important to the examinee.

The examiner should be cognizant of the evidence supporting efficacious and cost-effective care, whether physical, pharmacological, or surgical. The examiner also should be aware of the lack of evidence, or negative evidence, for many commonly used tests and treatments. Even effective treatments may lose their effectiveness for an individual after a period of time, or may have negative effects if prolonged too long. Pharmacological therapy and physical medicine in particular fall into this category.

A balanced health care perspective is important: First, placing precedence on medical or surgical therapy rather than other forms of therapy may prevent the examiner from considering the best treatment for the examinee's circumstances. Second, many of the factors that delay functional recovery and return to work are not purely physical.

The examiner must be skilled in applying medical logic to the data acquired in order to validate the diagnosis, suggest specific additional testing, affirm or recommend changes in treatment, and to reach reasonable conclusions about causation, impairment, and ability to work. Without this skill, and the ability to convey the steps in the analysis to the reader, the value of the data acquired will be largely unrealized. Knowledge and skill in answering the types of questions typically posed to independent medical examiners is also essential. Examiners rating permanent impairment must be familiar with the use of the often complex rating systems deployed in their particular jurisdiction.

An excellent examiner will maintain a neutral point of view as a medical expert. The examiner will render opinions consistent with the case and the evidence for causation, test and treatment effectiveness, and the reproducibility of impairment assessment. He or she should not issue "boilerplate" reports (that are generic rather than specific in nature), nor use a preconceived framework based on a pro-business or pro-labor philosophy rather than the objective facts of each case.

The examiner should be able to render an opinion that is "impartial, unbiased, and objective." The examiner should clearly differentiate between facts and opinions. Generally, it has been considered difficult for treating physicians to achieve this level of objectivity, especially in circumstances where some sort of dispute concerning their examinee is involved.

As stated previously, in some jurisdictions, independent medical reports are not in themselves admissible in legal disputes. Therefore, another important skill of medical examiners is the ability to testify clearly, logically, and in an informed way in a deposition or hearing on the issues and facts in the case. When testifying, the examiner should be able to assimilate contradictory information and consider it reasonably, even if it changes his or her prior opinion.

Referral Issues and the Independent Medical Examination (IME) Process

A referral request should specify the concerns to be addressed in the independent or expert assessment, including the relevant medical and nonmedical issues, diagnosis, causal relationship, prognosis, temporary or permanent impairment, work capability, clinical management, and treatment options. The appendix that appears at the end of this chapter provides an added level of detail to the sections below regarding the process and content of IMEs.

A consultation report or IME may contain these elements:

- History and physical findings
- Interpretation of test results
- Diagnosis
- Expected natural history of the disease or injury
- Causation
- Maximal medical improvement (MMI)
- Impairment
- If indicated, apportionment of the impairment
- Work capacity and its evaluation, including a physical capacity estimate (PCE), based on best medical evidence and restrictions
- Appropriateness of current course, treatment, or medical management
- Expected future medical care because of the specified exposure or injury

A. History

A comprehensive history in a consultation or IME should contain the following:

1. HISTORY OF THE PRESENT INJURY OR ILLNESS, INCLUDING:

- Description of the incident resulting in injury, body part affected, and onset of symptoms, obtained from both the injured worker and employer

- Mechanism of injury or illness
- Investigation and accident reports
- Summary of exposure monitoring data to quantify exposure
- Examinee's preinjury health status, including preexisting conditions, previous injuries, and the examinee's perceived preinjury functional status, for comparison
- Chronology of symptoms and response to treatment

2. CURRENT STATUS OF THE EXAMINEE'S HEALTH PROBLEM(S), INCLUDING:

- Nature, location, pattern, and quality of current symptoms, identifying the body part(s) involved and the specific type and location of the symptoms
- Change in function or capacity during the course of the problem
- Examinee's current perceived functional status, including the ability to carry out daily living, recreational and work activities, with consistencies and inconsistencies noted
- Aggravating and relieving factors
- Physician-imposed work restrictions
- Treatment history and response to treatment, particularly if the questions posed relate to treatment effectiveness or recommendations
- Work and disability status since the onset of the problem
- Examinee's perceptions about causation, satisfaction with care, and expectations for recovery from the condition
- Associated symptoms such as anxiety, depression, and sleep disturbances
- Effects on social function

3. REVIEW OF OTHER MEDICAL AND DISABILITY HISTORY, INCLUDING:

- Other past illnesses, injuries, surgeries, allergies, medications, and family history of illness, injury, and disability
- The effects of previous injuries or preexisting conditions
- Nonoccupational exposures
- Review of organ systems
- Absence history prior to the current health problem
- Disability history

4. REVIEW OF PERTINENT MEDICAL AND OTHER RECORDS, WHICH MAY INCLUDE:

- Preexisting conditions and previous similar illnesses or injuries
- Health problems reported by other examiners
- Diagnostic test results and functional capacity assessments and the methodology used
- Summary of other physicians' opinions
- Direct review of past test data, and imaging studies or electrodiagnostic study data.

The reviewer should note any questions he or she might have, as well as inconsistencies among tests or between test interpretations, and the history and physical examination in the analysis section (see below).

5. EMPLOYMENT HISTORY MAY INCLUDE:

- Examinee's occupational history including current and prior jobs, noting work tasks, exposures, and protection such as engineering controls, personal protective equipment, and ergonomic practices
- Review of job descriptions preferably agreed to by the worker and the supervisor
- Viewing of videotapes of actual job tasks
- Review of ergonomic evaluations of the worker's workstation
- Specific essential functions of the examinee's job and workplace exposures at the time of injury, or prior to the appearance of symptoms of a work-related illness, as obtained from both examinee and employer
- Examinee's job satisfaction, relationships with supervisors and co-workers, and recent performance evaluations, job satisfaction, task satisfaction, level of monotony and control, and opportunities for advancement

6. PSYCHOSOCIAL HISTORY

- Education, prior work experiences, and future goals and plans
- Description of a typical day and time use
- Family situation, and changes in that situation since injury
- Recreation, including related nonoccupational exposures
- Tobacco, alcohol, and other drug use
- Other psychosocial factors

A focused history for circumstances that predispose examinees to symptom magnification or chronic pain syndrome is recommended when:

*Table 7-1. Risk Factors for Potential Symptom Magnification, Somatization, or Malingering**

• Childhood history/dysfunction • School performance • Ability to form lasting relationships • Family emotional issues • Psychosomatic illness history • Litigation history	• Prior emotional or physical trauma • Emotional difficulties • Developmental transitions • Substance abuse • Past medical problems, disability

* Derived from Aranoff, Feldman, and Campion, 2000; Brigham and Ensalada, 2000; Ensalada, 2000; Proctor, Gatchel, and Robinson, 2000.

- Pain symptoms are impeding functional recovery
- There are questions of symptom magnification
- There are questions about the need for future treatment or vocational rehabilitation

The elements of such a history are shown in Table 7-1.

B. Physical Assessment

1. A general physical examination should be completed, including the examiner's general observation of:
   - examinee behavior, appropriateness, and affect
   - station, gait, posture, and body movements
   - cardiopulmonary function

2. A detailed examination of the body system involved is important and may require referral for specialized evaluation. For instance:
   - In cases of neuromusculoskeletal complaints or presumed nerve or nerve root compression, a complete neurologic examination of the affected area and related areas is mandatory. Sole use of physical examination maneuvers to make these diagnoses is inadequate. A neurological examination also may be indicated when there is evidence of other neurosensory findings when examining other body systems.
   - In cases of visual system or periorbital complaints, a comprehensive ocular examination is appropriate with the addition of specific laboratory procedures, as indicated by the examination findings.
   - Nonphysiologic findings should be noted. Such findings might include back pain with axial loading, inappropriate responses to stimuli, and other findings that do not correspond to known anatomic or physiologic problems.
   - Behavioral assessment, including the examinee's responses during the physical assessment should be noted and, in some cases, a formal mental status examination may be indicated.

C. Inventories

Pain and functional status inventories may supplement the evaluation of behavioral and psychological factors and provide information on the perceived level of function and disability. These questionnaires also can provide an indication of behavioral overlay and psychological problems that might contribute to delayed recovery or dysfunction at work or at home. The examiner can judiciously choose applicable inventories, considering their intended use, appropriateness to the examinee, and ecological and intrinsic validity and reliability within a work setting.

D. Surveillance

Examining physicians should use surveillance material only to reach medical conclusions and only if the surveillance materials allow them to reach their conclusions. Surveillance recordings and reports may assist in determining which activities are safe for the examinee. Surveillance is most useful when an individual is observed engaging in activities that cannot be reconciled with the claimed injury. An examinee's maximum abilities cannot be extrapolated reliably from surveillance data unless continuous strenuous or demanding activities are observed. Brief exertion can occur during the "best" days representing maximal performance assisted by premedication or subsequently requiring medication. It is reasonable to state whether the documented activities are consistent or inconsistent with documented functional capacity evaluations.

E. Analysis

A careful analysis of past medical history, history of the present illness or injury, work history, test results, and the physical examination as a group of data should yield answers to the questions posed, or reveal the need for further consultation or testing. Analyzing the following elements should enable the examiner to make a full assessment of diagnostic accuracy, work-relatedness, testing and treatment appropriateness, level of function, physical or psychological impairment, and motivation to return to work:

- Diagnosis of the underlying conditions or disorders, based on a synthesis of all available information, and diagnosis guidelines (i.e., those in this book). An accurate diagnosis is needed to formulate the most efficient and effective treatment plan.
- Comparison of specific treatments and results to usual or best-practice treatments outcomes for the most efficient and effective future treatment plan. The examiner should analyze past records in chronological order for diagnostic accuracy, test appropriateness and findings, treatment appropriateness and effectiveness, the appropriateness of work restrictions or accommodations, and the timing of return to work.

- Validation of impairment ratings. These are often incorrectly calculated.
- Opinion about causation, based on the scientific literature, to a reasonable degree of medical probability (more probable than not). The relationship of the diagnosis to the work-related event should be defined as clearly as possible. Factors supporting correlation of the diagnosis to the work-related event should be specifically stated. The frequently used statement, "in the absence of other factors, the complaint is related to work," has no scientific basis and is therefore unacceptable.
- Opinion about apportionment of causation or disability among various factors, including prior impairment or concurrent medical conditions. Apportionment is state or jurisdiction specific. When a permanent impairment results from adding or combining a prior impairment with the existing impairment from the industrial accident, then the permanent impairment is apportioned between the current injury and the prior impairment condition(s).
- Determination of whether the current medical problem is an exacerbation (flare-up of symptoms) of a preexisting or comorbid condition or an aggravation (ongoing worsening) of such a condition, based on high-grade scientific evidence.
- Determination of achievement of MMI, and functional status. MMI, medical stability, or fixed state of recovery refers to a date when the period of healing has ended and the examinee's impairment rating is not expected to materially improve or deteriorate as a result of further medical treatment. MMI should not preclude the provision of necessary maintenance care. The date of medical stability and the date when the examinee qualifies for an impairment rating do not have to be the same. The definition and timing of MMI is often state or jurisdiction specific. Evaluators should be familiar with the definition of the jurisdiction in which they are working.
- Opinion about current work capability and, if requested, the current objective functional capacity of the examinee. The examiner is responsible for determining whether the impairment results in functional limitations and to inform the examinee and the employer about the examinee's abilities and limitations. The physician should state whether the work restrictions are based on limited capacity, risk of harm, or subjective examinee tolerance for the activity in question. The employer or claim administrator may request functional ability evaluations, also known as functional capacity evaluations, to further assess current work capability. These assessments also may be ordered by the treating or evaluating physician, if the physician feels the information from such testing is crucial. Though functional capacity evaluations (FCEs) are widely used and promoted, it is important for physicians and others to understand the limitations and pitfalls of these evaluations. Functional capacity evaluations may establish physical abilities, and

also facilitate the examinee/employer relationship for return to work. However, FCEs can be deliberately simplified evaluations based on multiple assumptions and subjective factors, which are not always apparent to their requesting physician. There is little scientific evidence confirming that FCEs predict an individual's actual capacity to perform in the workplace; an FCE reflects what an individual can do on a single day, at a particular time, under controlled circumstances, that provide an indication of that individual's abilities. As with any behavior, an individual's performance on an FCE is probably influenced by multiple nonmedical factors other than physical impairments. For these reasons, it is problematic to rely solely upon the FCE results for determination of current work capability and restrictions. It is the employer's responsibility to identify and determine whether reasonable accommodations are possible to allow the examinee to perform the essential job activities.

- Opinion about prognosis (i.e., the predicted time of recovery and likelihood of recovery to achieve specified physical or functional levels), comparing the examinee's condition and recovery to date with the natural history of the disorder and consideration of workplace and psychosocial factors that may influence recovery. The relative role of each influencing factor in determining the clinical prognosis should be addressed. Reference to statistics about the median recovery time and guidelines on the period of benefit from various therapies can provide input toward the formation of an opinion about further recovery.
- Calculation or rating of permanent impairment, based on jurisdictional requirements or a consensus system such as the *American Medical Association Guides to the Evaluation of Permanent Impairment*, 5th (or latest available) edition, if called for in the state for which the examination is done. The examiner should show all calculations for later validation or replication.
- Identification, if requested, of specific effective medical treatment(s) that may be reasonably required in the future as a direct result of the industrial accident or illness.

The guidelines set forth in the bulleted paragraphs immediately above are deliberately reflective of high examination and documentation standards. It is of vital importance that the decision-making process that leads to recommendations for or against medical care be credible. Credibility requires not only that the evaluative process itself be fair, but also that in any given case the substance of the process was appropriate for that injured worker. Though a physician may believe that the attention given an injured worker in an independent medical examination was appropriate, those reviewing the report of the examination will not be able to reach the same conclusion without adequate documentation. The paragraphs above describe the documentation that reviewing tribunals frequently seek in their determination of the weight to give conflicting opinions. In a very real way, clear and complete documentation by independent medical examiners can produce substantial efficiency in the workers' compensation decision-making process. Regrettably, the absence of such documentation can hinder or completely stop the forward motion of a workers' compensation claim.

References

Able W. A system of impartial medical testimony. *J Indiana State Med Assoc.* 1966;59(4):357-8.

Adams W. *Impairment Rating Trends in the Texas Workers' Compensation System.* Austin, Texas: Research and Oversight Council on Workers' Compensation; 1999.

American Medical Association. *Guides to the Evaluation of Permanent Impairment.* 5th ed, revised. Chicago, Ill: AMA Press; 2001.

American Medical Association Council on Ethical and Judicial Affairs (CEJA) *Report: Patient-Physician Relationship in the Context of Work-Related and Independent Medical Examinations.* Issued December 1999, adopted June, 1999.

American Psychiatric Association. *Diagnostic and Statistical Manual of Mental Disorders*. 4th ed. Washington, DC: APA; 1994.

Aranoff GM, Feldman JB, Campion TS. Management of chronic pain and control of long-term disability. *Occup Med.* 2000;15:755-70.

Babitsky S, Mangraviti JJ Jr. *Understanding the AMA Guides in Workers' Compensation.* Gaithersburg, Md: Aspen Publishers, Inc.; 1997.

Bagley HM, Kniffen DC, Blackmon JG Jr, Griffeth PC. Workers' compensation. *Mercer Law Review.* Fall 1996. 48 Mercer L. Rev. 583.

Ballantyne DS, Mazingo CJ. *Measuring Dispute Resolution Outcomes—A Literature Review with Implications for Workers' Compensation.* Cambridge, Mass: Workers' Compensation Research Institute; 1999:WC-99-1.

Ballantyne DS. *Dispute Prevention and Resolution in Workers' Compensation: A National Inventory, 1997-1998.* Cambridge, Mass: Workers' Compensation Research Institute; 1998:WC-98-3.

Barth, Peter S. *Resolving Occupational Disease Claims—The Use of Medical Panels.* Cambridge, Mass: Workers' Compensation Research Institute; 1985:WC-85-1X and WC-1-85.

Baslam A, Zabin AP. *Disability Handbook.* New York, NY: McGraw-Hill; 1990.

Benoit BG, Marshall TD, Ivan LP, Forcier P, Evans KG. Legal issues in the practice of neurology and neurosurgery. *Can J Neurol Sci.* 1990;17(4):434-9.

Boden LI, Kern DE, Gardner JA. *Reducing Litigation—Using Disability Guidelines and State Evaluations in Oregon.* Cambridge, Mass: Workers' Compensation Research Institute; 1991:WC-91-3.

Boden LI. *Permanent Partial Disability in Tennessee: Similar Benefits for Similar Injuries?* Cambridge, Mass: Workers' Compensation Research Institute; 1997:WC-97-5.

Boden LI. *Use of Medical Evidence—Low-Back Permanent Partial Disability Claims in Maryland.* Cambridge, Mass: Workers' Compensation Research Institute; 1986:SP-86-1.

Boden LI. *Use of Medical Evidence—Low-Back Permanent Partial Disability Claims in New Jersey.* Cambridge, Mass: Workers' Compensation Research Institute; 1987:WC-87-2.

Boynton B. Independent medical examinations. Analyzing IME reports for workers compensation cases. *National Medico-legal J.* 1996;7:1,6-7.

Brigham CR, Ensalada LH. Perfecting the IME process: evaluation. *The Guides Newsletter.* March/April 2001:9-12.

Brigham CR. Perfecting the IME process. *The Guides Newsletter.* September/October 2000:6-7.

Brigham CR, Ensalada LH. Nonorganic findings. *The Guides Newsletter.* July/August 2000:4-8.

Brigham CR. Recommended reading list for impairment evaluation. *The Guides Newsletter*, May/June 2000;7-8.

Brigham CR, Babitsky S. Independent medical evaluations and impairment ratings. *Occup Med.* 1998;325-44.

Brigham CR. *The Comprehensive IME System.* Falmouth, Mass: SEAK, Inc; 1997.

Brigham CR, Babitsky S, Mangraviti JJ. *The Independent Medical Examination Report: A Step-by-Step Guide with Models.* Falmouth, Mass: SEAK, Inc; 1996.

Brigham CR. *How to Perform an Excellent Independent Medical Evaluation.* Falmouth, Mass: SEAK, Inc. Medical and Legal Information Systems; 1994.

Brigham CR, Boucher W, Engelberg AL. The independent medical evaluation. In: McCunney RJ, ed. *A Practical Approach to Occupational and Environmental Medicine.* 3rd ed. Philadelphia, Pa: Lippincott, Williams and Wilkins; 2003:86-96.

Brigham CR, Babitsky S. Independent medical evaluations and impairment ratings. *Occup Med STARS.* 1998;13(2):325-43.

Bunn WB, Johnson CL. Causation in workers' compensation. *Occup Med.* 1996; 11:113-20.

Campbell DC, Russell S. *The Texas Workers' Compensation Impairment Rating System: Variations and Features.* Austin, Texas: Research and Oversight Council on Workers' Compensation; 2000.

Canadian Medical Association. *The Physician's Role in Helping Patients Return to Work after an Illness or Injury.* (www.cma.ca/inside/policybase1997/3-1.htm). Ottawa, Ont: Canadian Medical Association; 1997.

Carnathan ST. Due process and the independent medical examiner system in the Maine Workers' Compensation Act. *Maine Law Review.* Fall/Winter 1993.45 Me. L. Rev. 123.

Chibnall JT, Tait RC, Merys SC. Disability management of low back injuries by employer-retained physicians: ratings and costs. *Am J Ind Med.* 2000;38:529-38.

Clark WL, Haldeman S, Johnson P, et al. Back impairment and disability determination. *Spine.* 1988;13(3):332-41.

Clark W, Haldeman S. The development of guideline factors for the evaluation of disability in neck and back injuries. *Spine.* 1993;18(13): 1736-45.

Colledge AL, Holmes EB, Soo Hoo R , Johns RE Jr, Kuhnlein J, DeBerard, S. Motivation determination (sincerity of effort): the performance APGAR model. *Dis Med.* 2001;1(2).

Colledge AL, Sewell J, Holbrook B. Impairment ratings in Utah, reduction of variability and litigation within workers' compensation: *Dis Med.* 2001;1(1).

Colledge AL, Johns RE Jr, Thomas MH, et al. Functional ability assessment: guidelines for the workplace. *J Occup Environ Med.* 1999;41(3):172-80.

Colledge AL, Johns RE Jr. Unified fitness report for the workplace. *Occup Med.* 2000;15:723-37.

Cox RAF, Edwards FC, Palmer K. *Fitness for Work: The Medical Aspects.* 3rd ed. Oxford: Oxford University Press; 2000.

Cumming GR. The independent medical examination: cardiology assessment. *Can J Cardiol.* 1996;12(12):1245-52.

Demeter SL. Disability evaluation. *Occup Med.* 1998;13:315-24.

Demeter SL, Andersson GBJ, Smith GM. *Disability Evaluation.* St. Louis, Mo: Mosby; 1996.

Department of Labor and Industries. *Your Independent Medical Exam.* (www.wa.gov/lni/pub/i245-224-00.htm) Olympia, Wash: State of Washington, Department of Labor and Industries; 2000.

Department of Labor and Industries. *Independent Medical Examinations. Report to the Legislature in Accordance with RCW 51.32.116.* Olympia, Wash: State of Washington, Department of Labor and Industries; 1998.

Doege TC, ed. *Guide to the Evaluation of Permanent Impairment.* 4th ed. Chicago, Ill: American Medical Association Press, 1994.

Doyle RL. *Healthcare Management Guidelines: Volume 2: Return to Work Planning.* New York, NY: Milliman & Robertson; 1991.

Drury DL, Vasudevan SV. Denied worker's compensation claims: what physicians can and cannot do. *WMJ.* 1998;97(11):20-2.

Eccleston SE, Yeager CM. *Managed Care and Medical Cost Containment in Workers' Compensation—A National Inventory, 1997-1998.* Cambridge, Mass: Workers' Compensation Research Institute; 1997:WC-97-6.

Ellis T. Multistate analysis. *Occup Health Safety.* April 1, 1999. www.ohsonline.com.

Employer Consultants—Consultation Services. *Doctor's Desk Reference on Early Return to Work for Injured Workers.* Seattle, Wash: Department of Labor and Industries, Region 2; 1995.

Engelberg AL. Disability and workers compensation. *Primary Care.* 1994;21:275-89.

Ensalada LH. The importance of illness behavior in disability management. *Occup Med.* 2000;15:739-54.

Fraser TM. *Fitness for Work.* Washington, DC: Taylor & Francis; 1992.

Gardner JA, Telles CA, Moss GA. *The 1991 Reforms in Massachusetts: An Assessment of Impact.* Cambridge, Mass: Workers' Compensation Research Institute; 1996:WC-96-3.

Geiringer SR. Evaluation and reporting requirements of the disability examiner. *Physical Med Rehabil Clin N Am.* 2001;12(3):543-57.

Gold JA. The occupational physician as expert witness. *Occup Med.* 1996;11:145-52.

Grace T. *Independent Medical Evaluations.* Rosemont, Ill: American Academy of Orthopaedic Surgery; 2001.

Grant D. Independent medical examinations and the fuzzy politics of disclosure. *CMAJ.* 1997;156(1):73-5.

Greenwood JG. Low-back impairment-rating practices of orthopedic surgeons and neurosurgeons in West Virginia. *Spine.* 1985;10:773-6.

Guidotti TL. Evidence-based medical dispute resolution in workers' compensation. *Occup. Med.* 1998;13:289-302.

Guidotti TL. Applying epidemiology to adjudication. *Occup Med.* 1998; 13:303-14.

Hadler NM. Criteria for screening workers for the establishment of disability. *J Occup Med.* 1986;28(10):940-5.

Hadler NM, Bunn WB. *Occupational Problems in Medical Practice.* New York, NY: Medical Publications; 1990.

Hansen J. Scientific decision-making in workers' compensation: a long overdue reform. *Southern Calif Law Rev.* 1986;59 S. Cal. L. Rev. 911.

Hardberger P. Texas workers' compensation: a ten-year survey—strengths, weaknesses, and recommendations. *St. Mary's Law J.* 2000. 32 St. Mary's L. J. 1.

Harris JS. Development, use and evaluation of clinical practice guidelines. *J Occup Environ Med.* 1997;39(1):23-34.

Harte D, Smith DA. Workers' compensation appeals systems in Canada and the United States. *Occup Med.* 1998;13(2):423-7.

Hayman FE. Toward making IMEs independent: balancing the source of work. *Pain Res Manage.* 2001;6(1):13-4.

Himmelstein JS. Worker fitness and risk evaluations in context. In: Himmelstein JS, Pransky GS, eds. *Worker Fitness and Risk Evaluations. Occup Med State Art Rev.* 1988;3:169.

Isernhagen SJ. Contemporary issues in functional capacity evaluation. In: Isernhagen SJ, ed. *The Comprehensive Guide to Work Injury Management.* Gaithersburg, Md: Aspen; 1995.

Joseph GP. Less than "certain" medical testimony. *Med Trial Technol.* 1978:25;10-20.

Kizer D. *Amended QME Regulations as Approved by the Office of Administrative Law.* South San Francisco, Calif: Industrial Medical Council; 2000.

Kizer D. *Sanction Guidelines for Qualified Medical Evaluators.* South San Francisco, Calif: Industrial Medical Council; 2000.

Kizer D, Searcy A, Lum JB, eds. *Industrial Medical Council Physician's Guide: Medical Practice in the California Worker's Compensation System.* 2nd ed. South San Francisco, Calif: Industrial Medical Council; 1997.

Klein Z. Applying assessment skills to analyzing medical-related cases. *National Medico-legal J.* 1997;8:3.

Kraus J. The independent medical examination and the functional capacity evaluation. *Occup Med.* 1997;12(3):525-56.

Luck JV, Florence DW. A brief history and comparative analysis of disability systems and impairment rating guides. *Orthop Clin North Am.* 1988;19(4):839-44.

Mayer TG, Gatchel RJ, Polatin PB. *Occupational Musculoskeletal Disorders: Function, Outcome and Evidence.* Philadelphia, Pa: Lippincott, Williams and Wilkins; 2000.

McGraw R, Ranavaya MI. Editorial: Perils of being an independent medical examiner: *Dis Med.* 2002;2(2).

Miller TR. *Evaluating Orthopedic Disability—A Commonsense Approach.* 2nd ed. Oradell, NJ: Medical Economics Books; 1987.

Moon SD, Sauter SL. *Beyond Biomechanics: Psychosocial Aspects of Musculoskeletal Disorders in Office Work.* Bristol, Pa: Taylor and Francis; 1996.

National Council of State Legislatures. *State of Workers' Compensation.* www.ncsl.org/public/cataglog/3302IN.htm.

Neuhauser F. *Report on the Quality of Treating Physician Reports and Cost-Benefit of Presumption in Favor of the Treating Physician.* San Francisco, Calif: Commission on Health, Safety and Workers' Compensation; 2000.

Nordin M, Andersson GBH, Pope M. *Musculoskeletal Disorders in the Workplace: Principles and Practice.* St. Louis, Mo: Mosby; 1997.

North DA, Higdon KM. Landmark survey: best practices in integrated disability management. *J Workers Comp.* 1998;7(2):9-26.

Pease SR. *Performance Indicators for Permanent Disability—Low Back Injuries in Texas.* Cambridge, Mass: Workers' Compensation Research Institute; 1988:WC-88-4.

Pease SR. *Performance Indicators for Permanent Disability—Low Back Injuries in Wisconsin.* Cambridge, Mass: Workers' Compensation Research Institute; 1987:WC-87-4.

Pease SR. *Performance Indicators for Permanent Disability—Low-Back Injuries in New Jersey.* Cambridge, Mass: Workers' Compensation Research Institute; 1987:WC-87-5.

Petersen DD. General Mills case study: the critical steps in managing workers compensation costs. *J Workers Comp.* 1994;3(3):22-30.

Peterson KW. The Americans with Disabilities Act. In: McCunney RJ, ed. *A Practical Approach to Occupational and Environmental Medicine.* Boston, Mass: Little, Brown and Company, 1994.

Pierce AS. The IME: what's in an acronym? *J Workers Comp.* 1998;8(1):28-35.

Proctor T, Gatchel RJ, Robinson RC. Psychosocial factors and risk of pain and disability. *Occup Med.* 2000;15:803-12.

Pryor ES. Flawed promises: a critical evaluation of the American Medical Association's "guides to the evaluation of permanent impairment." *Harv Law Rev.* 1990;103:964.

Pye H, Orris P. Workers' compensation in the United States and the role of the primary care physician. *Prim Care.* 2000;27(4):831-44.

Ranavaya MI, Talmadge JB. AMA guides to the evaluation of permanent impairment: what's new in the 5th edition? *Disability Med.* 2001;1(1).

Ranavaya MI, Ambroz A, Ambroz, C. The independent medical examinations: are they really needed? *Disability Med.* 2001;1(1).

Ransford AO, Cairns D, Mooney V. The pain drawing as an aid to the psychologic evaluation of patients with low-back pain. *Spine.* 1978;1(2):127-34.

Reiso H, Nygard JF, Brage S, Gulbrandesen P, Tellnes G. Work ability assessed by patients and their GPs in new episodes of sickness certification. (Norway). *Fam Pract.* 2000;17(2):139-44.

Rogers R. *Clinical Assessment of Malingering and Deception.* New York, NY: Guilford Press; 1988.

Rondinelli RD, Katz RT. *Impairment Rating and Disability Evaluation.* Philadelphia, Pa: WB Saunders; 2000.

Sandler HM. Trends in occupational and environmental disease claims. *J Workers Comp.* 1993;2(2):21-6.

Schulman B, Schwartz S, Boyle P. *Workers' Compensation/Occupational Health National Trends Study.* Seattle, Wash: University of Washington Department of Health Services; 1997.

Simon RI. The credible forensic psychiatric evaluation in multiple chemical sensitivity litigation. *J Am Acad Psychiatry Law.* 1998;26(3):361-74.

Smith GL. *How to Write a Winning Workers' Compensation Report: A Programmed Text.* Beverly Farms, Mass: OEM Press; 1995.

Snyder JW, Maier JC, Love BD, et al. Injury and causation on trial: the phenomenon of "multiple chemical sensitivities." *Widener Law Symp J.* 1997:2.

Social Security Administration. *Disability Evaluation under Social Security.* Washington, DC: US Department of Health and Human Services; Social Security Administration; 1986.

Soderstrom E, Stewart J. Adjudicating claims. *Occup Med.* 1998;13:273-8.

Solomon DF. Medical expert testimony in administrative hearings. *J Natl Assoc Admin Law Judges.* 1997.

Spieler EA, Barth PS, Burton JF Jr, Himmelstein J, Rudolph L. Recommendations to guide revision of the AMA guides to the evaluation of permanent impairment. *JAMA.* 2000;283:532-3.

Talmadge JB. Assessment and management of upper and lower extremity impairment and disability. *Occup Med.* 2000;15:771-88.

Telles CA, Fox SE. *Revisiting Workers' Compensation in Washington—Administrative Inventory.* Cambridge, Mass: Workers' Compensation Research Institute; 1996:WC-96-10.

Telles CA, Fox SE. *Workers' Compensation in Colorado—Administrative Inventory.* Cambridge, Mass: Workers' Compensation Research Institute; 1996:WC-96-8.

Telles CA, Shiman L. *Revisiting Workers' Compensation in Minnesota—*

Administrative Inventory. Cambridge, Mass: Workers' Compensation Research Institute; 1997:WC-97-3.

Texas Workers' Compensation Commission and Research and Oversight Council on Workers' Compensation. *An Analysis of Texas Workers with Permanent Impairments.* Austin, Texas: Research and Oversight Council on Workers' Compensation; 1996.

Turk DC. Evaluation of pain and disability. *J Disability.* 1991;2:24-33.

Turk DC, Melzack R. *Handbook of Pain Assessment.* New York, NY: Guilford Press; 1992.

UC Data. *Evaluating the Reforms of the Medical-Legal Process Using the WCIRB Permanent Disability Survey.* San Francisco, Calif: California Commission on Health and Safety and Workers' Compensation; 1997.

US Chamber of Commerce. *Analysis of Workers' Compensation Laws.* Washington, DC: US Chamber of Commerce; 2000.

Vasudevan SV, Drury DL. The independent medical examination: purpose and process. *WMJ.* 1999;98(2):10-12.

Welch EM. Independent medical exams. In: *Materials for Michigan State Claims Adjuster Course.* East Lansing: Michigan State University; 2000.

Wise LM. Ethical considerations for the IME. *Chiropractic J.* 1999. www.worldchiropracticalliance.org/tcj/199/sep/sep1999viewpoint.htm

*Appendix: Review of the Use and Attributes of Excellent Independent Medical Examinations**

According to the literature reviewed, IMEs have at least four accepted purposes. To be most effective in accomplishing these, IMEs must be complete, focused, rigorously and clearly reasoned, and impartial and must supply the information needed by persons requesting them.

Provision of Information for Adjudication of Workers' Compensation Claims

First, IMEs are intended to provide specific, relevant, and impartial information to guide adjudication of workers' compensation claims when required information has not been made available by other means or when existing information is believed to be inaccurate. Claims adjusters may use IMEs to provide guidance on entitlement issues such as the work relatedness of a medical condition, the need for further medical or income benefits, and the nature and extent of permanent impairments.

Guidance in Managing Medical Care, Disability, and Rehabilitation

Second, IMEs may be used to guide management of medical care, disability, and rehabilitation when the claims adjuster is concerned that the care may be inadequate or inappropriate or that return to work is unreasonably delayed. Case managers and rehabilitation specialists may need clarification of the diagnosis, appropriateness of treatment, or need for work modifications or absence. IMEs may also be used to elicit hitherto unknown facts in particular situations or to uncover reasons for delayed functional recovery. While an IME is not the preferred method for obtaining basic medical information, it can be an invaluable aid when a claims adjuster has questions and needs expert corroboration or guidance. This is particularly true when the health problem is unusual or the nature of, or need for, the proposed treatment is controversial.

*Reprinted with permission from *The OEM Report*, April and May, 2003. Copyright © 2003 OEM Health Information, Beverly Farms, Massachusetts.

The authors of this study—part of the Project to Improve the Quality of Independent Medical Examinations produced in 2002 under contract with the Washington Department of Labor and Industries—surveyed the literature and state regulations; interviewed workers' compensation officials, insurance personnel, and recognized experts on independent medical examinations; and synthesized the results. They found substantial consensus about best practices in the conduct and content of independent medical examinations (IMEs). These findings are also applicable to many consultations for work-related health problems.

Provision of Information for Compliance with Requirements of the Claims Adjustment Adjudication Process

IMEs may also be used to provide technical data and written opinions in order to comply with requirements of the claims adjudication process or to move even an uncontested claim to the next step. Statutes, regulations, organizational policies, or tradition often consider obtaining a signed doctor's report a pre-condition to moving to the next step—for example, work release, closing examination, MMI findings, or impairment rating. IMEs may provide these data if they are not provided by the treating physician.

Serving as a Source of Expert Medical Opinions

IMEs can be a source of expert medical opinions on issues of diagnosis, causality, treatment, or impairment for defense or claimants' attorneys and workers' compensation commissioners or judges. Attorneys, adjusters, and judges are generally seeking information to clarify a disputed point. In many states, the IME itself is not admissible evidence in a court of law; rather, the testimony of the examiner is the admissible evidence. The written report is considered hearsay unless both parties agree to the contrary or the administrative law judge allows the report to be entered into evidence (for example, in Kentucky).

Legal and Regulatory Requirements

Each state has legal and regulatory provisions governing the collection and use of medical information, the circumstances under which IMEs may be obtained, and the qualifications and selection process for medical examiners. In most states, the workers' compensation board is allowed to order physical examination of a claimant by a physician of its choice, and the insurer or employer is also allowed to order a physical examination of a claimant by a physician of its choice.

Some states allow IMEs to be conducted at the discretion of the employer or insurer or "as needed" (for example, Alaska). The majority of states allow IMEs to resolve disputes, especially those regarding treatment, the nature of the injury, and disability (for example, Arizona). Some states use IMEs primarily for permanent partial disability ratings (for example, Iowa). In other states, a hearing is required before the workers' compensation board can order an IME (for example, Hawaii).

Appropriate IME Issues by Phase of Claim

The best practice for obtaining and using an IME is linked to the phase of the claim. At a claim's inception, appropriate issues to evaluate include causality and diagnosis. In general, the study's interviewees felt that it is not necessary to obtain an IME to confirm a diagnosis in a new claim, unless fraud or malingering is suspected. An IME is sometimes obtained if the treating physician records an unusual or serious diagnosis. An accurate diagnosis is needed to correlate the existing injury or disease entity with studies linking it to occupational exposure.

During the course of the claim, an IME may be used to evaluate testing and treatment appropriateness or disability management. The best practice in cases of protracted treatment is to obtain an IME promptly after the recommended duration of care is declared if such duration exceeds that stated in the respective evidence-based guidelines or if the reasons that the case is different or unique are not available elsewhere. Many insurers obtain IMEs if there is prolonged or apparently ineffective treatment. The best practice in using IMEs to manage delayed recovery is contingent on the availability of information and the time at which it is available. If the necessary information is not available from the attending physician, the suggested best practice is to obtain an IME as soon as time-based benchmarks for return to function for the given diagnosis and treatment program are exceeded.

At closure of a claim, an IME is appropriate to obtain an opinion on maximal medical improvement (MMI), an assessment of impairment rating, and/or prediction of future medical needs if the information from the attending (AP) physician is not available, is felt to be biased or inaccurate, or is needed to resolve a dispute. If the claimant appears to be at maximal medical improvement, but the attending physician does not agree with this assessment, an IME may be appropriate.

Most states require an impairment assessment or rating at the conclusion of the claim if the AP states that the claimant has not recovered to a degree equivalent to his or her pre-injury status. In most states there is a treating physician presumption (official or unofficial), making the AP physician the preferred initial source of information. The best practice is to obtain an IME only if the AP declines to evaluate or rate the patient. Not all states require that the AP perform the rating calculations.

Requests for IMEs

Ideally, requests for IMEs include questions tailored to and addressing the specific issues or problems that are unclear or in dispute. Participants strongly recommend that the requestor include a detailed narrative summary of the case to date.

Choice of Examiner

The ideal method for selecting an examiner assures that the one chosen fits the needs of the evaluation. Different parties have different views of these needs, but a number of medical journal articles emphasize that the examiner must not only have medical expertise but also knowledge of IME methodology and report-writing skills.

Qualifications of Examiner

The examiner should be well trained and knowledgeable about the body systems and health problems that the injured worker appears to have and should know how to elicit and interpret key symptoms and signs. For example, if the worker complains of low back pain, the examiner should be knowledgeable about the anatomy and physiology of both the musculoskeletal and nervous systems as well as the diagnosis of disorders of the low back.

If causation is an issue, the examiner should be able to assess work and home exposure to ergonomic factors, chemicals, and other sources of work-related health problems. In addition, if asked to assess health issues other than evident direct trauma, the examiner should have a thorough knowledge of the evidence linking exposures and adverse health effects.

Good communication—that is, interpersonal and language skills—is a crucial component of the required skill set for conducting IMEs. Because the results of an IME may affect the worker's ability to obtain financially desired or needed benefits, the examination may be a threatening experience to the examinee. Furthermore, not all examinees are good "historians" without careful questioning and interpretation. One of examinees' main complaints about IMEs is examiners' failure to listen or to cover points that are important to the examinee.

The examiner should be cognizant of the evidence supporting effective and efficient therapies and self-care of all kinds, whether physical, pharmacological, or surgical. The examiner should also be aware of the limitations as well as the efficacy of many commonly used tests and treatments. Even normally effective treatments lose their efficacy in treating an individual after a period of time or may have negative effects if unnecessarily prolonged. Pharmacological therapy and physical medicine, in particular, fall into this category.

Having a balanced health care perspective is important for medical examiners. Placing precedence on surgical therapy rather than other forms of therapy may prevent the examiner from considering the best treatment for the patient's circumstances. Many of the factors that delay functional recovery and return to work are not purely physical.

To rate permanent impairment, examiners must be familiar with the use of the often complex rating systems used in their particular jurisdiction.

The examiner must be skilled in applying medical logic to the data acquired in order to validate the diagnosis, suggest specific additional testing, affirm or recommend changes in treatment, and reach reasonable conclusions about causation, impairment, and ability of the examinee to work. Without this skill, and the ability to convey the steps in the analysis to the reader, the value of the data acquired will be largely unrealized. Knowledge and skill in answering the types of questions they are typically asked by insurers, employers' attorneys, judges, and regulators is also essential for independent medical examiners.

An experienced and skilled examiner will maintain a neutral point of view as a medical expert and will thus render opinions consistent with the case and the evidence for causation, test and treatment effectiveness, and the reproducibility of impairment assessment. A competent examiner will not issue "boilerplate" reports (that are generic rather than specific in nature) or use a preconceived framework based on a pro-business or pro-labor philosophy rather than the objective facts of each case. The examiner should be able to render an opinion that is "impartial, unbiased, and objective" and should be able to clearly differentiate between facts and opinions. Third parties often consider it difficult for treating physicians to achieve this level of objectivity, especially in circumstances in which some sort of dispute concerning the patient is involved.

As previously mentioned, in many jurisdictions written IME reports per se are not admissible in legal disputes. Therefore, another important skill required of medical examiners is the ability to testify clearly, logically, and in an informed manner on the issues and facts of the case in a deposition or hearing. When testifying, the examiner should be able to assimilate contradictory information and consider it reasonably, even if it changes his or her prior opinion.

One indication of an examiner's training and skill is board certification in the area of inquiry. Another is Board Certification in Independent Medical Examination by the American Board of Independent Medical Examiners. While these certifications represent assurance of competence in the two key areas previously discussed, they may not be specific enough as a quality control mechanism. Several states have regulatory qualifications for medical experts. In New Jersey, for example, a medical expert is one who performs 25 or more workers' compensation exams per year.

Process and Content of High-quality IMEs

There is a clear consensus among published sources about the process that should be followed and the content to be collected or analyzed in conducting a fair, impartial, responsive, and complete IME. There is a fairly uniform process for the sequence and conduct of the examination summarized in the texts and articles reviewed but no statutory or regulatory requirements for the process or content of the written IME report itself.

The American Board of Independent Medical Examiners, the American Academy of Disability Evaluating Physicians, and the California Industrial Medical Commission have published lists of the items that should be present in an independent medical examination report. These lists contain similar items to those subsequently discussed in this article.

The consensus view starts with the conduct of the examiner. It includes a specific list of explanations, disclosures, and consents that should be made, or obtained and then recorded as "done" in the examination report. It also includes recommended behaviors for the examiner. Failure to behave in the ways subsequently described in this discussion has resulted in substantial numbers of complaints to state regulatory authorities and funds, and has been raised as an issue in our survey of injured workers who underwent IMEs.

Provision of Records for Review

Best practice dictates that all pertinent and available prior medical records accompany a request for an IME. These should be arranged in chronological order, with duplicates removed. Before the IME appointment, careful selection, duplication, assembly, and preparation of the file is key so that the examiner does not waste time fumbling through paper and can efficiently develop a solid understanding of the background and facts in the case as a basis for opinion. It is most useful to put all records in a single file but group them by type, i.e., clinic records, imaging reports, operative reports, and so on.

The examiner's ability to formulate a fresh opinion is reduced if he/she must rely on others' interpretations of the primary data. For example, when an IME has been ordered to clarify a diagnosis or evaluate adequacy of treatment, the ready availability of certain primary source documents is key—that is, all test results, surgical notes, and radiographic films. Likewise, if the examiner is to consider causality, details of the accident from the employer's or insurer's injury investigation along with medical records from the initial medical visit and acute injury care period provide the best historical source of "clues" as to causality.

Conduct of the Examination

Explanation and Consent

At the beginning of the examination, the examiner should clearly establish his or her identity and explain the purpose, nature, and scope of the examination. The examiner should inform the examinee that he or she has no relationship with the current attending (treating) physician. The nature of the IME precludes establishing a doctor-patient relationship or doctor-patient privilege. It follows that the examiner will not provide treatment to the injured worker as part of the examination or subsequent to it, except if specifically permitted by state statute or regulation. The examiner should obtain specific consent for the examination, as well as authorization to release the report if required in that state. Completion of all of the above procedural steps should be documented in the IME report.

Examiner Communication

The available literature recommends that the examiner establish rapport with the examinee to help ensure obtaining a complete and accurate history of exposures, the injury or illness, related issues, and factors that could affect functional recovery. One effective starting point is to have the examinee fill out a structured questionnaire before the examination, and then review it with the examinee.

Published sources also suggest that the examiner listen carefully, respectfully, and objectively to the examinee. They recommend that the examiner paraphrase the history back to the examinee to ensure that it is correct. In the most extensive, complex cases, several sources suggest that the examiner dictate at least the history and examination parts of the report in the presence of the examinee to ensure his/her agreement with the recorded history and physical findings.

The examiner should tell the examinee that the examination is not intended to be uncomfortable and ask to be informed immediately if a maneuver causes pain or discomfort. By extension, the examiner should perform maneuvers carefully and record limitations in the examination caused by the examinee's discomfort.

Historical Information

PAST RECORDS

The sources reviewed recommend reviewing past records of office visits, test results, physical medicine notes, surgical procedures, and scales and inventories in chronological order. It is important that the examiner have all pertinent records and that they be well arranged and easy to review.

The examiner should review primary records and not rely exclusively on summaries prepared by others. There are two views about when to do this. The predominant view is that it is preferable to review the materials prior to the examination in order to identify areas that require clarification during the history and allow the examiner to focus particular attention on key areas during the physical examination. Alternatively, to avoid creating any preconceptions during the history, the examiner can review the materials after the examinee leaves. The danger of this approach is that there may be no opportunity to clarify issues and inconsistencies directly with the examinee.

The examiner should also review past test reports and results such as radiographic or EMG findings directly. In workers' compensation cases, relevant tests in workers' compensation might include plain-film radiography, other imaging studies, electrophysiologic tests, laboratory tests, symptom inventories, functional capacity evaluations, and neuropsychological testing. The reviewer should note any questions he or she might have, as well as inconsistencies between or among tests or test interpretations and the history and physical examination.

The output of this review should be a summary of diagnoses, treatment to date, and progress toward functional recovery. It should also lead to an analysis of prior causal attribution, exposures or mechanism of injury, and the appropriateness and effectiveness of prior testing, treatment, and disability management, including time off work.

MEDICAL AND OCCUPATIONAL HISTORY

The first task in taking a history for an IME is to identify the examinee's current primary concern as well as other issues of concern to the examinee. These issues may or may not include the chief complaint, which also should be elicited.

The examiner should then explore the examinee's pre-injury status, including pre-existing conditions, previous injuries, and the examinee's pre-injury perceived functional status (the effects of pre-existing or previous injuries or conditions, which may be asymptomatic). The examinee's history of work absence prior to the current health problem should also be explored.

Particularly when the issue in question is causality, the examiner should review the examinee's occupational history for all jobs prior to the current complaint. The review should include work tasks, exposures, and protection such as engineering controls, personal protective equipment, and ergonomic practices. Nonoccupational exposures should be sought as well. It is often helpful to review mutually derived job descriptions agreed to by the worker and the supervisor, view videotapes of actual job tasks, review ergonomic evaluations of the worker's workstation or review, and summarize exposure monitoring data to quantify exposure.

In cases in which there is delayed return to work or persistent complaints out of proportion to the apparent illness or injury, the examiner should explore the examinee's task and job satisfaction as well as work relationships with co-workers and supervisors.

HISTORY OF PRESENT ILLNESS

Next, the examiner should elicit information about the mechanism of injury or illness. It is also helpful, particularly in cases of delayed return to work, to explore the worker's perceptions about the causation of the health problem and fault for the causative factor.

After ascertaining the mechanism of injury, the examiner should obtain information about the examinee's symptoms at the time of the injury or illness as well as progression of symptoms to date. This line of questioning should culminate with inquiry into the worker's current symptoms and functional limitations.

Part of the history to be assembled and assessed by the examiner is the treatment history and response to treatment, particularly if the questions posed in the IME request relate to treatment effectiveness or recommendations. Other key elements are the worker's disability history, functional and physician-imposed work restrictions, and effects on social function. The disability history reflects a combination of treatment effectiveness, health beliefs, and psychosocial factors.

PAIN AND SYMPTOM INVENTORIES

The review showed that medical experts emphasize the need to uncover psychological and behavioral components of an illness or injury episode because they believe that these problems must be acknowledged and addressed in order to facilitate functional recovery and return to work. (Employer and insurer materials were silent in this arena, presumably out of a presumed concern for possible complications of claim management.) Many jurisdictions no longer allow the question of pain to enter into rating systems, because of its subjectivity and susceptibility to distortion in response to system incentives.

Symptom inventories and drawings can provide a semi-quantitative measurement that can be scored against population norms. They are often useful to provide another view of the patient's level of symptoms and his or her perceived impairment. For states such as California that rate impairment caused by pain, pain scales, maps, and descriptions are also useful as direct sources of pain levels, locations, character, and frequency. Instruments for rating pain impairment include pain drawings, analog pain scales, and pain inventories. Personality inventories may be useful to understand some symptoms, the intensity and chronicity of symptoms, and absence from work. Depression scales are an effective way to identify and quantify depression, which may be the cause of delayed return to work or may be a result of loss of function or work status. When using inventories and scales, it is important to ensure accurate grading and interpretation.

SPECIAL DETAILED HISTORY FOR CASES WITH SEVERE PAIN COMPLAINTS IN EXCESS OF OBJECTIVE FINDINGS

For cases in which pain symptoms are impeding functional recovery, there is the possibility of symptom magnification, or there are questions about the need for future treatment or vocational rehabilitation, a focused history to identify circumstances that predispose patients to symptom magnification or the development of chronic pain syndromes may prove useful in answering these questions or guiding effective future treatment. A number of jurisdictions do not rate impairments attributed to pain. This discussion was directed at clarifying symptom "drivers," maximal medical improvement, and appropriate therapy.

Physical Examination

After collection of historical data that supports the focused inquiry called for by the person requesting the examination, which generally includes much or most of the information discussed above, the examiner should carefully perform a similarly focused physical examination, taking care not to cause discomfort for the examinee. If necessary, the examiner should note whenever a maneuver is terminated because of complaints of pain or discomfort.

The examination should focus on the area of injury, including related areas (e.g., the cervical spine in cases involving some upper extremity neurological complaints or the contralateral side in cases involving atrophy, deformity, or joint motion). The examination should be complete but focused and relevant. In the general assessment, the examiner should note habitus, gait, station, appearance, and affect, as well as the presence of assistive devices, stimulators, braces, and so on. In cases involving presumed nerve or nerve root compression, a complete neurological examination of the affected area and related areas is mandatory. Use of physical maneuvers alone to make these diagnoses is inadequate.

The IME report should include relevant measurements, bilaterally if possible. It should include all pertinent positives and negatives as well as the examinee's response to the examination and nonphysiologic findings such as Waddell's signs. Any symptom magnification should be noted. More specifics on the examination of various body areas can be found in the ACOEM *Occupational Medicine Practice Guidelines*, the AMA *Guides to the Evaluation of Permanent Impairment*, and medical texts.

Further Data

If clarification of the situation is necessary, which generally occurs in cases in which appropriate specialty evaluation or tests have not yet been obtained, the examiner may order or request specialty consultations or testing. Needed tests might include imaging, electrophysiological tests, inventories, functional capacity evaluations or neuropsychological testing, depending on the circumstances, the issue at hand, and the appropriateness and quality of previous tests.

Analysis and Report Content

A careful analysis of the past history, the history of the present illness or injury, the work history, tests results, and the physical examination (as a group of data) should yield answers to the questions posed or reveal the need for further consultation or testing. First, the examiner should analyze past records from all treaters and testers, in chronological order, for diagnostic accuracy, test appropriateness and findings, treatment appropriateness and effectiveness, the appropriateness of work restrictions or accommodations, and the timing of return to work. The examiner should also validate impairment ratings—they are often incorrectly calculated.

Next, the examiner should analyze the interpretation of past test results if qualified to do so. Again, at times, these are subject to misinterpretation. There are studies of the accuracy of test interpretation in various practice guidelines but none directly related to IMEs.

An important piece of data for accurate interpretation of the history obtained from the examinee is the examiner's assessment of his or her reliability and consistency as a historian. The examinee's cooperativeness with the examination, or lack thereof, should also be noted.

The examiner should then describe the logic, methods, and rationale for diagnoses and causality conclusions. Again, if there is evidence in the literature to support diagnosis or causality, other than obvious trauma, it should be cited. Similarly, the examiner should explain the logic used to conclude whether the worker has reached maximal medical improvement or further functional recovery can be reasonably expected.

If an impairment rating is called for, the rater should describe the method used to determine the rating and the rationale for the rating assigned. He or she should also describe the examinee's capacity for social and work functioning as it relates to the degree of physical impairment.

Making Recommendations

The consensus view is that examiners should make recommendations in response to questions posed by, or implied by, the examination request. Recommendations should be based on the available evidence, or if lacking evidence, consensus views of what is effective (with benefits outweighing risks). Such recommendations may include the need for further testing to define the condition in question, either to further the analysis of causation or to clarify the diagnosis. Recommendations may also be called for regarding further treatment, the prognosis for further improvement, physical or mental impairment, the examinee's current or future work capacity, the need for vocational rehabilitation, and the potential for employment.

Advice Given to Examinees Before Undergoing Independent Medical Examinations

A number of Web sites for injured workers have appeared in the last several years. The information provided falls into four general categories: rights and responsibilities, as determined by state workers' compensation agencies or occupational medicine organizations (for example, the Cleveland Clinic); expert medical advice in response to queries (again, the Cleveland Clinic); bad experiences with IMEs or the perceived results of IMEs; and quasi-legal or legal advice on conduct at an IME.

Making a recording of the examination in one way or another (e.g., videotape) might enhance the quality of the examinations. Some advice proferred by examiners, such as for the examinee to see the attending physician immediately after the examination to get another assessment, may contribute to conflict between medical professionals, that is, the "dueling docs" syndrome. Refusal to allow testing may compromise the accuracy of the IME.

References

Administrative Code 2:235-5.10. Conduct of formal hearings: (4)(m)(1).

Brigham CR. *The Comprehensive IME System.* Falmouth, Mass: SEAK; 1997.

Brigham CR, Babitsky S, Mangraviti JJ. *The Independent Medical Examination Report: A Step-by Step Guide with Models.* Falmouth, Mass: SEAK; 1996.

Brigham CR. Perfecting the IME process. *Guides Newsletter* 2000;Sept/Oct:6-7.

Harris JS, Brigham CR. Independent medical examinations. In: Harris JS, Blais BB, Brigham CR, Kuhnen A, eds. *Management of Common Health Problems and Functional Recovery in Workers: The ACOEM Occupational Medicine Practice Guidelines.* Beverly Farms, Mass: OEM Press; 1997.

Kraus J. The independent medical examination and the functional capacity evaluation. *Occup Med.* 1997;12(4):525-56.

Pierce AS. The IME—what's in an acronym? *J Workers' Comp.* 1998;8(1):28-35.

Smith GL. *How to Write a Winning Workers' Compensation Report: A Programmed Text.* Beverly Farms, Mass: OEM Press; 1995.

Literature Reviewed

Able W. A system of impartial medical testimony. *J Indiana State Med Assoc.* 1966;59(4):357-8.

Adams W. *Impairment Rating Trends in the Texas Workers' Compensation System.* Austin, Texas: Research and Oversight Council on Workers' Compensation; 1999.

Aranoff GM, Feldman JB, Campion TS. Management of chronic pain and control of long-term disability. *Occup Med.* 2000;1(4)5:755-70.

Austin A. *Independent Medical Examination Project. Focus Group and Interview Summary Report.* Olympia, Wash: State of Washington, Department of Labor and Industries; 2000.

Babitsky S, Mangraviti JJ Jr. *Understanding the AMA Guides in Workers' Compensation.* Gaithersburg, Md: Aspen; 1997.

Bagley HM, Kiffen DC, Blackmon JG Jr, Griffeth PC. Workers' compensation. *Mercer Law Rev.* Fall 1996. 48 Mercer L Rev 583.

Ballantyne DS, Mazingo CJ. *Measuring Dispute Resolution Outcomes—A Literature Review with Implications for Workers' Compensation.* Cambridge, Mass: Workers' Compensation Research Institute; 1999:WC-99-1.

Ballantyne DS. *Dispute Prevention and Resolution in Workers' Compensation: A National Inventory, 1997-1998.* Cambridge, Mass: Workers' Compensation Research Institute; 1998:WC-98-3.

Barth PS. *Resolving Occupational Disease Claims—The Use of Medical Panels.* Cambridge, Mass: Workers' Compensation Research Institute; 1985:WC-85-1X and WC-1-85.

Baslam A, Zabin AP. *Disability Handbook.* New York, NY: McGraw-Hill; 1990.

Benoit BG, Marshall TD, Ivan LP, et al. Legal issues in the practice of neurology and neurosurgery. *Can J Neurol Sci.* 1990;17(4):434-9.

Boden LI, Kern DE, Gardner JA. *Reducing Litigation: Using Disability Guidelines and State Evaluators in Oregon.* Cambridge, Mass: Workers' Compensation Research Institute; 1991.

Boynton B. Independent medical examinations: analyzing IME reports for workers' compensation cases. *National Medico-legal J.* 1996;7:1,6-7.

Brigham CR, Ensalada LH. Perfecting the IME process: evaluation. *Guides Newsletter.* 2001;March/April:9-12.

Brigham CR. Recommended reading list for impairment evaluation. *Guides Newsletter.* 2000;May/June:7-8.

Brigham CR, Ensalada LH. Non-organic findings. *Guides Newsletter.* 2000;July/Aug: 4-8.

Brigham CR, Babitsky S. Independent medical evaluations and impairment ratings. *Occup Med* 1998;13(2):325-44.

Bunn WB 3rd, Johnson CE. Causation in workers' compensation. *Occup Med.* 1996;11(1):113-20.

Campbell DC, Russell S. *The Texas Workers' Compensation Impairment Rating System: Variations and Features.* Austin, Texas: Research and Oversight Council on Workers' Compensation; 2000.

Canadian Medical Association. *The Physician's Role in Helping Patients Return to Work after an Illness or Injury.* Ottawa, Ont: Canadian Medical Association; 1997. www.cma ca/inside/policybase 1997/3-1.htm

Carnathan ST. Due process and the independent medical examiner system in the Maine Workers' Compensation Act. *Maine Law Rev.* Fall/Winter 1993. 45 Me L Rev 123.

Chibnall JT, Tait RC, Merys SC. Disability management of low back injuries by employer-retained physicians: ratings and costs. *Am J Ind Med.* 2000;38(5):529-38.

Colledge AL, Johns RE Jr. Unified fitness report for the workplace. *Occup Med.* 2000;15(4):723-37.

Colledge AL, Johns RF Jr, Thomas MH. Functional ability assessment: guidelines for the workplace. *J Occup Environ Med.* 1999;41(3):172-80.

Cox RAF, Edwards FC, McCallum RI. *Fitness for Work: The Medical Aspects.* Oxford, England: Oxford University Press; 1995.

Cumming GR. The independent medical examination: cardiology assessment. *Can J Cardiol.* 1996;12(12):1245-52.

Demeter SL. Disability evaluation. *Occup Med.* 1998;13(2):315-23.

Demeter SL. Andersson GBJ, Smith GM. *Disability Evaluation.* St. Louis, Mo: Mosby; 1996.

Department of Labor and Industries. *Your Independent Medical Exam.* Olympia, Wash: State of Washington, Department of Labor and Industries; 2000. www.wagov/lni/pub/i245-224-00-htm.

Department of Labor and Industries. *Independent Medical Examinations: Report to the Legislature in Accordance with RCW 51.32.116.* Olympia, Wash: State of Washington, Department of Labor and Industries; 1998.

Drury DL, Vasudevan SV. Denied worker's compensation claims: what physicians can and cannot do. *WMJ.* 1998;97(11):20-2.

Eccleston SE, Yeager CM. *Managed Care and Medical Cost Containment in Workers' Compensation—A National Inventory, 1997-1998.* Cambridge, Mass: Workers' Compensation Research Institute; 1997:WC-97-6.

Ellis T. Multistate analysis. *Occup Health Safety.* April 1999. www.ohsonline.com.

Employer Consultants-Consultation Services. *Doctor's Desk Reference on Early*

Return to Work for Injured Workers. Seattle, Wash: Department of Labor and Industries, Region 2; 1995.

Engelberg AL. Disability and workers' compensation. *Prim Care.* 1994; 21(2):275-89.

Ensalada LH. The importance of illness behavior in disability management. *Occup Med.* 2000;15(4):739-54.

Fraser TM. *Fitness for Work.* Washington, DC: Taylor & Francis; 1992.

Gardner JA, Telles CA, Moss GA. *The 1991 Reforms in Massachusetts: An Assessment of Impact.* Cambridge, Mass: Workers' Compensation Research Institute; 1996:WC-96-3.

Gold JA. The occupational physician as expert witness. *Occup Med.* 1996;11(1):145-51.

Grant D. Independent medical examinations and the fuzzy politics of disclosure. *CMAJ.* 1997;156(1):73-5.

Greenwood JG. Low-back impairment-rating practices of orthopedic surgeons and neurosurgeons in West Virginia. *Spine.* 1985;10(8):773-6.

Guidotti TL. Applying epidemiology to adjudication. *Occup Med.* 1998; 13(2):303-14.

Guidotti TL. Evidence-based medical dispute resolution in workers' compensation. *Occup Med.* 1998;13(2):289-302.

Hadler NM. Criteria for screening workers for the establishment of disability. *J Occup Med.* 1986;28(10):940-5.

Hansen J. Scientific decision-making in workers' compensation: a long overdue reform. *Southern Calif Law Rev.* May 1986. 59 S. Cal. L. Rev. 911.

Hardberger P. Texas workers' compensation: a ten-year survey—strengths, weaknesses, and recommendations. *St. Mary's Law J.* 2000:32. St Mary's L J 1.

Harber P, Harris JS. Work-relatedness. In: Harris JS, Blais BB, Brigham CR, Kuhnen A, eds. *Management of Common Health Problems and Functional Recovery in Workers: The ACOEM Occupational Medicine Practice Guidelines.* Beverly Farms, Mass: OEM Press; 1997.

Harris JS. Delayed recovery. In: Harris JS, Blais BB, Brigham CR, Kuhnen A, eds. *Management of Common Health Problems and Functional Recovery in Workers: The ACOEM Occupational Medicine Practice Guidelines.* Beverly Farms, Mass: OEM Press; 1997.

Harris JS. Development, use and evaluation of clinical practice guidelines. *J Occup Environ Med.* 1997;39(1):23-34.

Harte D, Smith DA. Workers' compensation appeals systems in Canada and the United States. *Occup Med.* 1998;13(2):423-7.

Joseph GP. Less than "certain" medical testimony. *Med Trial Technol.* 1978;25:10-20.

Kizer D. *Amended QME Regulations as Approved by the Office of Administrative Law.* South San Francisco, Calif: Industrial Medical Council; 2000.

Kizer D. *Sanction Guidelines for Qualified Medical Evaluators.* South San Francisco, Calif: Industrial Medical Council; 2000.

Kizer D, Searcy A, Lum JB, eds. *Industrial Medical Council Physician's Guide: Medical Practice in the California Worker's Compensation System.* 2nd ed. South San Francisco, Calif: Industrial Medical Council; 1997.

Klein Z. Applying assessment skills to analyzing medical-related cases. *National Medico-legal J.* 1997;8:3.

Mayer TG, Gatchel RJ, Polatin PB. *Occupational Musculoskeletal Disorders: Function, Outcome and Evidence.* Philadelphia, Pa: Lippincott, Williams & Wilkins; 2000.

Miller TR. *Evaluating Orthopedic Disability—A Commonsense Approach.* 2nd ed. Oradell, NJ: Medical Economics Books; 1987.

Moon SD, Sauter SL. *Beyond Biomechanics: Psychosocial Aspects of Musculoskeletal Disorders in Office Work.* Bristol, Pa: Taylor and Francis; 1996.

National Council of State Legislatures. *State of Workers' Compensation.* www.ncsl.org/public/cataglog/3302IN.htm

Neuhauser F. *Report on the Quality of Treating Physician Reports and Cost-Benefit of Presumption in Favor of the Treating Physician.* San Francisco, Calif: Commission on Health, Safety and Workers' Compensation; 2000.

Nordin M, Andersson GBH, Pope M. *Musculoskeletal Disorders in the Workplace: Principles and Practice.* St. Louis, Mo: Mosby; 1997.

North DA, Higdon KM. Landmark Survey: Best practices in integrated disability management. *J Workers' Comp.* 1998;7(2):9-26.

Pease SR. *Performance Indicators for Permanent Disability—Low Back Injuries in Texas.* Cambridge, Mass: Workers' Compensation Research Institute; 1988:WC-88-4.

Pease SR. *Performance Indicators for Permanent Disability—Low Back Injuries in Wisconsin.* Cambridge, Mass: Workers' Compensation Research Institute; 1987:WC-87-4.

Pease SR. *Performance Indicators for Permanent Disability—Low-back Injuries in New Jersey.* Cambridge, Mass: Workers' Compensation Research Institute; 1987:WC-87-5.

Petersen DD. General Mills case study: the critical steps in managing workers' compensation costs. *J Workers Comp.* 1994;3(3):22-30.

Proctor T, Gatchel RJ, Robinson RC. Psychosocial factors and risk of pain and disability. *Occup Med.* 2000;15(4):803-12.

Pryor ES. Flawed promises: a critical evaluation of the American Medical Association's "guides to the evaluation of permanent impairment." *Harv Law Rev.* Feb 1990. 103 Harv L Rev 964.

Reiso H, Nygard JF, Brage S, et al. Work ability assessed by patients and their GPs in new episodes of sickness certification (Norway). *Fam Pract.* 2000;17(2):139-44.

Rondinelli RD, Katz RT. *Impairment Rating and Disability Evaluation.* Philadelphia, Pa: W.B. Saunders; 2000.

Sandler HM. Trends in occupational and environmental disease claims. *J Workers' Comp.* 1993;2(2):21-6.

Schulman B, Schwartz S, Boyle P. *Workers' Compensation/Occupational Health National Trends Study.* Seattle, Wash: University of Washington Department of Health Services; 1997.

Simon RI. The credible forensic psychiatric evaluation in multiple chemical sensitivity litigation. *J Am Acad Psychiatry Law.* 1998;26(3):361-74.

Snyder JW, Maier JC, Love BD. Injury and causation on trial: the phenomenon of "multiple chemical sensitivities." *Widener Law Symposium*. Fall 1997. 2 Wid L Symp J 97.

Social Security Administration (SSA). *Disability Evaluation under Social Security.* Washington, DC: US Department of Health and Human Services, SSA; 1986.

Soderstrom E, Stewart J. Adjudicating claims. *Occup Med.* 1998;13(2):273-8.

Solomon DF. Medical expert testimony in administrative hearings. *J Natl Assoc Admin Law Judges.* 1997.

Spieler EA, Barth PS, Burton JF Jr, et al. Recommendations to guide revision of the AMA Guides to the Evaluation of Permanent Impairment. *JAMA.* 2000;283(4):519-23.

Talmage JB. Assessment and management of upper and lower extremity impairment and disability. *Occup Med.* 2000;15(4):771-88.

Telles CA, Fox SE. *Revisiting Workers' Compensation in Washington—Administrative Inventory.* Cambridge, Mass: Workers' Compensation Research Institute; 1996:WC-96-10.

Telles CA, Fox SE. *Workers' Compensation in Colorado—Administrative Inventory.* Cambridge, Mass: Workers' Compensation Research Institute; 1996:WC-96-8.

Telles CA, Shiman L. *Revisiting Workers' Compensation in Minnesota—Administrative Inventory.* Cambridge, Mass: Workers' Compensation Research Institute; 1997:WC-97-3.

Texas Workers' Compensation Commission and Research and Oversight Council on Workers' Compensation. *An Analysis of Texas Workers with Permanent Impairments.* Austin, Texas: Research and Oversight Council on Workers' Compensation; 1996.

UC Data. *Evaluating the Reforms of the Medical-Legal Process Using the WCIRB Permanent Disability Survey.* San Francisco, Calif: California Commission on Health and Safety and Workers' Compensation; 1997.

US Chamber of Commerce. *Analysis of Workers' Compensation Laws.* Washington, DC: US Chamber of Commerce; 2000.

Vasudevan SV, Drury DL. The independent medical examination: purpose and process. *Wisc Med J.* 1999;98(2):10-2. http://wismed.org/wkrscomp/wmjmarapr99-vasudevan.htm.

Welch EM. Independent medical exams. In: *Materials for Michigan State Claims Adjuster Course.* East Lansing: Michigan State University; 2000.

Wise LM. Ethical considerations for the IME. *Chiropractic J.* 1999. www.worldchiropracticalliance .org/tcj/1999/sep/sep1999viewpoint.htm.

Websites and Web-Published Materials

The references in this section include a wide variety of materials and come from a wide variety of sources. To make the context of each of these sources clearer, the references are presented in topical groups. URLs for virtually all references are provided. The specific web pages referenced below were of particular interest to us, but you can find other useful information on many of these sites by exploring them further, especially by going to their home pages.

MEDICAL AND HEALTH CARE ORGANIZATIONS

Physical Medicine Research Foundation, 1998. BC Whiplash Initiative: PMRF's Whiplash-Associated Disorders-A Comprehensive Syllabus. www.health-sciences.ubc.ca/whiplash.bc.

Cleveland Clinic Center for Corporate Health: www.clevelandclinic.org/corphealth/workcomp/pgime.htm.

HEALTH CARE SPECIALTY AND PROFESSIONAL SOCIETIES

American College of Chiropractic Consultants, Mission Statement: www.accc-chiro.com.

College of Physicians and Surgeons of British Columbia 1995. Policy Manual: The Independent Medical Examination. www.cpsbc.bc.ca/policymanual/i/i1.htm.

College of Physicians and Surgeons of Alberta 2000. Guideline: Medical Examinations by Non-treating Physicians (NTMEs). www.cpsa.ab.ca/policyguidelines/ntmes.html.

II. *Presenting Complaints*

Master Algorithm. *ACOEM Guidelines for Care of Acute and Subacute Occupational Neck and Upper Back Complaints*

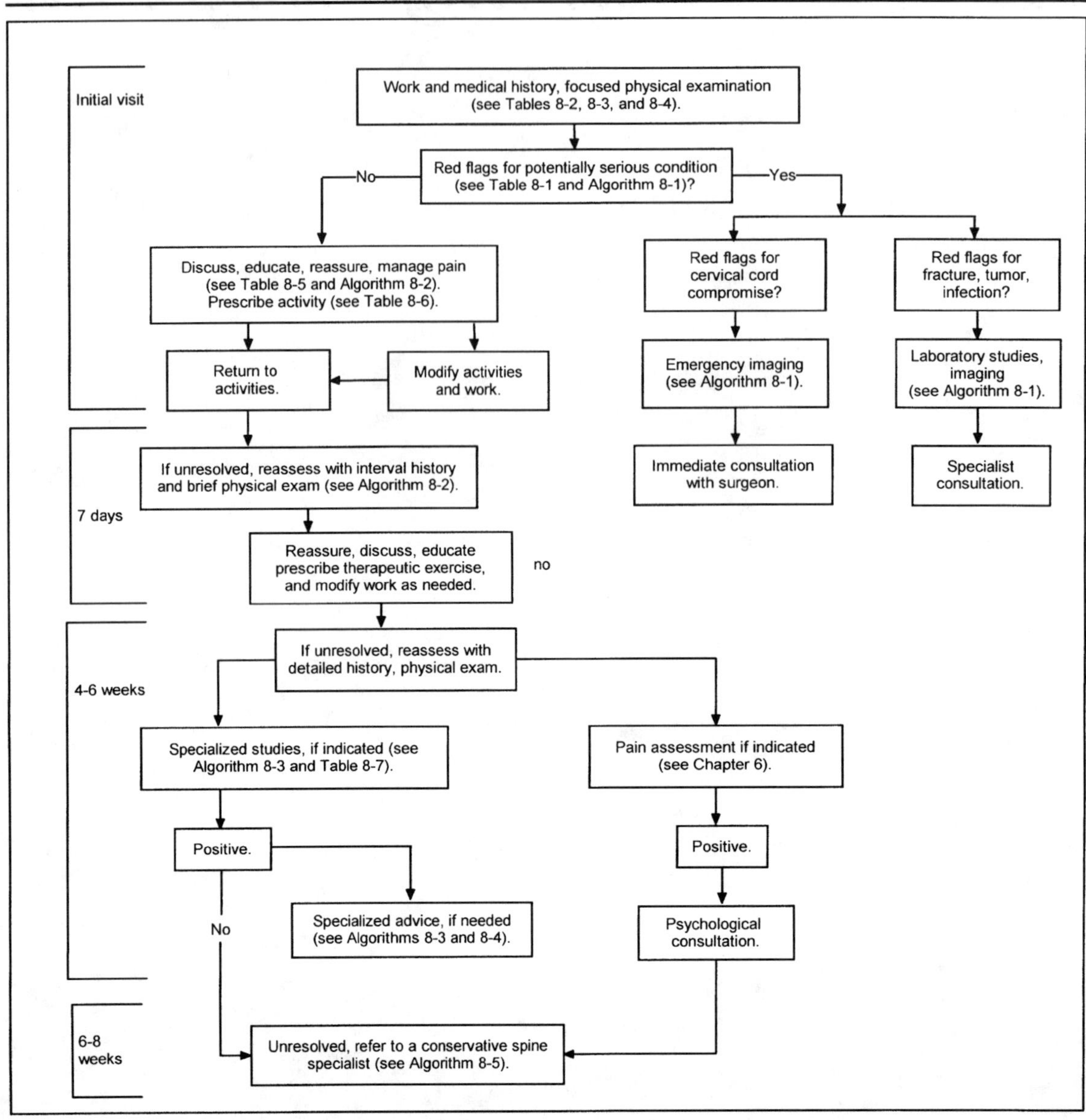

8 Neck and Upper Back Complaints

General Approach and Basic Principles

Neck and upper back complaints that may be work related are common problems presenting to occupational and primary care providers; such complaints are among the ten most common causes of reported occupational complaints and workers' compensation claims. These complaints account for about 6-8% of total lost workdays in workers' compensation and about 8% of claims, ranking them in the top ten for financial severity as well.

Recommendations on assessing and treating adults with potentially work-related neck and upper back complaints are presented in this chapter. Topics include the initial assessment and diagnosis of patients; identification of red flags that may indicate the presence of a serious underlying medical condition; initial management; diagnostic considerations and special studies for identifying clinical pathology, work-relatedness, return to work, modified duty and activity; and further management considerations, including the management of delayed recovery.

Algorithms for patient management are included. This chapter's master algorithm schematizes the manner in which primary care and occupational medicine practitioners generally can manage patients with acute and subacute neck and upper back complaints. The following text, tables, and numbered algorithms expand upon the master algorithm.

The principal recommendations for assessing and treating patients with neck and upper back complaints are as follows:

- The initial assessment focuses on detecting indications of potentially serious disease, termed red flags.
- In the absence of red flags, imaging and other tests are not usually helpful during the first four weeks of neck and upper back symptoms.
- Relieving discomfort can be accomplished most safely by nonprescription medication.
- Primary care or occupational physicians can effectively manage acute and subacute neck and upper back problems conservatively in the absence of red flags.

- While some activity or job modification may be necessary in the acute period, bed rest for more than two days is not helpful and may further debilitate the patient.
- Patients may engage in normal, preinjury activities to facilitate recovery from non-red-flag acute neck disorders such as whiplash-associated disorders (WAD), which is generally more effective than rest and immobilization.[1]
- Low-stress aerobic activities can be safely started immediately as tolerated to help avoid debilitation. Stretching exercises may be helpful to avoid further restriction of motion. Exercises to strengthen neck, upper back, and shoulder muscles are commonly delayed for several weeks.
- Patients recovering from acute and subacute neck and upper back problems should be encouraged to return to modified- or full-duty work as soon as possible.
- If symptoms persist (e.g., beyond four to six weeks), further evaluation may be indicated.
- Within the first three months of neck and upper back symptoms, the only patients who can be expected to benefit from surgery are those with evidence of severe spinovertebral disease (tumor, infection, major trauma, or progressive neurologic deficit) or with severe, debilitating symptoms and physiologic evidence of specific nerve root or spinal cord compromise, corroborated by appropriate imaging studies.
- Nonphysical factors (such as psychosocial, workplace, or socioeconomic problems) can be investigated and addressed in cases of delayed recovery or return to work.

Initial Assessment

Thorough medical and work histories and a focused physical examination (see Chapter 2) are sufficient for initially assessing a patient complaining of potentially work-related neck or upper back symptoms. Certain findings in this assessment raise suspicion of serious underlying medical conditions; these are referred to as red flags (see Table 8-1). Their absence rules out the need for special studies, referral, or inpatient care during the first four weeks, during which time spontaneous recovery is expected (provided any inciting workplace factors are mitigated). Findings of the medical history and physical examination also may alert the clinician to other pathology (not of neck or upper back

[1]The Quebec Task Force on Whiplash Associated Disorders (WAD) defines whiplash as an acceleration/deceleration mechanism of energy transferred to the neck and may result from rear end or side impact motor vehicle collisions but can also occur during diving or other mishaps. The impact may result in bony or soft tissue injuries, which in turn may lead to a variety of clinical manifestations called WAD. Neck pain, headache and decreased mobility of the cervical spine are the most common symptoms.

Table 8-1. Red Flags for Potentially Serious Neck and Upper Back Conditions

Disorder	Medical History	Physical Examination
Fracture	Direct blow to the head Excessive force to the neck, with pain postinjury Loss of consciousness Thrown from vehicle	Inability to move neck due to pain Severe cervical (midline vertebral) tenderness Patient observed to hold head for stability Possible neurologic deficits
Tumor	Age > 50 years Pain at rest Weight loss History of cancer	Tenderness to vertebral percussion Cachexia
Infection	Systemic symptoms of fever, chills Recent bacterial infection IV drug abuse Immune suppression or compromise (e.g., corticosteroids, HIV, diabetes) Pain at rest Fever and nuchal rigidity	Severe cervical spasm Systemic signs of sepsis (elevated temperature, chills, hypotension, tachycardia)
Possible cervical spinal cord compromise	Significant trauma to neck Paresthesias of upper (or upper and lower) extremities Weakness of upper/lower extremity Global weakness of upper extremities Difficulty walking	Severe cervical spasm Weakness of upper or lower extremity major muscle groups Bilateral decreased sensation in upper or lower extremities Disturbance of sphincter control Positive Babinski signs Hyperactive reflexes

origin) that can present as neck or upper back complaints. Neck and upper back complaints can then be classified into one of three working categories although common factors may be operative in all three, thus confounding this classification:

- Potentially serious neck or upper back disorders: fracture, dislocation, infection, tumor, progressive neurologic deficit, or cord compression
- Degenerative disorders: consequences of aging or repetitive use, or a combination thereof, such as degenerative disk disease and osteoarthritis
- Nonspecific disorders: including benign, self-limited disorders with unclear etiology, such as regional upper back and neck pain and shoulder pain adjacent to the neck

Medical History

Asking the patient open-ended questions, such as those listed below, allows the clinician to gauge the need for further discussion or specific inquiries to obtain more detailed information (see also Chapter 2):

1. WHAT ARE YOUR SYMPTOMS?
   - Do you have pain, numbness, weakness, or stiffness?
   - For traumatic injuries: Was the area deformed? Did you lose any blood or have an open wound?
   - Is the discomfort located primarily in your neck, upper back, or shoulder? Do you have pain or other symptoms elsewhere?
   - Are your symptoms constant or intermittent? What makes the problem worse or better?

2. HOW DO THESE SYMPTOMS LIMIT YOU?
   - How long can you sit, stand, walk, do overhead work?
   - Can you lift? How much weight?
   - When did your current limitations begin? Was there a specific inciting event?
   - How did the limitations develop?
   - How long have your activities been limited? More than four weeks?
   - Have your symptoms changed? How?
   - Have you had similar episodes previously?
   - Have you had previous testing or treatment? With whom?
   - What do you think caused the problem? How do you think it is related to work?
   - What are your specific job duties? Do you use your neck and upper back to perform them? How? How often?
   - What other activities (hobbies, workouts, sports) do you engage in at home or elsewhere? Do you use your neck and upper back to perform them? How? How often?
   - Are your symptoms affected by activities of daily living, such as grooming (combing your hair) or driving?
   - Do you have other medical problems?
   - What do you hope we can accomplish during this visit?

Determining the presence of cervical nerve root compromise (and, if so, the level of compromise) is critical. Pain or paresthesia, combined with muscle weakness, sensory deficits, and reflex loss suggests cervical nerve root compression. Clinical findings correlating with specific dermatomal levels of compression are shown in Table 8-2.

Physical Examination

Guided by the medical history, the physical examination includes:

- General observation of the patient, including stance and gait
- Regional examination of neck, proximal shoulder area, and upper back
- Neurologic screening
- Testing for cervical nerve root irritation

The objective parts of the examination are testing reflexes and circumferential measurements of the upper extremity for atrophy. All other findings require the patient's cooperation. If spasm is present, it is an objective finding, not simply an inferred manifestation of guarding by the patient.

A patient who has a neck or upper back disorder may present with a complaint of shoulder pain; he or she may point to the top of the shoulder or to the upper trapezius area, between the base of the neck and the point of the shoulder. This type of pain is most commonly related to the neck, and evaluation includes inspecting the neck and upper back, as noted in this guideline. Interscapular or scapular pain also is a common manifestation of neck abnormalities. Careful physical examination of the cervical area is indicated for patients with either shoulder or interscapular/scapular pain.

Table 8-2. Symptoms of Cervical Nerve Root Compromise

Root Level	Pain or Paresthesia	Motor Weakness
C3	Ear	Neck rotation, shoulder elevation, diaphragm
C4	Top of shoulders	Shoulder elevation, rotation
C5	Lower shoulder, lateral upper arm	Shoulder abduction, elbow flexion, and supination
C6	Lateral forearm, thumb, index finger	Radial wrist extension
C7	Neck or scapula radiating to index, middle, and ring fingers	Elbow extension, ulnar wrist flexion, and finger extension
C8	Neck, radiating to ring and small fingers	Finger flexion
T1	Upper medial forearm, medial arm	Finger abduction, adduction

Observation and Regional Neck Examination

Observing the patient's stance and gait is useful to guide the remainder of the examination. Uncoordination or abnormal use of the extremities may indicate the need for specific neurologic testing. Severe guarding of cervical motion in all planes may add credence to a suspected diagnosis of spinal or intrathecal infection, tumor, or fracture. However, because of the marked variation among persons with and without symptoms, range-of-motion measurements of the neck and upper back are of limited value except as a means to monitor recovery in cases of restriction of motion due to symptoms.

Vertebral-point tenderness to palpation, when associated with other signs or symptoms, is suggestive of, but not specific for, spinal fracture or infection. Palpable soft-tissue tenderness alone is an even less specific or reliable finding.

Neurologic Screening

The neurologic examination should focus on a few tests that reveal evidence of nerve root impairment, peripheral neuropathy, or spinal cord dysfunction. Most herniated disks in the cervical spine involve the C5-6 or the C6-7 levels and the C6 or C7 nerve roots, respectively. The C5 and C8 roots are less commonly involved. Table 8-3 summarizes the clinical features of cervical nerve root compression.

Table 8-3. Physical Examination Correlates of Cervical Nerve Root Dysfunction

Root Level	Sensory Deficit	Motor Weakness	Reflex Loss
C3	Ear, anterior neck, occiput, posterior temporal area	Neck rotation, shoulder elevation, diaphragm	None
C4	Shoulder, posterior upper arm, upper chest	Shoulder elevation, rotation	None
C5	Lateral shoulder, upper arm	Shoulder abduction, elbow flexion	Biceps (brachioradialis)
C6	Lateral forearm, thumb, index and lateral middle fingers	Radial wrist extension	Brachioradialis (biceps)
C7	Middle finger	Elbow extension, wrist flexion, finger extension	Triceps
C8	Distal forearm, ulnar ring, and small finger	Finger flexion	Triceps
T1	Medial upper forearm and arm	Long-finger flexion, finger abduction, and adduction	None

1. TESTING FOR MUSCLE STRENGTH

Nerve root compromise at the C5 level (C4-5 disk) can cause weakness of shoulder abduction as well as elbow flexion or supination. Compromise at the C6 level (C5-6 disk) can produce weakness of radial wrist extension. The C7 nerve root (C6-7 disk) innervates the triceps muscle; weakness of elbow extension and of ulnar wrist flexion indicates compromise at this level. Weak finger extension is a sign of C7 nerve root compromise as well. C8 (C7-8 disk) involvement is indicated by weakness of finger abduction and adduction, as the lumbrical muscles of the hand are affected.

2. CIRCUMFERENTIAL MEASUREMENTS

Muscle atrophy can be detected by bilateral circumferential measurements of the upper arms and forearms. The dominant upper extremity usually will have an increase of ¼ inch in circumference at the forearm and, possibly, also at the upper arm.

3. REFLEXES

The biceps reflex primarily tests the C5 root, and, to a lesser extent, the C6 root. The brachioradialis reflex tests the C6 root; the triceps reflex, the C7 root. The Hoffmann reflex in combination with clonus may indicate an upper motor neuron lesion.

4. SENSORY EXAMINATION

Testing light touch, pressure, and pinprick sensations in the forearm and hand is usually sufficient to detect common nerve root compromise, but sensory examination of the area from the neck to the forearm may be necessary to test for higher nerve root compromise. Decreased sensation over the lateral deltoid muscle is a sign of C5 nerve root or axillary nerve compromise. Loss of sensation in the area of the lateral thumb, index finger, and medial half of the middle finger indicates C6 nerve root involvement. Decreased sensation in the long (middle) finger may be a sign of C7 involvement, although it also is supplied occasionally by the C6 or C8 nerve root. The C8 root may show ring- and fifth-finger sensory findings; the ulnar side of the small (fifth) finger is the purest area of C8 innervation. The T1 nerve root can be tested by evaluating sensation in the upper medial forearm and medial arm.

Assessing Red Flags and Indications for Immediate Referral

Physical examination evidence of severe neurologic compromise that correlates with the medical history and test results may indicate a need for immediate consultation. The examination may further reinforce or reduce suspicions of tumor, infection, fracture, or dislocation. A medical history suggestive of pathology originating somewhere other than in the cervical area may warrant examination of the head, shoulder, or other areas.

Cervical nerve root irritation can be demonstrated by depressing the clavicle or deeply palpating the posterior triangle of the neck. This maneuver should reproduce the patient's symptoms and signs if the cervical nerves are the source of neurologic symptoms and signs.

Diagnostic Criteria

If the patient does not have red flags for serious conditions, the clinician can then determine which common musculoskeletal disorder is present. The criteria presented in Table 8-4 follow the clinical thought process, from the mechanism of illness or injury to unique symptoms and signs of a particular disorder, and finally to test results if any tests are needed to guide treatment at this stage.

Table 8-4. Diagnostic Criteria for Non-red-flag Conditions that Can Be Managed by Primary Care Physicians

Probable Diagnosis or Injury	Mechanism	Unique Symptoms	Unique Signs	Tests and Results
Regional neck pain (ICD-9 723.1, 723.3, 723.5, 723.7, 723.8, 723.9)	Not known	Diffuse pain	None	None indicated
Cervical strain (ICD-9 847.0)	Flexion-extension or rotation force Blow to head or neck	Neck pain Difficult or reduced motion	Limited range of motion due to pain	None indicated
Cervical nerve root compression with radiculopathy (ICD-9 722.71)	Degenerative condition Trauma	Dermatomal sensory changes Motor weakness	Specific motor, sensory, and reflex changes	None indicated for 4-6 weeks in the absence of progressive motor weakness
Spinal stenosis (ICD-9 723.0)	Older patients: degenerative condition Younger patients: congenital stenosis	Neck, shoulder, posterior arm pain Paresthesias in same distribution as pain	Weakness of shoulder girdle and upper arms Long tract signs Signs worse with extension, improved with flexion of neck	CT or MRI shows spinal stenosis
Postlaminectomy syndrome (ICD-9 722.81)	Complication of surgery	Pain and sensory complaints in nerve root distribution at level of surgery	Radicular signs corresponding to level of distribution of surgery	MRI with gadolinium shows scarring

Note: ICD-9 = *International Classification of Diseases*, 9th Ed.

Work-Relatedness

A thorough work history is crucial to establishing work-relatedness. See Chapter 2 for components of the work history.

Because neck and upper back complaints may be related to workstation factors, an accurate history of work- and non-work-related activities is imperative. Questioning about ergonomic positioning, use of a headset, computer screen placement, and many other factors is important. Reviews of epidemiologic studies have shown neck tension symptoms to be related to repetitive work and constrained postures. The work relatedness of the other neck and upper back conditions is not well delineated.

Initial Care

Comfort is often a patient's first concern. Nonprescription analgesics will provide sufficient pain relief for most patients with acute and subacute symptoms. If treatment response is inadequate (i.e., if symptoms and activity limitations continue), prescribed pharmaceuticals or physical methods can be added. Comorbid conditions, side effects, cost, and provider and patient preferences generally guide the clinician's choice of recommendations. Table 8-5 summarizes comfort options.

- Manipulation has been compared to various treatments, but not placebo or nontreatment, for patients with neck pain in nearly twenty randomized clinical trials. More than half favored manipulation, with one reporting better results in combination with exercise, while the remainder indicated treatments were equivocal. Cervical manipulation has not yet been studied in workers' compensation populations.

  In rare instances (estimated at 1.0-1.5 per million manipulations), manipulation has been associated with cerebrovascular accident. Some studies suggest that this risk is based on the position of the patient, not the act of manipulation itself. Serious side effects are extremely rare and far less frequent than those associated with commonly prescribed alternatives such as nonsteroidal anti-inflammatory drugs (NSAIDs), but the issue is currently under study and should be monitored.

  Using cervical manipulation may be an option for patients with occupationally related neck pain or cervicogenic headache. Consistent with application of any passive manual approach in injury care, it is reasonable to incorporate it within the context of functional restoration rather than for pain control alone. There is insufficient evidence to support manipulation of patients with cervical radiculopathy.

- There is no high-grade scientific evidence to support the effectiveness or ineffectiveness of passive physical modalities such as traction, heat/cold applications, massage, diathermy, cutaneous laser treatment, ultrasound, transcutaneous electrical neurostimulation (TENS) units, and

Table 8-5. Methods of Symptom Control for Neck and Upper Back Complaints

RECOMMENDED

Nonprescription Medications

- Acetaminophen (safest)
- NSAIDs (aspirin, ibuprofen)

Physical Modalities

- Adjustment or modification of workstation, job tasks, or work hours and methods
- Stretching
- Specific neck exercises for range of motion and strengthening
- At-home local applications of cold packs during first few days of acute complaints; thereafter, applications of heat packs
- Relaxation techniques
- Aerobic exercise
- 1-2 physical therapy visits for education, counseling, and evaluation of home exercise

Prescribed Pharmaceutical Methods

Other NSAIDs

OPTIONS

Cervical Disk Displacement with Radiculopathy	Cervical Strain	Central Cord Compression
Short-term immobilization of the cervical spine if severe	Brief immobilization of the cervical spine if severe	Collar or brace for stabilization until emergent surgery performed
Spinal Stenosis	**Postlaminectomy Syndrome**	**Regional Neck Symptoms**
Brief immobilization of the cervical spine if severe	Immobilization of the cervical spine if severe	Brief immobilization of the cervical spine if severe

biofeedback. These palliative tools may be used on a trial basis but should be monitored closely. Emphasis should focus on functional restoration and return of patients to activities of normal daily living.

- There is limited evidence that electromagnetic therapy may be effective to reduce pain in mechanical neck disorders. If used, there should be a trial period with objective signs of functional progress.
- Invasive techniques (e.g., needle acupuncture and injection procedures, such as injection of trigger points, facet joints,[2] or corticoste-

[2]There is limited evidence that radio-frequency neurotomy may be effective in relieving or reducing cervical facet joint pain among patients who had a positive response to facet injections. Lasting relief (eight to nine months, on average) from chronic neck pain has been achieved in about 60% of cases across two studies, with an effective success rate on repeat procedures, even though sample sizes generally have been limited (n = 24, 28). Caution is needed due to the scarcity of high-quality studies.

roids, lidocaine, or opioids in the epidural space) have no proven benefit in treating acute neck and upper back symptoms. However, many pain physicians believe that diagnostic and/or therapeutic injections may help patients presenting in the transitional phase between acute and chronic pain.

- Injecting botulinum toxin (type A and B) has been shown to be effective in reducing pain and improving range of motion (ROM) in cervical dystonia (a disorder that is non-traumatic and non-work-related). Mild side effects were fairly common and dose dependent, including dry mouth and dysphagia. While existing evidence shows injecting botulinum toxin to be safe, caution is needed due to the scarcity of high-quality studies. There are no high quality studies that support its use in whiplash-associated disorder.
- Cervical epidural corticosteroid injections are of uncertain benefit and should be reserved for patients who otherwise would undergo open surgical procedures for nerve root compromise.
- Other miscellaneous therapies have been evaluated and found to be ineffective or minimally effective. For example, cervical collars have not been shown to have any lasting benefit, except for comfort in the first few days of the clinical course in severe cases; in fact, weakness may result from prolonged use and will contribute to debilitation. Immobilization using collars and prolonged periods of rest are generally less effective than having patients maintain their usual, "preinjury" activities.

Activity Alteration

To avoid neck or upper back irritation and debilitation due to inactivity, recommendations for alternative activity can be helpful. As a general principle, acutely avoid activities that precipitate symptoms, but general activities and motion may be continued. Therapeutic exercise, including strengthening, should start as soon as it can be done without aggravating symptoms. Most patients with neck pain do not require bed rest. The most severe cases of neck pain (primarily those with arm pain) may be treated with one to two days of bed rest. Prolonged bed rest (more than two days) has potential debilitating effects, and its efficacy in treating acute neck pain is unproved.

Activities causing an increase in stress on the neck tend to increase neck symptoms. These activities can be reviewed with the patient and modifications advised. Activities and postures that increase stress on the neck (e.g., driving, workstation position, telephone use, repetitive motions, and other activities) may require modification. Patients who work with video-display terminals should be sure the keyboard and monitor are at a comfortable height and angle because misadjustment of terminals as well as awkward use of laptop computers are common causes of neck symptoms. Sitting posture and support are important as well. For example, cradling a telephone receiver on the shoulder can cause neck symptoms and indicates the need for a headset. Frequent changes in position become important in many cases of neck and upper back problems. Work activities involving crouching, stooping, working under automobiles or dashboards, working in confined spaces, and the like may require modification to maximize the patient's activities and allow early return to work.

Work Activities

Table 8-6 provides recommendations on activity modification and duration of absence from work. Intended for patients without comorbidity or complicating factors, including employment or legal issues, these guidelines are targets

*Table 8-6. Guidelines for Modification of Work Activities and Disability Duration**

		Recommended Target for Disability Duration**		NHIS Experience Data***	
Disorder	**Activity Modifications and Accommodation**	**With Modified Duty**	**Without Modified Duty**	**Median (cases with lost time)**	**Percent No Lost Time**
Cervical strain	Avoid extremes of motion, prolonged periods in one position, and any other aggravating activities	5-7 days	7-14 days	13 days	19%
Cervical disk displacement, with radiculopathy	Same as for cervical strain, with avoidance of activities that aggravate arm symptoms as well	5-7 days	7-14 days	30 days	28%
Spinal stenosis	Same as for cervical radiculopathy, with generalized accommodation of life-style activities	5-7 days	7-14 days	6 days	58%
Postlaminectomy syndrome	Same as for radiculopathy, with surgical referral if limitations are ineffective	5-7 days	7-14 days	29 days	38%
Regional neck pain	Avoid aggravating circumstances; maximize safe activities	2-4 days	7-10 days	5 days	43%

* These are general guidelines based on consensus or population sources and are never meant to be applied to an individual case without consideration of workplace factors, concurrent disease or other social or medical factors that can affect recovery.

** These parameters for disability duration are "consensus optimal" targets as determined by a panel of ACOEM members in 1996, and reaffirmed by a panel of ACOEM members in 2002. In most cases persons with one nonsevere injury can return to modified duty immediately.

*** Based on the CDC NHIS (National Health Interview Survey), as compiled and reported in the eighth annual edition of *Official Disability Guidelines (ODG)*, © 2002 Work Loss Data Institute, all rights reserved.

providing a guide from the perspective of physiologic recovery. Key factors to consider in disability duration are age and type of job, especially if the regular work includes activities likely to worsen the condition. The clinician can make clear to patients and employers that:

- Even moderately heavy lifting, carrying, or working in awkward positions may aggravate neck symptoms from cervical strain, cervical nerve root irritation, etc.
- Any restrictions are intended to allow for spontaneous recovery or for time to build activity tolerance through exercise.

Measures to assist the patient in avoiding aggravating activities include reviewing work duties to decide whether modifications can be accomplished and to determine whether modified duty is available. Make every attempt to maintain the patient at maximal levels of activity, including work activities.

Follow-up Visits

Patients whose neck or upper back complaints may be work related should receive follow-up care every three to five days by a midlevel practitioner, who can counsel them about avoiding static positions, medication use, activity modification, and other concerns. Take care to answer questions and make these sessions interactive so that patients are fully involved in their recovery. If the patient has returned to work, these interactions may be done on site or by telephone to avoid interfering with modified- or full-work activities.

Physician follow-up generally occurs when a release to modified, increased, or full duty is needed, or after appreciable healing or recovery can be expected, on average. Physician follow-up might be expected every four to seven days if the patient is off work and every seven to fourteen days if the patient is working.

Special Studies and Diagnostic and Treatment Considerations

For most patients presenting with true neck or upper back problems, special studies are not needed unless a three- or four-week period of conservative care and observation fails to improve symptoms. Most patients improve quickly, provided any red-flag conditions are ruled out.

Criteria for ordering imaging studies are:

- Emergence of a red flag
- Physiologic evidence of tissue insult or neurologic dysfunction

- Failure to progress in a strengthening program intended to avoid surgery
- Clarification of the anatomy prior to an invasive procedure

Physiologic evidence may be in the form of definitive neurologic findings on physical examination, electrodiagnostic studies, laboratory tests, or bone scans. Unequivocal findings that identify specific nerve compromise on the neurologic examination are sufficient evidence to warrant imaging studies if symptoms persist. When the neurologic examination is less clear, however, further physiologic evidence of nerve dysfunction can be obtained before ordering an imaging study. Electromyography (EMG), and nerve conduction velocities (NCV), including H-reflex tests, may help identify subtle focal neurologic dysfunction in patients with neck or arm symptoms, or both, lasting more than three or four weeks. The assessment may include sensory-evoked potentials (SEPs) if spinal stenosis or spinal cord myelopathy is suspected. If physiologic evidence indicates tissue insult or nerve impairment, consider a discussion with a consultant regarding next steps, including the selection of an imaging test to define a potential cause (magnetic resonance imaging [MRI] for neural or other soft tissue, compute tomography [CT] for bony structures). Additional studies may be considered to further define problem areas. The recent evidence indicates cervical disk annular tears may be missed on MRIs. The clinical significance of such a finding is unclear, as it may not correlate temporally or anatomically with symptoms.

Diskography is frequently used prior to cervical fusions and certain disk-related procedures. There is significant scientific evidence that questions the usefulness of diskography in those settings. While recent studies indicate diskography to be relatively safe and have a low complication rate, some studies suggest the opposite to be true. In any case, clear evidence is lacking to support its efficacy over other imaging procedures in identifying the location of cervical symptoms, and, therefore, directing intervention appropriately. Tears may not correlate anatomically or temporally with symptoms. Because this area is rapidly evolving, clinicians should consult the latest available studies.

Table 8-7 provides a general comparison of the abilities of different techniques to identify physiologic insult and define anatomic defects. In the following circumstances, an imaging study may be appropriate for a patient whose limitations due to consistent symptoms have persisted for four to six weeks or more:

- When surgery is being considered for a specific anatomic defect
- To further evaluate the possibility of potentially serious pathology, such as a tumor

Reliance on imaging studies alone to evaluate the source of neck or upper back symptoms carries a significant risk of diagnostic confusion (false-positive test results) because it's possible to identify a finding that was present before symptoms began and, therefore, has no temporal association with the symptoms.

Table 8-7. Ability of Various Techniques to Identify and Define Neck and Upper Back Pathology

Technique	Identify Physiologic Insult	Identify Anatomic Defect
History	+	+
Physical examination		
Circumference	+	+
Reflexes	+ +	+ +
Motor	+ +	+ +
Sensory	+ +	+ +
Physiologic studies	+ +	0
Laboratory studies		
Bone scan[1]	+ + +	+ +
Electromyography/sensory evoked potentials (EMG/SEPs)	+ + +	+ +
Imaging		
Radiography[1]	0	+ (+ + +)[2]
Computed tomography (CT)[1]	0	+ + + +[3]
Magnetic resonance imaging (MRI)	0	+ + + +[3]
Myelo-CT [1]	0	+ + + +[3]
Myelography [1]	0	+ + + +[3]

[1]Risk of complications (e.g., infection, radiation) highest for myelo-CT; second highest for myelography; relatively less for bone scan, radiography, and CT.
[2]Cervical radiographs are most appropriate for patients with acute trauma associated with midline vertebral tenderness, head injury, drug or alcohol intoxication, or neurologic compromise. (*American College of Surgeons. Advanced Trauma and Life Support: A Manual for Instructors.* Chicago: ACS; 1993.)
[3]False-positive diagnostic findings in up to 30% of people without symptoms at age 30.
Note: Number of plus signs indicates relative ability to identify or define pathology.

Surgical Considerations

Within the first three months of onset of potentially work-related acute neck and upper back symptoms, consider surgery only if the following are detected:

- Severe spinovertebral pathology
- Severe, debilitating symptoms with physiologic evidence of specific nerve root or spinal cord dysfunction corroborated on appropriate imaging studies that did not respond to conservative therapy

A disk herniation, characterized by protrusion of the central nucleus pulposus through a defect in the outer annulus fibrosis, may impinge on a nerve root, causing irritation, shoulder and arm symptoms, and nerve root dysfunction. The presence of a herniated cervical or upper thoracic disk on an imaging study, however, does not necessarily imply nerve root dysfunction. Studies of asymptomatic adults commonly demonstrate intervertebral disk herniations that apparently do not cause symptoms.

Referral for surgical consultation is indicated for patients who have:

- Persistent, severe, and disabling shoulder or arm symptoms
- Activity limitation for more than one month or with extreme progression of symptoms
- Clear clinical, imaging, and electrophysiologic evidence, consistently indicating the same lesion that has been shown to benefit from surgical repair in both the short- and long-term
- Unresolved radicular symptoms after receiving conservative treatment

The efficacy of cervical fusion for patients with chronic cervical pain without instability has not been demonstrated. If surgery is a consideration, counseling and discussion regarding likely outcomes, risks and benefits, and especially expectations is essential. Patients with acute neck or upper back pain alone, without findings of serious conditions or significant nerve root compromise, rarely benefit from either surgical consultation or surgery. If there is no clear indication for surgery, referring the patient to a physical medicine and rehab (PM&R) specialist may help resolve symptoms. Based on extrapolating studies on low back pain, it also would be prudent to consider a psychological evaluation of the patient prior to referral for surgery.

Many patients with strong clinical findings of nerve root dysfunction due to disk herniation recover activity tolerance within one month; there is no evidence that delaying surgery for this period worsens outcomes in patients without progressive neurologic findings. Spontaneous improvement in MRI-documented cervical disk pathology has been demonstrated with a high rate of resolution. Surgery increases the likelihood that patients will have to have future procedures with higher complication rates. A 12% reoperation rate was reported in one large series. Patients with comorbid conditions, such as cardiac or respiratory disease, diabetes, or mental illness, may be poor candidates for surgery. Comorbidity can be judged and discussed carefully with the patient.

A. Cervical Nerve Root Decompression

Cervical nerve root decompression may be accomplished in one of two major ways. Some practitioners prefer cervical laminectomy and disk excision with nerve root decompression, especially for posterolateral or lateral disk ruptures or foraminal osteophytes. However, anterior disk excision is performed more often, especially for central herniations or osteophytes. Possible complications of decompression include wound infections, diskitis, recurrent disk material or graft slippage (requiring return to surgery either immediately or subacutely), and cervical cord damage. Thoroughly discussing the risks, benefits, and realistic expectations of surgery with the patient is warranted. For instance, in one study, patients with radiation of pain to the arm(s) and hand(s) had better relief of pain with surgery than those with neck pain alone. Pre-surgical screening should include consideration of psychological evaluation.

B. Other Procedures

Chemonucleolysis with chymopapain is less efficacious and has rare but serious complications. Percutaneous diskectomy is not recommended because the effectiveness of this procedure has not been demonstrated.

Summary of Recommendations and Evidence

See Table 8-8.

Table 8-8. Summary of Recommendations for Evaluating and Managing Neck and Upper Back Complaints

Clinical Measure	Recommended	Optional	Not Recommended
History and physical exam	Basic history and exam (C) History of cancer infection (B) History of significant trauma (D) Neurologic exam (C)		
Medication (See Chapter 3)	Acetaminophen (C) NSAIDs (B)	Muscle relaxants (C) Opioids, short course (C)	Use of opioids for more than 2 weeks (C)
Physical treatment methods		Physical manipulation for neck pain early in care only (B) At-home applications of heat or cold (D) Radio-frequency neurotomy (C)	Traction (B) TENS (C) Other modalities (D)
Injections		Epidural injection of corticosteroids to avoid surgery (D) Botulinum toxin (dystonia only) (B)	Facet injection of corticosteroids (D) Diagnostic blocks (D)
Rest and immobilization		1 or 2 days' partial bed rest for severe pain (D)	Bed rest longer than 1 or 2 days (B) Cervical collar more than 1 or 2 days

Table 8-8. (continued)

Clinical Measure	Recommended	Optional	Not Recommended
Activity and exercise	Maintenance of activity levels while recovering (B) Office instruction on exercises after initial pain decreases (D) Low-stress conditioning and aerobic exercises to avoid debilitation (D)		
Detection of neurologic abnormalities	EMG to clarify nerve root dysfunction in cases of suspected disk herniation preoperatively or before epidural injection (D)	SEPs if spinal stenosis or myelopathy suspected (D)	EMG for diagnosis of nerve root involvement if findings of history, physical exam, and imaging study are consistent (D)
Radiography	Initial studies when red flags for fracture, or neurologic deficit associated with acute trauma, tumor, or infection are present (D)		Routine use in first 4 to 6 weeks if red flags are absent (D)
Other imaging procedures	MRI or CT to evaluate red-flag diagnoses as above (D)		Imaging before 4 to 6 weeks in absence of red flags (C, D)
	MRI or CT to validate diagnosis of nerve root compromise, based on clear history and physical examination findings, in preparation for invasive procedure (D). If no improvement after 1 month, bone scan if tumor or infection possible (D)		Preoperative diskography (D)

Table 8-8. (continued)

Clinical Measure	Recommended	Optional	Not Recommended
Surgical considerations	Careful preoperative education of the patient regarding expectations, complications, and short- and long-term sequelae of surgery (D) Indications clear for failed conservative treatment and history, exam, and imaging consistent for specific lesion (D)		Diskectomy or fusion without conservative treatment 4 to 6 weeks minimum (D) Diskectomy or fusion for nonradiating pain or in absence of evidence of nerve root compromise (D)

A = Strong research-based evidence (multiple relevant, high-quality scientific studies).
B = Moderate research-based evidence (one relevant, high-quality scientific study or multiple adequate scientific studies).
C = Limited research-based evidence (at least one adequate scientific study of patients with neck and upper back disorders).
D = Panel interpretation of information not meeting inclusion criteria for research-based evidence.

Algorithm 8-1. *Initial Evaluation of Occupational Neck and Upper Back Complaints*

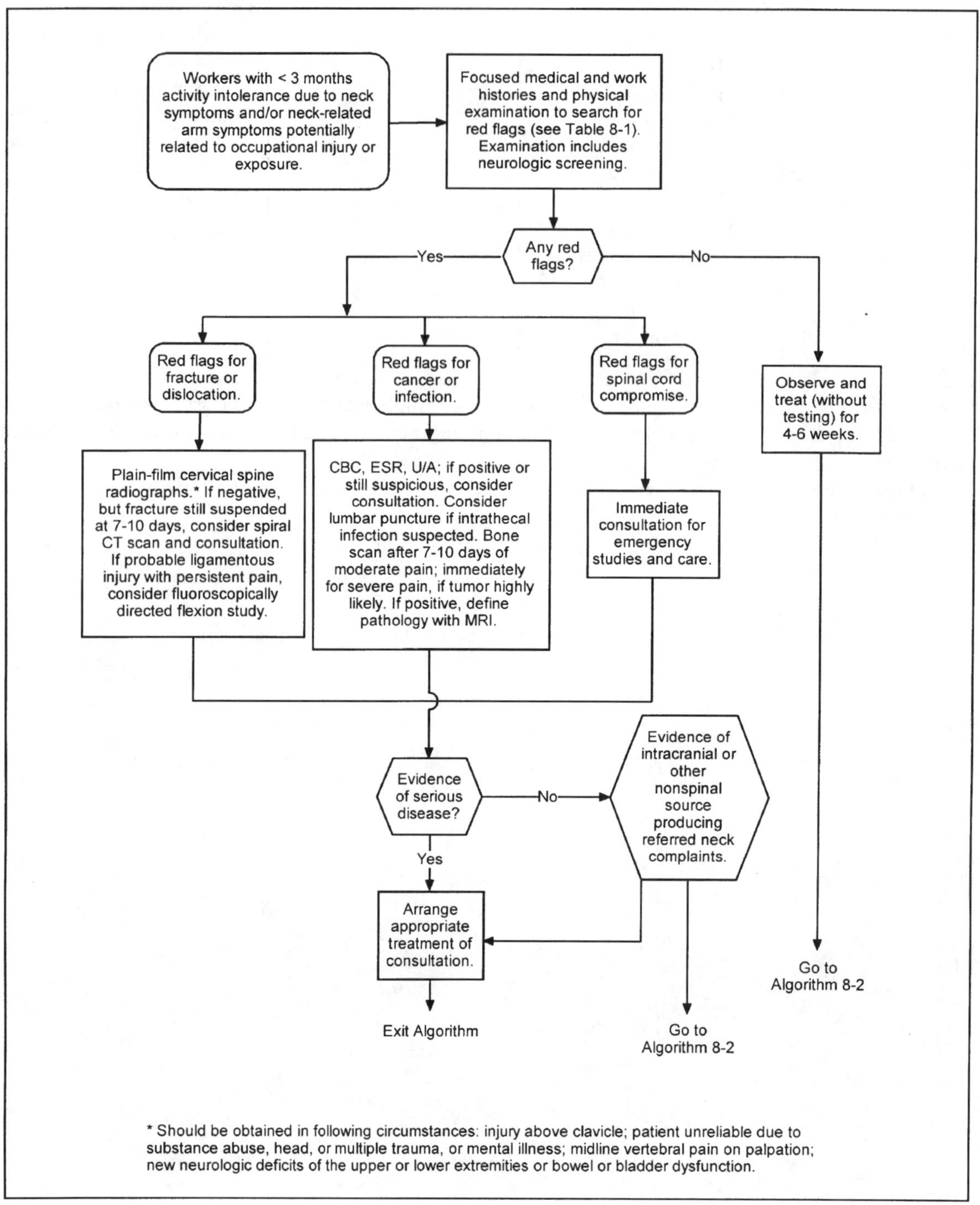

* Should be obtained in following circumstances: injury above clavicle; patient unreliable due to substance abuse, head, or multiple trauma, or mental illness; midline vertebral pain on palpation; new neurologic deficits of the upper or lower extremities or bowel or bladder dysfunction.

Algorithm 8-2. *Initial and Follow-up Management of Occupational Neck and Upper Back Complaints*

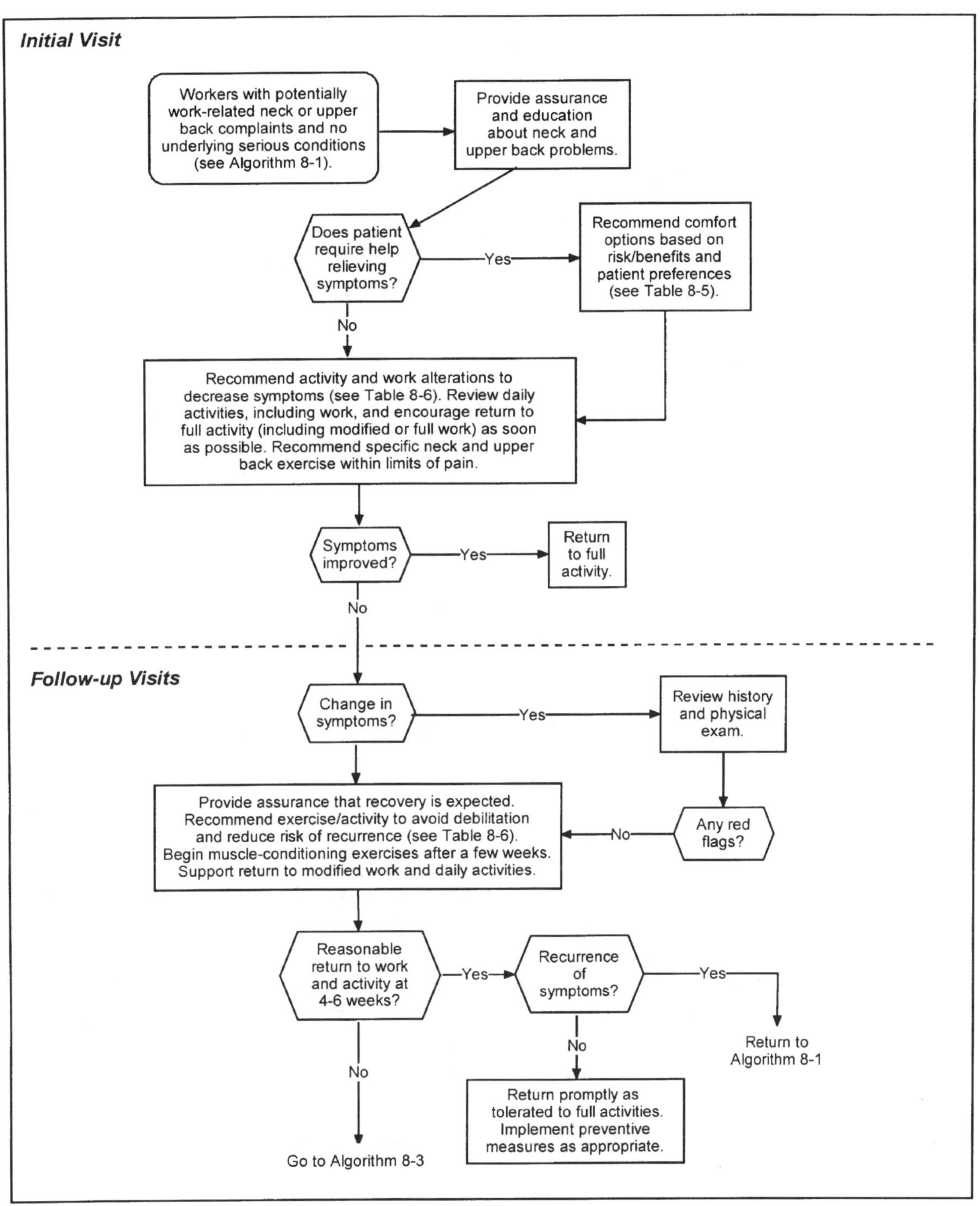

Algorithm 8-3. *Evaluation of Slow-to-recover Patients with Occupational Neck or Upper Back Complaints (Symptoms > 4 Weeks)*

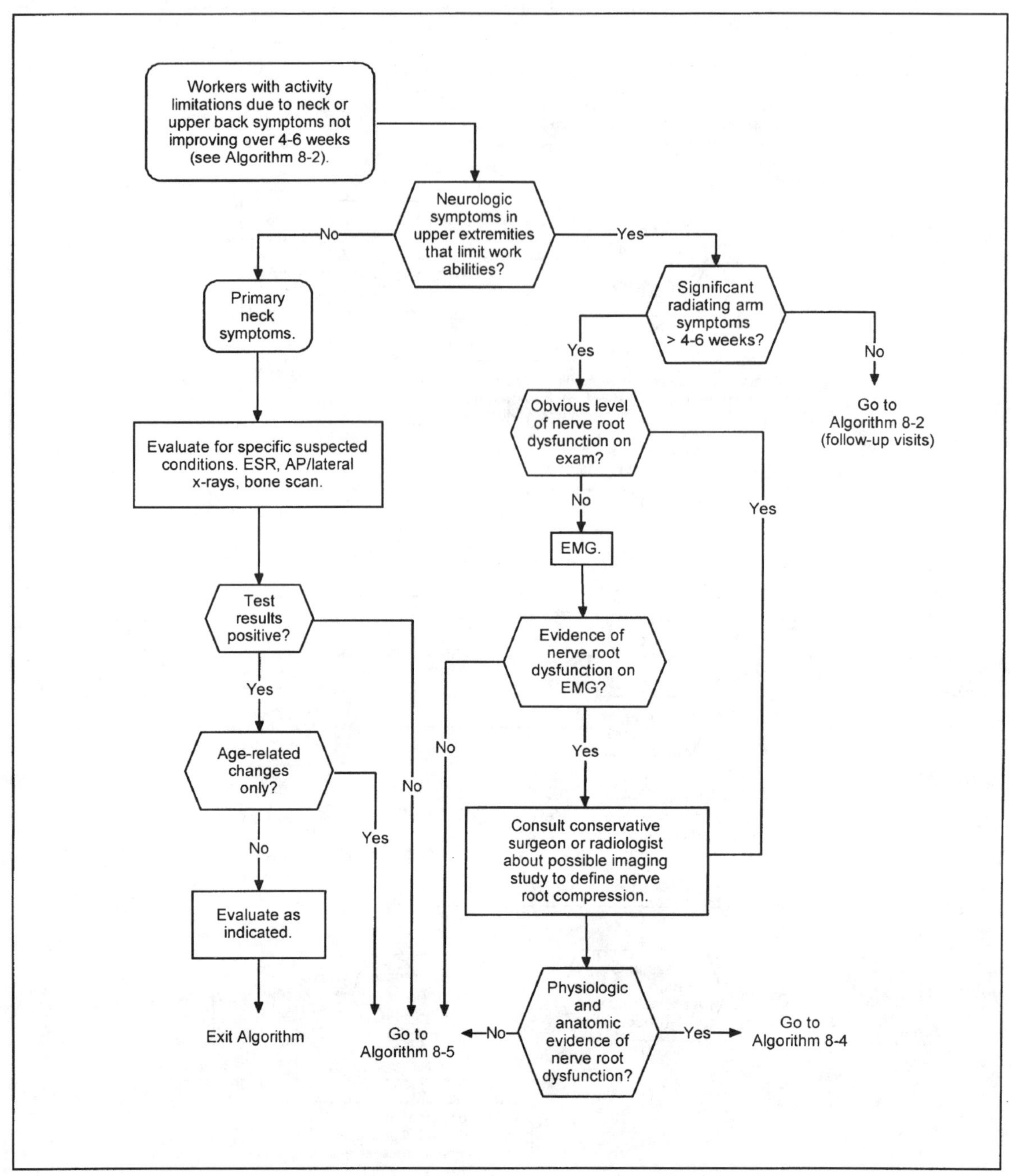

Algorithm 8-4. *Surgical Considerations for Patients with Persistent Radiating Arm Pain*

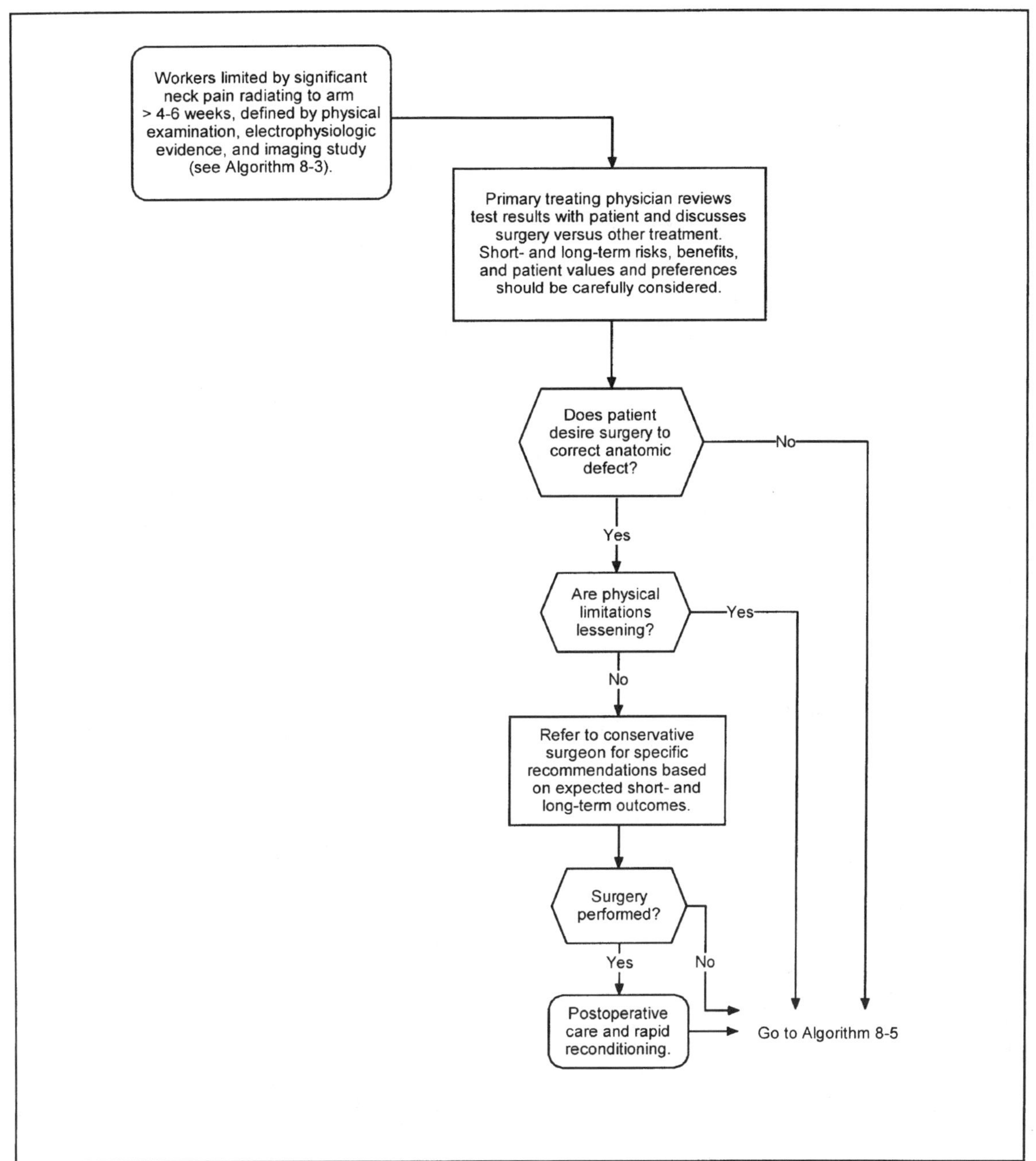

Algorithm 8-5. *Further Management of Occupational Neck and Upper Back Complaints*

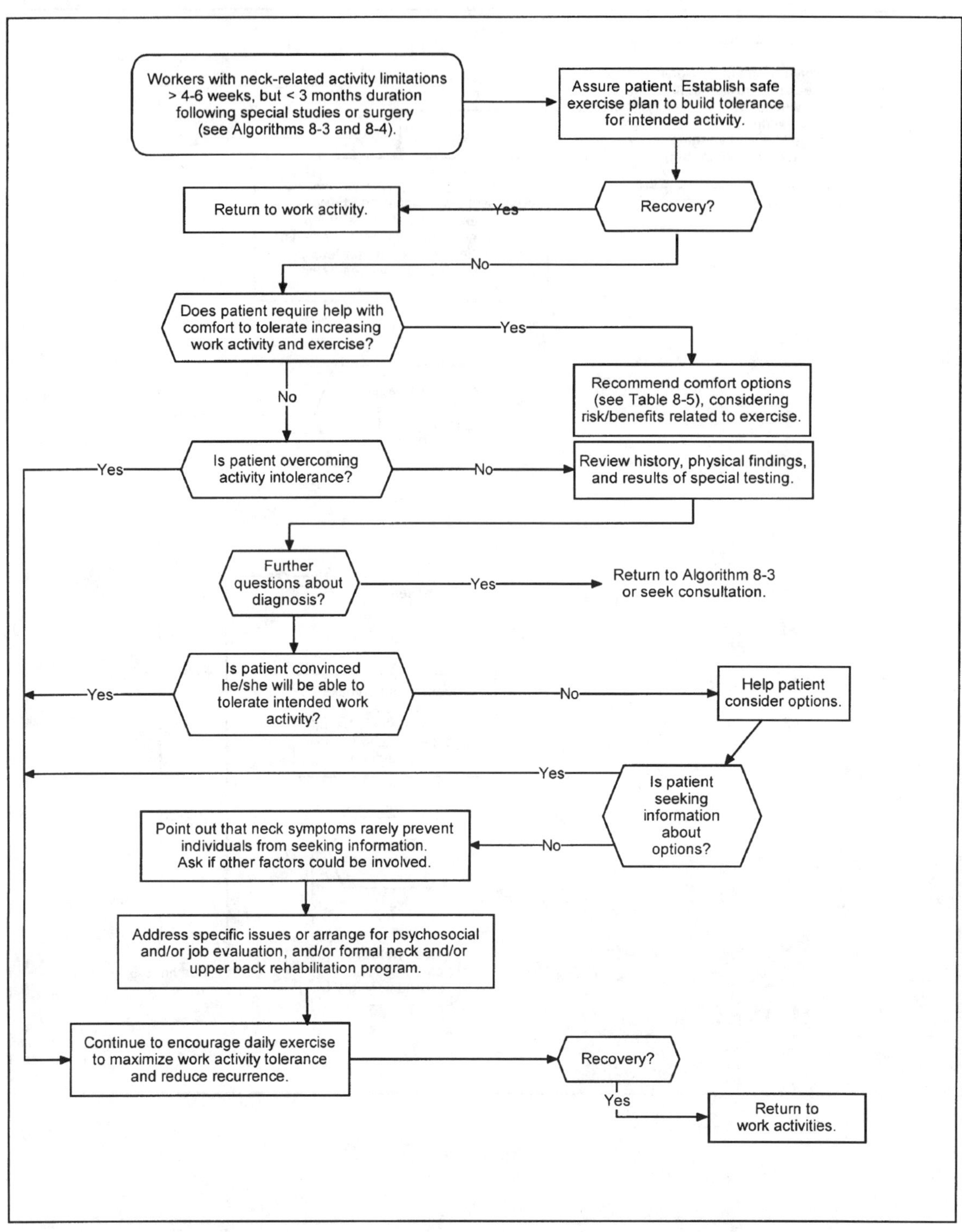

HISTORY AND PHYSICAL EXAMINATION

Bickerstaff ER. *Neurological Examination in Clinical Practice.* Oxford: Blackwell Scientific; 1975.

Davis JW, Phreaner DL, Hoyt DB, et al. The etiology of missed cervical spine injuries. *J Trauma.* 1993;34:342-6.

Denniston PL, ed. *OSHA Durations Report: Return-to-Work by State, Industry, & Age (plus Diagnosis, Body Part, Event, Gender and Length of Service).* Corpus Christi, Texas: Work Loss Data Institute; 2002.

Devinsky O, Feldmann E. *Examination of the Cranial and Peripheral Nerves.* New York, NY: Churchill Livingstone; 1988.

Hills MW, Deane SA. Head injury and facial injury: is there an increased risk of cervical spine injury? *J Trauma.* 1993;34:549-53.

Hoppenfeld S. *Orthopaedic Neurology: A Diagnostic Guide to Neurologic Levels.* Philadelphia, Pa: J.B. Lippincott; 1977.

Joynt RJ. *Clinical Neurology, Volume 1.* Philadelphia, Pa: Lippincott-Raven; 1995.

Krapac L, Krmpotic A, Pavicevic L, et al. Cervicobrachial syndrome—work and disability. *Arh Hig Rada Toksikol.* 1992;43:255-62.

Roberge RJ, Wears RC. Evaluation of neck discomfort, neck tenderness, and neurologic deficits as indicators. *J Emerg Med.* 1992;10:539-44.

Ross SE, O'Malley KF, DeLong WG, et al. Clinical predictors of unstable cervical spinal injury in multiply injured patients. *Injury.* 1992;23:317-9.

Ryan GA, Taylor GW, Moore VM, et al. Neck strain in car occupants: injury status after 6 months and crash-related factors. *Injury.* 1994;25:533-7.

Waldvogel FA, Vasey H. Osteomyelitis: the past decade. *N Engl J Med.* 1980;303:360-70.

MEDICATION

See Chapter 3 references.

PHYSICAL TREATMENT METHODS

Bronfort G. Spinal manipulation: current state of research and its indications. *Neurol Clin.* 1999;17(1):91-111.

Bronfort G, Evans R, Nelson B, Aker PD, Goldsmith CH, Vernon H. A randomized clinical trial of exercise and spinal manipulation for patients with chronic neck pain. *Spine.* 2001;26(7):788-97.

Cassidy JD, Lopes AA, Yong-Hing K. The immediate effect of manipulation versus mobilization on pain and range of motion in the cervical spine: a randomized controlled trial. *J Manipulative Physiol Ther.* 1992;15:570-5.

Graff-Radford SB, Reeves JL, Baker RL, et al. Effects of transcutaneous electrical nerve stimulation on myofascial pain and trigger point sensitivity. *Pain.* 1989;37:1-5.

Gross AR, Aker PD, Goldsmith CH, Peloso P. Physical medicine modalities for mechanical neck disorders (Cochrane Review). In: *The Cochrane Library.* Issue 3; 2002. Oxford: Update Software.

Haldeman S, Kohlbeck FJ, McGregor M. Risk factors and precipitating neck movements causing vertebrobasilar artery dissection after cervical trauma and spinal manipulation. *Spine.* 1999;24:785-94.

Hurwitz EL, Morgenstern H, Harber P, Kominski GF, Yu F, Adams AH. A randomized trial of chiropractic manipulation and mobilization for patients with neck pain: clinical outcomes from the UCLA neck-pain study. *Am J Public Health.* 2002;92(10):1634-41.

Kjellman GV, Skargren EI, Oberg BE. A critical analysis of randomised clinical trials on neck pain and treatment efficacy. A review of the literature. *Scand J Rehabil Med.* 1999;31(3):139-52.

Koes BW, Bouter LM, van Mameren H, et al. The effectiveness of manual therapy, physiotherapy, and treatment by the general practitioner for nonspecific back and neck complaints. *Spine.* 1992;17:28-35.

Lehmann TR, Russell DW, Spratt KF. The impact of patients with nonorganic physical findings on a controlled trial of transcutaneous electrical nerve stimulation and electroacupuncture. *Spine.* 1983;8:625-34.

Levoska S, Keinanen-Kiukaanniemi S. Active or passive physiotherapy for occupational cervicobrachial disorders? A comparison of two treatment methods with a 1-year follow-up. *Arch Phys Med Rehabil.* 1993;74:425-30.

Lord SM, Barnsley L, Wallis BJ, McDonald GJ, Bogduk N. Percutaneous radio-frequency neurotomy for chronic cervical zygapophyseal-joint pain. *N Engl J Med.* 1996;335:1721-6.

McDonald GJ, Lord SM, Bogduk N. Long-term follow-up of patients treated with cervical radiofrequency neurotomy for chronic neck pain. *Neurosurgery.* 1999;45(1):61-7; discussion 67-8.

Philadelphia Panel. Philadelphia Panel evidence-based clinical practice guidelines on selected rehabilitation interventions for neck pain. *Phys Ther.* 2001;81(10):1701-17.

Rothwell DM, Bondy SJ, Williams JI. Chiropractic manipulation and stroke: a population-based case-control study. *Stroke.* 2001;32(5):1054-60.

Thorsteinsson G, Stonnington HH, Stillwell GK, et al. The placebo effect of transcutaneous electrical stimulation. *Pain.* 1978;5:31-41.

van der Heijden GJMG, Beurskens AJHM, Koes BW, et al. The efficacy of traction for back and neck pain: a systematic, blinded review of randomized clinical trial methods. *Phys Ther.* 1995;75:93-104.

Vernon HT. Spinal manipulation and headaches: an update. *Top Clin Chiropr.* 1995;2(3):34-47.

Vernon HT. Spinal manipulation in the management of tension-type migraine and cervicogenic headaches: state of the evidence. *Top Clin Chiropr.* 2002;9(1):14-20.

INJECTIONS

Barnsley L, Lord S, Wallis B, et al. False-positive rates of cervical zygapophyseal joint blocks. *Clin J Pain.* 1993;9:124-30.

Barnsley L, Lord SM, Wallis BJ, et al. Lack of effect of intraarticular corticosteroids for chronic pain in the cervical zygapophyseal joints. *N Engl J Med.* 1994;330:1047-50.

Catchlove RF, Braha R. The use of cervical epidural nerve blocks in the management of chronic head and neck pain. *Can Anaesth Soc J.* 1984;31:188-91.

Cicala RS, Thoni K, Angel JJ. Long-term results of cervical epidural steroid injections. *Clin J Pain.* 1989;5:10-5.

Freund BJ, Schwartz M. Treatment of whiplash associated neck pain corrected with botulinum toxin-A: a pilot study. *J Rheumatol.* 2000;27(2):481-4.

Frost FA, Jessen B, Siggaard-Andersen J. A control, double-blind comparison of mepivacaine injection versus saline injection for myofascial pain. *Lancet.* 1980;8167:499-501.

Lew MF, Adornato BT, Duane DD, et al. Botulinum toxin type B: a double-blind, placebo-controlled, safety and efficacy study in cervical dystonia. *Neurology.* 1997;49:701-7.

Stav A, Ovadia L, Sternberg A, et al. Cervical epidural steroid injection for cervicobrachialgia. *Acta Anaesthesiol Scand.* 1993;37:562-6.

Warfield CA, Biber MP, Drews DA, et al. Epidural steroid injection as a treatment for cervical radiculitis. *Clin J Pain.* 1988;4:201-4.

ACTIVITY AND EXERCISE

Borchgrevink GE, Kaasa A, McDonagh D, Stiles TC, Haraldseth O, Lereim I. Acute treatment of whiplash neck sprain injuries. *Spine.* 1998;23:25-31.

Gennis P, Miller L, Gallagher J, Giglio J, Carter W, Nathanson N. The effect of soft cervical collars on persistent neck pain in patients with whiplash injury. *Acad Emerg Med.* 1996;568-73.

Kraut RM, Anderson TP. Role of anterior cervical muscles in production of neck pain. *Arch Phys Med Rehabil.* 1966;47:603-11.

Rodriquez AA, Bilkey WJ, Agre JC. Therapeutic exercise in chronic neck and back pain. *Arch Phys Med Rehabil.* 1992;73:870-5.

Silverman JL, Rodriquez AA, Agre JC. Quantitative cervical flexor strength in healthy subjects and in subjects with mechanical neck pain. *Arch Phys Med Rehabil.* 1991;72:679-81.

Verhagen AP, Peeters GGM, de Bie RA, Oostendorp RAB. Conservative treatment for whiplash (Cochrane Review). In: *The Cochrane Library.* Issue 3; 2002. Oxford: Update Software.

RADIOGRAPHY

Andrew CT, Gallucci JG, Brown AS, et al. Is routine cervical spine radiographic evaluation indicated in patients with mandibular fractures? *Am Surg.* 1992;58:369-72.

Beirne JC, Butner PE, Brady FA. Cervical spine injuries in patients with facial fractures: a 1-year prospective study. *Int J Oral Maxillofac Surg.* 1995;24:26-9.

Daffner RH. Evaluation of cervical vertebral injuries. *Semin Roentgenol.* 1992;27:239-53.

Hoffman JR, Schriger DL, Mower W, et al. Low-risk criteria for cervical-spine radiography in blunt trauma: a prospective study. *Ann Emerg Med.* 1992;21:1454-60.

Lindsey RW, Dilberti TC, Doherty BJ, et al. Efficacy of radiographic evaluation of the cervical spine in emergency situations. *South Med J.* 1993;86:1253-5.

Malomo AO, Shokunbi MT, Adeloye A. Evaluation of the use of plain cervical spine radiography in patients with head injury. *East Afr Med J.* 1995;72: 186-81.

Montgomery JL, Montgomery ML. Radiographic evaluation of cervical spine trauma: procedures to avoid catastrophe. *Postgrad Med.* 1994;95:173-4, 177-9, 182-4, passim.

Roth BJ, Martin RR, Foley K, et al. Roentgenographic evaluation of the cervical spine: a selective approach. *Arch Surg.* 1994;129:643-5.

Woodring JH, Lee C. Limitations of cervical radiography in the evaluation of acute cervical trauma. *J Trauma.* 1993;34:32-9.

Woodring JH, Lee C, Duncan V. Transverse process fractures of the cervical vertebrae: are they insignificant? *J Trauma.* 1993;34:797-802.

OTHER IMAGING PROCEDURES

Carragee EJ, Chen Y, Tanner CM, Hayward C. Rossi M, Hagle C. Can diskography cause long-term back symptoms in previously asymptomatic subjects? *Spine.* 2000;25(14):1803-8.

Colorado Division of Workers' Compensation. *Medical Treatment Guidelines, Rule XVII.* Cervical Spine Injury, 12 December 1, 2001.

Connor PM, Darden BV II. Cervical diskography complications and clinical efficacy. *Spine.* 1993;18:2035-8.

Grubb SA, Kelly CK. Cervical diskography: clinical implications from 12 years of experience. *Spine.* 2000;25:1382-9.

Kuroki T, Kumano K, Hirabayashi S. Usefulness of MRI in the preoperative diagnosis of cervical disk herniation. *Arch Orthop Trauma.* 1993;112:180-4.

Lehto IJ, Tertti MO, Komu ME, et al. Age-related MRI changes at 0.1 T in cervical disks in asymptomatic subjects. *Neuroradiology.* 1994;36:49-53.

Schellhas KP, Smith MD, Gundry CR, Pollei SR. Cervical discogenic pain: prospective correlation of magnetic resonance imaging and diskography in asymptomatic subjects and pain sufferers. *Spine.* 1996;21:300-12.

Siebenrock KA, Aebi M. Cervical diskography in discogenic pain syndrome and its predictive value for cervical fusion. *Arch Orthop Trauma Surg.* 1994;113:199-203.

Silberstein M, Tress BM, Hennessy O. Prevertebral swelling in cervical spine injury: identification of ligament injury with magnetic resonance imaging. *Clin Radiol.* 1992;46:318-23.

Tehranzadeh J, Bonk RT, Ansari A, et al. Efficacy of limited CT for nonvisualized lower cervical spine in patients with blunt trauma. *Skeletal Radiol.* 1994;23:349-52.

Woodring JH, Lee C. The role and limitations of computed tomographic scanning in the evaluation of cervical trauma. *J Trauma.* 1992;33:698-708.

Zeidman SM, Thompson K, Ducker TB. Complications of cervical diskography: analysis of 4400 diagnostic disc injections. *Neurosurgery.* 1995;37: 414-7.

SURGERY

Fouyas IP, Statham PFX, Sandercock PAG, Lynch C. Surgery for cervical radiculomyelopathy (Cochrane Review). In: *The Cochrane Library.* Issue 3; 2002.

Hubach PC. A prospective study of anterior cervical spondylodesis in intervertebral disc disorders. *Eur Spine J.* 1994;3:209-13.

Maigne JY, Deligne L. Computed tomographic follow-up study of 21 cases of nonoperatively treated cervical intervertebral soft disc herniation. *Spine.* 1994;19:189-91.

Perrin G, Lapras C, Goutelle A. Results of surgical treatment for cervicobrachial neuralgia: a retrospective study of 122 patients with long-term follow-up. *J Neuroradiol.* 1992;19:204-10.

Shinomiya K, Okamoto A, Kamikozuru M, et al. An analysis of failures in primary cervical anterior spinal cord decompression and fusion. *J Spinal Disorders.* 1993;6:277-88.

Spitzer WO, Skovron ML, Salmi LR, et al. Scientific monograph of the Quebec Task Force on whiplash associated disorders. *Spine.* 1995;20(8S):1S-73S.

Ullman JS, Camins MB, Post KD. Complications of cervical disc surgery. *M Sinai J Med.* 1994;61:276-9.

Master Algorithm. *ACOEM Guidelines for Care of Acute and Subacute Occupational Shoulder Complaints*

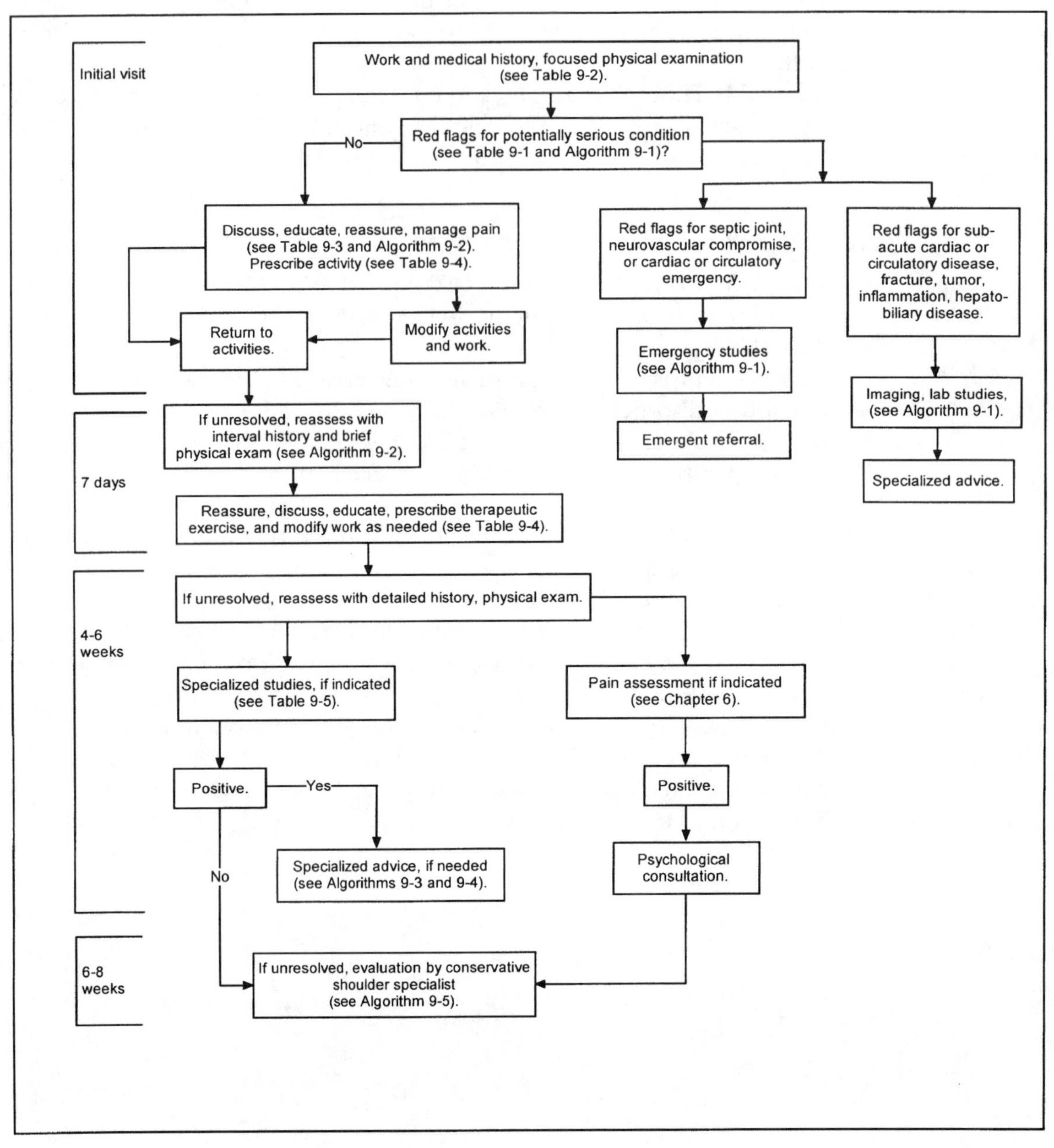

9 Shoulder Complaints

General Approach and Basic Principles

Occupational and primary care providers commonly see shoulder complaints that are potentially work related; they are among the five most common causes of reported work-related health complaints in workers' compensation claims. These complaints account for about 3-5% of total lost workdays and 10-11% of claims and costs in workers' compensation, ranking them in the top five for financial severity, although much of the total expense is incurred for surgical procedures.

This clinical practice guideline presents recommendations on assessing and treating adults with potentially work-related shoulder complaints. Topics include the initial assessment and diagnosis of patients with acute and subacute shoulder complaints that are potentially work related, identification of red flags that may indicate the presence of a serious underlying medical condition, initial management, diagnostic considerations, and special studies for identifying clinical pathology, work-relatedness, return to work, modified duty and activity, and further management considerations, including the management of delayed recovery.

Algorithms for patient management are included. This chapter's master algorithm schematizes the manner in which primary care and occupational medicine practitioners generally can manage patients with acute and subacute shoulder problems. The following text, tables, and numbered algorithms expand upon the master algorithm.

The principal recommendations for assessing and treating patients with shoulder complaints are as follows:

- The initial assessment focuses on detecting indications of potentially serious disease, termed red flags, and making an accurate diagnosis.
- In the absence of red flags, work-related shoulder complaints can be safely and effectively managed by occupational or primary care providers. The focus is on monitoring for complications, facilitating the healing process, and facilitating return to work in a modified- or full-duty capacity.

- Relief of discomfort can be accomplished most safely by activity modification and systemic nonprescription analgesics.
- Patients recovering from acute and subacute shoulder injury or infection are encouraged to return to modified work as their condition permits.
- If symptoms persist for more than 4-6 weeks, referral for specialty care may be indicated.
- Nonphysical factors (such as psychosocial, workplace, or socioeconomic problems) should be addressed in an effort to resolve delayed recovery.

Initial Assessment

Thorough medical and work histories and a focused physical examination (see Chapter 2) are sufficient for the initial assessment of the worker complaining of potentially work-related shoulder symptoms. The medical history and examination include evaluation for serious underlying conditions. This evaluation can consider the possibility of referred shoulder pain due to a disorder in another part of the body (most commonly from the cervical spine). Certain findings on the history and physical examination raise suspicion of serious underlying medical conditions, referred to as red flags (see Table 9-1). The absence of red flags rules out the need for special studies, referral, or inpatient care during the first four to six weeks, when spontaneous recovery is expected (provided any contributory workplace factors are mitigated). Shoulder complaints can then be classified into one of four working categories:

- **Potentially serious bone conditions,** including fractures, glenohumeral dislocation, infection, or serious nerve or circulation conditions, including referred neck, cardiac, or intraabdominal pain, thoracic outlet syndrome (TOS), or brachial plexus injury
- **Mechanical disorders:** derangements of the shoulder related to acute trauma, such as acute rotator cuff tear, acromioclavicular (AC) joint strain or separation, or a recently reduced dislocation
- **Degenerative disorders:** consequences of aging or repetitive use, such as impingement syndrome, rotator cuff tendinitis, degenerative rotator cuff tear, adhesive capsulitis (frozen shoulder), tendonopathy, bursitis, or recurrent dislocation
- **Nonspecific shoulder disorders:** suggesting neither internal derangement nor referred pain

Medical History

Asking the patient open-ended questions, such as those listed on pages 198-199, allows the clinician to gauge the need for further discussion or specific inquiries to obtain more detailed information (see also Chapter 2):

Table 9-1. Red Flags for Potentially Serious Shoulder Conditions

Disorder	Medical History	Physical Examination
Fractures	History of significant trauma (direct, deceleration)	Significant bruising or hemarthrosis Deformity consistent with displaced fracture (with fracture, check for pulmonary injury and rib fracture as well) Significant swelling
Dislocation (glenohumeral joint)	Severe pain and inability to move the shoulder History of significant trauma History of prior dislocation History of deformity, with spontaneous reduction or self-reduction	Deformity consistent with unreduced dislocation
Infection	Diabetes Persistent, severe shoulder pain History of systemic symptoms of infection History of immunosuppression (transplant, chemotherapy, HIV)	Limited range of motion due to severe pain Systemic signs of sepsis (elevated temperature, chills, hypotension, tachycardia)
Tumor	Pain at rest History of smoking History of cancer (especially lung) History of immunosuppression (transplant, chemotherapy, HIV)	Palpable mass Tumor vessels
Progressive neurologic compromise	History of neurologic disease History of diabetes Degenerative disk disease Trauma	Decreased upper-extremity sensation, motor strength, and/or reflexes
Progressive vascular compromise	History of vascular disease History of diabetes History of atherosclerotic History of syphilis History of dislocation, fracture, etc. History of high-impact collision	Decreased pulses in the upper extremities Cold, pulseless extremity Pain-free full range of motion Differential blood pressure in upper extremities Bruit (with thoracic aortic aneurysm)

Table 9-1. (continued)

Disorder	Medical History	Physical Examination
Cardiac condition	History of angina or coronary disease History of cardiac risk factors (smoking, high cholesterol, high blood pressure, obesity) Family history of heart disease	S3 or S4 heart sounds Arrhythmia Cold, clammy skin Apprehension Hypotension Pain-free full ROM
Subdiaphragmatic conditions	History of subdiaphragmatic condition (gallbladder or liver disorder, perihepatitis, PID, or cervicitis)	Tender right upper quadrant Palpable mass in right upper quadrant Evidence of pelvic infection
Acute rotator cuff tear in a young worker	Heavy lifting Sudden pull Pain in shoulder with overhead work Fall on outstretched arm	Weakness of abduction with thumbs down Weakness of external rotation Weakness on supra- and infraspinatus tests Weakness on elevation and external rotation

1. PREVIOUS SHOULDER PROBLEMS

   - Have you had similar episodes previously (prior to the recent episode of this condition)?
   - What investigations were conducted with prior episodes of this shoulder condition.
   - What treatment did you have with prior episodes of this shoulder condition.

2. SYMPTOM ONSET

   - When did your current limitations begin?
   - Do you recall a specific inciting event?
   - Was there an acute event that triggered the pain or limitation of motion?
   - How did it occur?
   - How did the limitations develop?

3. PROGRESS OF SHOULDER CONDITION

   - Have your symptoms changed?
   - How long have your activities been limited?
   - What investigations and x-rays have you had?
   - Have you had specialist consultations.
   - What treatments have you had so far, including medication?

4. PRESENT SYMPTOMS

- Are you experiencing pain, weakness, popping, or limited motion in your shoulder?
- Are your symptoms located primarily in the shoulder joint?
- Do you have pain or other symptoms elsewhere (e.g., neck, chest, or abdomen?
- Are your symptoms constant or intermittent?
- What makes the problem worse or better?
- Is your shoulder pain associated with pain, numbness, tingling, swelling, or color change in the hand or arm?

5. PRESENT SHOULDER CAPABILITIES

- Can you do overhead work?
- For how long can you perform overhead work?
- How much weight can you lift?
- Can you move your shoulder without pain?
- Can you sleep on the affected shoulder?
- Do you have weakness in your hand, arm, or shoulder?
- Have you noticed any loss of muscle mass?

6. JOB DEMANDS

- What are your specific job duties.
- Shoulder activities at work:
    - What postures and activities are required at work.
    - Are there job duties requiring shoulder activity.
    - How often are shoulder activities required?

7. OFF-THE-JOB ACTIVITIES (AVOCATIONAL ACTIVITIES)

- What other activities (hobbies, workouts, sports) do you do at home or elsewhere?
- Do you use your shoulder to perform these activities?
- Do you do any overhead arm actions? How? How Often?

8. DO YOU HAVE OTHER MEDICAL PROBLEMS?

- Do you have heart disease?
- Do you have gallbladder disease or any other digestive or liver disorder?
- Do you have vaginal discharge (in women)?
- Do you have neck pain or trauma?
- Have you ever had cancer?
- Do you smoke?

9. WHAT ARE YOUR GOALS IN RELATION TO THIS SHOULDER PROBLEM?

Physical Examination

Based on the medical history, the physical examination includes:

- General observation of the patient
- General level of fitness and physical condition
- Regional examination of the neck and shoulder girdle
- Neurovascular screening

The examination is mostly subjective, because the patient must exert voluntary effort or state a response to the sensory findings on the examination. In many cases of shoulder problems, there are no objective findings, but only painful range of motion (ROM), tenderness, or stiffness in the shoulder. Frozen shoulder or signs of infection or deformity due to fracture or dislocation may be present, but these causes are much less common than nonspecific pain, impingement syndrome, rotator cuff tendinitis, or rotator cuff tears (in that order). The clinician needs to be aware that a patient with a shoulder complaint but painless full range of motion of the shoulder may be experiencing referred pain.

A. Regional Shoulder Examination

A shoulder examination includes the neck region as well as the shoulder. Ask the patient to point to the area of discomfort with one finger. The range of motion of the shoulder should be determined actively and passively. The examiner may determine passive ROM by eliminating gravity in the pendulum position or by using the other arm to aid elevation. Atrophy of the deltoid or scapular muscles is an objective finding but arises only after weeks to months of symptoms. Deformities due to AC separations are visible, objective findings, as are signs of infection (elevated temperature, redness, heat, fluctuance) or gross tumor (visible vessels, palpable mass). The impingement sign of Neer and the modified impingement sign of Hawkins can be used to test for rotator cuff impingement. The apprehension test can be used to help detect dislocation (a positive test indicates glenohumeral instability, often due to previous dislocation). Strength of the supraspinatus and infraspinatus can be tested to diagnose rotator cuff tear or tendonopathy.

B. Neurologic and Vascular Screening

The neurologic and vascular status of the shoulder, proximal upper extremity, and neck can be assessed. Peripheral pulses in neutral and stress positions, edema and or color changes are assessed. The motor and sensory status of the shoulder and surrounding structures also can be assessed. Because C5 or C6 radiculopathy can present as shoulder pain or dysfunction, and soft tissue disorders of the neck also sometimes present as shoulder pain, examining the neck and cervical nerve root function is also required. Thoracic outlet syndrome (TOS) has signs and symptoms of scalene tenderness, positive Tinel's sign over the brachial plexus, and positive maneuvers that provoke neurovascular signs and symptoms. Tests for TOS are of questionable value. Once all other diagnoses have been ruled out and TOS is suspected, referral to a specialist is recommended if invasive treatment is entertained as an option.

C. Assessing Red Flags

Physical examination evidence of septic arthritis, neurologic compromise, cardiac disease, or intra-abdominal pathology that correlates with the medical history and test results may indicate a need for immediate consultation. The consultations may further reinforce or reduce suspicions of tumor, infection, fracture, or dislocation. A medical history that suggests pathology originating in a part of the body other than the shoulder may warrant examining the cardiovascular and respiratory systems, abdomen, or other areas. Painless full ROM of the shoulder suggests referred pain.

Diagnostic Criteria

If no red flags for serious conditions are present, then determine which common musculoskeletal disorder is present. The criteria presented in Table 9-2 follow the clinical thought process, from the mechanism of illness or injury to unique symptoms and signs of a particular disorder, and to test results, if any tests are needed to guide treatment at this stage.

Work-Relatedness

A thorough work history is crucial to establishing work-relatedness. (See Chapter 2 for components of the work history.) Repetitive overhead work contributes to shoulder tendinitis or tendonopathy (see Table 9-1). Evidence of the work-relatedness of other entities discussed in this chapter, such as adhesive capsulitis, is not well delineated. Acute work-related trauma can be associated with rotator cuff tears, AC ligament strains, and AC separations.

Initial Care

Pain relief is often a patient's first concern. Nonprescription analgesics may provide sufficient pain relief for most patients with acute and subacute symptoms. If treatment response is inadequate (i.e., if symptoms and activity limitations continue), prescribed pharmaceuticals or physical methods can be added. Comorbid conditions, side effects, cost, and provider and patient preferences

Table 9-2. Diagnostic Criteria for Non-red-flag Shoulder Conditions that Can Be Managed by Primary Care Physicians

Probable Diagnosis or Injury	Mechanism	Unique Symptoms	Unique Signs	Tests and Results
Nonspecific shoulder pain (ICD-9 719.41, 719.51, 726.0, 729.89)	No known specific mechanism Overuse relative to physical conditioning	Pain in shoulder	None	None indicated
Rotator cuff tear (ICD-9 727.61 [chronic], 727.61 [acute])	Heavy lifting Sudden pull Fall on outstretched arm especially in > 30-year-old workers with preexisting degenerative changes Spontaneous in onset	Pain over the deltoid area with overhead work Weakness on elevation and external rotation of shoulder	Weakness of shoulder in "thumbs down" abduction Weak external rotation	MRI positive for acute tears in younger workers (preoperatively only) Arthrography positive for full-thickness tears (preoperatively only if MRI unavailable) MRI may show partial-thickness tears
Labral tear (ICD-9 718.01)	Direct trauma laterally to shoulder	Pain with movement	Instability	MRI positive for lateral tear
Impingement (ICD-9 718.91, 726.10, 726.11, 726.12, 726.19, 726.2)	Chronic rotator cuff degenerative changes May be exacerbated by repeated overhead work Acute irritation	Night pain in shoulder joint Nonradiating pain in deltoid area	Positive impingement sign Positive modified impingement sign	None indicated
Shoulder instability (ICD-9 718.81)	Congenital anatomic problem Trauma (rare)	Slipping Popping Feeling of instability "Dead arm" syndrome	Positive apprehension test Positive relocation test of Job	Positive stress films (weight bearing)
Recurrent dislocation (ICD-9 718.31) (nonacute)	Previous dislocation due to a fall or direct impact	Recurrent dislocation Fear of dislocation when shoulder is abducted in external rotation	Positive apprehension test	Radiographic films positive for dislocation if acute
AC joint strain (ICD-9 840.0)	Fall on top of shoulder	Pain over AC joint	Tender over AC joint	None indicated

Table 9-2. (continued)

Probable Diagnosis or Injury	Mechanism	Unique Symptoms	Unique Signs	Tests and Results
AC joint separation (ICD-9 831.04)	Fall on top of shoulder	Severe pain over AC joint	Deformity over AC joint (i.e., high-riding distal clavicle)	Weighted films show separation > 5 mm (typically not performed, because the disorder is clinically obvious and the test is painful)
Adhesive capsulitis (ICD-9 726.0)	Failed treatment or inactivity Idiopathic	Night pain in shoulder joint Lack of range of motion	Limited passive range of motion	MRI if diagnosis unclear (frozen shoulder)
Bursitis (ICD-9 727.3)	Overuse	Night pain	Tenderness over subacromial bursa	None indicated

Note: ICD-9 = International Classification of Diseases, 9th Edition.

guide the clinician's choice of recommendations. Table 9-3 summarizes comfort options.

- Instruction in home exercise. Except in cases of unstable fractures, acute dislocations, instability or hypermobility, patients can be advised to do early pendulum or passive ROM exercises at home. Instruction in proper exercise technique is important, and a few visits to a good physical therapist can serve to educate the patient about an effective exercise program.
- Manipulation by a manual therapist has been described as effective for patients with frozen shoulders. The period of treatment is limited to a few weeks, because results decrease with time. Scalene-stretching and trapezius-strengthening exercises have been found effective in relieving thoracic outlet compression symptoms.
- Physical modalities, such as massage, diathermy, cutaneous laser treatment, ultrasound treatment, transcutaneous electrical neurostimulation (TENS) units, and biofeedback are not supported by high-quality medical studies, but they may be useful in the initial conservative treatment of acute shoulder symptoms, depending on the experience of local physical therapists available for referral. Some medium quality evidence supports manual physical therapy, ultrasound, and high-energy extracorporeal shock wave therapy for calcifying tendinitis of the shoulder. Patients' at-home applications of heat or cold packs may be used before or after exercises and are as effective as those performed by a therapist. Initial use of less-invasive techniques provides an opportunity for the clinician to monitor progress before referral to a specialist.

Table 9-3. Methods of Symptom Control for Patients with Shoulder Complaints

RECOMMENDED
Nonprescription Medications
Acetaminophen (safest) NSAIDs (aspirin, ibuprofen)
Nonprescribed Physical Methods
Adjust or modify workstation after ergonomic assessment, job tasks, or work hours Stretching Specific shoulder exercises for ROM and strengthening Home, local application of cold during first few days of acute complaint; thereafter, then heat application Relaxation techniques
Prescribed Pharmaceutical Methods
NSAIDs Short course of narcotic analgesics for AC separation, if needed
Prescribed Physical Methods
Initial and follow-up visits for education, counseling, and evaluation of home exercise

OPTIONS

Impingement Syndrome	Nonspecific Shoulder Pain	Rotator Cuff Tear
Corticosteroid injection into subacromial bursa Global shoulder strengthening	Global shoulder strengthening Aerobic exercise	Refer young active workers with acute tears for surgical repair Sling for acute pain
Recurrent Dislocation	**Shoulder Instability**	**AC Joint Strain or Separation**
Rotator muscle strengthening	Global shoulder girdle strengthening	Sling for comfort

- Invasive techniques have limited proven value. If pain with elevation significantly limits activities, a subacromial injection of local anesthetic and a corticosteroid preparation may be indicated after conservative therapy (i.e., strengthening exercises and nonsteroidal anti-inflammatory drugs) for two to three weeks. The evidence supporting such an approach is not overwhelming. The total number of injections should be limited to three per episode, allowing for assessment of benefit between injections.
- Some small studies have supported using acupuncture, but referral is dependent on the availability of experienced providers with consistently good outcomes.

- If response to exercise is protracted, anterior scalene block has been reported to be efficacious in relieving acute thoracic outlet symptoms, and as an adjunct to diagnosis.
- Significant differences between traditional approaches and various alternative and multidisciplinary intervention programs for shoulder pain have not been demonstrated in the medical literature to date. Recommendations, prescription, or referral regarding such multidisciplinary programs or alternative care can be based on the practitioner's professional judgment and the patient's individual situation or condition. For example, the success of chiropractic manipulation is highly dependent on the patient's previous successful experience with chiropractors.

Activity Modification

Shoulder disorders may lead to joint stiffness more often than other joint disorders. Because patients with shoulder disorders tend to have stiffness followed by weakness and atrophy, careful advice regarding maximizing activities within the limits of symptoms is imperative, once red flags have been ruled out. If indicated, the joint can be kept at rest in a sling. Gentle exercise even during this time is desirable. Patients acutely should avoid activities that precipitate symptoms, but should continue general activities and motion. Therapeutic exercise, including strengthening, should start as soon as it can be done without aggravating symptoms. Patients usually can tolerate pendulum exercises even when discomfort is pronounced, and this method can preserve ROM.

Activities and postures that increase stress on the shoulder and contribute to structural damage tend to aggravate symptoms. Lifting and working at 90 degrees forward or sideways, as well as overhead work, can be proscribed or restricted during the first few weeks after onset of problems due to acute rotator cuff tear, AC joint strain or separation, and impingement syndrome.

Work Activities

Occupational clinicians often are asked to make specific recommendations about work activities for patients with acute limitations due to acute shoulder problems. Table 9-4 provides a guide for recommendations about activity modification. These guidelines are intended for patients without comorbidity or complicating factors, including employment or legal issues. They are targets to provide a guide from the perspective of physiologic recovery. The clinician can make it clear to patients and employers that:

- Even moderately heavy (more than 20 pounds) unassisted lifting or repeated work at "shoulder level" (90 degrees forward or sideways) or overhead may aggravate shoulder symptoms due to rotator cuff tears, inflammatory conditions, ligament damage, and impingement syndrome.

*Table 9-4. Guidelines for Modification of Work Activities and Disability Duration**

Disorder	Activity Modifications and Accommodation	Recommended Target for Disability Duration**		NHIS Experience Data***	
		With Modified Duty	Without Modified Duty	Median (cases with lost time)	Percent No Lost Time
Acute tears in rotator cuff in younger workers	Refer for possible repair. Avoid work at a 90-degree forward or sideway position, pushing, pulling, and heavy lifting if patient wishes to avoid surgical repair.	1-2 days	21 days	27 days	66%
Chronic tear in rotator cuff	Avoid work at a 90-degree forward or sideway position, pushing, pulling, and heavy lifting.	1-2 days	21 days	27 days	66%
Impingement syndrome	Avoid overhead work, pushing, pulling, and heavy lifting.	1 day	3-7 days	14 days	65%
Shoulder instability	Avoid pushing, pulling, and heavy lifting.	0 days	21 days	9 days	50%
Recurrent dislocation	Avoid overhead work, pushing, and pulling.	0 days	21 days	12 days	35%
AC joint strain	Avoid overhead work, pushing, and pulling.	1 day	3-7 days	14 days	23%
AC joint separation	Allow activity as tolerated, with arm in immobilizer.	7 days	21 days	14 days	18%
Regional shoulder pain	Allow all activities as tolerated; avoid those that aggravate symptoms but start range-of-motion exercises and conditioning.	0 days	3-7 days	4 days	49%

* These are general guidelines based on consensus or population sources and are never meant to be applied to an individual case without consideration of workplace factors, concurrent disease or other social or medical factors that can affect recovery.
** These parameters for disability duration are "consensus optimal" targets as determined by a panel of ACOEM members in 1996, and reaffirmed by a panel of ACOEM members in 2002. In most cases persons with one nonsevere extremity injury can return to modified duty immediately. Restrictions should take into consideration the opposite extremity also to prevent strain injuries to the uninjured extremity.
*** Based on the CDC NHIS (National Health Interview Survey), as compiled and reported in the 8th annual edition of *Official Disability Guidelines (ODG)*, © 2002 Work Loss Data Institute, all rights reserved.

- Any restrictions are intended to allow for spontaneous recovery or time to build activity tolerance through exercise.

Assist the patient in avoiding aggravating activities by reviewing work activities and responsibilities to decide whether modifications can be accomplished and to determine whether modified activity is an option. To aid recovery, make every attempt to maintain the patient at sufficient levels of activity, including work, hobbies, and sports activities.

Follow-up Visits

Patients with shoulder complaints can have follow-up every three to five days by an appropriate health professional who can counsel them about avoiding static positions, medication use, activity modification, and other concerns. The practitioner should take care to answer questions and make these sessions interactive so that the patient is fully involved in his or her recovery. If the patient has returned to work, these interactions may be done on site or by telephone.

Physician follow-up generally occurs when a release to modified, increased, or full activity is needed, or after appreciable healing or recovery can be expected, on average. Physician follow-up might be expected every four to seven days if the patient is off work and every seven to fourteen days if the patient is working.

Special Studies and Diagnostic and Treatment Considerations

For most patients with shoulder problems, special studies are not needed unless a four- to six-week period of conservative care and observation fails to improve symptoms. Most patients improve quickly, provided red-flag conditions are ruled out. There are a few exceptions:

- Stress films of the AC joints (views of both shoulders, with and without patient holding 15-lb weights) may be indicated if the clinical diagnosis is AC joint separation. Care should be taken when selecting this test because the disorder is usually clinically obvious, and the test is painful and expensive relative to its yield.
- If an initial or recurrent shoulder dislocation presents in the dislocated position, shoulder films before and after reduction are indicated.
- Persistent shoulder pain, associated with neurovascular compression symptoms (particularly with abduction and external rotation), may indicate the need for an AP cervical spine radiograph to identify a cervical rib.

Routine testing (laboratory tests, plain-film radiographs of the shoulder) and more specialized imaging studies are not recommended during the first month to six weeks of activity limitation due to shoulder symptoms, except when a red flag noted on history or examination raises suspicion of a serious shoulder condition or referred pain. Cases of impingement syndrome are managed the same regardless of whether radiographs show calcium in the rotator cuff or degenerative changes are seen in or around the glenohumeral joint or AC joint. Suspected acute tears of the rotator cuff in young workers may be surgically repaired acutely to restore function; in older workers, these tears are typically treated conservatively at first. Partial-thickness tears should be treated the same as impingement syndrome regardless of magnetic resonance imaging (MRI) findings. Shoulder instability can be treated with stabilization exercises; stress radiographs simply confirm the clinical diagnosis. For patients with limitations of activity after four weeks and unexplained physical findings, such as effusion or localized pain (especially following exercise), imaging may be indicated to clarify the diagnosis and assist reconditioning. Imaging findings can be correlated with physical findings.

Primary criteria for ordering imaging studies are:

- Emergence of a red flag (e.g., indications of intra-abdominal or cardiac problems presenting as shoulder problems)
- Physiologic evidence of tissue insult or neurovascular dysfunction (e.g., cervical root problems presenting as shoulder pain, weakness from a massive rotator cuff tear, or the presence of edema, cyanosis or Raynaud's phenomenon)
- Failure to progress in a strengthening program intended to avoid surgery.
- Clarification of the anatomy prior to an invasive procedure (e.g., a full-thickness rotator cuff tear not responding to conservative treatment)

Laboratory studies, such as liver function tests, tests of gallbladder function, and tests for pelvic disease may be useful to determine if pain is being referred to the shoulder from a subdiaphragmatic source. Electrocardiography, and possibly cardiac enzyme studies, may be needed to clarify apparent referred cardiac pain. Chest radiographs may be needed to elucidate shoulder pain that could be the result of pneumothorax, apical lung tumor, or other apical disease such as tuberculosis. An erythrocyte sedimentation rate (ESR), complete blood count (CBC), and tests for autoimmune diseases (such as rheumatoid factor) can be useful to screen for inflammatory or autoimmune sources of joint pain. All of these tests can be used to confirm clinical impressions, rather than purely as screening tests in a "shotgun" attempt to clarify reasons for unexplained shoulder complaints.

Anatomic definition by means of imaging is commonly required to guide surgery or other procedures. A discussion with a specialist on selecting the most clinically valuable study can often help the primary care physician avoid duplication. Table 9-5 compares the abilities of different imaging techniques to identify physiologic insult and define anatomic defects. Selecting an imaging test takes into consideration any patient allergies to contrast materials (used in arthrography or contrast computer tomography [CT]), or concerns about claustrophobia (sometimes a problem in patients undergoing MRI), and costs.

Imaging may be considered for a patient whose limitations due to consistent symptoms have persisted for one month or more, i.e., in cases:

- When surgery is being considered for a specific anatomic defect (e.g., a full-thickness rotator cuff tear). Magnetic resonance imaging and arthrography have fairly similar diagnostic and therapeutic impact and comparable accuracy although MRI is more sensitive and less specific.

Table 9-5. Ability of Various Techniques to Identify and Define Shoulder Pathology

Technique	Impingement Syndrome	Rotator Cuff Tear	Instability	Recurrent Dislocation	Regional Pain	Tumor	Infection
History	+ +	+	+ +	+ + +	+	0	+ +
Physical examination	+ + +	+ +	+ + +	+ +	+	0	+ + +
Laboratory studies	0	0	0	0	0	+ +	+ + +
Imaging studies							
Radiography[1]	+	+	+	+ +	0	+ +	+ +
Bone scan[1]	0	0	0	0	0	+ + + +	+ + +
Arthrography[1]	0	+ + + +	0	+	0	0	+
Computed tomography (CT)[1]	0	0	0	+ +	0	+ +	+ +
Magnetic resonance imaging (MRI)[1]	+	+ + + +	0	+ +	0	+ + +	+ + +

[1] Risk of complications, e.g., infection, radiation, highest for contrast CT or arthrography; second highest for, and relatively less for, bone scan, radiography, and CT; lowest for MRI.

Note: Number of plus signs indicates relative ability to identify or define pathology.

Magnetic resonance imaging may be the preferred investigation because it demonstrates soft tissue anatomy better.

- To further evaluate the possibility of potentially serious pathology, such as a tumor.

Selecting specific imaging equipment and procedures will depend on the availability and experience of local referrals.

Relying only on imaging studies to evaluate the source of shoulder symptoms carries a significant risk of diagnostic confusion (false-positive test results) because of the possibility of identifying a finding that was present before symptoms began (for example, degenerative partial thickness rotator cuff tears), and therefore has no temporal association with the symptoms.

Surgical Considerations

Referral for surgical consultation may be indicated for patients who have:

- Red-flag conditions (e.g., acute rotator cuff tear in a young worker, glenohumeral joint dislocation, etc.)
- Activity limitation for more than four months, *plus* existence of a surgical lesion
- Failure to increase ROM and strength of the musculature around the shoulder even after exercise programs, *plus* existence of a surgical lesion
- Clear clinical and imaging evidence of a lesion that has been shown to benefit, in both the short and long term, from surgical repair

Surgical considerations depend on the working or imaging-confirmed diagnosis of the presenting shoulder complaint. If surgery is a consideration, counseling regarding likely outcomes, risks and benefits, and expectations, in particular, is very important. If there is no clear indication for surgery, referring the patient to a physical medicine practitioner may help resolve the symptoms.

For postsurgical rehabilitation, key indicators for further assessment and treatment include:

- Prolonged course
- Multiple surgical procedures
- Use of narcotic medications

A. Acromioclavicular (AC) Joint Separation

Patients with AC joint separation may be treated conservatively. The expected period of pain is three weeks, with the pain gradually decreasing. If pain persists after recovery and return to activities, resection of the outer clavicle may be indicated after six months to one year, although local cortisone injections can be tried. The initial deformity decreases as healing and scar contracture take place. In one series, 79% of patients with moderate-to-severe AC separations had good-to-excellent late results with nonoperative treatment, and of the remainder, 90% had good-to-excellent results with simple excision of the outer clavicle.

B. Rotator Cuff Tear

Rotator cuff repair is indicated for significant tears that impair activities by causing weakness of arm elevation or rotation, particularly acutely in younger workers. Rotator cuff tears are frequently partial-thickness or smaller full-thickness tears. For partial-thickness rotator cuff tears and small full-thickness tears presenting primarily as impingement, surgery is reserved for cases failing conservative therapy for three months. The preferred procedure is usually arthroscopic decompression, which involves debridement of inflamed tissue, burring of the anterior acromion, lysis and, sometimes, removal of the coracoacromial ligament, and possibly removal of the outer clavicle. Surgery is not indicated for patients with mild symptoms or those whose activities are not limited.

Lesions of the rotator cuff are a continuum, from mild supraspinatus tendon degeneration to complete ruptures. Studies of normal subjects document the universal presence of degenerative changes and conditions, including full avulsions without symptoms. Conservative treatment has results similar to surgical treatment but without surgical risks. Studies evaluating results of conservative treatment of full-thickness rotator cuff tears have shown an 82-86% success rate for patients presenting within three months of injury. The efficacy of arthroscopic decompression for full-thickness tears depends on the size of the tear; one study reported satisfactory results in 90% of patients with small tears. A prior study by the same group reported satisfactory results in 86% of patients who underwent open repair for larger tears. Surgical outcomes of rotator cuff tears are much better in younger patients than in older patients who may be suffering from degenerative changes in the rotator cuff.

C. Shoulder Dislocation

Multiple traumatic shoulder dislocations indicate the need for surgery if the shoulder has limited functional ability and if muscle strengthening fails. In the acute phase, shoulder dislocations can be immobilized for up to three weeks although recommendations for immobilization for a period as short as three days have appeared in the literature. If shoulder instability is present only with violent forceful overhead activity, activity modification is recommended. Surgery can be considered for patients who are symptomatic with all overhead activities and patients who have had two or three episodes of dislocation and instability that limited their activity between episodes. Rates of instability recurrence after surgery have been reported as 8% after open repair for anterior instability and 10% after arthroscopic anterior repair. A high incidence of rotator cuff tears accompanying anterior shoulder dislocations occurs in patients 40 years old or older. Although the dislocation recurrence rate is very low, persistent weakness several weeks after a primary dislocation dictates further study to define the anatomy of the rotator cuff.

D. Impingement Syndrome

Surgery for impingement syndrome is usually arthroscopic decompression. This procedure is not indicated for patients with mild symptoms or those who have no activity limitations. Conservative care, including cortisone injections, can be carried out for at least three to six months before considering surgery. Because this diagnosis is on a continuum with other rotator cuff conditions, including rotator cuff syndrome and rotator cuff tendinitis, also refer to the previous discussion of rotator cuff tears.

E. Ruptured Biceps Tendon

Ruptures of the proximal (long head) of the biceps tendon are usually due to degenerative changes in the tendon. It can almost always be managed conservatively because there is no accompanying functional disability. Surgery may be desired for cosmetic reasons, especially by young bodybuilders, but is not necessary for function.

F. Thoracic Outlet Compression Syndrome

Most patients with acute thoracic outlet compression symptoms will respond to a conservative program of global shoulder strengthening (with specific exercises) and ergonomic changes. While not well supported by high-grade scientific studies, cases with progressive weakness, atrophy, and neurologic dysfunction are sometimes considered for surgical decompression. A confirmatory response to electromyography (EMG)-guided scalene block, confirmatory electrophysiologic testing and/or magnetic resonance angiography with flow studies is advisable before considering surgery.

Summary of Recommendations and Evidence

See Table 9-6.

Table 9-6. Summary of Recommendations for Evaluating and Managing Shoulder Complaints

Clinical Measure	Recommended	Optional	Not Recommended
History and physical exam	Focused history and exam Search for red flags (e.g., for tumor, infection, angina) (C)		
Patient education	Patient education regarding condition or disorder, expectations of treatment, side effects, etc. (D)		
Medication (See Chapter 3)	Acetaminophen (C) NSAIDs (B)	Opioids, short course (C)	Use of opioids for more than 2 weeks (C) Muscle relaxants (D)
Physical treatment methods, activities and exercise	Maintain activities of other parts of body while recovering (D) Maintain passive range of motion of the shoulder with pendulum exercises and wall crawl (D) Treat initially with strengthening or stabilization exercises for impingement syndrome, rotator cuff tear, instability, and recurrent dislocation (C, D)	At-home applications of heat or cold packs to aid exercises (D) Short course of supervised exercise instruction by a therapist (D)	Passive modalities by a therapist (unless accompanied by teaching the patient exercises to be carried out at home) (D)

Table 9-6. (continued)

Clinical Measure	Recommended	Optional	Not Recommended
Injections	Two or three sub-acromial injections of local anesthetic and cortisone preparation over an extended period as part of an exercise rehabilitation program to treat rotator cuff inflammation, impingement syndrome, or small tears (C, D) Diagnostic lidocaine injections to distinguish pain sources in the shoulder area (e.g., impingement) (D)		Prolonged or frequent use of cortisone injections into the sub-acromial space or the shoulder joint (D)
Rest and immobilization	Brief use of a sling for severe shoulder pain (1 to 2 days), with pendulum exercises to prevent stiffness in cases of rotator cuff conditions (D) Three weeks use, or less, of a sling after an initial shoulder dislocation and reduction (C) Same for AC separations or severe sprains (D)		Prolonged use of a sling only for symptom control (D)
Detection of physiologic abnormalities	Rarely, nerve conduction time of the suprascapular nerve for cases of severe cuff weakness unaccompanied by signs of a rotator cuff tear (D)		EMG or NCV studies as part of a shoulder evaluation for usual diagnoses (D)

Table 9-6. (continued)

Clinical Measure	Recommended	Optional	Not Recommended
Radiography		For acute AC joint separations, stress films (views of both shoulders, with and without patient holding 15-lb weights) (D)	Routine radiographs for shoulder complaints before 4 to 6 weeks of conservative treatment (D) Stress films for instability (D)
Other imaging procedures	MRI for preoperative evaluation of partial-thickness or large full-thickness rotator cuff tears (C, D)	Arthrography for preoperative evaluation of small full-thickness tears (C) Bone scan for detection of AC joint arthritis (D)	Routine MRI or arthrography for evaluation without surgical indications (D) Ultrasonography for evaluation of rotator cuff (C)
Surgical considerations	Anterior repair for recurrent dislocation after 2 to 3 dislocations (D) Resection of outer clavicle for chronic disabling AC joint pain after conservative care of acute separation (C) Rotator cuff repair after firm diagnosis is made and rehabilitation efforts have failed (D) Capsular shift surgery for disabling instability (D) Subacromial decompression after failure of non-operative care (C)		Anterior repair for initial shoulder dislocation (C) Acute repair of AC separation (C) Acute repair of rotator cuff tears, except for massive acute tears (C) Surgery for recurrent dislocation of instability before rehabilitation efforts (C)

A = Strong research-based evidence (multiple relevant, high-quality scientific studies).
B = Moderate research-based evidence (one relevant, high-quality scientific study or multiple adequate scientific studies).
C = Limited research-based evidence (at least one adequate scientific study of patients with shoulder disorders).
D = Panel interpretation of information not meeting inclusion criteria for research-based evidence.

Algorithm 9-1. *Initial Evaluation of Occupational Shoulder Complaints*

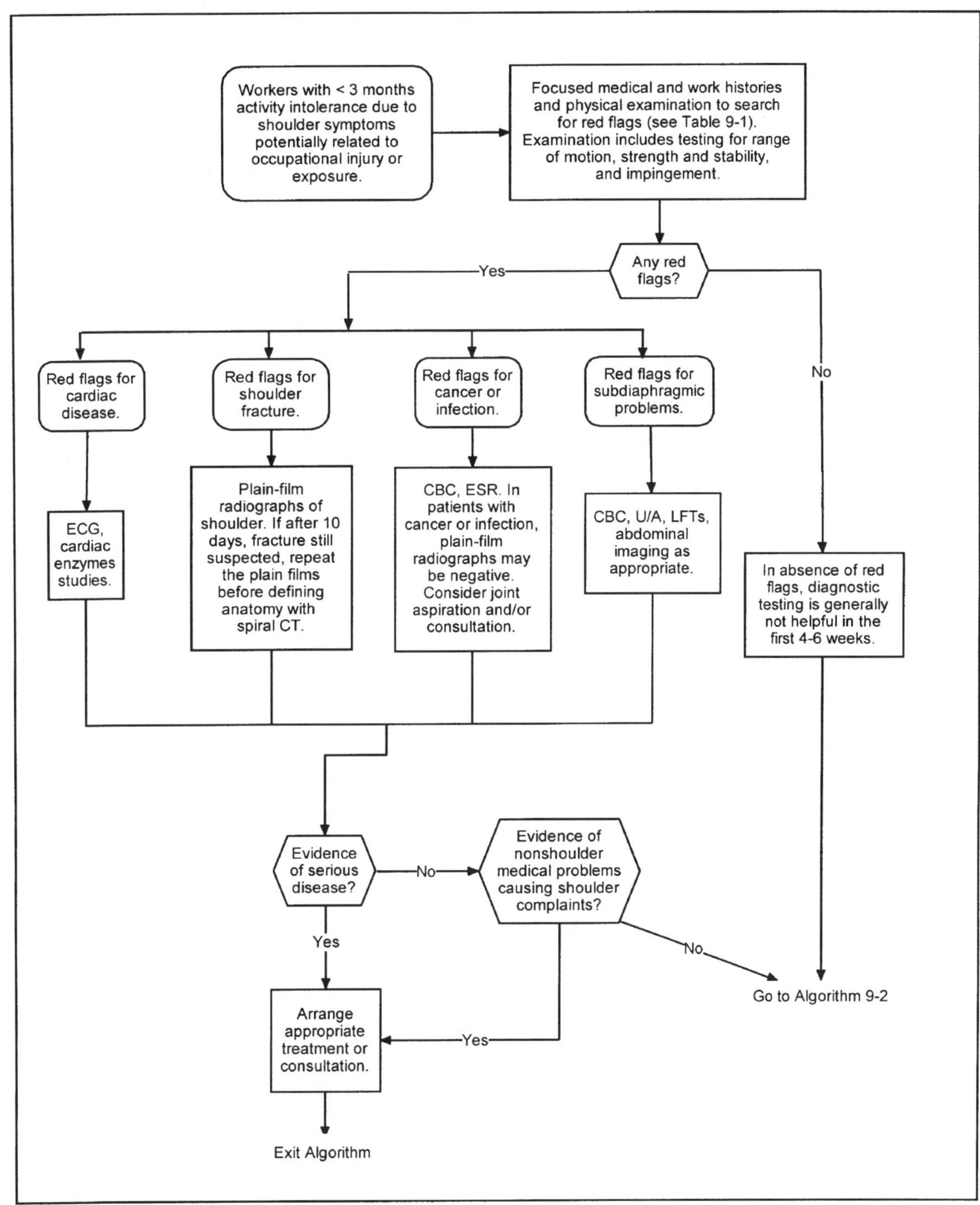

Algorithm 9-2. *Initial and Follow-up Management of Occupational Shoulder Complaints*

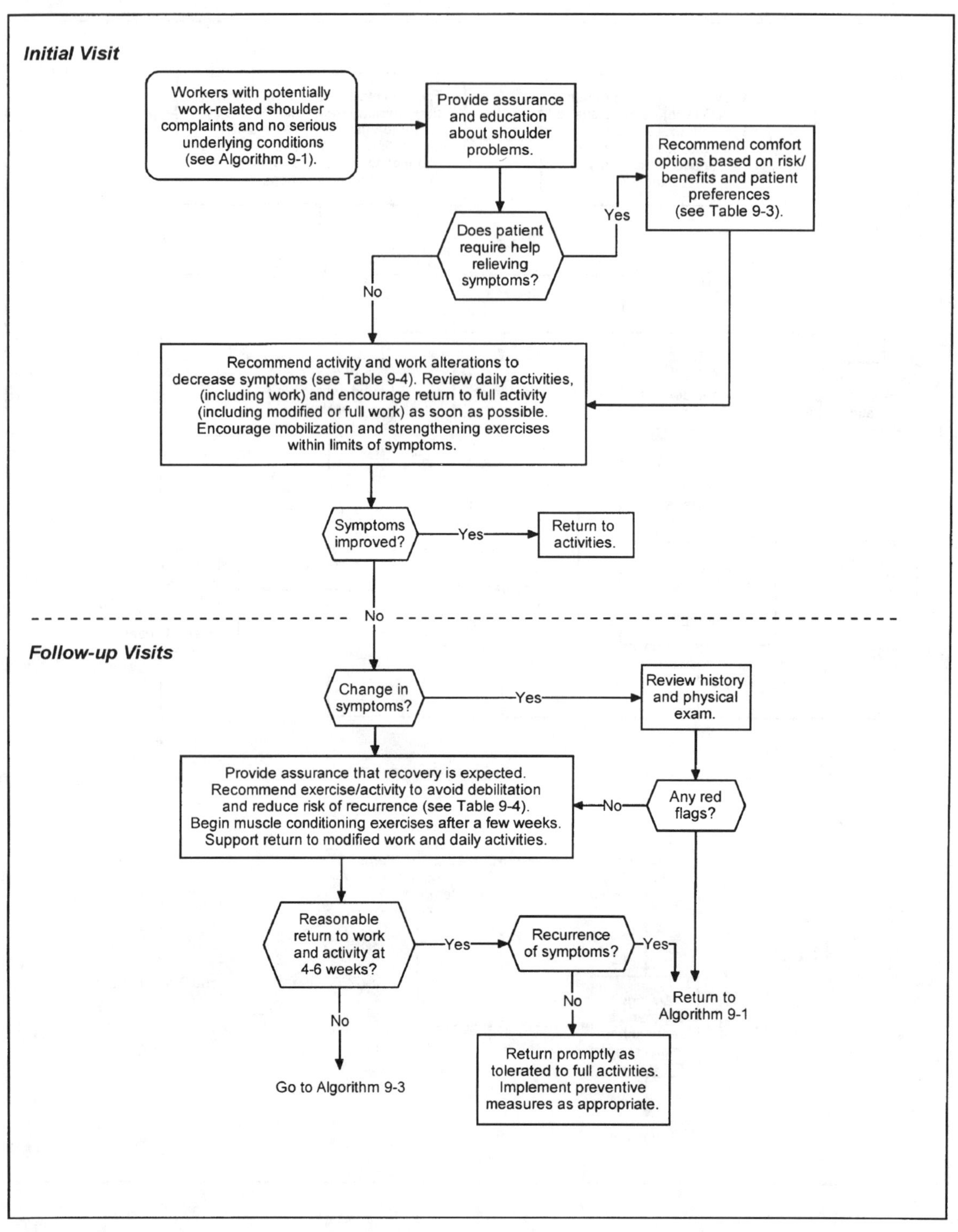

Algorithm 9-3. *Evaluation of Slow-to-recover Patients with Occupational Shoulder Complaints (Symptoms > 4 Weeks)*

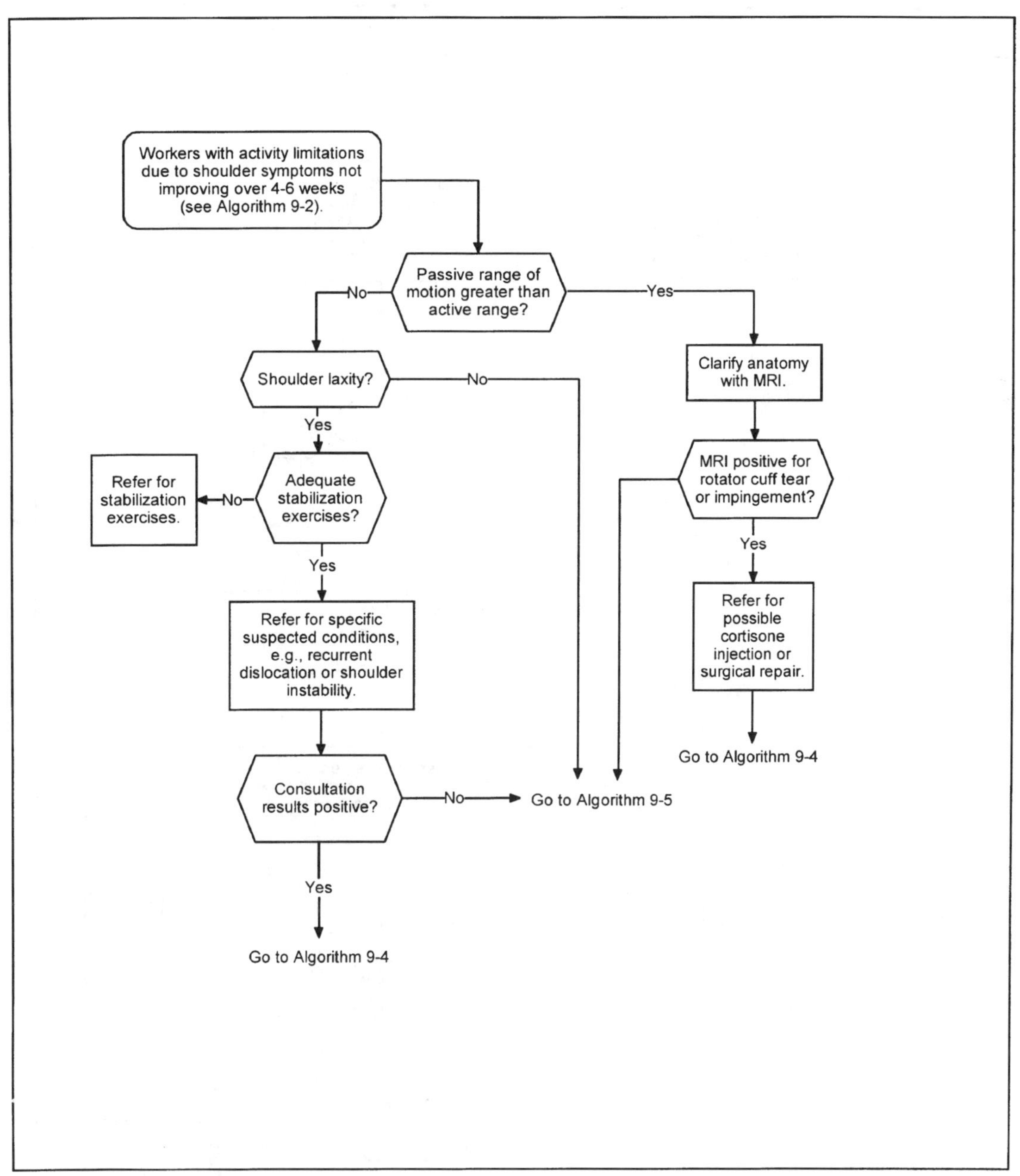

Algorithm 9-4. *Surgical Considerations for Patients with Anatomic and Physiologic Evidence of Shoulder Instability, Complete Rotator Cuff Tear, or Impingement Syndrome Coupled with Persistent Complaints*

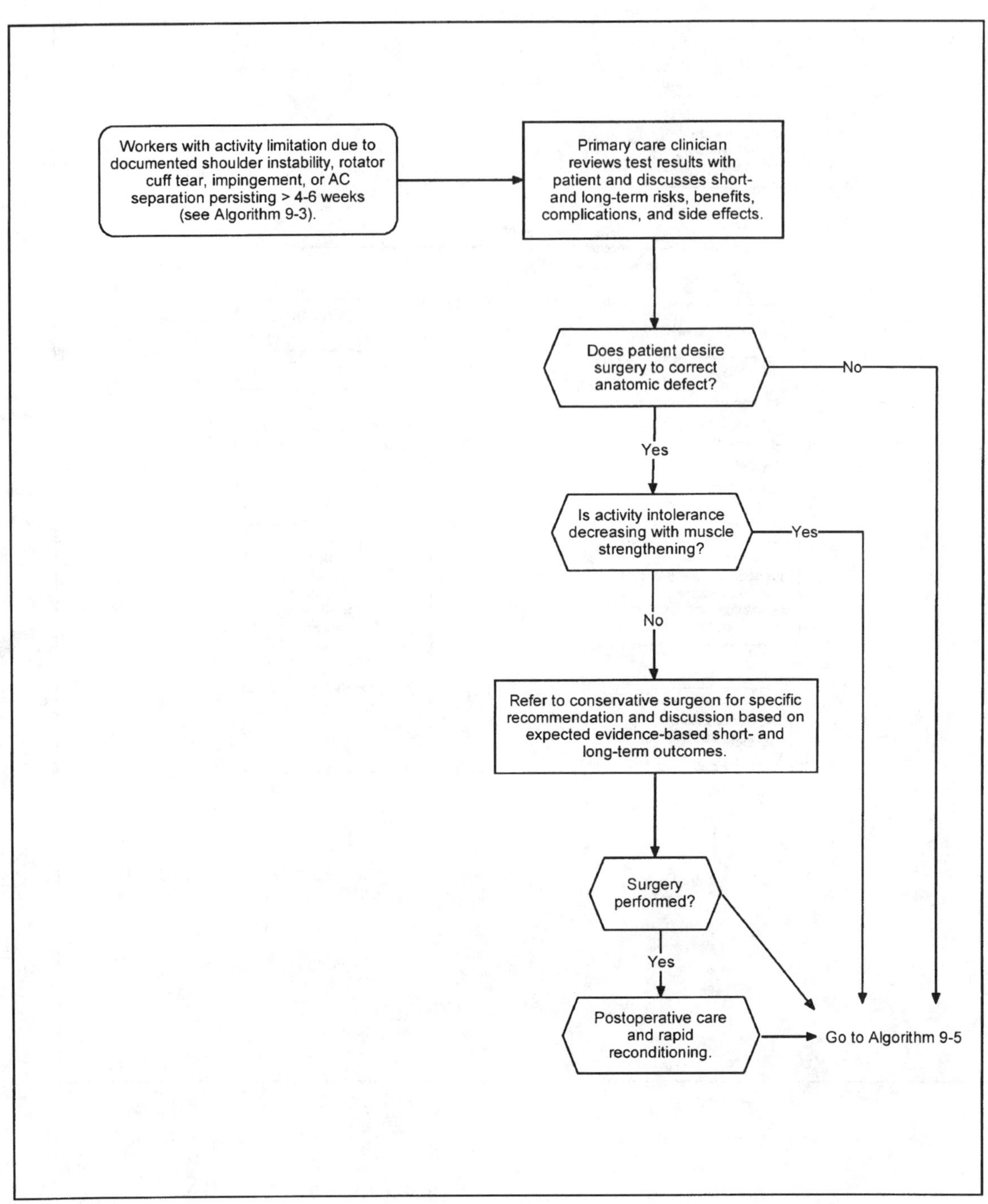

Algorithm 9-5. *Further Management of Occupational Shoulder Complaints*

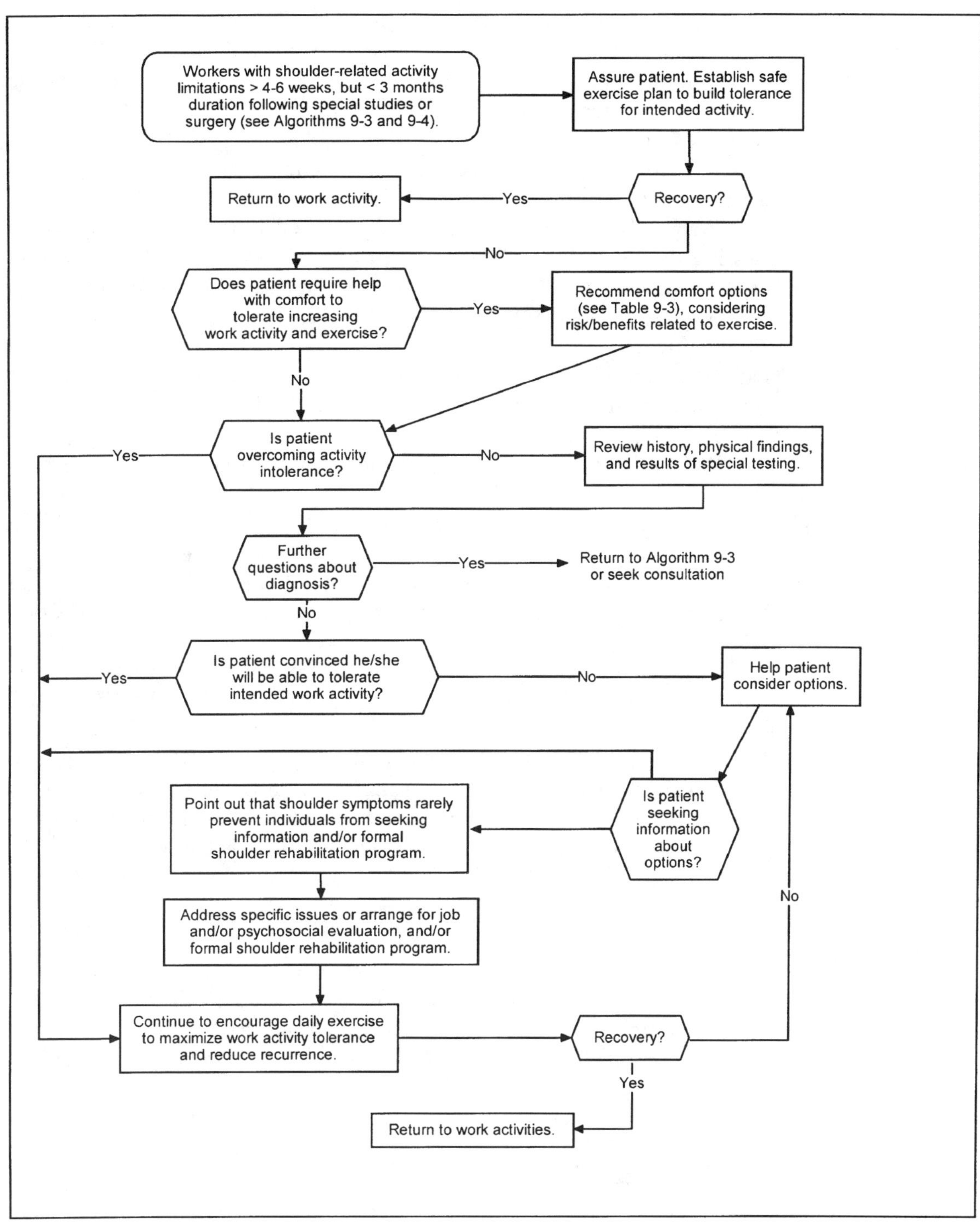

HISTORY AND PHYSICAL EXAMINATION

Boon AJ, Smith J. Manual scapular stabilization: its effect on shoulder rotational range of motion. *Arch Phys Med Rehabil.* 2000;81(7):978-83.

Gockel M, Lindholm H, Vastamaki M, Lindqvist A, Viljanen A. Cardiovascular functional disorder and distress among patients with thoracic outlet syndrome. *J Hand Surg [Br].* 1995;20(1):29-33.

Hawkins RJ, Abrams JS. Impingement syndrome in the absence of rotator cuff tear (stages 1 and 2). *Orthop Clin North Am.* 1987;18:375.

Hayes K, Walton JR, Szomor ZR, Murrell GA. Reliability of five methods for assessing shoulder range of motion. *Aust J Physiother.* 2001;47(4):289-94.

Jordan SE, Machleder HI. Diagnosis of thoracic outlet syndrome using electrophysiologically guided anterior scalene blocks. *Ann Vasc Surg.* 1998;12(3): 260-4.

Laursen B, Jensen BR. Shoulder muscle activity in young and older people during a computer mouse task. *Clin Biomech (Bristol, Avon).* 2000;15; Suppl;1:S30-3.

Lyons, AR, Tomlinson JE. Clinical diagnosis of tears of the rotator cuff. *J Bone Joint Surg [Br].* 1992;74(3):414-5.

Neer CS, Welsh RP. The shoulder in sports. *Orthop Clin North Am.* 1977;8: 583-91.

Pascarelli EF, Hsu YP. Understanding work-related upper extremity disorders: clinical findings in 485 computer users, musicians, and others. *J Occup Rehabil.* 2001;11(1):1-21.

Plewa MC, Delinger M. The false-positive rate of thoracic outlet syndrome shoulder maneuvers in healthy subjects. *Acad Emerg Med.* 1998;5(4):337-42.

Roddey TS, Olson SL, Cook KF, Gartsman GM, Hanten W. Comparison of the University of California–Los Angeles shoulder scale and the simple shoulder test with the shoulder pain and disability index: single-administration reliability and validity. *Phys Ther.* 2000;80(8):759-68.

MEDICATION

See Chapter 3 references.

van der Windt DA, van der Heijden GJ, Scholten RJ, Koes BW, Bouter LM. The efficacy of nonsteroidal anti-inflammatory drugs (NSAIDs) for shoulder complaints. A systematic review. *J Clin Epidemiol.* 1995;48(5): 691-704.

PHYSICAL TREATMENT METHODS

Anderson NH, Sojbjerg JO, Johannsen HV, Sneppen O. Self-training versus physiotherapist-supervised rehabilitation of the shoulder in patients treated with arthroscopic subacromial decompression: a clinical randomized study. *J Shoulder Elbow Surg.* 1999;8(2):99-101.

Aronen JG, Regan K. Decreasing the incidence of recurrence of first-time anterior shoulder dislocations with rehabilitation. *Am J Sports Med.* 1984; 12:382-91.

Bang MD, Deyle GD. Comparison of supervised exercise with and without manual physical therapy for patients with shoulder impingement syndrome. *J Orthop Sports Phys Ther.* 2000;30(3):126-37.

Bartolozzi A, Andreychik D, Ahmad S. Determinants of outcome in the treatment of rotator cuff disease. *Clin Orthop.* 1994;308:90-7.

Brox JI, Staff PH, Ljunggren AE. Arthroscopic surgery compared with supervised exercises in patients with rotator cuff disease (stage II impingement syndrome). *Br Med J.* 1993;307:899-903.

Ebenbichler GR, Erdogmus CB, Resch KL, et al. Ultrasound therapy for calcific tendinitis of the shoulder. *N Engl J Med.* 1999;340(20):1533-8.

Hagberg M, Harms-Ringdahl K, Nisell R, Hjelm EW. Rehabilitation of neck-shoulder pain in women industrial workers: a randomized trial comparing isometric shoulder endurance training with isometric shoulder strength training. *Arch Phys Med Rehabil.* 2000;81(8):1051-8.

Horneij E, Hemborg B, Jensen I, Ekdahl C. No significant differences between intervention programmes on neck, shoulder and low back pain: a prospective randomized study among home-care personnel. *J Rehabil Med.* 2001;33(4):170-6.

Jensen I, Nygren A, Gamberale F, Goldie I, Westerholm P, Jonsson E. The role of the psychologist in multidisciplinary treatments for chronic neck and shoulder pain: a controlled cost-effectiveness study. *Scand J Rehabil Med.* 1995;27(1):19-26.

Karjalainen K, Malmivaara A, van Tulder M, et al. Multidisciplinary biopsychosocial rehabilitation for neck and shoulder pain among working age adults: a systematic review within the framework of the Cochrane Collaboration Back Review Group. *Spine.* 2001;26(2):174-81.

Kivimaki J, Pohjolainen T. Manipulation under anesthesia for frozen shoulder with and without steroid injection. *Arch Phys Med Rehabil.* 2001;82(9): 1188-90.

Kleinhenz J, Streitberger K, Windeler J, Gussbacher A, Mavridis G, Martin E. Randomised clinical trial comparing the effects of acupuncture and a newly designed placebo needle in rotator cuff tendinitis. *Pain.* 1999; 83(2):235-41.

Philadelphia Panel. Philadelphia Panel evidence-based clinical practice guidelines on selected rehabilitation interventions for shoulder pain. *Phys Ther.* 2001;81(10):1719-30.

Sun KO, Chan KC, Lo SL, Fong DY. Acupuncture for frozen shoulder. *Hong Kong Med J.* 2001;7(4):381-91.

van der Heijden GJ, Leffers P, Wolters PJ, et al. No effect of bipolar interferential electrotherapy and pulsed ultrasound for soft tissue shoulder disorders: a randomised controlled trial. *Ann Rheum Dis.* 1999;58(9):530-40.

van der Windt DA, Koes BW, Deville W, Boeke AJ, de Jong BA, Bouter LM. Effectiveness of corticosteroid injections versus physiotherapy for treatment of painful stiff shoulder in primary care: randomised trial. *BMJ* 1998;317(7168):1292-6.

van der Windt DA, van der Heijden GJ, van den Berg SG, ter Riet G, de Winter AF, Bouter LM. Ultrasound therapy for musculoskeletal disorders: a systematic review. *Pain.* 1999;81(3):257-71.

Winters JC, Jorritsma W, Groenier KH, Sobel JS, Meyboom-de Jong B, Arendzen HJ. Treatment of shoulder complaints in general practice: long term results of a randomised, single-blind study comparing physiotherapy, manipulation, and corticosteroid injection. *BMJ.* 1999;318(7195):1395-6.

INJECTIONS

Arslan S, Celiker R. Comparison of the efficacy of local corticosteroid injection and physical therapy for the treatment of adhesive capsulitis. *Rheumatol Int.* 2001;21(1):20-3.

Bokor DJ, Hawkins RJ, Huckell GH, et al. Results of nonoperative management of full-thickness tears of the rotator cuff. *Clin Orthop.* 1993;294:103-10.

Dahan TH, Fortin L, Pelletier M, Petit M, Vadeboncoeur R, Suissa S. Double-blind randomized clinical trial examining the efficacy of bupivacaine suprascapular nerve blocks in frozen shoulder. *J Rheumatol.* 2000;27(6):1464-9.

Green S, Buchbinder R, Glazier R, Forbes A. Interventions for shoulder pain (Cochrane Review). In: *The Cochrane Library.* Issue 1; 2002. Oxford: Update Software.

Itoi E, Tabata S. Conservative treatment of rotator cuff tears. *Clin Orthop.* 1992;275:165-73.

Jones DS, Chattopadhyay C. Suprascapular nerve block for the treatment of frozen shoulder in primary care: a randomized trial. *Br J Gen Pract.* 1999;49(438):39-41.

Pons S, Gallardo C, Caballero J, Martinez T. Transdermal nitroglycerin versus corticosteroid infiltration for rotator cuff tendinitis [Article in Spanish]. *Aten Primaria.* 2001;28(7):452-5.

Rovetta G, Monteforte P. Intraarticular injection of sodium hyaluronate plus steroid versus steroid in adhesive capsulitis of the shoulder. *Int J Tissue React.* 1998;20(4):125-30.

van der Heijden GJ, van der Windt DA, Kleijnen J, Koes BW, Bouter LM. Steroid injections for shoulder disorders: a systematic review of randomized clinical trials. *Br J Gen Pract.* 1996;46(406):309-16.

REST AND IMMOBILIZATION

Henry JH, Genung JA. Natural history of glenohumeral dislocation—revisited. *Am J Sports Med.* 1982;10:135-7.

IMAGING

Blanchard TK, Bearcroft PW, Constant CR, Griffin DR, Dixon AK. Diagnostic and therapeutic impact of MRI and arthrography in the investigation of full-thickness rotator cuff tears. *Eur Radiol.* 1999;9(4):638-42.

Milgrom C, Schaffler M, Gilbert S, et al. Rotator-cuff changes in asymptomatic adults. *J Bone Joint Surg [Br].* 1995;77:296-8.

Oh CH, Schweitzer ME, Spettell CM. Internal derangements of the shoulder: decision tree and cost-effectiveness analysis of conventional arthrography, conventional MRI, and MR arthrography. *Skeletal Radiol.* 1999;28(12):670-8.

Paavolainen P, Ahovuo J. Ultrasonography and arthrography in the diagnosis of tears of the rotator cuff. *J Bone Joint Surg [Am].* 1994;76:335-40.

Robertson PL, Schweitzer ME, Mitchell DG, et al. Rotator cuff disorders: interobserver and intraobserver variation in diagnosis with MR imaging. *Radiology.* 1995;194(3):831-5.

Sher JS, Uribe JW, Posada A, et al. Abnormal findings on magnetic resonance images of asymptomatic shoulders. *J Bone Joint Surg [Am].* 1995;77:10-5.

Traughber PD, Goodwin TE. Shoulder MRI: arthroscopic correlation with emphasis on partial tears. *J Comput Assist Tomogr.* 1992;16:129-33.

Wang YM, Shih TT, Jiang CC, et al. Magnetic resonance imaging of rotator cuff lesions. *J Formos Med Assoc.* 1994;93:234-9.

SURGERY

Adolfsson L, Lysholm J. Results of arthroscopic acromioplasty related to rotator cuff lesion. *Int Orthop.* 1993;17:228-31.

Brostrom LA, Kronberg M, Nemeth G, et al. The effect of shoulder muscle training in patients with recurrent shoulder dislocations. *Scand J Rehabil Med.* 1992;24:11-5.

Brox JI, Gjengedal E, Uppheim G, et al. Arthroscopic surgery versus supervised exercises in patients with rotator cuff disease (stage II impingement syndrome): a prospective, randomized, controlled study in 125 patients with a 2-year follow-up. *J Shoulder Elbow Surg.* 1999;8(2):102-11.

Cordasco FA, McGinley BJ, Charlton T. Rotator cuff repair as an outpatient procedure. *J Shoulder Elbow Surg.* 2000;9(1):27-30.

Gartsman GM. All arthroscopic rotator cuff repairs. *Orthop Clin North Am.* 2001;32(3):501-10, x.

Gartsman GM, Roddey TS, Hammerman SM. Arthroscopic treatment of bidirectional glenohumeral instability: two- to five-year follow-up. *J Shoulder Elbow Surg.* 2001;10(1):28-36.

Goldberg BJ, Nirschl RP, McConnell JP, et al. Arthroscopic transglenoid suture capsulolabral repairs: preliminary results. *Am J Sports Med.* 1993;21:656-64; discussion 664-5.

Haake M, Deike B, Thon A, Schmitt J. Exact focusing of extracorporeal shock wave therapy for calcifying tendinopathy. *Clin Orthop.* 2002;397:323-31.

Jorgensen U, Svend-Hansen H, Bak K, Pedersen I. Recurrent post-traumatic anterior shoulder dislocation—open versus arthroscopic repair. *Knee Surg Sports Traumatol Arthrosc.* 1999;7(2):118-24.

Kirkley A, Griffin S, Richards C, Miniaci A, Mohtadi N. Prospective randomized clinical trial comparing the effectiveness of immediate arthroscopic stabilization versus immobilization and rehabilitation in first traumatic anterior dislocations of the shoulder. *Arthroscopy.* 1999;15(5):507-14.

Loew M, Daecke W, Kusnierczak D, Rahmanzadeh M, Ewerbeck V. Shockwave therapy is effective for chronic calcifying tendinitis of the shoulder. *J Bone Joint Surg [Br].* 1999;81(5):863-7.

MacDonald PB, Alexander MJ, Frejuk J, Johnson GE. Comprehensive functional analysis of shoulders following complete acromioclavicular separation. *Am J Sports Med.* 1988;16:475-80.

Ogilvie-Harris DJ, Demaziere A. Arthroscopic debridement versus open repair for rotator cuff tears: a prospective cohort study. *J Bone Joint Surg [Br].* 1993;75:416-20.

Rompe JD, Burger R, Hopf C, Eysel P. Shoulder function after extracorporeal shock wave therapy for calcific tendinitis. *J Shoulder Elbow Surg.* 1998;7(5):505-9.

Rompe JD, Zoellner J, Nafe B. Shock wave therapy versus conventional surgery in the treatment of calcifying tendinitis of the shoulder. *Clin Orthop.* 2001;387:72-82.

Speed CA, Richards C, Nichols D, et al. Extracorporeal shock-wave therapy for tendinitis of the rotator cuff. A double-blind, randomised, controlled trial. *J Bone Joint Surg [Br].* 2002;84(4):509-12.

Sperber A, Hamberg P, Karlsson J, Sward L, Wredmark T. Comparison of an arthroscopic and an open procedure for posttraumatic instability of the shoulder: a prospective, randomized multicenter study. *J Shoulder Elbow Surg.* 2001;10(2):105-8.

Taft TN, Wilson FC, Oglesby JW. Dislocation of the acromioclavicular joint: an end-result study. *J Bone Joint Surg [Am].* 1987;69:1045-51.

Warner JJ, Miller MD, Marks P, Fu FH. Arthroscopic Bankart repair with the Suretac device. Part I: clinical observations. *Arthroscopy.* 1995;11:2-13.

Zvijac JE, Levy JH, Lemak LJ. Arthroscopic subacromial decompression in the treatment of full-thickness rotator cuff tears: a 3- to 6-year follow-up. *Arthroscopy.* 1994;10:518-23.

***Master Algorithm**. ACOEM Guidelines for Care of Acute and Subacute Occupational Neck and Upper Back Complaints*

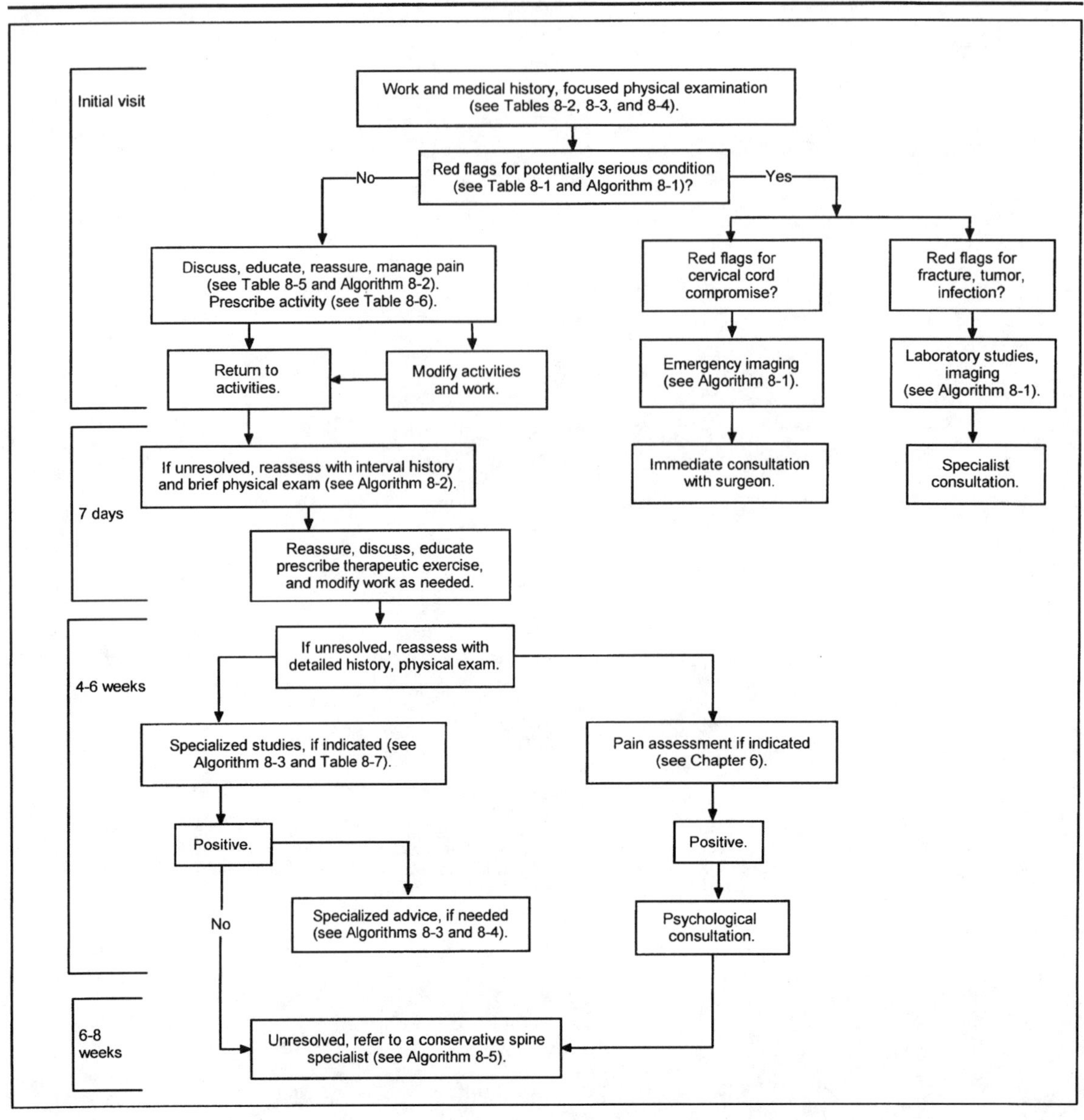

10 Elbow Complaints

General Approach and Basic Principles

Physicians often encounter work-related elbow complaints, which are among the most common causes of reported occupational injuries and workers' compensation claims. Elbow complaints account for about 2-3% of total lost workdays and 5-6% of claims and costs in workers' compensation, ranking them in the top ten for financial severity. Surgical procedures account for much of the total elbow-related expense, even though quality medical literature, summarized in this book, does not support the efficacy of such procedures.

This chapter presents recommendations on assessing and treating adults with elbow complaints that may be work related. Topics include the initial assessment and diagnosis of patients with acute and subacute elbow complaints; identifying red flags that may indicate the presence of a serious underlying medical condition; initial management; diagnostic considerations; and special studies for identifying clinical pathology, work relatedness, return to work, modified duty and activity; and further management considerations, including managing delayed recovery.

Algorithms for patient management are included. This chapter's master algorithm shows how physicians should generally manage patients with acute and subacute elbow complaints. The following text, tables, and numbered algorithms expand upon the master algorithm.

The principal recommendations for assessing and treating patients with elbow complaints are as follows:

- The initial assessment of patients with acute and subacute elbow problems should focus on detecting indications of potentially serious disease, termed red flags, and determining an accurate diagnosis.
- In the absence of red flags, occupational or primary care providers can safely and effectively manage work-related elbow complaints. Management focuses on monitoring patients for complications, facilitating the healing process and return to work in modified or full duty.
- Relieving discomfort can be accomplished most safely by temporarily decreasing activities, immobilization if necessary, and systemic nonprescription analgesics.

- Patients recovering from acute and subacute elbow problems may be encouraged to return to modified work as soon as their condition permits.
- If symptoms persist beyond 4-6 weeks, referral for specialty care may be indicated.
- Nonphysical factors (such as psychosocial, workplace, or socioeconomic problems) should be investigated and addressed in cases of delayed recovery or return to work.

Initial Assessment

Thorough medical and work histories and a focused physical examination (see Chapter 2) are sufficient for the initial assessment of workers complaining of potentially work-related elbow symptoms. This evaluation should consider the possibility that the elbow pain is due to a disorder in another part of the body, particularly the neck, shoulder, or forearm. Certain findings on the history and physical examination raise suspicion of serious underlying medical conditions; these are referred to as red flags (see Table 10-1). Their absence rules out the need for special studies, referral, or inpatient care during the first four weeks when spontaneous recovery is expected (provided any inciting workplace factors are mitigated). Then, elbow complaints can be classified into one of four working categories:

- **Potentially serious elbow condition:** fractures, acute dislocation, infection, or neurovascular compromise, which usually have preceding trauma;
- **Mechanical disorders:** derangements of the elbow related to acute trauma, such as ligament strain or tears; or repetitive use conditions leading to inflammation, nerve entrapment, and other problems;
- **Degenerative disorders:** consequences of aging or repetitive use, or a combination thereof, such as bursitis or tendinitis;
- **Nonspecific disorders:** occurring in the elbow and suggesting neither internal derangement nor referred pain.

Medical History

Asking the patient open-ended questions, such as those listed below, allows the clinician to gauge the need for further information. Discussion, or more specific inquiries, will usually produce the detail necessary for clinical decision-making:

1. WHAT ARE YOUR SYMPTOMS?
    - Do you have pain, weakness, limited motion, or locking?
    - For traumatic injuries: Was the area deformed? Did you lose any blood or have an open wound?

Table 10-1. Red Flags for Potentially Serious Elbow Conditions

Disorder	Medical History	Physical Examination
Fracture	History of significant trauma Fall on outstretched hand	Disturbance in the triangular relationship between the olecranon and the epicondyles Significant bruising, if subacute (unusual)
Dislocation	History of deformity with or without spontaneous or self reduction	Deformity consistent with dislocation Hemarthrosis
Infection	Diabetes History of immunosuppression (e.g., transplant, chemotherapy, HIV) History of systemic symptoms	Systemic signs of sepsis Localized heat, swelling, erythema
Tumor	History of cancer Weight loss	Palpable mass not consistent with usual diagnoses Tumor vessels
Inflammation	History of gout or pseudo-gout History of rheumatoid arthritis History of inflammatory arthritis	Effusion Findings of inflammatory arthritis
Rapidly progressive neurologic deficit	History of neurologic disease	Abnormal neurologic examination
Vascular compromise	History of diabetes History of fracture or dislocation	Decreased peripheral pulses

- Are your symptoms located primarily in the elbow? Do you have pain or other symptoms elsewhere, e.g., shoulder, forearm, hand?
- Are your symptoms constant or intermittent? What makes the problem worse or better?

2. HOW DO THESE SYMPTOMS LIMIT YOU?

- Can you flex your elbow to work? For how long?
- Do you have trouble turning a door knob or using a screwdriver (pronation/supination)?
- Can you lift? How much weight?

3. WHEN DID YOUR CURRENT LIMITATIONS BEGIN?

- Was there an event that precipitated the symptoms? How did they start?
- How long have your activities been limited? More than four weeks?

- Have your symptoms changed? How?
- Have you had similar episodes previously?
- Have you had previous testing or treatment? With whom?
- What do you think caused the problem? How do you think it is related to work?
- What are your specific job duties? Do you use your elbow to perform them? How? How often?
- What are your hobbies (tennis, golf, etc.)? Do you use your elbow to perform them? How? How often?

4. DO YOU HAVE OTHER MEDICAL PROBLEMS?

- Do you have any autoimmune, infectious, or metabolic diseases such as rheumatoid arthritis or gout?
- Do you have arthritis in any other joint?
- Do you have diabetes or HIV?
- Have you ever had cancer?

5. WHAT DO YOU HOPE WE CAN ACCOMPLISH DURING THIS VISIT?

Elbow complaints, as described by the patient, can sometimes be consistent with radiating symptoms from the neck or shoulder, and the examining physician's diagnostic judgment is important in determining the source. For instance, mid-upper-arm pain on arm elevation is most likely related to a problem originating in the rotator cuff area, not the elbow, although patients may have pain in both areas. A complaint of painful numbness in the fourth and fifth fingers is usually due to ulnar nerve impingement at the elbow, but may be due to impingement of that nerve at the level of the wrist. In cases of complaints that are not clear disorders, a diagnosis of nonspecific pain should be used. Note that lateral elbow pain can be due to cervical disk disease, radial nerve entrapment, synovitis due to degeneration, or true epicondylitis (enthesitis).

Physical Examination

Guided by the medical history, the physical examination includes:

- General observation of the patient
- Focused examination of the forearm, arm, and elbow (on the affected side)
- Neurovascular screening

Though it may seem a point too obvious to warrant mention, the physician should specifically note which elbow—left or right—is the subject of the patient's complaints. Not infrequently, injured workers have prior workers' compensation claims that involve the opposite elbow. Any ambiguity in documentation can lead to delay in acceptance of the patient's workers' compensation claim, delay in the authorization of time-loss benefits, delay in the authorization of payment of medical care, or even outright denial of the workers' compensation claim.

The physician should seek objective evidence of pathology that is consistent with the patient's subjective complaints. In many cases, careful examination will reveal one or more truly objective findings, such as swelling, deformity, atrophy, reflex changes, or spasm. Any such findings should be thoroughly documented in the medical record both for reference during future visits, and for the value the information will have in the patient's workers' compensation claim. For some patients with elbow complaints, however, there are no objective findings. Meticulous documentation of the patient's complaints at each visit is of the utmost importance in such cases.

A. Focused Elbow Examination

Examining the elbow also includes examining the forearm. The elbow's range of motion should be determined both actively and passively. Limitation of motion or pain at the extremes of flexion or extension suggest an intraarticular abnormality. Atrophy of the muscles of the ulnar or radial hand intrinsics is an objective finding, but it arises only after weeks to months of problems. Deformities due to fractures are often subtle; dislocations may be associated with visible, objective findings of abnormalities. Signs of infection (redness, heat, swelling, tenderness, etc.) or gross tumor (vessels, palpable mass) may also be obvious. A medical history suggestive of pathology originating somewhere other than in the elbow may warrant examination of the neck, shoulder, forearm, or other areas.

B. Neurovascular Screening

Physicians should assess the neurologic and vascular status of the elbow and distal upper extremity, especially following dislocation. They also should seek evidence of cervical disc disease associated with radiculopathy that radiates to the elbow. C5 radiculopathy may result in weakness of elbow flexion, and T1 lesions may weaken the hand intrinsics in a manner that is similar to entrapment of the ulnar nerve. C6 radiculopathy can cause lateral elbow pain.

C. Assessing Red Flags

Physical examination evidence of neurovascular compromise, fracture, unreduced dislocation, infection, or tumor that correlates with the medical history and with test results may indicate a need for immediate consultation. The examination may further reinforce or reduce suspicions of tumor, infection, fracture, or dislocation.

Diagnostic Criteria

If the patient does not have red flags for serious conditions, the clinician can then determine which common musculoskeletal elbow disorder is present. The criteria presented in Table 10-2 follow the clinical thought process, from

Table 10-2. Diagnostic Criteria for Non-red-flag Elbow Conditions that Can Be Managed by Primary Care Physicians

Probable Diagnosis or Injury	Mechanism	Unique Symptoms	Unique Signs	Test and Results
Lateral epicondylitis (ICD-9 726.32)	Repetitive overload (Possible) acute trauma	Pain in lateral elbow with resisted extension of wrist or gripping	Tenderness over epicondyle Normal elbow ROM Diffuse lateral elbow pain with repetitive wrist dorsiflexion	Positive resistance test results: pain with resisted extension of the wrist and fingers, resisted supination
Medial epicondylitis (ICD-9 726.31)	Repetitive overload (Possible) acute trauma	Pain in medial elbow with resisted flexion of wrist or gripping	Diffuse medial elbow pain with repeated wrist volarflexion Tenderness over epicondyle Normal elbow ROM	Positive resistance test results: pain with resisted flexion of the wrist and fingers, resisted pronation
Olecranon bursitis (noninfectious) (ICD-9 712.2, 712.3, 712.8, 726.32)	Leaning on elbow (Possible) acute trauma Repetitive flexion and extension Chronic irritation	Pain over olecranon bursa Swelling of bursa	Effusion/mass effect in bursa	Crystals if gout or pseudogout
Olecranon bursitis (infectious) (ICD-9 726.33)	Trauma Systemic infection	Progressive painful swelling Systemic symptoms	Erythema, heat and/or surrounding cellulitis Tenderness over bursa	Purulent tap, positive gram-stain results, positive culture results
Ulnar nerve entrapment (ICD-9 354.2)	(Possible) overuse or leaning on elbow	Pain or paresthesias in ulnar ring and all small fingers (palm-up position)	Reproduction of symptoms with percussion or compression of cubital tunnel Pain in ulnar ring and all of small fingers on full elbow flexion Weakness/atrophy of ulnar hand intrinsics and interosseous muscles (unusual/late)	NCV < 50 msec elbow to hand (depending on lab)

Table 10-2. (continued)

Probable Diagnosis or Injury	Mechanism	Unique Symptoms	Unique Signs	Test and Results
Radial nerve entrapment (ICD-9 354.3) (radial tunnel syndrome)	Repetitive use (very unusual)	Aching pain in extensor/supinator area of forearm Pain/paresthesias in thumb and index finger	Reproduction of symptoms by percussion or compression of radial tunnel Pain on stressing extended middle finger Maximum tenderness four fingerbreadths below lateral epicondyle	Positive EMG
Contusion (ICD-9 923.11)	Direct blow Fall	Local pain	Normal range of motion Soft tissue swelling Ecchymosis	None
Nondisplaced radial head fracture (ICD-9813.05)	Fall on outstretched hand	Pain on pronation and supination of hand	Maximal tenderness over radial head	Positive fat-pad sign on radiograph Fracture on radiograph
Nonspecific elbow pain (ICD-9 726.39)	Possibly overuse	None	None	None

Note: ICD-9 = *International Classification of Diseases*, 9th Ed.

the mechanism of illness or injury to unique symptoms and signs of a particular disorder and finally to test results, if any tests are needed to guide treatment at this stage.

Work-Relatedness

Work-related symptoms commonly involve elbow complaints. A thorough work history is crucial to establishing work-relatedness. See Chapter 2 for components of the work history.

Repetitive work is currently thought to contribute to regional elbow pain and perhaps epicondylitis, although the strength of the association is not great. The association of repetitive or malpositioned work with nerve entrapment in the area of the elbow is not at all epidemiologically clear.

Epicondylitis and forearm tendinitis as well as nerve entrapments and olecranon bursitis have been attributed by some to employment activities. Such a conclusion requires a careful history about work tasks, non-work activities, and other risk factors, as well as a thoughtful, careful assessment of the relative contribution each makes to the patient's problem.

Acute work-related trauma can be associated with olecranon bursitis. Workstation modifications may be important to resolving the problem, and understanding the worksite and the employer's willingness to modify the workstation are crucial to maintaining the employee at work or minimizing disability time.

Initial Care

Comfort is often a patient's first concern. Nonprescription analgesics will provide sufficient pain relief for most patients with acute and subacute elbow symptoms. If treatment response is inadequate, i.e., if symptoms and activity limitations continue, prescribed pharmaceuticals or physical methods can be added. Comorbid conditions, side effects, cost, and provider and patient preferences should guide the clinician's choice of recommendations. Table 10-3 summarizes comfort options.

Conservative care consists of activity modification, using epicondylitis

Table 10-3. Methods of Symptom Control for Elbow Complaints

RECOMMENDED
Nonprescription Medications
Acetaminophen (safest) NSAIDs (aspirin, ibuprofen)
Physical Modalities
Adjustment or modification of workstation, job tasks, or work hours and methods Specific elbow exercises for range of motion and strengthening At-home local applications of cold packs during first few days of acute complaint; thereafter application of heat packs, or cold packs as the patient prefers Arobic exercise to maintain general conditioning Initial and follow-up visits for education, counseling, and evaluation of home exercise
Prescribed Pharmaceutical Methods
Other NSAIDs (not recommended for nerve entrapment syndromes)

OPTIONS

Epicondylitis	Olecranon Bursitis	Nonspecific Elbow Pain
Tennis elbow band Corticosteroid injection Wrist splint	Splint in extension if needed Elbow padding Activity modification Broad-spectrum antibiotics if elbow is infected	None
Ulnar Nerve Entrapment	**Radial Nerve Entrapment**	
Night extension splints	Cock-up wrist splint	

supports (tennis elbow bands), and using nonsteroidal anti-inflammatory drugs (NSAIDs) with the usual precautions and education. A cock-up wrist splint and NSAIDs are helpful in many cases of radial tunnel syndrome.

Most cases of sterile effusion of the olecranon bursa may be treated by padding the elbow and modifying activities. If the bursa is infected, aspiration or drainage as well as systemic antibiotics may be needed.

Physical Methods

Any one or more of a variety of physical methods may be appropriate in the treatment of a patient's elbow condition. These methods include:

- Instruction in home exercise. Except for cases of unstable fractures or acute dislocations, physicians should advise patients to do early range-of-motion exercises at home. Instruction in proper exercise technique is important, and a few visits to a good physical therapist can serve to educate the patient about an effective exercise program.
- Patient's at-home applications of heat or cold packs may be used before or after exercises and are as effective as those performed by therapists.
- Published randomized clinical trials are needed to provide better evidence for the use of many physical modalities that are commonly employed. Some therapists use a variety of procedures; conclusions regarding their effectiveness may be based on anecdotal reports or case studies. Included among these modalities are massage, diathermy, extracorporeal shockwave therapy (ESWT), low-level laser therapy (LLLT), ultrasonography, transcutaneous electrical neurostimulation (TENS), electrical stimulation (E-STIM), iontophoresis, and biofeedback. In general, if tied to signs of objective progress within two to three weeks, it may be acceptable to use these modalities as an adjunct to a program of evidence-based functional restoration.
- The efficacy of needle acupuncture is not yet clearly supported by quality medical evidence. While limited existing studies support needle acupuncture for short-term relief of lateral elbow pain, clear evidence currently is insufficient to either support or refute using needle acupuncture to treat lateral epicondylitis; and discovery of potential adverse effects is inadequate. More trials, using adequate sample sizes, are needed before conclusions can be drawn regarding the effect of needle acupuncture on lateral epicondylitis.
- Physicians may consider referring the patient to a specialist for local anesthetic and corticosteroid injections into tender areas of epicondylitis and, possibly, injection in the area of the radial tunnel in the forearm for distal symptoms. In most cases, physicians should carry out conservative measures for four to six weeks before considering injections. Corticosteroid injections have been shown to be effective, at least in the short term; however, the evidence on long-term effects

is mixed, some studies show high recurrence rate among injection groups.

Activity Alteration

Careful advice regarding maximizing activities within the limits of symptoms is imperative once red flags have been ruled out. If a sling is needed for treatment of an elbow condition, the use of the sling should be for as short a time as necessary, and gentle exercise is desirable, even at this stage. Wrist supports to limit pronation and supination may be used in the acute management of lateral epicondylitis or tendinosis.

Activities and postures that increase stress on the elbow tend to aggravate symptoms. Consequently, consideration may be given to restrictions on lifting and repetitive flexion or extension following the onset of epicondylitis. Those with olecranon bursitis should limit direct pressure on the olecranon.

Conditioning exercises for muscles above and below the elbow are more mechanically stressful than aerobic exercise. To avoid debilitation, regular aerobic exercise may be appropriate. Elbow conditioning exercises are generally not advisable during the first few weeks of symptoms. Later, such exercises may help patients regain and maintain activity tolerance, particularly patients with epicondylitis and regional elbow pain. There is no evidence to indicate that elbow-specific or adapted exercise machines are effective for treating acute elbow problems.

Work Activities

Table 10-4 provides recommendations on activity modification and duration of absence from work. These guidelines are intended for patients without comorbidity or complicating factors, including legal or employment issues. The guidelines are targets. They provide a guide, from the perspective of physiologic recovery. Key factors to consider in disability duration are the patient's age and type of job. Workplace factors can be paramount, especially if the patient's regular work includes activities that are likely to worsen the condition. The clinician should make it clear to patients and employers that:

- Repetitive motions, or even moderately heavy unassisted lifting and carrying, may aggravate elbow symptoms caused by epicondylitis or bursitis.
- Any restrictions are intended to allow for spontaneous recovery or for the time necessary for the development of activity tolerance through exercise.

Measures to assist the patient in avoiding aggravating activities should include a review of work duties to decide whether modifications can be accomplished,

Table 10-4. *Guidelines for Modification of Work Activities and Disability Duration**

Disorder	Activity Modifications and Accommodation	Recommended Target for Disability Duration**		NHIS Experience Data***	
		With Modified Duty	**Without Modified Duty**	**Median (cases with lost time)**	**Percent (no lost time)**
Epicondylitis	Avoid symptom-aggravating activities, e.g., lifting, carrying, keyboard work. Also workstation assessment to insure optimal ergonomics, as appropriate.	1 day	7 days	22 days	66%
Olecranon bursitis	Avoid the above activities, but more importantly, avoid direct pressure on the olecranon area.	1 day	3 days	22 days	66%
Ulnar nerve entrapment	Avoid the above activities, especially direct pressure on the ulnar groove. Also workstation assessment to insure optimal ergonomics, as appropriate.	1 day	7 days	21 days	33%
Radial nerve entrapment	See Epicondylitis above	1 day	7 days	13 days	58%
Regional elbow pain	Avoid any aggravating activities	0 days	3 days	4 days	50%

* These are general guidelines based on consensus or population sources and are never meant to be applied to an individual case without consideration of workplace factors, concurrent disease, or other social or medical factors that can affect recovery.
** These parameters for disability duration are "consensus optimal" targets as determined by a panel of ACOEM members in 1996, and reaffirmed by a panel of ACOEM members in 2002. In most cases persons with one non-severe extremity injury can return to modified duty immediately. Restrictions should take into consideration the opposite extremity also to prevent strain injuries to the uninjured extremity.
*** Based on the CDC NHIS (National Health Interview Survey), as compiled and reported in the 8th annual edition of *Official Disability Guidelines (ODG)*, © 2002 Work Loss Data Institute, all rights reserved.

and to determine whether modified duty is available. Every attempt should be made to maintain the patient at maximal levels of activity, including work activities.

Follow-up Visits

Patients with potentially work-related elbow complaints should have follow-up visits every three to five days by a midlevel practitioner who can counsel the patient about avoiding static positions, medication use, activity modification, and other concerns. Practitioners should take care to answer questions and make these sessions interactive so the patient is involved in his or her recovery. If the patient has returned to work, these interactions may be done on site or by telephone to avoid interfering with modified or full-work activities.

Follow-up by the physician should occur when a release to modified, increased, or full duty is needed, or after appreciable healing or recovery can be expected, on average. Physician follow-up might be expected every four to seven days if the patient is off work and every seven to fourteen days if the patient is working.

Special Studies and Diagnostic and Treatment Considerations

Criteria for ordering imaging studies are:

- Emergence of a red flag
- Physiologic evidence of tissue insult or neurologic dysfunction
- Failure to progress in a strengthening program intended to avoid surgery

For most patients presenting with true elbow problems, special studies are not needed unless a four-week period of conservative care and observation fails to improve symptoms. Most patients improve quickly, provided red-flag conditions are ruled out. There are a few exceptions:

- Plain-film radiography to rule out osteomyelitis or joint effusion in cases of significant septic olecranon bursitis
- Electromyography (EMG) and nerve conduction velocity (NCV) study if cervical radiculopathy is suspected as a cause of lateral arm pain
- Nerve conduction velocity study and, possibly, EMG if severe nerve entrapment is suspected on the basis of physical examination and denervation atrophy is likely

For patients with limitations of activity after four weeks and unexplained physical findings such as effusion or localized pain (especially following exercise), imaging may be indicated to clarify the diagnosis and assist reconditioning. Imaging findings should be correlated with physical findings.

In general, an imaging study may be an appropriate consideration for a patient whose limitations due to consistent symptoms have persisted for one month or more, as in the following cases:

- When surgery is being considered for a specific anatomic defect, e.g., preoperative plain-film radiography when incision and drainage of an infected olecranon is indicated
- To further evaluate potentially serious pathology, such as a possible tumor, when the clinical examination suggests the diagnosis

Surgical Considerations

The timing of a referral for surgery should be consistent with the condition that has been diagnosed. Conditions that produce objective evidence of nerve entrapment and that do not respond to non-surgical treatment can be considered for surgery when treatment failure has been documented. Conditions of inflammatory nature may take many months to heal and the timing of a surgical consultation referral should take into consideration the normal healing time.

Referral for surgical consultation may be indicated for patients who have:

- Limitations of activity for more than six months
- Failed to improve with exercise programs to increase range of motion and strength of the musculature around the elbow
- Clear clinical and electrophysiologic, or imaging evidence of a lesion that has been shown to benefit in both the short and long term from surgical repair

Emergency consultation is reserved for patients who require drainage or aspiration of acute septic effusions or hematomas and/or drainage of infected bursitis or who have severe acute nerve impingement. Table 10-5 provides a general comparison of the abilities of different techniques to identify physiologic insult and define anatomic defects.

If surgery is a consideration, counseling regarding likely outcomes, risks and benefits, and especially expectations is very important. If there is no clear indication for surgery, referring the patient to a physical medicine practitioner may help resolve the symptoms.

Table 10-5. Ability of Various Techniques to Identify and Define Elbow Pathology

Technique	Identify Physiologic Insult	Define Anatomic Defect
History	+ +	+ +
Physical examination		
Motor	+ + +	+ +
Sensory	+ + +	+ +
Palpation (tendinitis, bursitis)	+ +	+ + + +
Laboratory studies	+ + + + (infection)	0
EMG/NCN	+ + + +	0
Imaging studies (osteomyelitis or fracture)		
Radiography[1]	0	+ + +
Bone scan[1]		+ + +
Arthrography[1]	0	+
Computed tomography (CT)[1]	0	+ + + +
Magnetic resonance imaging (MRI)[1]	0	+ + + +

[1] Risk of complications (e.g., infection, radiation) highest for contrast CT or arthrography; second highest for myelography; relatively less for bone scan, radiography, and CT; lowest for MRI.

Note: Number of plus signs indicates relative ability to identify or define pathology.

A. Ulnar Nerve Entrapment

There are two main areas for entrapment of the ulnar nerve at the elbow. The first is in the condylar groove and the more distal is in the cubital tunnel. Many cases of condylar groove ulnar neuropathy are mistakenly labeled as cubital tunnel syndrome without a localization of the problem. Surgery for ulnar nerve entrapment is indicated after establishing a firm diagnosis on the basis of clear clinical evidence and positive electrical studies that correlate with clinical findings. A decision to operate presupposes that a significant problem exists, as reflected in significant activity limitations due to the specific problem and that the patient has failed conservative care, including use of elbow pads, removing opportunities to rest the elbow on the ulnar groove, workstation changes (if applicable), and avoiding nerve irritation at night by preventing elbow flexation while sleeping. Before proceeding with surgery, patients must be apprised of all possible complications, including wound infections, anesthetic complications, nerve damage, and the possibility that surgery will not relieve symptoms.

B. Radial Nerve Entrapment (Radial Tunnel Syndrome)

This condition, which causes proximal forearm aching and pain, and sometimes dysesthesias in the hand, only rarely requires surgical release. A decision to operate presupposes that a significant problem exists, as reflected in significant activity limitations due to the specific problem, and that the patient has failed conservative care. Possible complications of surgery for radial nerve entrapment are the same as those for entrapment of the ulnar nerve, with the exception of nerve dislocation. Scarring also may be a factor.

C. Olecranon Bursa Excision

Although it is a rare consequence of the condition, persistent olecranon bursal effusions may interfere with activities to a degree that warrants surgical excision. Once again, education the patient regarding expectations from surgery and complications is necessary.

D. Lateral Epicondylitis

Lateral epicondylitis is a painful condition of the elbow, the etiology of which is not fully understood. There is currently a debate regarding whether it is an inflammatory condition or an enthesopathy. Consequently, there is a debate as to whether treatment with anti-inflammatories is appropriate. Conservative care should be maintained for a minimum of six to twelve months. At this time there are no published randomized controlled studies that indicate that surgery is warranted for this condition.

Summary of Guideline Recommendations

See Table 10-6.

Table 10-6. Summary of Recommendations for Evaluating and Managing Elbow Complaints

Clinical Measure	Recommended	Optional	Not Recommended
History and physical exam	Basic history and exam (search for red flags for tumor, infection, systemic disease) (D) Occupational and nonoccupational activity history (C, D)		
Patient education	Patient education regarding diagnosis, prognosis, expectations of treatment, etc. (D)		
Medication (See Chapter 3)	Acetaminophen (C) NSAIDs (B)	Opioids (D) Topical medications (C, D)	
Physical treatment methods	Physician recommendations for range-of-motion instruction and strengthening exercises in epicondylitis patients (D)	Exercise instruction by a therapist for epicondylitis (D) At-home applications of heat or cold packs (D) Other physical modalities based on objective results for a 2-3-week trial (D)	Use of passive modalities by a therapist (D)
Injections		Acupuncture based on objective results after a 2-3-week trial (D) Local corticosteroid injection for epicondylitis (C, D)	Corticosteroid injection into olecranon bursa (C)
Rest and immobilization	Immobilization with a sling for a brief period for severe symptoms (D)	Trial of casting for severe recalcitrant epicondylitis (D) Tennis elbow bands for conservative treatment (D)	

Table 10-6. (continued)

Clinical Measure	Recommended	Optional	Not Recommended
Activity and exercise	Stretching (D) Aerobic exercise (D) Activity modification (D)		
Detection of neurologic abnormalities	NCV to confirm ulnar nerve entrapment if conservative treatment fails (D)	EMG to distinguish radial entrapment from lateral epicondylitis if history and physical exam are equivocal (D)	EMG/NCV before conservative treatment (D)
Radiography and other imaging studies	Plain-film radiography for red-flag cases (D)	MRI for suspected ulnar collateral ligament tears (C)	Repeat plain-film radiography for readings with "fat pad sign" (D) MRI for epicondylitis (D)
Surgical considerations	Ulnar nerve transposition for patients with significant activity limitation and delayed NCV (D) Debridement of inflammatory or scarred tissue for patients with epicondylitis if conservative treatment fails (C) Excision and closure over drains for infected olecranon bursitis not responsive to IV antibiotics (D) Radial tunnel decompression for failure of conservative treatment and positive EMG (D)		Excision of olecranon bursa due to metabolic arthritis (rather than medical treatment) (D) Ulnar or radial nerve surgery in the presence of normal electrical studies (D)

A = Strong research-based evidence (multiple relevant, high-quality scientific studies).
B = Moderate research-based evidence (one relevant, high-quality scientific study or multiple adequate scientific studies).
C = Limited research-based evidence (at least one adequate scientific study of patients with elbow disorders).
D = Panel interpretation of information not meeting inclusion criteria for research-based evidence or consensus.

Algorithm 10-1. *Initial Evaluation of Occupational Elbow Complaints*

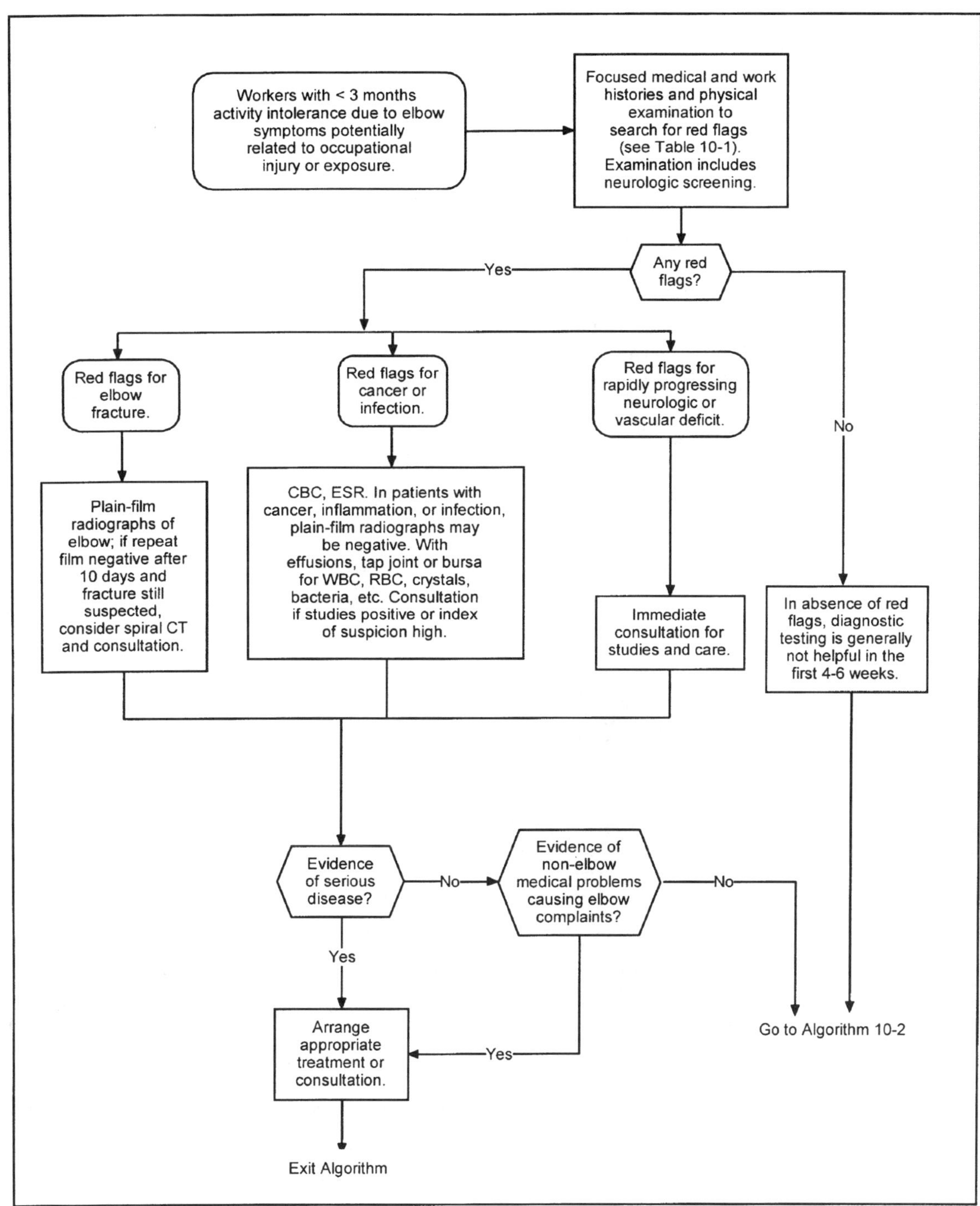

Algorithm 10-2. *Initial and Follow-up Management of Occupational Elbow Complaints*

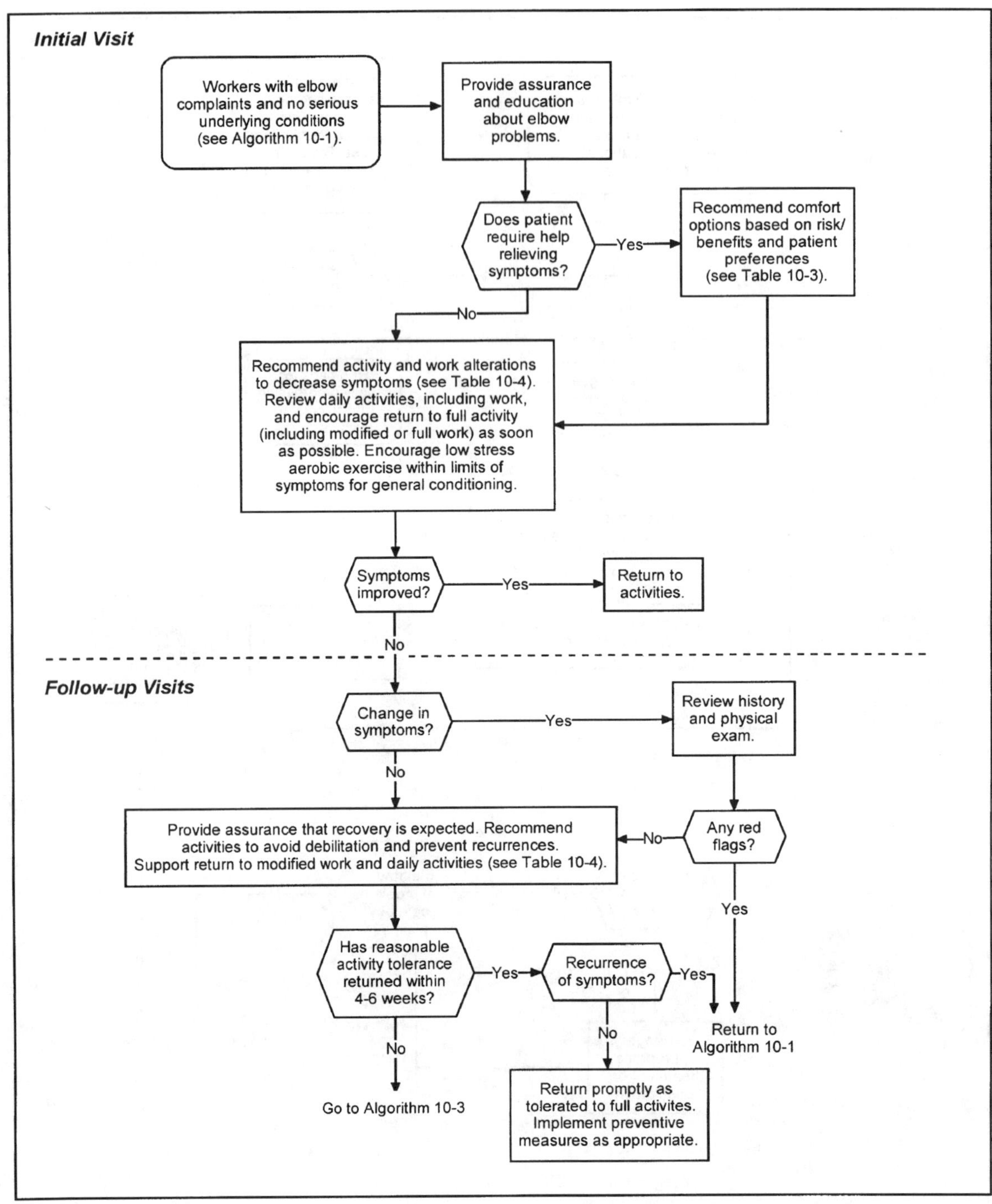

Algorithm 10-3. *Evaluation of Slow-to-recover Patients with Occupational Elbow Complaints (Symptoms > 4 Weeks)*

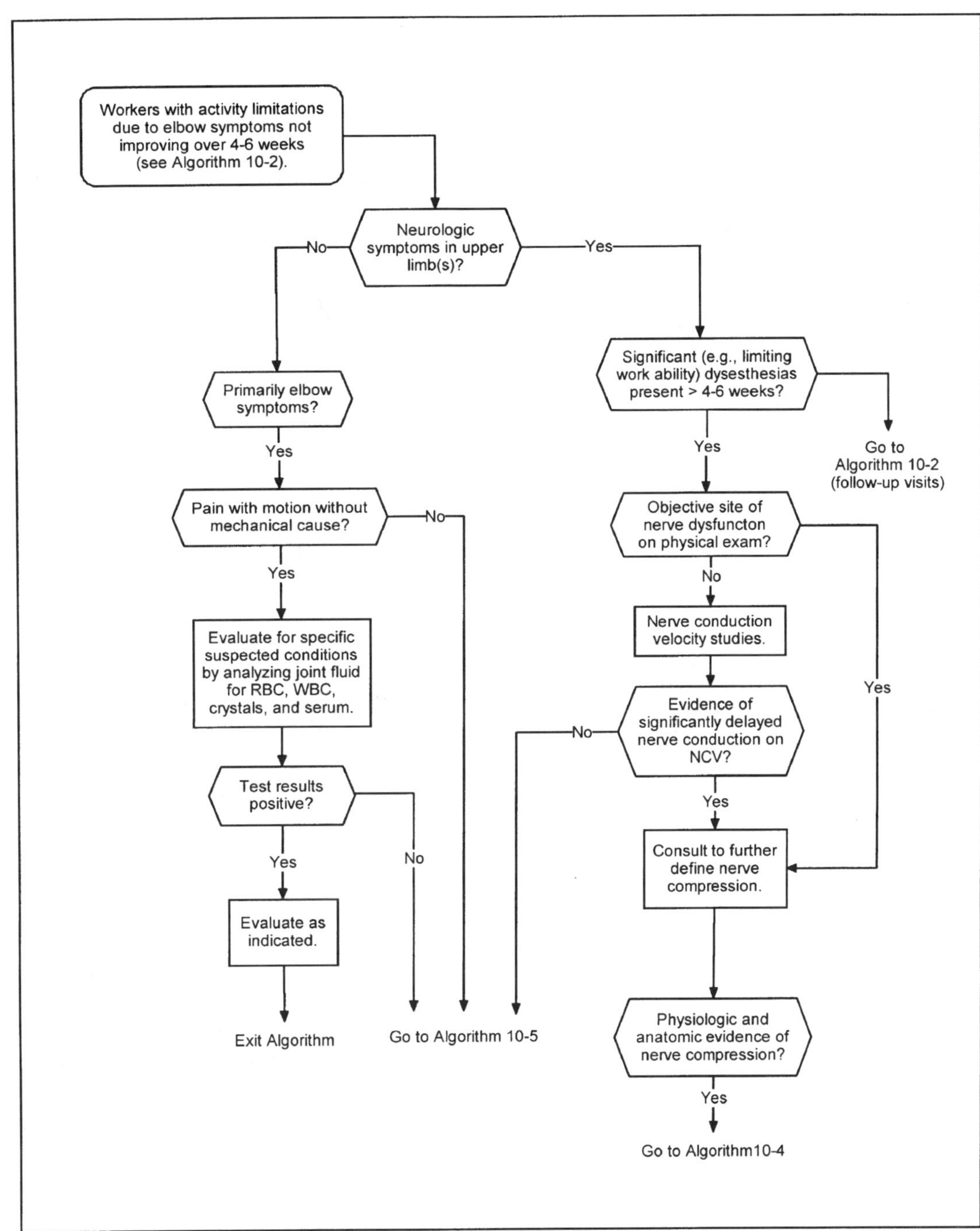

Algorithm 10-4. *Surgical Considerations for Patients with Anatomic and Physiologic Evidence of Nerve Compression Coupled with Persistent Elbow Complaints*

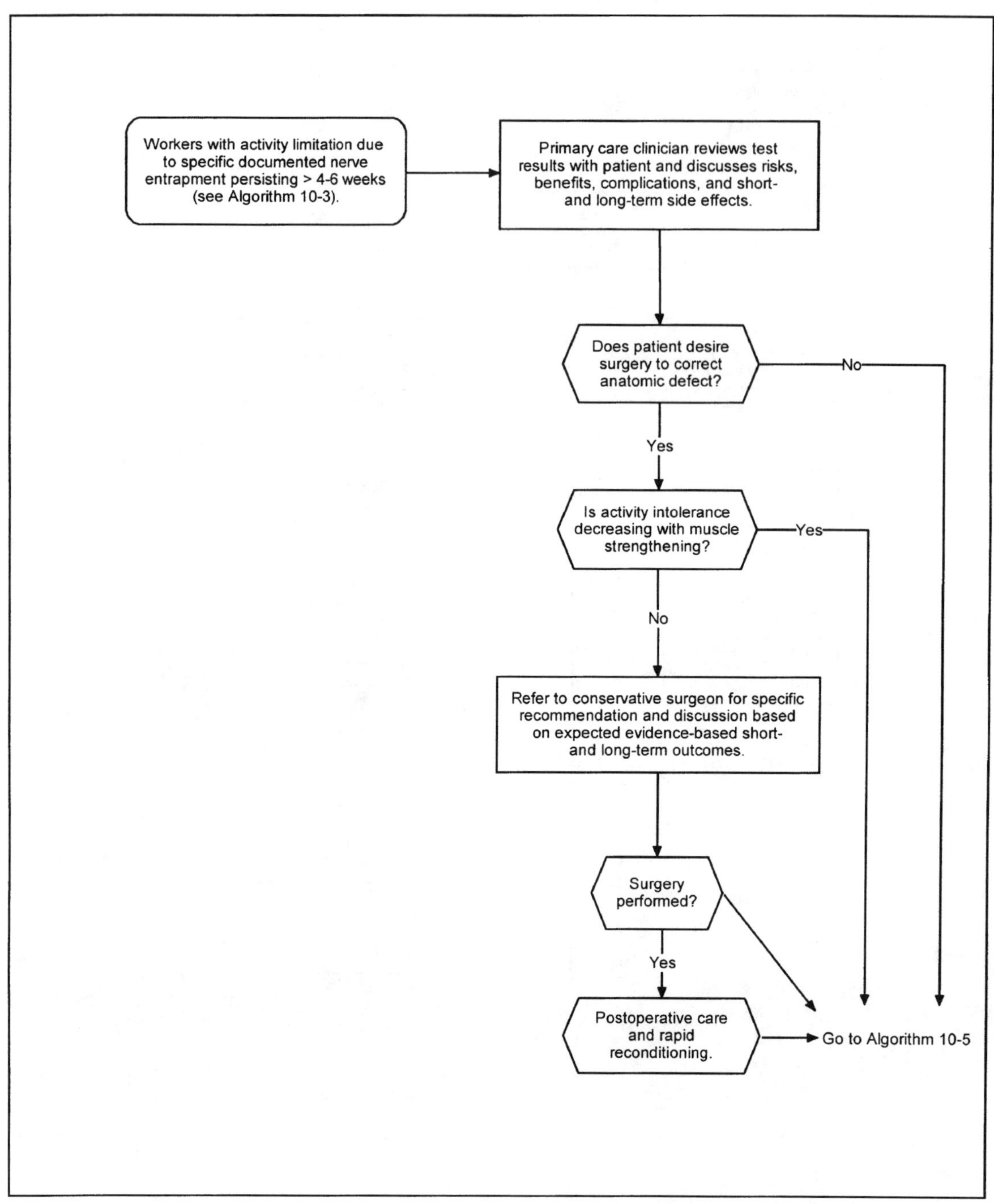

Algorithm 10-5. *Further Management of Occupational Elbow Complaints*

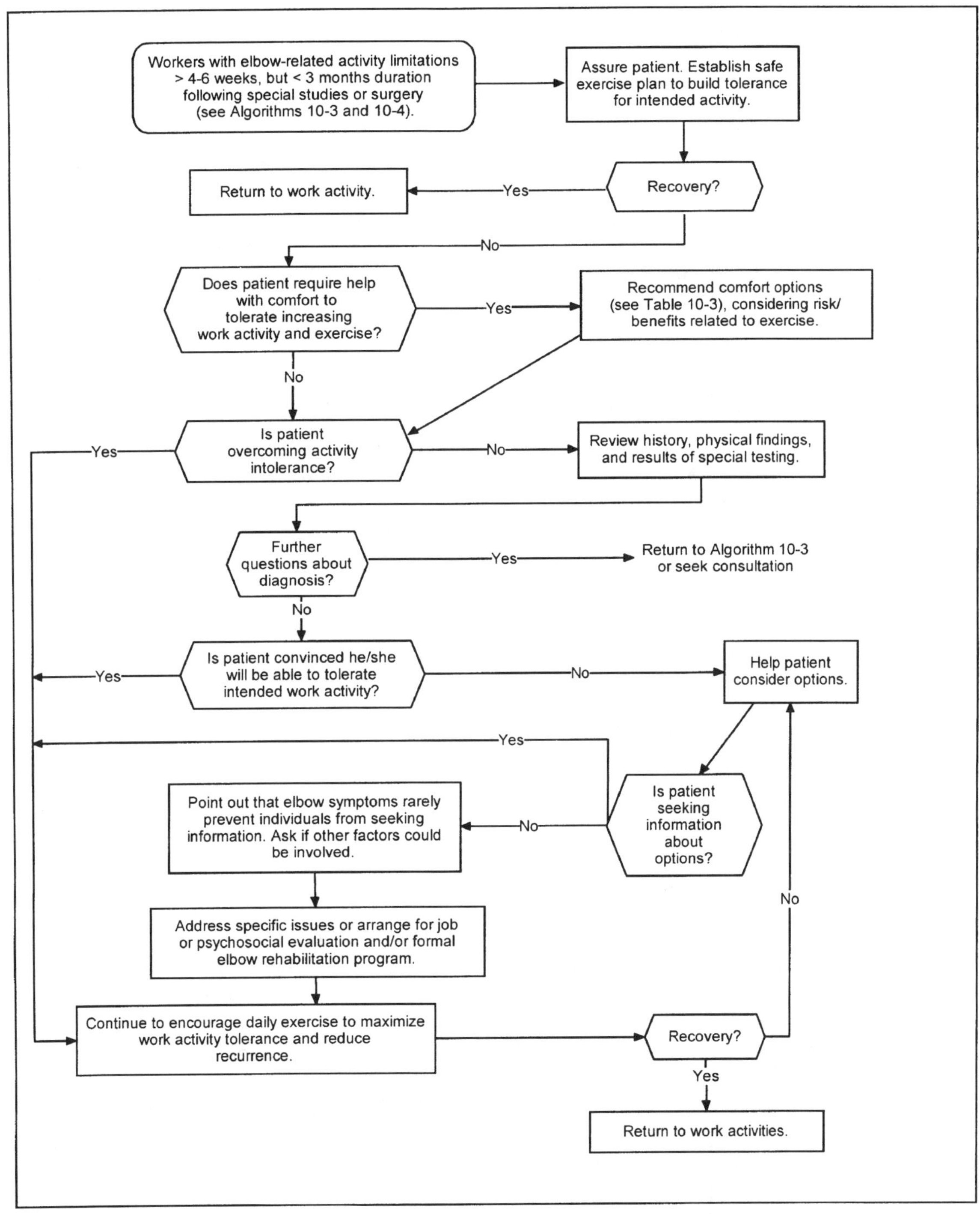

EPIDEMIOLOGY

Khan KM, Cook JL, Kannus P, Maffulli N, Bonar SF. Time to abandon the "tendinitis" myth. *BMJ*. 2002;324(7338):626-7.

Kivi P. Rheumatic disorders of the upper limbs associated with repetitive occupational tasks in Finland in 1975-1979. *Scand J Rheumatol*. 1984;13: 101-7.

Kurppa K, Viikari-Juntura E, Kuosma E, et al. Incidence of tenosynovitis or peritendinitis and epicondylitis in a meat-processing factory. *Scand J Work Environ Health*. 1991;17:32-7.

Viikari-Juntura E, Kurppa K, Kuosma E, et al. Prevalence of epicondylitis and elbow pain in the meat-processing industry. *Scand J Work Environ Health*. 1991;17:38-45.

HISTORY AND PHYSICAL EXAMINATION

American Academy of Orthopaedic Surgeons. *Athletic Training and Sports Medicine*. 2nd ed. Rosemont, Ill: American Academy of Orthopaedic Surgeons; 1994.

Green D. *Operative Hand Surgery*. New York, NY: Churchill Livingstone; 1982.

MEDICATION

See also Chapter 3 references.

Green S, Buchbinder R, Barnsley L, et al. Nonsteroidal anti-inflammatory drugs (NSAIDs) for treating lateral elbow pain in adults (Cochrane Review). In: *The Cochrane Library*. Issue 2; 2002. Oxford: Update Software.

INJECTIONS

Hay EM, Paterson SM, Lewis M, Hosie G, Croft P. Pragmatic randomised controlled trial of local corticosteroid injection and naproxen for treatment of lateral epicondylitis of elbow in primary care. *BMJ*. 1999;9;319(7215): 964-8.

Nevelos AB. The treatment of tennis elbow with triamcinolone acetonide. *Curr Med Res Opin*. 1980;6:507-9.

Newcomer KL, Laskowski ER, Idank DM, McLean TJ, Egan KS. Corticosteroid injection in early treatment of lateral epicondylitis. *Clin J Sport Med*. 2001;11(4):214-22.

Smidt N, van der Windt DA, Assendelft WJ, Deville WL, Korthals-de Bos IB, Bouter LM. Corticosteroid injections, physiotherapy, or a wait-and-see policy for lateral epicondylitis: a randomised controlled trial. *Lancet*. 2002;359(9307):657-62.

Weinstein PS, Canoso JJ, Wohlgethan JR. Long-term follow-up of corticosteroid injection for traumatic olecranon bursitis. *Ann Rheum Dis.* 1984;43: 44-6.

ACTIVITY AND EXERCISE

Viikari-Juntura E. Tenosynovitis, peritendinitis and the tennis elbow syndrome. *Scand J Work Environ Health.* 1984;10:443-9.

RADIOGRAPHY AND OTHER IMAGING PROCEDURES

de Beaux AC, Beattie T, Gilbert F. Elbow fat pad sign: implications for clinical management. *J R Coll Surg Edinb.* 1992;37:205-6.

Sugimoto H, Ohsawa T. Ulnar collateral ligament in the growing elbow: MR imaging of normal development and throwing injuries. *Radiology.* 1994;192:417-22.

Timmerman LA, Schwartz ML, Andrews JR. Preoperative evaluation of the ulnar collateral ligament by magnetic resonance imaging and computed tomography arthrography: evaluation in 25 baseball players with surgical confirmation. *Am J Sports Med.* 1994;22:26-31; discussion 32.

SURGICAL CONSIDERATIONS

Buchbinder R, Green S, Bell S, Barnsley L, Smidt N, Assendelft WJJ. Surgery for lateral elbow pain (Cochrane Review). In: *The Cochrane Library.* Issue 2; 2002. Oxford: Update Software.

Foster RJ, Edshage S. Factors related to the outcome of surgically managed compressive ulnar neuropathy at the elbow level. *J Hand Surg.* 1981;6: 181-92.

Mowlavi A, Andrews K, Lille S, Verhulst S, Zook EG, Milner S. The management of cubital tunnel syndrome: a meta-analysis of clinical studies. *Plast Reconstr Surg.* 2000;106(2):327-34.

Vangsness CT Jr, Jobe FW. Surgical treatment of medial epicondylitis: results in 35 elbows. *J Bone Joint Surg [Br].* 1991;73:409-11.

PHYSICAL TREATMENT METHODS

Basford JR, Sheffield CG, Cieslak KR. Laser therapy: a randomized, controlled trial of the effects of low intensity Nd:YAG laser irradiation on lateral epicondylitis. *Arch Phys Med Rehabil.* 2000;81(11):1504-10.

Boddeker I, Haake M. Extracorporeal shockwave therapy in treatment of epicondylitis humeri radialis. A current overview. *Orthopade.* 2000;29(5): 463-9.

Buchbinder R, Green S, White M, Barnsley L, Smidt N, Assendelft WJJ. Shock wave therapy for lateral elbow pain (Cochrane Review). In: *The Cochrane Library.* Issue 2; 2002. Oxford: Update Software.

Demirtas RN, Oner C. The treatment of lateral epicondylitis by iontophoresis of sodium salicylate and sodium diclofenac. *Clin Rehabil.* 1998;12(1):23-9.

Fink M, Wolkenstein E, Karst M, Gehrke A. Acupuncture in chronic epicondylitis: a randomized controlled trial. *Rheumatology (Oxford).* 2002;41(2):205-9.

Green S, Buchbinder R, Barnsley L, et al. Acupuncture for lateral elbow pain (Cochrane Review). *Cochrane Database Syst Rev.* 2002;(1):CD003527.

Klaiman MD, Shrader JA, Danoff JV, Hicks JE, Pesce WJ, Ferland J. Phonophoresis versus ultrasound in the treatment of common musculoskeletal conditions. *Med Sci Sports Exerc.* 1998;30(9):1349-55.

Simunovic Z, Trobonjaca T, Trobonjaca Z. Treatment of medial and lateral epicondylitis—tennis and golfer's elbow—with low level laser therapy: a multicenter double blind, placebo-controlled clinical study on 324 patients. *J Clin Laser Med Surg.* 1998;16(3):145-51.

***Master Algorithm**. ACOEM Guidelines for Care of Acute and Subacute Occupational Forearm, Wrist, and Hand Complaints*

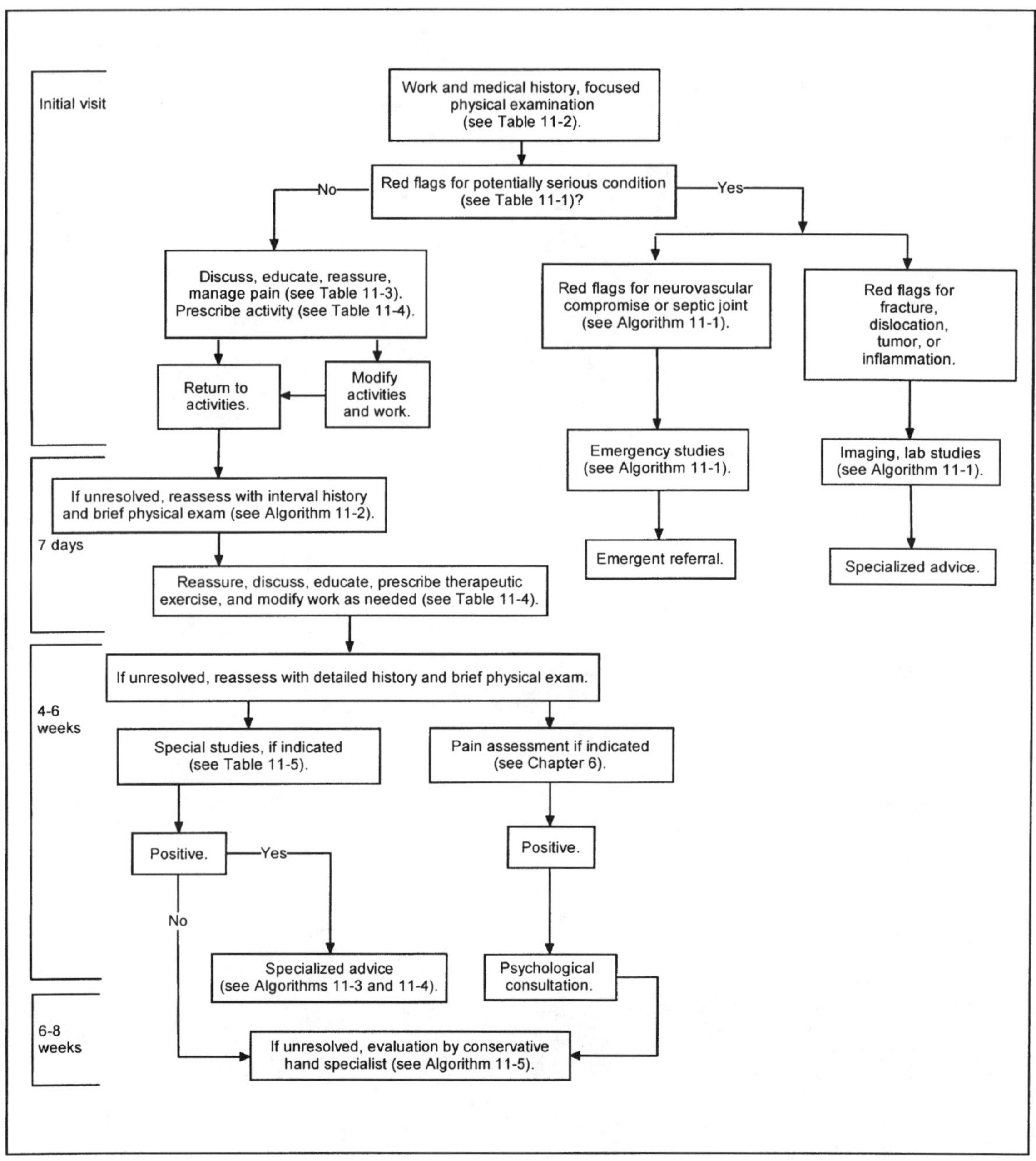

11 Forearm, Wrist, and Hand Complaints

General Approach and Basic Principles

Forearm, wrist, and hand complaints that may be work related are common problems presenting to occupational and primary care providers; they are among the five most common causes of reported work-related health complaints of workers' compensation claims. These complaints account for about 7 to 8% of total lost workdays in workers' compensation and 17-23% of cases and claims, ranking them in the top five for financial severity, much of the total expense is incurred for surgical procedures.

Recommendations on assessing and treating adults with work-related forearm, wrist, or hand complaints are presented in this clinical practice guideline. Topics include the initial assessment and diagnosis of patients with acute and subacute forearm, wrist, or hand complaints that may be work related, identification of red flags that may indicate the presence of a serious underlying medical condition, initial management, diagnostic considerations and special studies for identification of clinical pathology, work-relatedness, modified duty and activity, and return to work, as well as further management considerations, including the management of delayed recovery.

Algorithms for patient management are included. This chapter's master algorithm schematizes how primary care and occupational medicine practitioners may generally manage patients with acute and subacute forearm, wrist, and hand complaints. The following text, tables, and numbered algorithms expand upon the master algorithm.

The principal recommendations for assessing and treating patients with acute and subacute forearm, wrist, and hand complaints are as follows:

- The initial assessment focuses on detecting indicators of potentially serious disease, termed red flags.
- In the absence of red flags, occupational or primary care providers can safely and effectively manage work-related forearm, hand, and wrist complaints. The focus is on monitoring for complications, facilitating the healing process, and facilitating return to work in a modified- or full-duty capacity.

- Relieving discomfort can be accomplished most safely by modifying activities, temporary immobilization, and systemic nonprescription analgesics.
- Encourage patients recovering from acute or subacute forearm, hand, or wrist problems to return to modified work as their condition permits.
- Referral for specialty care may be indicated if symptoms persist beyond four to six weeks.
- Address nonphysical factors (such as psychosocial, workplace, or socioeconomic problems) in an effort to resolve delayed recovery.

Initial Assessment

Thorough medical and work histories as well as a focused physical examination (see Chapter 2) are sufficient for the initial assessment of a patient complaining of potentially work-related forearm, wrist, or hand symptoms. The medical history and examination include evaluation for serious underlying conditions. This evaluation may consider the possibility of referred pain to the forearm, wrist, and/or hand due to a disorder in another part of the body (e.g., cervical nerve root). Certain findings on the history and physical examination raise suspicion of serious underlying medical conditions; these are referred to as red flags (see Table 11-1). Their absence rules out the need for special studies, referral, or inpatient care during the first four weeks, during which time spontaneous recovery is expected (provided any inciting workplace factors are addressed). Forearm, hand, and wrist complaints can then be classified into one of four working categories:

- Potentially serious forearm, hand, or wrist condition: fracture, acute dislocation, infection, neurovascular compromise or injury, or tumor, in rare cases.
- Mechanical disorders: derangements of the forearm, hand, or wrist related to acute trauma, such as ligament or tendon strain.
- Degenerative disorders: resulting from aging or repetitive use, or a combination thereof, such as arthritis, tendinitis, or tenosynovitis.
- Nonspecific disorders: occurring in the hand or wrist and suggesting neither internal derangement nor referred pain.

Medical History

Asking the patient open-ended questions, such as those listed on page 256, allows the clinician to gauge the need for further discussion or specific inquiries to obtain more detailed information (see also Chapter 2):

Table 11-1. Red Flags for Potentially Serious Forearm, Wrist, or Hand Conditions

Disorder	Medical History	Physical Examination
Fracture	History of significant trauma History of deformities with or without spontaneous reduction or self-reduction Point pain	Significant swelling Deformity with displaced fracture Point tenderness Swelling, hematoma Point tenderness Ecchymosis
Dislocation	History of significant trauma History of deformities with or without spontaneous or self-reduction Inability to use the joint	Deformity present Tenderness and instability with history of deformity with reduction Hemarthrosis
Infection	History of systemic symptoms: chills, fever, dizziness History of immunosuppression (e.g., transplant, chemotherapy, HIV) Diabetes Painful, red, swollen areas	Tenderness with motion Systemic signs of sepsis Local heat, swelling, erythema Drainage of a sinus
Tumor	History of rapidly growing, painful mass of hand or wrist, not consistent with ganglion History of immunosuppression (e.g., transplant, chemotherapy, HIV)	Mass of forearm, hand, or wrist, not consistent with ganglion or other benign lesion
Inflammation	History of inflammatory arthritis or consistent with inflammatory arthritis Painful, swollen joints, usually without systemic symptoms	Swelling and deformity
Rapidly progressive neurologic compromise	Rapidly progressive numbness, paresthesias, or weakness in radial, ulnar, or median nerve distribution Progressive atrophy	Sensory deficit in ulnar, median, or radial distribution Loss of grip strength when picking up objects
Vascular compromise	History of vascular disease History of diabetes Cold, cool, or pale hand	Decreased pulses Decreased capillary filling
Osteoarthritis	History of sudden onset, or worsening of symptoms	Redness, heat, or tenderness
Severe carpal tunnel syndrome	Indications of causality (see Table 11-2) Dysesthesias in median nerve distribution	Muscle atrophy and severe weakness of thenar muscles

WHAT ARE YOUR SYMPTOMS?

- Do you have pain, numbness, tingling, weakness, or limited motion?
- For traumatic injuries: Was the area deformed? Did you lose any blood or have an open wound?
- Are your symptoms located primarily in the hand or wrist? Do you have pain or other symptoms elsewhere (e.g., forearm, neck)?
- Are your symptoms constant or intermittent? What makes the problem worse or better?
- Is the pain better or worse at any particular time of day?

HOW DO THESE SYMPTOMS LIMIT YOU?

- Can you do hand intensive activities? For how long?
- What stops you from working? Are the symptoms worse at work?
- Can you grasp? How much? Are you dropping things?
- Are the symptoms worse at night? Do they wake you up? How often?
- What have you tried to make it better? Does it work?

WHEN DID YOUR CURRENT LIMITATIONS BEGIN? WAS THERE A SPECIFIC INCITING EVENT? HOW DID THE LIMITATIONS DEVELOP?

- How long have your activities been limited? More than four weeks?
- Have your symptoms changed? How?
- Have you had similar episodes previously?
- Have you had previous testing or treatment? With whom?
- What do you think caused the problem? How do you think it is related to work?
- What are your specific job duties? Do you use your forearm, wrist, or hand to perform them? How? How often?
- What are your hobbies? Do you use your forearm, wrist, or hand to perform them? How? How often?
- Do you use vibrating tools or devices at work or at home (anything from air guns to blow dryers)? What effect, if any, do these devices have on your symptoms?
- Do you have other medical problems? For example, pregnancy, diabetes, or hypothyroidism.[1]

WHAT DO YOU HOPE WE CAN ACCOMPLISH DURING THIS VISIT?

[1]If pregnant and has carpal tunnel syndrome, the problem will likely go away after delivery. Work reassignment or modification may be indicated for any of these comorbid conditions.

Physical Examination

Guided by the medical history, the physical examination includes:

- General observation of the patient
- Regional examination of forearms, wrists, and hands as well as neck evaluation, if indicated by the history
- Neurologic screening

In most cases, the examination is subjective because the patient must exert voluntary effort or state a response to the sensory examination. In some cases of forearm, wrist, or hand problems, there are no objective findings. Strictly objective findings do not in any way require the patient's cooperation for determination. A palpable trigger finger is an objective finding, but any sensory findings are subjective because the patient reports the finding. Thenar atrophy is objective, while tenderness over a ligament or tendon is subjective. The presence of a visible ganglion is objective, though not necessarily work related, but whether pain is associated with it or there is tenderness on examination is subjective.

Though it may seem a point too obvious to warrant mention, the physician should specifically note which forearm, wrist, or hand—left or right—is the subject of the patient's complaints. Not infrequently, injured workers have prior workers' compensation claims that involve the opposite forearm, wrist, or hand. Any ambiguity in documentation can lead to delay in acceptance of the patient's workers' compensation claim, delay in the authorization of time-loss benefits, delay in the authorization of payment of medical care, or even outright denial of the workers' compensation claim.

The physician should seek objective evidence of pathology that is consistent with the patient's subjective complaints. In many cases, careful examination will reveal one or more truly objective findings, such as swelling, deformity, atrophy, reflex changes or spasm. Any such findings should be thoroughly documented in the medical record both for reference during future visits, and for the value the information will have in the patient's workers' compensation claim. For some patients with forearm, wrist, or hand, complaints, however, there are no objective findings. Meticulous documentation of the patient's complaints at each visit is of the utmost importance in such cases.

A. Regional Examination of Forearm, Hand, and Wrist

Because they are interrelated structures, the forearm, wrist, and hand can be examined together for observation of any swelling, masses, redness, deformity, or other abnormality. This examination may be followed by evaluating active and passive range of motion within the patient's limits of comfort with the area as relaxed as possible. Local tenderness may be accentuated by specific motions or stresses on specific joints, and active muscle contraction may produce pain, indicating a specific tendinitis. If this latter finding is on the radial side of the wrist, it suggests a diagnosis of DeQuervain's tenosynovitis. Specific areas of decreased pinprick sensation may indicate median or ulnar nerve compression; tapping the area of the nerve may produce dysesthesias in its distribution (a positive Tinel's sign). If the patient's flexing the wrist for a period of 60 seconds elicits dysesthesias in the median innervated digits, then this is a positive Phalen's test.

Several traditional findings of carpal tunnel syndrome (CTS) have limited specific diagnostic value. The various tests for CTS show a broad range of sensitivity, depending on the patient population. Clinicians should depend on more than one test. The most sensitive screening methods seem to be an abnormal Katz hand diagram, abnormal sensibility by Semmes-Weinstein testing, and night discomfort. Hypalgesia in the median nerve distribution and thumb abduction strength testing also have been found to be helpful in establishing the diagnosis of CTS. The flick sign is another diagnostic tool. (The sign is positive when a patient reports shaking his or her hand in an effort to relieve parathesias.) Table 11-3 lists various tests for CTS along with estimated sensitivity and specificity based on metaanalysis of existing studies.

Trigger finger nodules may be palpable both actively and passively. There may be only palmar tenderness over proximal interphalangeal joints. The presence of a ganglion is easily determined, but the severity of any symptoms is the basis for a decision to aspirate or, in persistent cases, to excise the cyst.

B. Neurovascular Screening

The neurologic and vascular status of the hand, wrist, forearm, and elbow, including peripheral pulses, and the motor, reflex, and sensory status of the forearm, hand, and wrist as well as the more proximal surrounding structures, can be assessed. Examining the neck and cervical nerve root function is also in order because C6 radiculopathy can affect the wrist extensors and T1 radiculopathy can present as dysfunction of the intrinsic muscles of the hand (see Table 8-3).

C. Assessing Red Flags

The forearm, wrist, and hand area may present with signs of serious infection or tumor (rarely metastatic) or manifest symptoms and signs of serious systemic disease (e.g., inflammatory arthritis, vascular disease), or neurologic conditions. Significant trauma requires evaluation for fracture or crush injury, while a history of deformity consistent with dislocation and spontaneous reduction requires surgical (preferably hand surgery) consultation.

Diagnostic Criteria

If there are no red flags present to indicate serious conditions, the clinician can then determine which common musculoskeletal disorder is present. The criteria presented in Table 11-2 follow the clinical thought process, from the

Table 11-2. Diagnostic Criteria for Non-red-flag Forearm, Wrist, or Hand Conditions that Can Be Managed by Primary Care Physicians

Probable Diagnosis or Injury	Unique Mechanism	Unique Symptoms	Unique Signs	Tests and Results
Ligament/tendon strain (ICD-9 842.00-.19)	Acute excess loading, worse with motion	Pain in tendon/ ligament area	Tenderness over tendon(s) or ligament(s) Pain or weakness on strength testing of the affected tendon	None
Tendinitis/ tenosynovitis (ICD-9 727.05)	Repetitive, forceful, awkward motion Direct pressure (*unusual*) Blunt trauma (*rare*)	Pain localized to muscle-tendon unit Triggering	Tenderness over tendon unit Synovial thickening Triggering or locking Crepitus Pain or weakness on strength testing of the affected tendon	None
DeQuervain's tenosynovitis (ICD-9 727.04)	Idiopathic Repetitive, forceful wrist or thumb motion Direct pressure (*unusual*) Blunt trauma (*rare*)	Pain over radial styloid or first dorsal compartment	Tenderness over radial styloid Mass over radial styloid Crepitus Thick tendon sheath Pain upon passive abduction Triggering Pain worse with ulnar deviation, thumb flexion, adduction, stretch of first dorsal compartment (Finkelstein test)	None
Trigger finger (ICD-9 727.03)	Idiopathic Repetitive, forceful, awkward motion (*unusual*) Blunt trauma (*rare*)	Triggering Pain at proximal interphalangeal joint Locked finger	Triggering Direct pressure Tender volar metacarpal crease Synovial thickening of specific parts of flexor retinaculum	None

Table 11-2. (continued)

Probable Diagnosis or Injury	Unique Mechanism	Unique Symptoms	Unique Signs	Tests and Results
Carpal tunnel syndrome (ICD-9 354.0)	Idiopathic Repetitive/ awkward grasp or pinch at the wrist Vibration Tenosynovitis	Numbness/ tingling in thumb, index, middle fingers, especially at night or with activity Hand pain radiating into the forearm Decreased grip strength Difficulty picking up small objects	Atrophy or decreased strength of abductor pollicis brevis, opponens (advanced cases) Decreased sensation in median nerve distribution + Semmes-Weinstein monofilament test + Durkan's test + Katz hand diagram	Median sensory latency > 3.2 msec Denervation potentials in abductor pollicis brevis possible (advanced cases) Median motor latency >4.5 msec
Nonspecific pain (ICD-9 719.43, 719.44, 719.5)	Idiopathic Possible occult trauma Other pathology Overuse	Varying if any underlying disorder	Varying if any underlying disorder	Plain films Coned in views if suspicion of bone chip, small fracture, etc. Bone scan positive after 72 hours if an occult fracture is present
Ganglion aggravation (ICD-9 727.41)	Unknown	Painful mass on wrist or hand	Tender mass over dorsal or volar wrist or hand	None

Note: ICD-9 = *International Classification of Diseases*, 9th Edition.

mechanism of illness or injury to unique symptoms and signs of a particular disorder and, finally, to test results if any tests are needed to guide treatment at this stage.

Carpal Tunnel Syndrome

CTS does *not* produce hand or wrist pain. It most often causes digital numbing or tingling primarily in the thumb, index, and long finger or numbness in the wrist. Symptoms of pain, numbness, and tingling in the hands are common in the general population, but based on studies, only about one in five symptomatic subjects would be expected to have CTS based on clinical examination and electrophysiologic testing.

Clinical testing may include:

- Administration of a Katz hand diagram: The patient is provided with a form that shows outlines of the arms, and the palmar and dorsal surfaces of the hands. The patient identifies areas of discomfort—characterizing them as pain, numbness, tingling, or other—on each of the diagrams the patient finds necessary. The results are termed "probable," "possible," or "unlikely," depending upon specified criteria.

- Testing for Tinel's sign: Up to six taps to the soft tissue overlying the carpal tunnel. A positive test occurs when the taps cause paresthesias in the median nerve distribution.
- Performing the Semmes-Weinstein test: A test involving nylon monofilaments that collapse at specific amounts of force when pushed perpendicularly against the palm or fingers. A positive test results when a filament of greater than normal size is required in order for its application to be perceived by the patient.
- Durkan's test: The examiner holds the supinated wrist in both hands and applies direct, even pressure over the transverse carpal ligament with both thumbs for up to 30 seconds. A positive test is indicated by tingling or paresthesia into the thumb, index finger, and middle and lateral half of the ring finger within 30 seconds.
- Testing for Phalen's sign: Prolonged, forced hyperflexion of the wrist is produced by requesting the patient to push the dorsa of both hands together, and to hold that position with the wrists in 90 degrees of flexion for sixty seconds. A positive test produces paresthesias in the distribution of the affected median nerve.
- Checking for the square wrist sign: The square wrist sign is positive if the ratio of the thickness of the wrist divided by the width of the wrist is greater than 0.7.

Appropriate electrodiagnostic studies (EDS) may help differentiate between CTS and other conditions, such as cervical radiculopathy. These may include nerve conduction studies (NCS), or in more difficult cases, electromyography (EMG) may be helpful. NCS and EMG may confirm the diagnosis of CTS but may be normal in early or mild cases of CTS. If the EDS are negative, tests may be repeated later in the course of treatment if symptoms persist.

The American Association of Electrodiagnostic Medicine, the American Academy of Neurology, and the American Academy of Physical Medicine and Rehabilitation jointly published a practice parameter for electrodiagnostic studies in CTS. In patients with suspected CTS, the following EDS studies are recommended:

1. Perform a median sensory NCS across the wrist with a conduction distance of 13 to 14 centimeters. If the result is abnormal, compare the result of the median sensory NCS to the result of a sensory NCS of one other adjacent sensory nerve in the symptomatic limb.

2. If the initial median sensory NCS across the wrist has a conduction distance greater than 8 cm and the result is normal, one of the following additional studies is recommended:
   a. Comparison of median-sensory- or mixed-nerve conduction across the wrist over a short (7 to 8 cm) conduction distance with ulnar-sensory-nerve conduction across the wrist over the same 7- to 8-cm conduction distance
   b. Comparison of median-sensory conduction across the wrist with radial- or ulnar-sensory conduction across the wrist in the same limb
   c. Comparison of median-sensory or mixed-nerve conduction through the carpal tunnel to sensory- or mixed-nerve conduction velocity of proximal (forearm) or distal (digit) segments of the median nerve in the same limb

Many other in-office tests and symptoms have varying predictive value for CTS, as summarized in Table 11-3.

Work-Relatedness

A thorough work history is crucial to establishing work-relatedness. (See Chapter 2 for components of the work history.) Determining whether a complaint of a hand, wrist, or forearm disorder is related to work requires a careful analysis and weighing of all associated or apparently causal factors operative at the time. A predominance of work factors suggests that worksite intervention would be appropriate. A cluster of cases in a work group suggests a greater probability of associated work design or management factors.

Repetitive work, especially pinch grasping and, possibly, keyboard work, is currently thought to have the potential to contribute to wrist or hand tendinitis. Problems with workstations have been associated with CTS and DeQuervain's tenosynovitis. The strength of these associations is not clear. Identification and ameliorization of other factors may be important, including compression at the wrist, awkward posture interacting with force, and the effect of sustained head and shoulder postures for office workers and computer users. Acute trauma at work can be associated with tendon and ligament strains.

The clinician may recommend work and activity modifications or ergonomic redesign of the workplace to facilitate recovery and prevent recurrence. The employer's role in accommodating activity limitations and preventing further problems through ergonomic changes is key to hastening the employee's return to full activity. In some cases it may be desirable to conduct a detailed ergonomic analysis of activities that may be contributing to the symptoms. A broad range of ergonomic surveys and instruments is available for measuring range of activity, strain, weights, reach, frequency of motion, flexion, and extension, as well as psychological factors such as organizational relationships and job satisfaction. Such detailed measures may be necessary or useful for

*Table 11-3. Sensitivity and Specificity of Diagnostic Tests for Carpal Tunnel Syndrome Measured Against Nerve Conduction Studies**

Test	Sensitivity	Specificity
Combination of abnormal Katz hand diagram, abnormal Semmes-Weinstein test, positive Durkan's test, and night pain	96%	99%
Katz hand diagram scores	96%	76%
Night pain symptoms	96%	80%
Flick sign (shaking hand)	93%	96%
Durkan's compression test	89%	90%
Semmes-Weinstein monofilament test	83%	59%
Nocturnal paresthesias	77%	33%
Weak thumb abduction strength	66%	66%
Closed fist sign	61%	92%
Phalen sign	55%	45%
Hypoalgesia in the median nerve territory	51%	85%
Square wrist sign	47%	83%
Tinel's sign	42%	67%
Static 2-point discrimination > 6 mm**	32%	99%
Tourniquet test	21%	36%
Thenar atrophy**	20%	91%

* Reported sensitivity and specificity values have varied markedly. Combining tests may increase the positive predictive value. The above values are adapted from Light TR, *Hand Surgery Update 2*, American Society for Surgery of the Hand Staff, September 1, 1999; Szabo RM, Slater RR Jr, Farver TB, Stanton DB, Sharman WK. The value of diagnostic testing in carpal tunnel syndrome. *J Hand Surg [Am]*. 1999;24(4):704-14; and D'Arcy CA, McGee S. The rational clinical examination. Does this patient have carpal tunnel syndrome? *JAMA* 2000;283(23):3110-7, including *Cochrane Review.*
** While the 2-point discrimination test and thenar atrophy do not have high sensitivity in isolating the diagnosis of carpal tunnel syndrome, they are useful in distinguishing severe CTS from mild or moderate CTS.

modifying activity, for redesigning the workstation, or for suggesting organizational and management relief. Such cases may call for referral to a certified human factors engineer or ergonomist, either through the patient or the employer.

Initial Care

Comfort is often a patient's first concern. Nonprescription analgesics will provide sufficient pain relief for most patients with acute and subacute symptoms. If treatment response is inadequate (that is, if symptoms and activity limitations continue), prescribed pharmaceuticals or physical methods may be added. Clinicians should consider the presence of medical diseases such as diabetes, hypothyroidism, Vitamin B complex deficiency, and arthritis. Side effects, cost, and provider and patient preferences should guide the clinician's choice of recommendations. Initial treatment of CTS should include night splints. Day splints can be considered for patient comfort as needed to reduce pain, along with work modifications. For patients with mild-to-moderate CTS who opt for conservative treatment, studies show that corticosteroids may be of greater benefit than nonsteroidal anti-inflammatory drugs (NSAIDs), but side effects prevent their general recommendation. Vitamin B6 is often used in CTS when it is perceived to be deficient, but this practice is not consistently supported by the medical evidence. Table 11-4 summarizes comfort options.

Table 11-4. Methods of Symptom Control for Forearm, Wrist, and Hand Complaints

RECOMMENDED
Nonprescription Medications
Acetaminophen (safest) NSAIDs (aspirin, ibuprofen) (secondary choice)
Physical Modalities
Adjust or modify workstation, job tasks, or work hours and methods Stretching Specific hand and wrist exercises for range of motion and strengthening At-home local applications of cold packs first few days of acute complaints; thereafter, applications of heat packs Aerobic exercise to maintain general conditioning Initial and follow-up visits for education, counseling, and evaluating home exercise
Prescribed Pharmaceutical Methods
Other NSAIDs

OPTIONS

Ligament/Tendon Strain	**Tendinitis/Tenosynovitis**	**DeQuervain's Syndrome**
Limit motion that causes pain	Limit motion of inflamed structures Injections of lidocaine and corticosteroids	Limit motion of inflamed structures with wrist and thumb splint
Trigger Finger	**Carpal Tunnel Syndrome**	**Ganglion**
Injection of lidocaine and corticosteroids	Splinting of wrist in neutral position at night & day Injections of lidocaine and corticosteroids	Corticosteroid injection Aspiration

Nonspecific Hand or Wrist Pain
None

Physical Methods

- Instruction in home exercise. Except in cases of unstable fractures or acute dislocations, patients should be advised to do early range-of-motion exercises at home. Instruction in proper exercise technique is important, and a physical therapist can serve to educate the patient about an effective exercise program.
- Manipulation has not been proven effective for patients with pain in the hand, wrist, or forearm. Studies show that therapeutic touch is no better than placebo in influencing median-motor-nerve distal latencies, pain scores, and relaxation scores. Using a magnet for reducing pain attributed to CTS is no more effective than using the placebo device.
- Physical modalities, such as massage, diathermy, cutaneous laser treatment, "cold" laser treatment, transcutaneous electrical neurostimulation (TENS) units, and biofeedback have no scientifically proven efficacy in treating acute hand, wrist, or forearm symptoms. Limited studies suggest there are satisfying short- to medium-term effects due to ultrasound treatment in patients with mild to moderate idiopathic CTS, but the effect is not curative. Patients' at-home applications of heat or cold packs may be used before or after exercises and are as effective as those performed by a therapist.
- Most invasive techniques, such as needle acupuncture and injection procedures, have insufficient high quality evidence to support their use. The exception is corticosteroid injection about the tendon sheaths or, possibly, the carpal tunnel in cases resistant to conservative therapy for eight to twelve weeks. For optimal care, a clinician may always try conservative methods before considering an injection. DeQuervain's tendinitis, if not severe, may be treated with a wrist-and-thumb splint and acetaminophen, then NSAIDs, if tolerated, for four weeks before a corticosteroid injection is considered. CTS may be treated for a similar period with a splint and medications before injection is considered, except in the case of severe CTS (thenar muscle atrophy and constant paresthesias in the median innervated digits). Outcomes from carpal tunnel surgery justify prompt referral for surgery in moderate to severe cases, though evidence suggests that there is rarely a need for emergent referral. Thus, surgery should usually be delayed until a definitive diagnosis of CTS is made by history, physical examination, and possibly electrodiagnostic studies. Symptomatic relief from a cortisone/anesthetic injection will facilitate the diagnosis; however, the benefit from these injections is short-lived. Trigger finger, if significantly symptomatic, is probably best treated with a cortisone/anesthetic injection at first encounter, with hand surgery referral if symptoms persist after two injections by the primary care or occupational medicine provider (see Table 11-4).
- When treating with a splint in CTS, scientific evidence supports the efficacy of neutral wrist splints. Splinting should be used at night, and may be used during the day, depending upon activity.

- Support for iontophoresis and phonophoresis is limited.
- Activity alteration.

Careful advice regarding maximizing activities within the limits of symptoms is imperative once red flags have been ruled out. Any splinting or limitations placed on hand, wrist, and forearm activity should not interfere with total body activity in a major way. Strict elevation can be done for a short period of time at regular intervals.

Activities that increase stress on the hand or wrist may contribute to structural damage and tend to aggravate symptoms. Limitations of keyboard work or pinch-grasping may be necessary during the first few weeks after onset of acute tendinitis, tenosynovitis, nerve impingement, or irritation around a ganglion.

Evidence shows that keyboard users may experience a reduction in hand pain after several months of using some alternative geometry keyboards, although the benefit appears to be dependent upon user preference.

Job Analysis

While not all CTS or other hand and wrist complaints are occupational in origin, complaints of workplace discomfort should be evaluated for ergonomic modifications as part of the treatment program. Careful ergonomic re-analysis of the job is indicated if the individual fails to improve. Delayed recovery or return of symptoms may suggest an association between job tasks or motions and the presenting complaint.

Work Activities

Table 11-5 provides recommendations on activity modification and duration of absence from work. These guidelines are intended for patients without

*Table 11-5. Guidelines for Modification of Work Activities and Disability Duration**

		Recommended Target for Disability Duration**		NHIS Experience Data***	
Disorder	**Activity Modifications and Accommodation**	**With Modified Duty**	**Without Modified Duty**	**Median (cases with lost time)**	**Percent (no lost time)**
Tendon strain	Modification of activities involving the muscle-tendon unit, i.e., those that cause significant symptoms. Also workstation assessment to insure optimal ergonomics, as appropriate.	0-3 days	7-14 days	10 days	46%

Table 11-5. (continued)

Disorder	Activity Modifications and Accommodation	Recommended Target for Disability Duration**		NHIS Experience Data***	
		With Modified Duty	Without Modified Duty	Median (cases with lost time)	Percent (no lost time)
Tenosynovitis	Same as for tendon strain	0-3 days	7-14 days	15 days	58%
DeQuervain's syndrome	Same as for tendon strain	0-3 days	7-14 days	15 days	58%
Trigger finger	After injection (see Table 11-3), allow all activity	0-3 days	7-14 days	15 days	58%
Carpal tunnel syndrome	Same as for tendon strain. Also workstation adjustments, night splints, avoidance of prolonged periods in wrist flexion or extension	0-3 days	7-14 days	14 days	43%
Ganglion (aggravation)	Same as for tendon strain but allow full activity after aspiration	0-3 days	7-14 days	10 days	65%
Regional hand and wrist pain	Allow all activities as tolerated Modification of activities that aggravate symptoms, but range-of-motion and conditioning exercises should be performed by patient	0-3 days	7-14 days	9 days	43%

* These are general guidelines based on consensus or population sources and are never meant to be applied to an individual case without consideration of workplace factors, concurrent disease or other social or medical factors that can affect recovery.

** These parameters for disability duration are *consensus optimal* targets as determined by a panel of ACOEM members in 1996, and reaffirmed by a panel of ACOEM members in 2002. In most cases, persons with one non-severe extremity injury can return to modified duty immediately. Restrictions should take into consideration the opposite extremity also to prevent strain injuries to the uninjured extremity. Additional limitations of the frequency or pressure of keyboard use or pinch grasp may be warranted.

*** Based on the CDC NHIS (National Health Interview Survey), as compiled and reported in the 8th annual edition of *Official Disability Guidelines (ODG)*, © 2002 Work Loss Data Institute, all rights reserved.

comorbidity or complicating factors, including employment or legal issues. They are targets to provide a guide from the perspective of physiologic recovery.

Key factors to consider in disability duration are age and type of job, especially if the regular work includes activities that may aggravate the condition. By communicating with patients and employers, clinicians can make it clear that:

- Even moderate pinch-grasping or extension and flexion may aggravate forearm, hand, and wrist symptoms.
- Restrictions may allow for recovery or time to build activity tolerance through exercise

Follow-up Visits

Patients with potentially work-related forearm, wrist, and hand complaints should have follow-up every three to five days by a midlevel practitioner, or by a physical or hand therapist who can counsel them about avoiding static positions, medication use, activity modification, and other concerns. Take care to answer questions and make these sessions interactive so that the patient is duly involved in his or her recovery. If the patient has returned to work, these interactions may be done on site or by telephone, to avoid interfering with modified- or full-work activities.

Physician follow-up can occur when the patient needs a release to modified, increased, or full duty, or after appreciable healing or recovery can be expected, on average. Physician follow-up might be expected every four to seven days if the patient is off work and seven to fourteen days if the patient is working.

Special Studies and Diagnostic and Treatment Considerations

For most patients presenting with true hand and wrist problems, special studies are not needed until after a four- to six-week period of conservative care and observation. Most patients improve quickly, provided red flag conditions are ruled out. Exceptions include the following:

- In cases of wrist injury, with snuff box (radial-dorsal wrist) tenderness, but minimal other findings, a scaphoid fracture may be present. Initial radiographic films may be obtained but may be negative in the presence of scaphoid fracture. A bone scan may diagnose a suspected scaphoid fracture with a very high degree of sensitivity, even if obtained within 48 to 72 hours following the injury.
- An acute injury to the metacarpophalangeal joint of the thumb, accompanied by tenderness on the ulnar side of the joint and laxity when that side of the joint is stressed (compared to the other side), may

indicate a gamekeeper thumb or rupture of the ligament at that location. Radiographic films may show a fracture; stress views, if obtainable, may show laxity. The diagnosis may necessitate surgical repair of the ligament; therefore, a surgical referral is warranted.

- In cases of peripheral nerve impingement, if no improvement or worsening has occurred within four to six weeks, electrical studies may be indicated. The primary treating physician may refer for a local lidocaine injection with or without corticosteroids.
- Recurrence of a symptomatic ganglion that has been previously aspirated or a trigger finger that has been previously treated with local injections (see Table 11-4) is usually an indication for re-aspiration or referral, based on the treating physician's judgment.
- A number of patients with hand and wrist complaints will have associated disease such as diabetes, hypothyroidism, Vitamin B complex deficiency and arthritis. When history indicates, testing for these or other comorbid conditions is recommended.
- If symptoms have not resolved in four to six weeks and the patient has joint effusion, serologic studies for Lyme disease and autoimmune diseases may be indicated. Imaging studies to clarify the diagnosis may be warranted if the medical history and physical examination suggest specific disorders. Table 11-6 provides a general comparison of the abilities of different imaging techniques to identify physiologic insult and define anatomic defects.

Table 11-6. Ability of Various Techniques To Identify and Define Forearm, Wrist, and Hand Pathology

Technique	Ligament/ Tendon Strain	Tendinitis/ Tenosynovitis	DeQuervain's Tendonitis	Trigger Finger	Carpal Tunnel Syndrome	Ganglion	Infection
History	+ + +	+ + +	+ + +	+ + + +	+ + + +	+ +	+ + + +
Physical examination	+ + + +	+ + + +	+ + + +	+ + + +	+ + +	+ + + +	+ + + +
Laboratory studies	0	0	0	0	0	0	+ + + +
Electromyography/ nerve conduction velocity (EMG/ NCV) testing	0	0	0	0	+ + + +	0	0
Imaging studies							Lytic lesions
Radiography[1]	0	0	0	0	+	+ +	+ + +
Bone scan[1]	0	0	0	0	0	0	+ + + +
Arthrography[1]	0	0	0	0	0	0	0
Computed tomography (CT)[1]	0	0	0	0	0	0	+ + + +
Magnetic resonance imaging (MRI)[1]	0	0	0	0	+	0	+ + + +

[1] Risk of complications (e.g., infection, radiation) highest for contrast CT or arthrography; second highest for myelography; relatively less for bone scan, radiography, and CT; lowest for MRI.

Note: Number of plus signs indicates relative ability to identify or define pathology.

Surgical Considerations

Referral for hand surgery consultation may be indicated for patients who:

- Have red flags of a serious nature
- Fail to respond to conservative management, including worksite modifications
- Have clear clinical and special study evidence of a lesion that has been shown to benefit, in both the short and long term, from surgical intervention

Surgical considerations depend on the confirmed diagnosis of the presenting hand or wrist complaint. If surgery is a consideration, counseling regarding likely outcomes, risks and benefits, and, especially, expectations is very important. If there is no clear indication for surgery, referring the patient to a physical medicine practitioner may aid in formulating a treatment plan.

A. Carpal Tunnel Syndrome

Surgical decompression of the median nerve usually relieves CTS symptoms. High-quality scientific evidence shows success in the majority of patients with an electrodiagnostically confirmed diagnosis of CTS. Patients with the mildest symptoms display the poorest postsurgery results; patients with moderate or severe CTS have better outcomes from surgery than splinting. CTS must be proved by positive findings on clinical examination and the diagnosis should be supported by nerve-conduction tests before surgery is undertaken. Mild CTS with normal electrodiagnostic studies (EDS) exists, but moderate or severe CTS with normal EDS is very rare. Positive EDS in asymptomatic individuals is not CTS. Studies have not shown portable nerve conduction devices to be effective diagnostic tools. Surgery will not relieve any symptoms from cervical radiculopathy (double crush syndrome). Likewise, diabetic patients with peripheral neuropathy cannot expect full recovery and total abatement of symptoms after nerve decompression.

Risks of surgical decompression include complications of anesthesia, wound infection, and damage to the median nerve. Incomplete decompression or recurrence of symptoms can lead to the need for further surgery. Based on the data from the randomized controlled trials, endoscopic carpal tunnel release seems to be an effective procedure compared to open surgery; however, greater emphasis must be given to training surgeons in this technique to avoid major complications such as median nerve injuries. With proper training and equipment, endoscopic carpal tunnel release can be done safely, with complication rates comparable to those for the open technique and with high patient satisfaction. Early return to work after either type carpal tunnel surgery is more dependent on the willingness of the employer and patient than on the surgical technique. Two prospective randomized studies show no beneficial effect from postoperative splinting after carpal tunnel release when compared to a bulky dressing alone. In fact, splinting the wrist beyond 48 hours following CTS release may be largely detrimental, especially compared to a home therapy program.

B. Trigger Finger

One or two injections of lidocaine and corticosteroids into or near the thickened area of the flexor tendon sheath of the affected finger are almost always sufficient to cure symptoms and restore function. A procedure under local anesthesia may be necessary to permanently correct persistent triggering.

C. DeQuervain's Syndrome

The majority of patients with DeQuervain's syndrome will have resolution of symptoms with conservative treatment. Under unusual circumstances of persistent pain at the wrist and limitation of function, surgery may be an option for treating DeQuervain's tendinitis. Surgery, however, carries similar risks and complications as those already mentioned above (see A, "Carpal Tunnel Syndrome"), including the possibility of damage to the radial nerve at the wrist because it is in the area of the incision.

D. Ganglion

Only symptomatic wrist ganglia merit or excision, if aspiration fails. Recurrences may be spontaneous or related to inadequate removal of the communication with the carpal joints or to satellite ganglia that the surgeon failed to excise.

Summary of Recommendations and Evidence

See Table 11-7.

Table 11-7. Summary of Recommendations for Evaluating and Managing Forearm, Wrist, and Hand Complaints

Clinical Measure	Recommended	Optional	Not Recommended
History and physical exam	Basic history, focused exam, and search for red flags (C)		
Patient education	Patient education regarding prevention, diagnosis, prognosis, and expectations of medical treatment (D)		
Medication (See Chapter 3)	Acetaminophen (C) NSAIDs (B)	Opioids, short course (C) Rarely, cortcosteroids (C)	Use of opioids for more than 2 weeks (C)
Physical treatment methods	Instructions for home exercises	At-home applications of heat or cold packs (D)	Passive modalities TENS units (C) Biofeedback (D)

Table 11-7. (continued)

Clinical Measure	Recommended	Optional	Not Recommended
Injections	Injection of corticosteroids into carpal tunnel in mild or moderate cases of CTS after trial of splinting and medication (C) Initial injection into tendon sheath for clearly diagnosed cases of DeQuervain's syndrome, tenosynovitis, or trigger finger (D)	Initial injection of corticosteroids in moderate cases of tendinitis (D)	Repeated or frequent injection of corticosteroids into carpal tunnel, tendon sheaths, ganglia, etc. (D)
Rest and immobilization	Splinting as first-line conservative treatment for CTS, DeQuervain's, strains, etc. (C)	Prolonged splinting (leads to weakness and stiffness) (D) Prolonged post-operative splinting (C)	
Activity and exercise	Stretching Aerobic exercise Maintaining strength and mobility of all remaining body parts while recovering from wrist problems (C)		Reduced general activities while recovering (D)
Detection of neurologic abnormalities	NCV for median (B) or ulnar (C) impingement at the wrist after failure of conservative treatment		Routine use of NCV or EMG in diagnostic evaluation of nerve entrapment or screening in patients w/o symptoms (D) Use of vibrometry for screening (C)
Radiography	Plain films for suspected scaphoid fractures, repeat films in 7-10 days (D)	Limited bone scan to detect fractures if clinical suspicion exists (C)	Routine use for evaluation of forearm, wrist, and hand (D)
Other imaging procedures		Use of arthrography, MRI, or CT scans prior to history and physical examination by a qualified specialist (D)	

Table 11-7. (continued)

Clinical Measure	Recommended	Optional	Not Recommended
Surgical considerations	Early surgical intervention for severe CTS confirmed by NCV may be indicated (B) Tendinitis (DeQuervain's), ganglion, or trigger finger: referral to surgeon only after patient education and conservative treatment, including splinting and injection, have failed (C, D)		
Psychosocial factors	Consider counseling for severe hand injuries (D) Awareness by treating practitioner of interplay between physical, economic, and psychological factors in patients with MSDs (C, D)		

A = Strong research-based evidence (multiple relevant, high-quality scientific studies).
B = Moderate research-based evidence (one relevant, high-quality scientific study or multiple adequate scientific studies).
C = Limited research-based evidence (at least one adequate scientific study of patients with forearm, wrist, or hand disorders).
D = Reviewer or consensus interpretation of evidence not meeting inclusion criteria for research-based evidence.

Algorithm 11-1. *Initial Evaluation of Occupational Forearm, Wrist, and Hand Complaints*

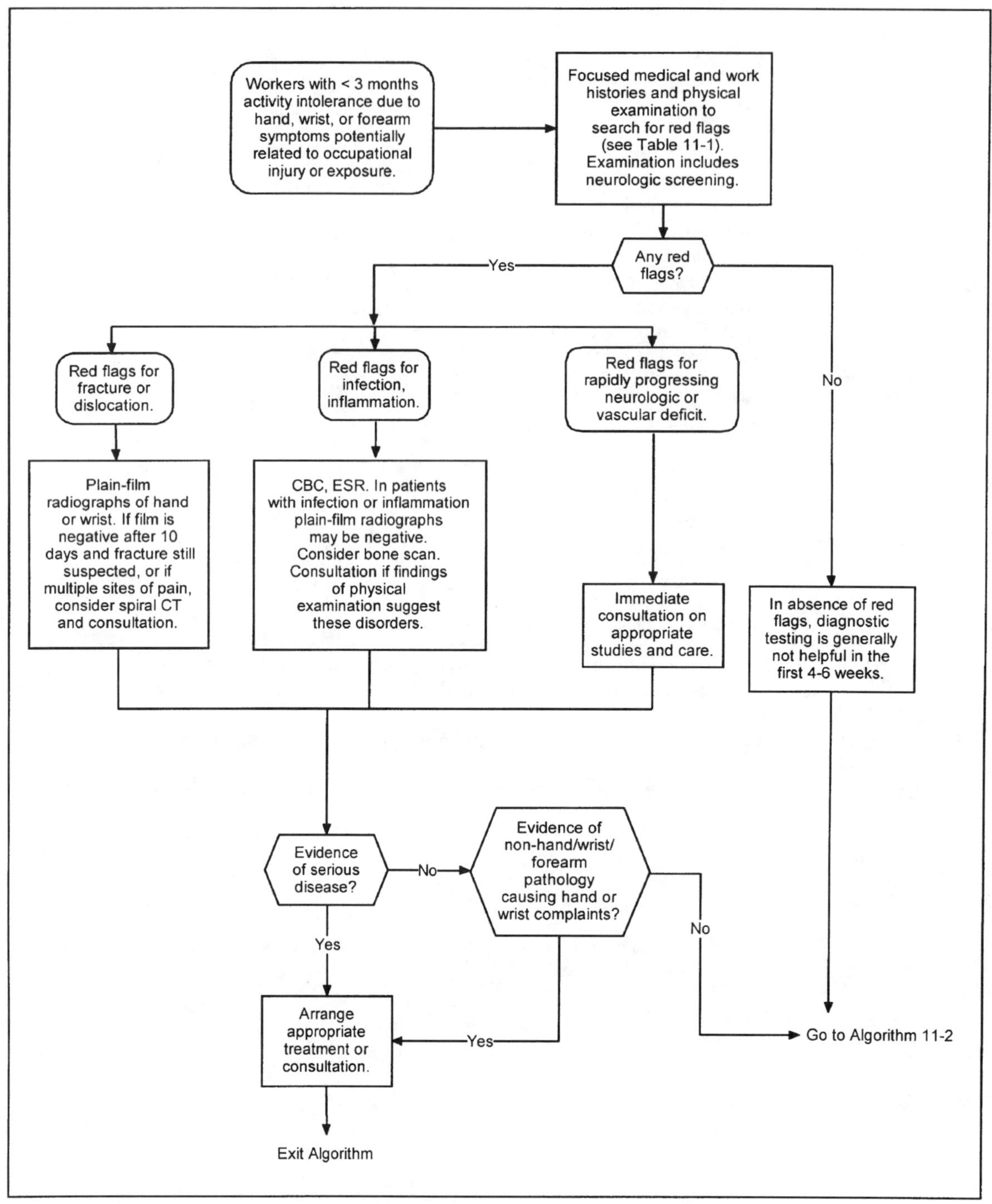

Algorithm 11-2. *Initial and Follow-up Management of Occupational Forearm, Wrist, and Hand Complaints*

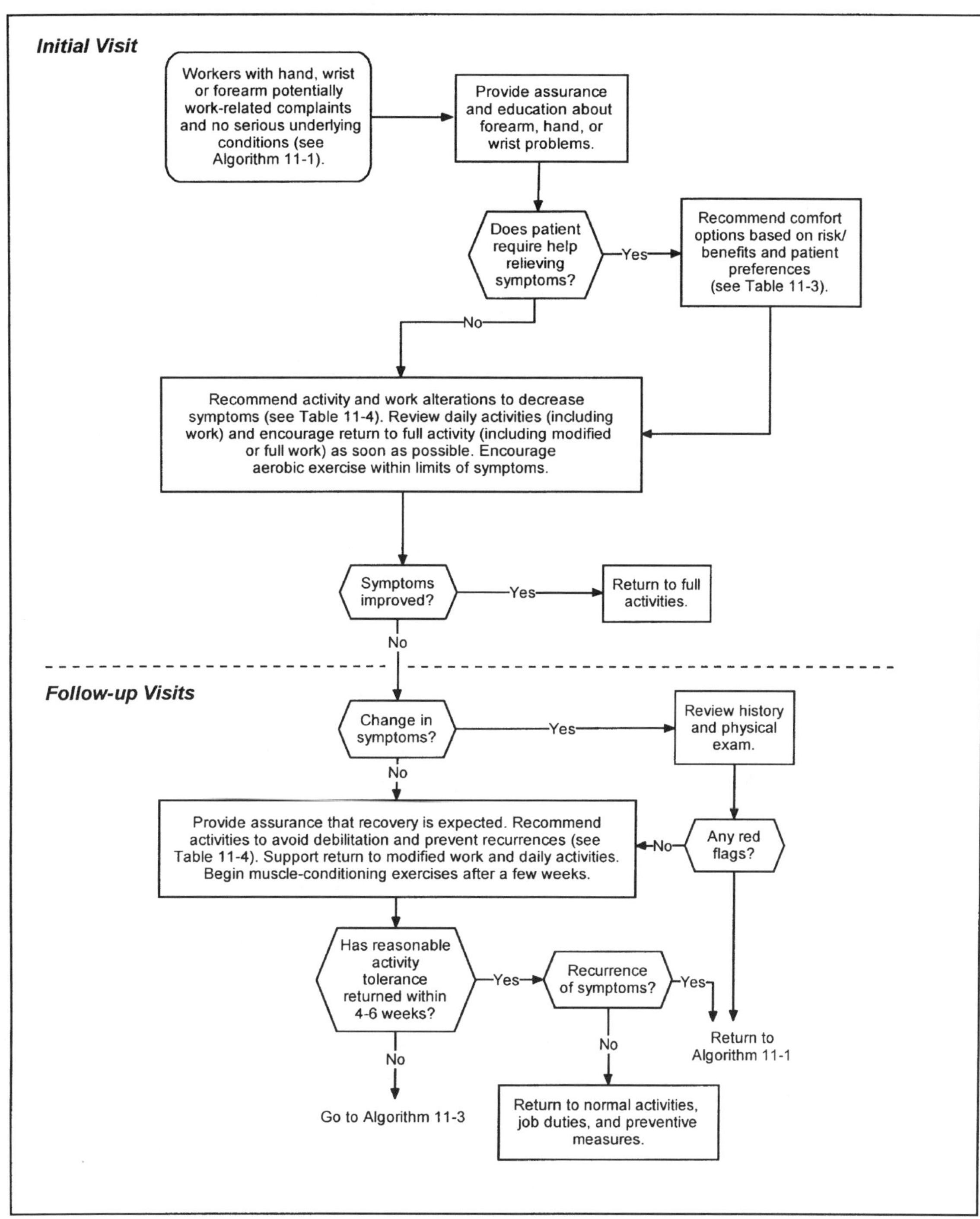

Algorithm 11-3. *Evaluation of Slow-to-recover Patients with Occupational Forearm, Wrist, and Hand Complaints (Symptoms > 4 Weeks)*

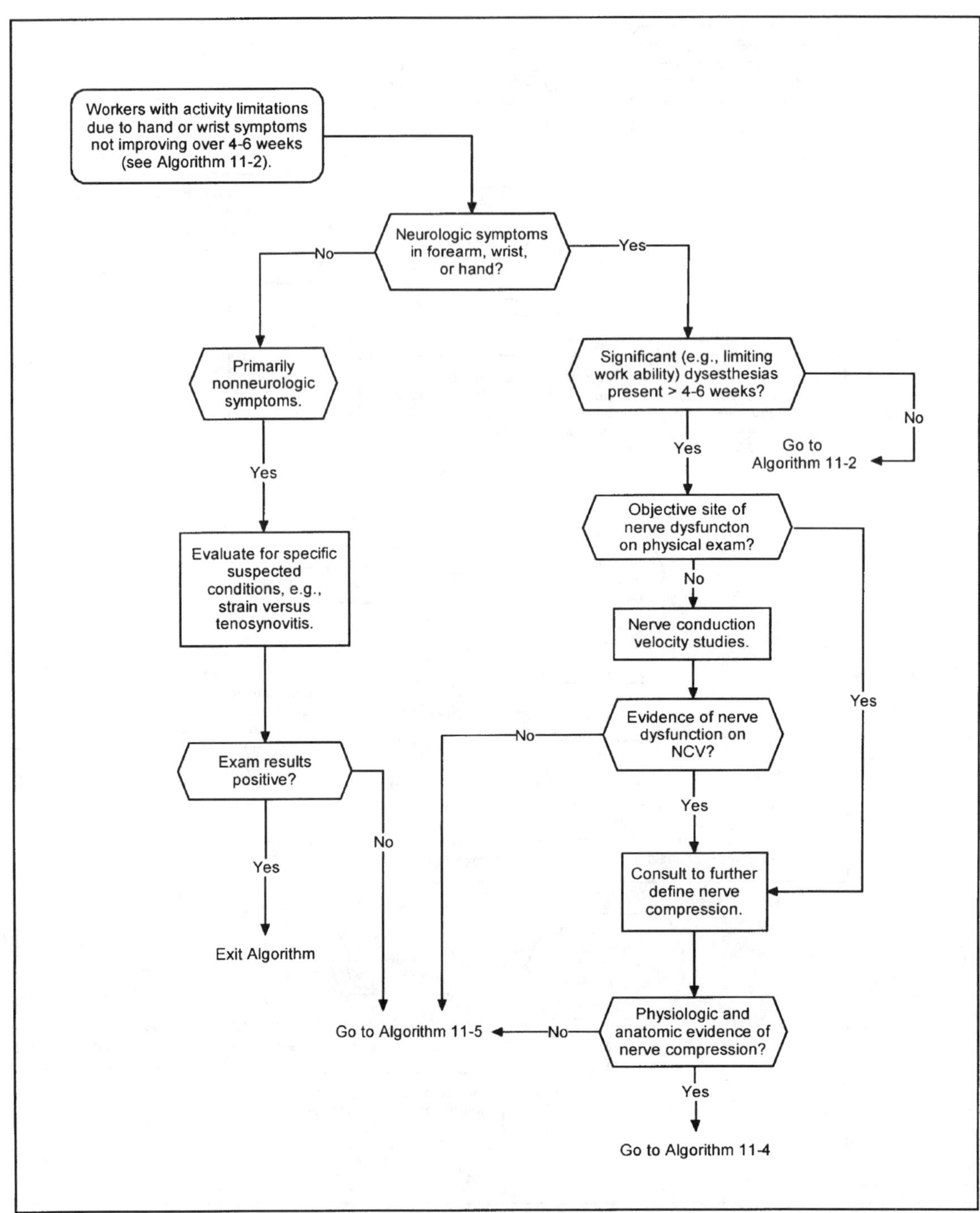

Algorithm 11-4. *Surgical Considerations for Patients with Anatomic and Physiologic Evidence of Nerve Root Compression and Persistent Forearm, Wrist, and Hand Symptoms*

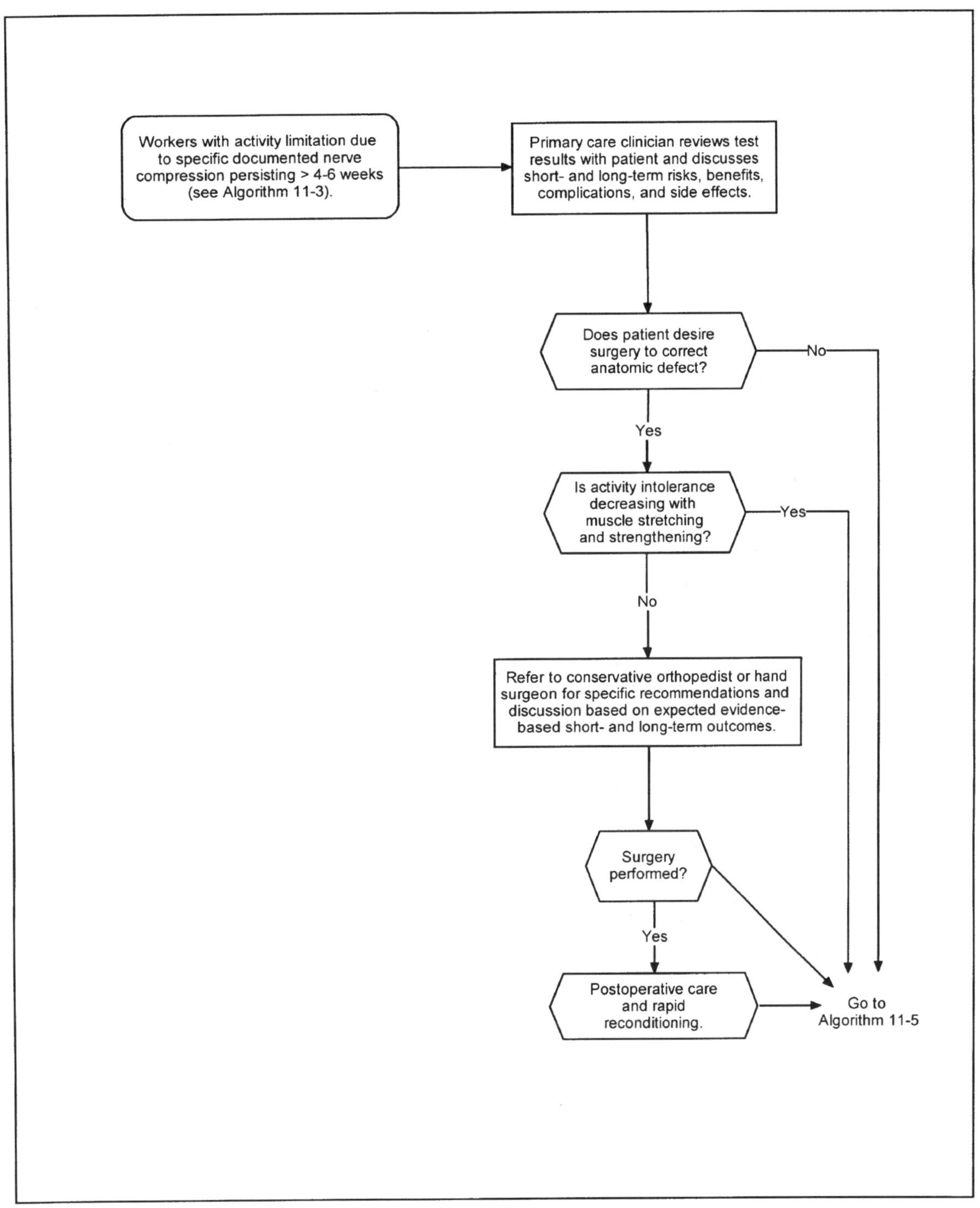

Algorithm 11-5. *Further Management of Occupational Forearm, Wrist, and Hand Complaints*

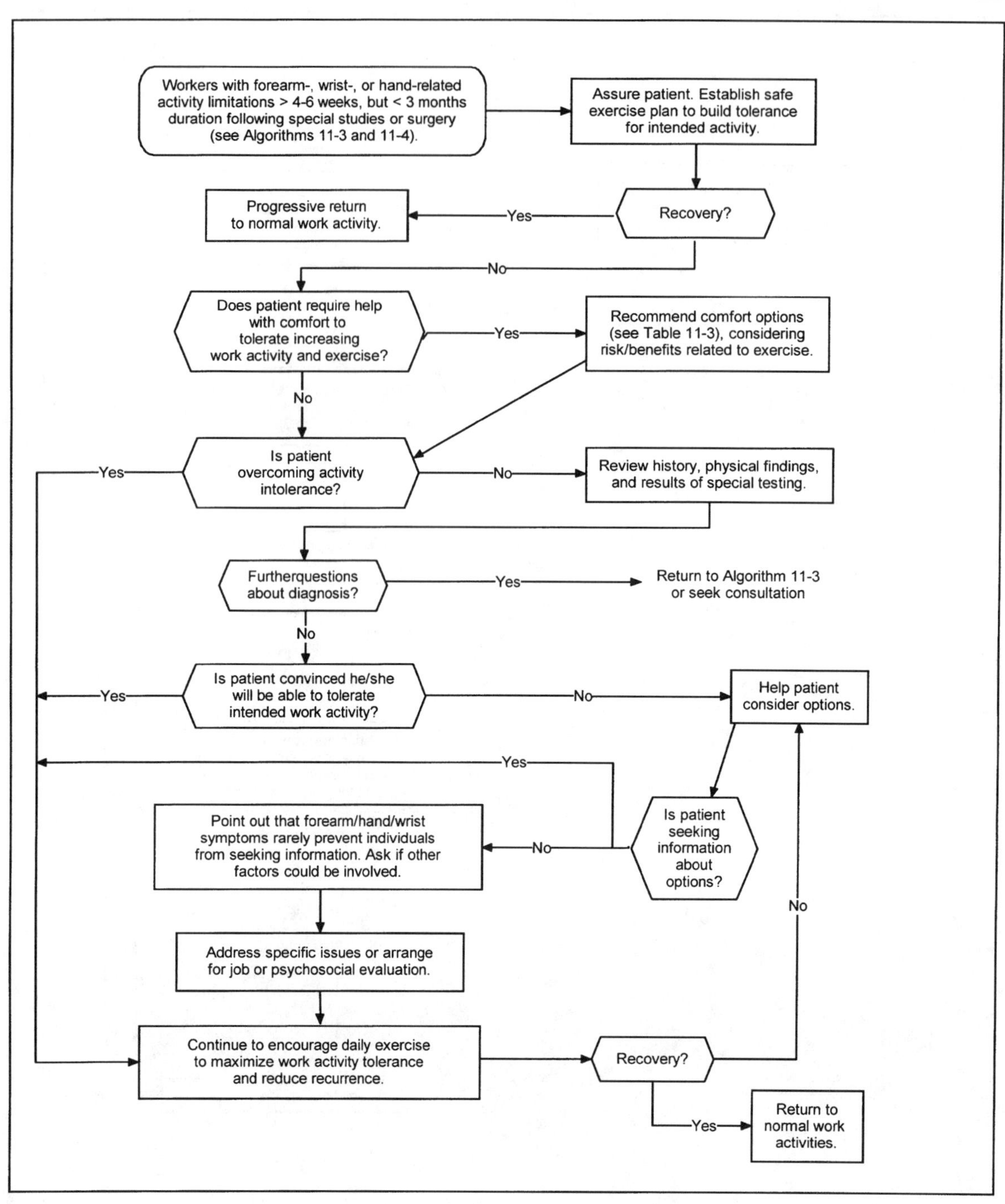

References

EPIDEMIOLOGY

Atroshi I, Gummesson C, Johnsson R, Ornstein E, Ranstam J, Rosen I. Prevalence of carpal tunnel syndrome in a general population. *JAMA.* 1999;282(2):153-8.

Denniston PL, Ranavaya MI, Kennedy CW, et al. Return-to-work best practice guidelines. In: Denniston PL, ed. *Official Disability Guidelines* 2003. 8th ed. Encinitas, Calif: Work Loss Data Institute; 2002.

Pransky G, Benjamin K, Himmelstein J, et al. Work-related upper-extremity disorders: prospective evaluation of clinical and functional outcomes. *J Occup Environ Med.* 1999;41(10):884-92.

HISTORY AND PHYSICAL EXAMINATION

Buch-Jaeger N, Foucher G. Correlation of clinical signs with nerve conduction tests in the diagnosis of carpal tunnel syndrome. *J Hand Surg [Br].* 1994;19:720-4.

D'Arcy CA, McGee S. The rational clinical examination. Does this patient have carpal tunnel syndrome? *JAMA.* 2000;283(23):3110-7.

deKrom MC, Knipschild PG, Kester AD, et al. Efficacy of provocative tests for diagnosis of carpal tunnel syndrome. *Lancet.* 1990;335:393-5.

Dunnan JB, Waylonis GW. Wrist flexion as an adjunct to the diagnosis of carpal tunnel syndrome. *Arch Phys Med Rehabil.* 1991;72:211-3.

Durkan JA. A new diagnostic test for carpal tunnel syndrome. *J Bone Joint Surg [Am].* 1991;73:535-8.

Hoppenfeld S. *Orthopaedic Neurology: A Diagnostic Guide to Neurologic Levels.* Philadelphia, Pa: Lippincott; 1977.

Katz JN, Larson MG, Fossel AH, Liang MH. Validation of a surveillance case definition of carpal tunnel syndrome. *Am J Public Health.* 1991;81(2): 189-93.

Katz JN, Larson MG, Sabra A, et al. The carpal tunnel syndrome: diagnostic utility of the history and physical examination findings. *Ann Intern Med.* 1990;112:321-7.

Katz JN, Stirrat CR. A self-administered hand diagram for the diagnosis of carpal tunnel syndrome. *J Hand Surgery [Am].* 1990;15:360-3.

Katz JN, Stirrat CR, Larson MG, Fossel AH, Eaton HM, Liang MH. A self-administered hand symptom diagram for the diagnosis and epidemiologic study of carpal tunnel syndrome. *J Rheumatol.* 1990;17(11):1495-8.

Katz JN, Simmons BP. Clinical practice. Carpal tunnel syndrome. *N Engl J Med.* 2002;346(23):1807-12.

Kuschner SH, Ebramzadeh E, Johnson D, et al. Tinel's sign and Phalen's test in carpal tunnel syndrome (review). *Orthopedics.* 1992;15:1297-302.

LaStayo PC, Wheeler DL. Reliability of passive wrist flexion and extension goniometric measurements: a multicenter study. *Phys Ther.* 1994;74:162-74; discussion 174-6.

Levine DW, Simmons BP, Koris MJ, et al. A self-administered questionnaire for the assessment of severity of symptoms and functional status in carpal tunnel syndrome. *J Bone Joint Surg [Am].* 1993;75:1585-92.

Light TR, ed. *Hand Surgery Update 2.* Rosemont, Ill: American Society for Surgery of the Hand; 1999.

Lutz RB. Acute carpal tunnel syndrome secondary to septic arthritis of the wrist. *J Am Osteopath Assoc.* 1989;89:933-4.

Novak CB, Mackinnon SE, Brownlee R, et al. Provocative sensory testing in carpal tunnel syndrome. *J Hand Surg [Br].* 1992;17:204-8.

Roquer J, Cano JF. Carpal tunnel syndrome and hyperthyroidism: a prospective study. *Acta Neurol Scand.* 1993;88:149-52.

Stevenson J, Anderson IW. Hand infections: an audit of 160 infections treated in an accident and emergency department. *J Hand Surg [Br].* 1993;18:115-8.

Szabo RM, Slater RR Jr, Farver TB, Stanton DB, Sharman WK. The value of diagnostic testing in carpal tunnel syndrome. *J Hand Surg [Am].* 1999;24(4):704-14.

Tittiranonda P, Rempel D, Armstrong T, Burastero S. Effect of four computer keyboards in computer users with upper extremity musculoskeletal disorders. *Am J Ind Med.* 1999;35(6):647-61.

Werner RA, Armstrong TJ. Reverse Phalen's maneuver as an aid in diagnosing carpal tunnel syndrome. *Arch Phys Med Rehabil.* 1994;75:783-6.

Williams TM, Mackinnon SE, Novak CB, et al. Verification of the pressure provocative test in carpal tunnel syndrome. *Ann Plast Surg.* 1992;29:8-11.

PATIENT EDUCATION

Monsivais DB, Monsivais JJ, Christensen M. Treatment for clients with cumulative trauma disorders: using an educational model to communicate choices. *AAOHN J.* 1993;41:587-91.

MEDICATION

See Chapter 3 references.

Chang MH, Chiang HT, Lee SS, Ger LP, Lo YK. Oral drug of choice in carpal tunnel syndrome. *Neurology.* 1998;51(2):390-3.

Franzblau A, Rock CL, Werner RA, Albers JW, Kelly MP, Johnston EC. The relationship of vitamin B6 status to median nerve function and carpal tunnel syndrome among active industrial workers. *J Occup Environ Med.* 1996;38(5):485-91.

Herskovitz S, Berger AR, Lipton RB. Low-dose, short-term oral prednisone in the treatment of carpal tunnel syndrome. *Neurology.* 1995;45(10):1923-5.

Keniston RC, Nathan PA, Leklem JE, Lockwood RS. Vitamin B6, vitamin C, and carpal tunnel syndrome. A cross-sectional study of 441 adults. *J Occup Environ Med.* 1997;39(10):949-59.

PHYSICAL TREATMENT METHODS

Agency for Healthcare Research and Quality (AHRQ), Evidence Report/Technology Assessment: Number 62, *Diagnosis and Treatment of Worker-Related Musculoskeletal Disorders of the Upper Extremity*, 2003.

Banta CA. A prospective, nonrandomized study of iontophoresis, wrist splinting, and anti-inflammatory medication in the treatment of early-mild carpal tunnel syndrome. *J Occup Med.* 1994;36(2):166-8.

Blankfield RP, Sulzmann C, Fradley LG, Tapolyai AA, Zyzanski SJ. Therapeutic touch in the treatment of carpal tunnel syndrome. *J Am Board Fam Pract.* 2001;14(5):335-42.

Carter R, Aspy CB, Mold J. The effectiveness of magnet therapy for treatment of wrist pain attributed to carpal tunnel syndrome. *J Fam Pract.* 2002;51(1):38-40.

Davis PT, Hulbert JR, Kassak KM, Meyer JJ. Comparative efficacy of conservative medical and chiropractic treatments for carpal tunnel syndrome: a randomized clinical trail. *J Manipulative Physiol Ther.* 1998;21(5):317-26.

Ebenbichler GR, Resch KL, Nicolakis P, et al.Ultrasound treatment for treating the carpal tunnel syndrome: randomised "sham" controlled trial. *BMJ.* 1998;316(7133):731-5.

Hochberg J. A randomized prospective study to assess the efficacy of two cold-therapy treatments following carpal tunnel release. *J Hand Ther.* 2001;14(3):208-15.

Oztas O, Turan B, Bora I, Karakaya MK. Ultrasound therapy effect in carpal tunnel syndrome. *Arch Phys Med Rehabil.* 1998;79(12):1540-4.

INJECTIONS

Dammers JW, Veering MM, Vermeulen M. Injection with methylprednisolone proximal to the carpal tunnel: randomised double blind trial. *BMJ.* 1999;319(7214):884-6.

Gelberman RH, Aronson D, Weisman M. Carpal-tunnel syndrome. *J Bone Joint Surg.* 1980;62A:1181-4.

Harter BT Jr, McKiernan JE, Kirzinger SS, et al. Carpal tunnel syndrome: surgical and nonsurgical treatment. *J Hand Surg.* 1993;18A:734-9.

Helwig AL. Treating carpal tunnel syndrome. *J Fam Pract.* 2000;49(1):79-80.

Marshall S, Tardif G, Ashworth N. Local corticosteroid injection for carpal tunnel syndrome (Cochrane Review). In: *The Cochrane Library.* Issue 1; 2002. Oxford: Update Software.

Murphy D, Failla JM, Koniuch MP. Steroid versus placebo injection for trigger finger. *J Hand Surg [Am].* 1995;20(4):628-31.

Weiss AP, Sachar K, Gendreau M. Conservative management of carpal tunnel syndrome: a reexamination of steroid injection and splinting. *J Hand Surg [Am].* 1994;19:410-5.

Wong SM, Hui AC, Tang A, et al. Local vs systemic corticosteroids in the treatment of carpal tunnel syndrome. *Neurology.* 2001;56(11):1565-7.

REST AND IMMOBILIZATION

Bury TF, Akelman E, Weiss AP. Prospective, randomized trial of splinting after carpal tunnel release. *Ann Plast Surg.* 1995;35(1):19-22.

Ekman-Ordeberg G, Salgeback S, Ordeberg G. Carpal tunnel syndrome in pregnancy: a prospective study. *Acta Obstet Gynecol Scand.* 1987;66:233-5.

Kaplan SJ, Glickel SZ, Eaton RG. Predictive factors in the non-surgical treatment of carpal tunnel syndrome. *J Hand Surg [Br].* 1990;15:106-8.

Mclean L, Tingley M, Scott RN, Rickards J. Computer terminal work and the benefit of microbreaks. *Appl Ergon.* 2001;32(3):225-37.

Richie DH Jr, Olson WR. *Orthoses for Athletic Overuse Injuries: Comparison of Two Component Materials.* Seal Beach, Calif: American Academy of Podiatric Sports Medicine, 1994.

Saitoh H. A flexible dorsal wrist splint. *J Hand Ther.* 1993;6:323-5.

Walker WC, Metzler M, Cifu DX, Swartz Z. Neutral wrist splinting in carpal tunnel syndrome: a comparison of night-only versus full-time wear instructions. *Arch Phys Med Rehabil.* 2000;81(4):424-9.

ACTIVITY AND EXERCISE

Cook AC, Szabo RM, Birkholz SW, King EF. Early mobilization following carpal tunnel release. A prospective randomized study. *J Hand Surg [Br].* 1995;20(2):228-30.

Garfinkel MS, Singhal A, Katz WA, Allan DA, Reshetar R, Schumacher HR Jr. Yoga-based intervention for carpal tunnel syndrome: a randomized trial. *JAMA.* 1998;280(18):1601-3.

DETECTION OF PHYSIOLOGIC ABNORMALITIES

Andersson GBJ, Cocchiarella L. *AMA Guides to the Evaluation of Permanent Impairment.* 5th ed. Chicago, Ill: AMA Press, 2001.

Boniface SJ, Morris I, Macleod A. How does neurophysiological assessment influence the management and outcome of patients with carpal tunnel syndrome? *Br J Rheumatol.* 1994;33:1169-70.

Braun RM, Jackson WJ. Electrical studies as a prognostic factor in the surgical treatment of carpal tunnel syndrome. *J Hand Surg [Am].* 1994;19A:893-900.

Jablecki CK, Andary MT, Floeter MK, et al. Practice parameter: electrodiagnostic studies in carpal tunnel syndrome. Report of the American Association of Electrodiagnostic Medicine, American Academy of Neurology, and the American Academy of Physical Medicine and Rehabilitation. *Neurology.* 2002;58(11):1589-92.

Kirschberg GJ, Fillingim R, Davis VP, et al. Carpal tunnel syndrome: classic clinical symptoms and electrodiagnostic studies in poultry workers with hand, wrist, and forearm pain. *South Med J.* 1994;87:328-31.

Pransky G, Long R, Hammer K, Schulz LA, Himmelstein J, Fowke J. Screening for carpal tunnel syndrome in the workplace. An analysis of portable nerve conduction devices. *J Occup Environ Med.* 1997;39(8):727-33.

Smith NJ. Nerve conduction studies for carpal tunnel syndrome: essential prelude to surgery or unnecessary luxury? *J Hand Surg [Br].* 2002;27(1): 83-5.

Werner RA, Albers JW. Relation between needle electromyography and nerve conduction studies in patients with carpal tunnel syndrome. *Arch Phys Med Rehabil.* 1995;76:246-9.

RADIOGRAPHY

Abdel-Salam A, Eyers KS, Cleary J. Detecting fractures of the scaphoid: the value of comparative x-rays of the uninjured wrist. *J Hand Surg [Br].* 1992;17:28-32.

Watson H, Ottoni L, Pitts EC, et al. Rotary subluxation of the scaphoid: a spectrum of instability. *J Hand Surg [Br].* 1993;18:62-4.

SURGICAL CONSIDERATIONS

Adams ML, Franklin GM, Barnhart S. Outcome of carpal tunnel surgery in Washington State workers' compensation. *Am J Ind Med.* 1994;25:527-36.

Agee JM, Peimer CA, Pyrek JD, et al. Endoscopic carpal tunnel release: a prospective study of complications and surgical experience. *J Hand Surg [Am].* 1995;20:165-71; discussion 172.

Agee JM, McCarroll HR Jr, Tortosa RD, et al. Endoscopic release of the carpal tunnel: a randomized prospective multicenter study. *J Hand Surg [Am].* 1992;17:987-95.

Al-Qattan MM, Bowen V, Manktelow RT. Factors associated with poor outcome following primary carpal tunnel release in non-diabetic patients. *J Hand Surg [Br].* 1994;19:622-5.

Boeckstyns ME, Sorensen AI. Does endoscopic carpal tunnel release have a higher rate of complications than open carpal tunnel release? An analysis of published series. *J Hand Surg [Br].* 1999;24(1):9-15.

Chang B, Dellon AL. Surgical management of recurrent carpal tunnel syndrome. *J Hand Surg [Br].* 1993;18:467-70.

Chow JC. The Chow technique of endoscopic release of the carpal ligament for carpal tunnel syndrome: four years of clinical results. *Arthroscopy.* 1993;9: 301-14.

Chung KC, Walters MR, Greenfield ML, Chernew ME. Endoscopic versus open carpal tunnel release: a cost-effectiveness analysis. *Plast Reconstr Surg.* 1998;102(4):1089-99.

Feuerstein M, Burrell LM, Miller VI, Lincoln A, Huang GD, Berger R. Clinical management of carpal tunnel syndrome: a 12-year review of outcomes. *Am J Ind Med.* 1999;35(3):232-45.

Gerritsen AA, de Vet HC, Scholten RJ, Bertelsmann FW, de Krom MC, Bouter

LM. Splinting vs. surgery in the treatment of carpal tunnel syndrome: a randomized controlled trial. *JAMA*. 2002;288:1245-51.

Gerritsen AA, Uitdehaag BM, van Geldere D, Scholten RJ, de Vet HC, Bouter LM. Systematic review of randomized clinical trials of surgical treatment for carpal tunnel syndrome. *JAMA*. 2002;288:1245-51.

Goodman RC. An aggressive return-to-work program in surgical treatment of carpal tunnel syndrome: a comparison of costs. *Plast Reconstr Surg*. 1992;89:715-7.

Jimenez DF, Gibbs SR, Clapper AT. Endoscopic treatment of carpal tunnel syndrome: a critical review. *J Neurosurg*. 1998;88(5):817-26.

Katz JN, Keller RB, Simmons BP, et al. Maine Carpal Tunnel Study: outcomes of operative and nonoperative therapy for carpal tunnel syndrome in a community-based cohort. *J Hand Surg [Am]*. 1998;23(4):697-710.

Leach WK, Esler C, Scott TD. Grip strength following carpal tunnel decompression. *J Hand Surg [Br]*. 1993;18:750-2.

Lottgen J, Pawlik G. Long-term results of carpal tunnel decompression: assessment of 60 cases. *J Hand Surg [Br]*. 1993;18:471-4.

Mackenzie DJ, Hainer R, Wheatley MJ. Early recovery after endoscopic vs. short-incision open carpal tunnel release. *Ann Plast Surg*. 2000;44(6):601-4.

Melhorn, JM. Upper extremity restrictions and guides: why early return to work. In: *Twenty-second Annual National Workers' Compensation and Occupational Medicine Seminar*. Falmouth, Mass: SEAK, Inc.; 2002: 335-68.

Padua L, Padua R, Aprile I, Pasqualetti P, Tonali P. The Italian CTS Study Group. Carpal tunnel syndrome, multiperspective follow-up of untreated carpal tunnel syndrome: a multicenter study. *Neurology*. 2001;56(11): 1459-66.

Shin AY, Perlman M, Shin PA, Garay AA. Disability outcomes in a worker's compensation population: surgical versus nonsurgical treatment of carpal tunnel syndrome. *Am J Orthop*. 2000;29(3):179-84.

Singh I, Khoo KM, Krishnamoorthy S. The carpal tunnel syndrome: clinical evaluation and results of surgical decompression. *Ann Acad Med Singapore*. 1994;23:94-7.

Stephen AB, Lyons AR, Davis TR. A prospective study of two conservative treatments for ganglia of the wrist. *J Hand Surg [Br]*. 1999;24(1):104-5.

Topper SM, Jones DE, Klajnbart JO, Friedel SP. Trigger finger: the effect of partial release of the first annular pulley on triggering. *Am J Orthop*. 1997; 26(10):675-7.

Uchiyama S, Toriumi H, Nakagawa H, Kamimura M, Ishigaki N, Miyasaka T. Postoperative nerve conduction changes after open and endoscopic carpal tunnel release. *Clin Neurophysiol*. Jan, 2002;113(1):64-70.

Verdugo RJ, Salinas RS, Castillo J, Cea JG. Surgical versus non-surgical treatment for carpal tunnel syndrome (Cochrane Review). In: *The Cochrane Library*. Issue 2; 2002. Oxford: Update Software.

Young VL, Logan SE, Fernando B, et al. Grip strength before and after carpal tunnel decompression. *South Med J.* 1992;85:897-900.

Yu GZ, Firrell JC, Tsai TM. Pre-operative factors and treatment outcome following carpal tunnel release. *J Hand Surg [Br].* 1992;17:646-50.

PSYCHOSOCIAL FACTORS

Crossman MW, Gilbert CA, Travlos A, Craig KD, Eisen A. Nonneurologic hand pain versus carpal tunnel syndrome: do psychological measures differentiate? *Am J Phys Med Rehabil.* 2001;80(2):100-7.

Grunert BK, Devine CA, Matloub HS, et al. Psychological adjustment following work-related hand injury: 18-month follow-up. *Ann Plast Surg.* 1992;29:537-42.

Grunert BK, Devine CA, Smith CJ, et al. Graded work exposure to promote work return after severe hand trauma: a replicated study. *Ann Plast Surg.* 1992;29:532-6.

Helliwell PS, Mumford DB, Smeathers JE. Work-related upper limb disorder: the relationship between pain, cumulative load, disability, and psychological factors. *Ann Rheum Dis.* 1992;51:1325-9.

Higgs PE, Edwards D, Martin DS, Weeks PM. Carpal tunnel surgery outcomes in workers: effects of workers' compensation status. *J Hand Surg.* 1995;20A:354-60.

Karjalainen K, Malmivaara A, van Tulder M, et al. Biopsychosocial rehabilitation for upper limb repetitive strain injuries in working age adults (Cochrane Review). In: *The Cochrane Library.* Issue 2; 2002. Oxford: Update Software.

Katz JN, Keller RB, Fossel AH, Punnett L, Bessette L, Simmons BP, Mooney N. Predictors of return to work following carpal tunnel release. *Am J Ind Med.* 1997;31(1):85-91.

Pransky G, Benjamin K, Himmelstein J, et al. Work-related upper-extremity disorders: prospective evaluation of clinical and functional outcomes. *J Occup Environ Med.* 1999;41(10):884-92.

Master Algorithm. *ACOEM Guidelines for Care of Acute and Subacute Occupational Low Back Complaints*

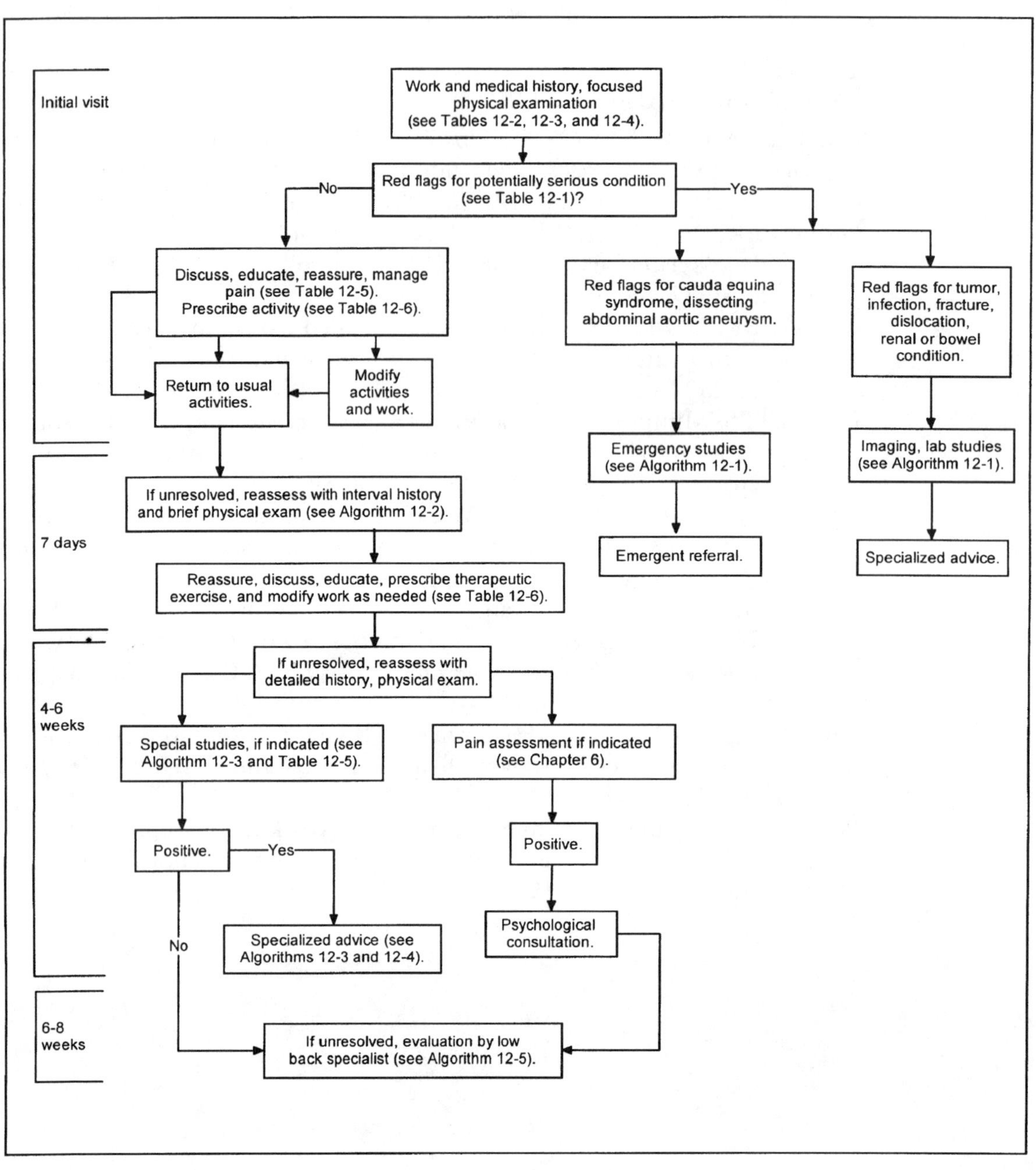

12 Low Back Complaints

General Approach and Basic Principles

Low back complaints that may be work related are the most common problems presented to occupational health and primary care providers. They are the most common cause of reported occupational complaints and workers' compensation claims. These complaints account for about 30% of both cases reported to the Bureau of Labor Statistics and workers' compensation claims. They are disproportionately expensive, accounting for 30-40% of costs as well.

Recommendations on assessing and treating adults with potentially work-related low back problems (i.e., activity limitations due to symptoms in the low back of less than three months duration) are presented in this clinical practice guideline. Topics include the initial assessment and diagnosis of patients with acute and subacute low back complaints that are potentially work related, identification of red flags that may indicate the presence of a serious underlying medical condition, initial management, diagnostic considerations and special studies to identify clinical pathology, work-relatedness, modified duty and activity, and return to work as well as further management considerations, including the management of delayed recovery.

Algorithms for patient management are included. This chapter's master algorithm schematizes how primary care and occupational medicine practitioners generally can manage acute or subacute low back complaints. The following text, tables, and numbered algorithms expand upon the master algorithm.

The principal recommendations for assessing and treating patients with low back complaints are as follows:

- The initial assessment of patients with low back problems focuses on detecting indications of potentially serious disease, termed red flags.
- In the absence of red flags, imaging and other tests are not usually helpful during the first four to six weeks of low back symptoms.
- Relieving discomfort can be accomplished most safely by nonprescription medication or an appropriately selected nonsteroidal anti-

inflammatory drug (NSAID), appropriate adjustment of activity, and use of thermal modalities such as ice and/or heat.

- Primary care or occupational physicians can effectively manage acute and subacute low back problems conservatively in the absence of red flags.
- To avoid undue back irritation and debilitation from inactivity, some activity or job modification may be helpful in the acute period. Most patients will not require bed rest. Bed rest may lead to a slower recovery and result in longer periods of sick leave. Bed rest has potential debilitating effects, and its efficacy in treating acute low back pain is unproven. Maintaining ordinary activity, as tolerated, leads to the most rapid recovery.
- Low-stress aerobic activities can be safely started after the first two weeks of symptoms to help avoid debilitation. Careful stretching exercises within the normal range of motion may be helpful to avoid further restriction of motion. Exercises to strengthen low back and abdominal muscles are commonly delayed for several weeks, but early stage lumbar stabilization exercises can be used without aggravation of symptoms.
- Encourage patients recovering from acute and subacute low back problems to return to modified- or full-duty work as soon as possible. Having patients continue their normal activities, within limits permitted by pain, leads to more rapid recovery than either bed rest or back-mobilizing exercises.
- The strongest medical evidence regarding potential therapies for low back pain indicates that having the patient return to normal activities has the best long-term outcome. Many invasive and noninvasive therapies are intended to cure the pain, but no strong evidence exists that they accomplish this as successfully as therapies that focus on restoring functional ability without focusing on the pain. In these cases, the traditional medical model of "curing" the patient does not work well. Furthermore, the patient should be aware that returning to normal activities most often aids recovery. Patients should be encouraged to accept responsibility for their recovery rather than expecting the provider to provide an easy "cure." This process will promote using activity rather than pain as a guide, and it will make the treatment goal of return to work more obvious in the occupational setting.
- If symptoms persist, further evaluation may be indicated.
- Within the first three months of low back symptoms, only patients with evidence of severe spinal disease or severe, debilitating symptoms, and physiologic evidence of specific nerve root compromise, confirmed by appropriate imaging studies, can be expected to benefit from surgery.
- More than 80% of patients with symptoms of lumbosacral nerve root irritation due to herniated disks (nucleus pulposus) eventually recover with or without surgery.
- Nonphysical factors (such as psychosocial, workplace, or socioeconomic problems) can be investigated and addressed in cases of delayed recovery or return to work.

- Clinicians can greatly improve the patient's response to back symptoms by providing assurance, encouraging activity, and emphasizing that more than 90% of low back pain complaints resolve without any specific therapies. While patients may be looking for a clear-cut diagnosis for their low back pain, the risk to them of a suggested "cure" for this assumed diagnosis may be worse than their symptoms.

Initial Assessment

Thorough medical and work histories and a focused physical examination (see Chapter 2) are sufficient for the initial assessment of a patient complaining of potentially work-related low back symptoms. In this assessment, certain findings, referred to as red flags, raise suspicion of serious underlying medical conditions (Table 12-1). Their absence rules out the need for special studies, referral, or inpatient care during the first four weeks, during which time spontaneous recovery is expected (provided any associated workplace factors are mitigated). Findings of the medical history and physical examination may also alert the clinician to other pathology (not of low back origin) that can present as low back complaints. Low back complaints can then be classified into one of three working categories, although common factors may be operative in all three and, thus, confound this classification:

- Potentially serious low back disorders, including acute fractures, acute dislocations, infection, tumor, progressive neurologic deficit, or cauda equina syndrome

Table 12-1. Red Flags for Potentially Serious Low Back Conditions

Disorder	Medical History	Physical Examination
	SPINAL DISORDERS	
Fracture	Major trauma, such as vehicular accident or fall from height Minor trauma or strenuous lifting, in older or potentially osteoporotic patients Percussion tenderness over specific spinous processes	
Tumor	Severe localized pain over specific spinal processes History of cancer Age > 50 years Constitutional symptoms, such as recent unexplained weight loss Pain that worsens when patient is supine Pain at night or at rest	Tenderness over spinous process and percussion tenderness Decreased range of motion due to protective muscle spasm

Table 12-1. (continued)

Disorder	Medical History	Physical Examination
Infection	Risk factors for spinal infection: recent bacterial infection (e.g., urinary tract infection); IV drug abuse; diabetes; or immune suppression (due to corticosteroids, transplant, or HIV) Constitutional symptoms, such as recent fever, chills, or unexplained weight loss	Tenderness over spinous processes Decreased range of motion Vital signs consistent with systemic infection (late): • Tachycardia • Tachypnea • Hypotension • Elevated temperature • Pelvic or abdominal mass or tenderness
Cauda equina syndrome Saddle anesthesia	Direct blow or fall, with axial loading Perianal/perineal sensory loss Recent onset of bladder dysfunction, such as urinary retention, increased frequency, or overflow incontinence Severe or progressive neurologic deficit in lower extremities	Unexpected laxity of the bladder* or anal sphincter Major motor weakness: quadriceps (knee extension weakness); ankle plantar flexors, evertors, and dorsiflexors (foot drop) Spastic (thoracic) or flaccid (lumbar) paraparesis Increased (thoracic) or decreased (lumbar) reflexes
Progressive neurologic deficit	Severe low back pain Progressive numbness or weakness	Significant progression of weakness Significant increased sensory loss New motor weakness Radicular signs
	EXTRASPINAL DISORDERS	
Dissecting abdominal aortic aneurysm	Excruciating low back pain History of atherosclerotic disease History of hypertension	Pulsatile midline abdominal mass
Renal colic	Excruciating pain from costovertebral angle to testis or labia History of urolithiasis	Possible tenderness at costovertebral angle
Retrocecal appendix	Constipation Subacute onset without inciting event	Low grade fever
Pelvic inflammatory disease	Vaginal discharge Pelvic pain Prior episode	Uterine tenderness Pelvic mass Cervical discharge
Urinary tract infection	Dysuria History of UTIs	Suprapubic tenderness

* Adapted from Bigos: by history.

- Degenerative disorders, including consequences of aging or repetitive use, or a combination thereof, such as degenerative disk disease and osteoarthritis
- Nonspecific disorders, including benign, self-limited disorders with unclear etiology, such as regional low back pain

Medical History

Asking the patient open-ended questions, such as those listed below, allows the clinician to gauge the need for further discussion or specific inquiries to obtain more detailed information (see also Chapter 2).

WHAT EXACTLY WERE YOU DOING WHEN SYMPTOMS BEGAN?

(It is important to obtain all information necessary to document the biomechanical forces of injury.)

- Did symptoms develop immediately, gradually, or after a period of delay?

WHAT ARE YOUR SYMPTOMS?

- Do you have pain, numbness, weakness, stiffness?
- For traumatic injuries: Was the area deformed? Did you lose any blood or have an open wound?
- Is the discomfort located primarily in your low back? Do you have pain or other symptoms elsewhere?
- Have you lost control of your bowel or bladder? Are you soiling your undergarments?
- Do you have fever, night sweats, or weight loss?
- When did your symptoms begin? Have you ever had symptoms like this before? Are your symptoms constant or intermittent? What makes the problem worse or better?
- What is the day pattern to your pain? Better in the morning or evening? Worse as the day progresses? Do you have a problem sleeping? What position is most comfortable? Is there any pain with cough, sneezing, deep breathing, or laughing?
- How do these symptoms limit you?
- How long can you sit, stand, walk, bend?
- Can you lift? How much weight (use items such as gallons of milk, groceries, etc. as examples)?
- Does your pain prevent you from sleeping?

Table 12-2. Symptoms of Lumbar Nerve Root Compromise

Root Level	Pain or Paresthesia	Motor Weakness
L1	Back, radiating to upper anterior thigh and groin	Hip flexion
L2	Back, radiating to anterior mid-thigh	Hip flexion and adduction, knee extension
L3	Back, radiating to anterior thigh and inner knee	Hip flexion and adduction, knee extension
L4	Back, radiating to lateral thigh, front and medial leg, and medial foot	Hip adduction, knee extension, foot inversion
L5	Back, radiating to lateral leg and dorsal foot (especially first web space)	Hip abduction, foot and great toe extension
S1	Back, radiating to back of thigh and lateral leg and foot	Knee flexion, plantar flexion

WHEN DID YOUR CURRENT LIMITATIONS BEGIN? WAS THERE A SPECIFIC INCITING EVENT? HOW DID THE LIMITATIONS DEVELOP?

- How long have your activities been limited? More than four weeks?
- Have your symptoms changed? How?
- Have you had similar episodes previously?
- Have you had previous testing or treatment? With whom?
- What do you think caused the problem? How do you think it is related to work?
- What are your specific job duties? How long do you spend performing each duty on a daily basis?
- What other activities (hobbies, workouts, sports) do you engage in? At home or elsewhere? Do you use your back to perform them? Any heavy lifting? How? How often?
- Do you have other medical problems?
- What do you hope we can accomplish during this visit?

Determining whether or not there is lumbosacral nerve root compromise (and if so, the level of compromise) is critical. Symptoms correlating with specific dermatomal levels of compression and possible motor weakness are shown in Table 12-2.

Physical Examination

Guided by the medical history, the physical examination includes:

- General observation of the patient, including stance and gait
- Regional examination of the low back

- Examination of organ systems related to appropriate differential diagnosis
- Neurologic screening
- Testing for lumbosacral nerve root tension
- Monitoring pain behavior during range-of-motion and while seated as a clue to origin of the problem

The objective parts of the low back examination are testing reflexes and circumferential measurements for atrophy. All other findings require the patient's cooperation. Patients who present with a complaint of leg pain may, in fact, have a disorder of the low back.

A. Observation and Regional Back Examination

Observing the patient's stance and gait is useful to guide the regional low back examination. Incoordination or abnormal use of the extremities may indicate the need for specific neurologic testing. Severe guarding of low-back motion in all planes may add credence to a suspected diagnosis of spinal or intrathecal infection, tumor, or fracture. However, because of the marked variation among persons with symptoms and those without, range-of-motion measurements of the low back are of limited value.

Vertebral point tenderness to palpation, when associated with other signs or symptoms, is suggestive but not specific for spinal fracture or infection. Palpable soft-tissue tenderness, by itself, is an even less specific, less reliable finding.

B. Neurologic Screening

The neurologic examination focuses on a few tests that reveal evidence of nerve root impairment, peripheral neuropathy, or spinal cord dysfunction. Most herniated disks in the lumbar spine involve the L5 nerve root (L4-5 disk) and the S1 nerve root (L5-S1 disk). The clinical features of lumbosacral nerve root compression are summarized in Table 12-3.

1. TESTING FOR MUSCLE STRENGTH

There are no specific muscle tests for the L1 to L3 nerve roots. The iliopsoas, the main flexor of the hip, is innervated by L1, L2, and L3 and is tested by asking the patient to flex the hip against resistance. The L4 nerve root can best be tested by evaluating the strength of ankle inversion and the strength of the quadriceps, which also is innervated by L2 and L3. The L5 nerve root, when compromised, may cause weakness of the great toe extensor on the affected side. In severe cases, the ankle dorsiflexors also may be weak and, if so, the patient will have foot drop during gait. The S1 root generally supplies the plantar flexors of the foot and ankle, but motor weakness is harder to detect due to the bulk and normal strength of these muscles (gastrocnemius,

Table 12-3. Physical Examination Correlates of Lumbosacral Nerve Root Dysfunction

Root Level	Sensory Deficit	Motor Weakness	Reflex Loss
L1	Upper anterior thigh below inguinal ligament to groin	Hip flexion	
L2	Anterior mid-thigh	Hip flexion and adduction; knee extension	
L3	Anterior lower thigh and inner knee	Hip flexion and adduction; knee extension	
L4	Back, radiating to lateral thigh and front and medial leg	Hip adduction; knee extension	Knee jerk
L5	Back, radiating to lateral leg and dorsal and lateral foot	Foot and great toe extension; hip abduction	
S1	Back, radiating to back of thigh and lateral leg and foot	Knee flexion; plantar flexion	Ankle jerk

soleus). The recommended test to detect S1 root compromise is repeated toe raises. Hamstring weakness may also be detected by this test.

2. CIRCUMFERENTIAL MEASUREMENTS

Muscle atrophy can be detected by bilateral circumferential measurements of the calf and thigh. Differences of less than 2 centimeters in measurement of the two limbs at the same level can be a normal variation. Symmetric muscle bulk and strength are expected unless the patient has a relatively long-standing neurologic impairment or disorder of the lower extremity muscle or joint.

3. REFLEXES

Loss of, or decrease in, the ankle jerk reflex indicates interruption of the reflex arc, as may be found in S1 nerve root compromise, such as L5-S1 disk herniation. For the other nerve root level commonly involved, L5 (the L4-L5 disk), there is no reflex change except for the posterior tibial tendon reflex, which is difficult to elicit. When abnormal, the knee jerk reflex indicates an L4 root problem (L3-L4 disk). This level of involvement is much less common.

4. SENSORY EXAMINATION

Sensory examination for nerve root compromise in the low back includes pinprick and light-touch testing. In general, the dorsal foot (especially the first web space), ankle, and calf areas are correlated with the L5 root, and the lateral foot is correlated with the S1 root. It is important to keep in mind the subjective nature of sensory testing and the influence that past exams may have on a patient with a history of back problems. Light pinprick should not elicit a painful response. If it does, ask patients if this replicates their typical low back pain and ask if the pain is superficial or deep. If the pain *is* typical of their low back pain or if it is described as deep, this suggests a non-organic basis for the pain.

5. PHYSICAL EXAMINATION TESTS

To be successful, the treatment of low back pain generally must be based upon a correct diagnosis. For a variety of reasons, a patient's response on any single test may not be reflective of the presence of identifiable, underlying pathology. When ambiguity or inconsistency in test results prompts a concern regarding the correct diagnosis or the appropriate treatment approach, corroborative testing may be indicated.

A number of tests are commonly employed to distinguish between physiologic and nonphysiologic responses:

- Most common among these are axial loading simulation, fixed pelvic rotation, exaggerated pain response, distraction simulation testing, and evaluation for nondermatomal and myotomal symptoms, referred to collectively as "Waddell's signs."
- The straight-leg-raising test is meant to detect irritation of the lumbar nerve roots by mechanically pulling on the sciatic nerve, and thus the root, as it goes around the posterior hip. Straight-leg raising should be tested in both sitting and lying positions. When sitting, extend and flex the knee while asking if there is any knee pain. The knee should then be left fully extended and the patient asked if there is ankle pain with plantar and dorsiflexion. If a true radicular component is present the patient should not easily tolerate full extension of the knee with dorsiflexion of the ankle in the sitting position—the typical response would be instead for the patient to lean back and complain of radiating pain. If there is no such response in the sitting position but there is a positive-lying straight-leg raise, a non-organic basis for the pain is suggested.
- Other tests, such as popliteal (posterior knee) compression, are designed for the same purpose.

These tests are subjective and can be confusing if the patient is simply having generalized pain that is increased by raising the leg. Results of the test are also influenced by repeated examinations in patients with a recurrent history of back problems. A negative test is generally a good prognostic sign. A positive test for lumbar nerve root irritation generally produces pain that radiates below the knee, and that follows a precise radicular distribution consistent with the nerve root involved. Crossed-straight-leg raises are the most highly specific test of sciatic nerve tension.

C. Assessing Red Flags and Indications for Immediate Referral

Physical-examination evidence of severe neurologic compromise that correlates with the medical history and test results may indicate a need for immediate consultation. The examination may further reinforce or reduce suspicions of tumor, infection, fracture, or dislocation. A history of tumor, infection, abdominal aneurysm, or other related serious conditions, together with positive findings on examination, warrants further investigation or referral. A medical history that suggests pathology originating somewhere other than in the lumbosacral area may warrant examination of the knee, hip, abdomen, pelvis or other areas.

Diagnostic Criteria

If the patient does not have red flags for serious conditions, the clinician can then determine which common musculoskeletal disorder is present. The criteria presented in Table 12-4 follow the clinical thought process, from the mechanism of illness or injury to unique symptoms and signs of a particular disorder and, finally, to test results, if any tests are needed to guide treatment at this stage. The ICD-9 coding system assigns codes based upon pathophysiologic mechanisms. Specific ICD-9 codes are frequently required for reimbursement for medical services. However, for at least 90% of low back pain cases,

Table 12-4. Diagnostic Criteria for Non-red-flag Conditions that Can Be Managed by Primary Care Physicians

Probable Diagnosis or Injury	Mechanism	Unique Symptoms	Unique Signs	Tests and Results
Acute lumbar strain (ICD-9 846.0, 846.1, 846.2, 846.3, 846.8, 846.9, 847.1, 847.2, 847.4, 847.9)	Lifting under load/ significant force Twisting, turning Bending Fall Direct blow	Low back pain that does not radiate below the knee Loss of range of motion	Paraspinous muscle spasm Nonrotational scoliosis of lumbar spine	None indicated for 4-6 weeks
Lumbosacral nerve root compression, with radiculopathy (ICD-9 722.1, 722.2, 722.5, 722.6, 722.7, 722.9)	Degenerative changes Possible aggravating factors	Leg pain Numbness Weakness, all in specific distribution Abnormal gait	Reflex changes Motor weakness in specific distribution Sensory changes in specific distribution Positive straight-leg raising Positive crossed straight-leg raising	None indicated for 4-6 weeks unless compression is severe or progressive

Table 12-4. (continued)

Probable Diagnosis or Injury	Mechanism	Unique Symptoms	Unique Signs	Tests and Results
Sciatica (ICD-9 724.3)	Possibility of traumatic or idiopathic origin	Pain and dysesthesias in the distribution of the sciatic nerve	None	None
Spinal stenosis (ICD-9 724.0, 724.01, 724.02) (aggravation)	Degenerative changes Congenital disorder	Nonspecific low back and leg pain Leg pain worse with activity (pseudo-claudication)	Straight-leg-raising test negative Symptoms reproduced by patient's sustained hyper-extension of spine while standing Straight-leg-raising test may be positive if performed immediately after patient has exercised	CT or MRIpositive for stenosis
Postlaminectomy syndrome (ICD-9 722.81, 722.83)	Scarring after surgery or other invasive procedures	Pain and dysesthesias at level of nerve root operated on (see Table 12-2)	Specific neurologic findings at level of nerve root operated on (see Table 12-2)	MRI with gactolinium positive for scarring
Regional low back pain (ICD-9 721.2, 721.3, 721.57, 724.1, 724.2, 724.5, 724.6, 724.7, 724.8, 756.1, 756.11, 756.12, 756.17, 307.89)	Unknown (idiopathic)	Nonspecific low back pain	None	None

ICD9 = *International Classification of Diseases*, 9th Edition.

the ICD-9 codes utilized are overly specific. The pathophysiologic correlates for lumbar sprain and strain, for example, have not been determined.

Work-Relatedness

Low back complaints, most of which are multifactorial in origin, can be related to work in a variety of ways (see Chapter 1). Physical factors that can contribute to regional low back pain include heavy physical work (especially with rapid lifting), bending, stretching and reaching, pushing or pulling, and prolonged sitting or standing. Employment-related factors such as task enjoyment, monotony, job satisfaction, and emotional distress also have been shown to correlate with the incidence of low back pain. There are no known factors that correlate with radiculopathy. Heavy lifting in bent or twisted postures, exposure to vibration, and driving for extended periods have been correlated with herniated disks, as has smoking. Sciatica has been associated with cumulative work stress. Age, cardiovascular fitness, obesity, and non-work stress are other factors that have been correlated with low back pain. Many cases are idiopathic, as the mechanism of regional back pain has not yet been elucidated. It also should be noted that the existence of a correlation between various factors and low back pain does NOT indicate that a causal relationship has actually been demonstrated, as association is not equivalent to causation. Very specific description of work-duty repetitions, and the length of time they take to perform would be needed to ascertain the probable relationship between work and these conditions.

There is no evidence for the effectiveness of lumbar supports in preventing back pain in industry. Proper lifting techniques and discussion of general conditioning should be emphasized, although teaching proper lifting mechanics and even eliminating strenuous lifting fails to prevent back injury claims and back discomfort, according to some high-quality studies.

Recurrence of regional low back pain is not uncommon, regardless of whether or not the pain is work related. In fact, a prior history of low back pain or sciatica is a powerful predictor of a future episode. It is not clear, however, whether a recurrence of the complaint represents a recurrence of a quantifiable physical injury, because pain is a subjective experience, and the anatomic pathology of regional low back pain has not been well documented. If an underlying condition is aggravated at work, it is important to document the course of pain and activity limitation due to the aggravating factors. Restoration to the prior activity level is the goal. When that level has been reached, the effects of the aggravation can be said to have ceased. At that point, cure and relief have been accomplished.

Initial Care

Comfort is often a patient's first concern. Nonprescription analgesics will provide sufficient pain relief for most patients with acute and subacute symptoms. If treatment response is inadequate (i.e., if symptoms and activity limitations continue), prescribed pharmaceuticals or physical methods can be added. Comorbid conditions, side effects, cost, and provider and patient preferences guide the clinician's choice of recommendations. Table 12-5 summarizes comfort options.

Physical Methods

- Manipulation appears safe and effective in the first few weeks of back pain without radiculopathy. Of note is that most studies of manipulation have compared it with interventions other than therapeutic exer-

Table 12-5. Methods of Symptom Control for Low Back Complaints

RECOMMENDED
Nonprescription Medications
Acetaminophen (safest) NSAIDs (aspirin, ibuprofen)
Physical Therapeutic Interventions
Adjustment or modification of workstation, job tasks, or work hours and methods Stretching Specific low back exercises for range of motion and strengthening At-home local applications of cold in first few days of acute complaint; thereafter, applications of heat or cold Relaxation techniques Aerobic exercise 1-2 visits for education, counseling, and evaluation of home exercise for range of motion and strengthening
Prescribed Pharmaceutical Methods
Other nonsteroidal anti-inflammatory drugs (NSAIDs) Short-term muscle relaxants for acute spasms Short-term opiates are rarely recommended, but may be used if symptoms are severe and accompanied by objective findings, for no more than two weeks

OPTIONS

Lumbar Disk Protrusion with Radiculopathy	Lumbar Strain	Sciatica
2 days bed rest if symptoms are severe	1-2 days rest if symptoms are severe	1-2 days rest if symptoms are severe
Spinal Stenosis	**Postlaminectomy Syndrome**	**Regional Low Back Symptoms**
Instruction in body mechanics	2 days bed rest if symptoms are severe	1-2 days rest if symptoms are severe

cise, hence its value as compared with active, rather than passive, therapeutic options is unclear. Nonetheless, in the acute phases of injury manipulation may enhance patient mobilization. If manipulation does not bring improvement in three to four weeks, it should be stopped and the patient reevaluated. For patients with symptoms lasting longer than one month, manipulation is probably safe but efficacy has not been proved.

- A trial of manipulation for patients with radiculopathy may also be an option. There is consensus on its utility among practitioners who perform it, when radiculopathy is not progressive, and large series and cohort studies suggest value for some forms of manipulation.

Randomized trials are under way. As with any promising intervention in the absence of definitive high-quality evidence, careful attention to patient response to treatment is critical. Many passive and palliative interventions can provide relief in the short term but may risk treatment dependence without meaningful long-term benefit. Such interventions may be used to the extent they are aimed at facilitating return to normal functional activities, particularly work.

- Manipulation under anesthesia (MUA) cannot be recommended at the present time because high quality studies do not exist and the procedure has significant associated risks.
- Traction has not been proved effective for lasting relief in treating low back pain. Because evidence is insufficient to support using vertebral axial decompression for treating low back injuries, it is not recommended.
- Physical modalities such as massage, diathermy, cutaneous laser treatment, ultrasound, transcutaneous electrical neurostimulation (TENS) units, percutaneous electrical nerve stimulation (PENS) units, and biofeedback have no proven efficacy in treating acute low back symptoms. Insufficient scientific testing exists to determine the effectiveness of these therapies, but they may have some value in the short term if used in conjunction with a program of functional restoration. Insufficient evidence exists to determine the effectiveness of sympathetic therapy, a noninvasive treatment involving electrical stimulation, also known as interferential therapy. At-home local applications of heat or cold are as effective as those performed by therapists.
- Acupuncture has not been found effective in the management of back pain, based on several high-quality studies, but there is anecdotal evidence of its success.
- Invasive techniques (e.g., local injections and facet-joint injections of cortisone and lidocaine) are of questionable merit. Although epidural steroid injections may afford short-term improvement in leg pain and sensory deficits in patients with nerve root compression due to a herniated nucleus pulposus, this treatment offers no significant long-term functional benefit, nor does it reduce the need for surgery. Despite the fact that proof is still lacking, many pain physicians believe that diagnostic and/or therapeutic injections may have benefit in patients presenting in the transitional phase between acute and chronic pain.
- There are conflicting studies concerning the effectiveness of prolotherapy, also known as sclerotherapy, in the low back. Lasting functional improvement has not been shown. The injections are invasive, may be painful to the patient, and are not generally accepted or widely used. Therefore, using prolotherapy for low back pain is not recommended.
- There is good quality medical literature demonstrating that radiofrequency neurotomy of facet joint nerves in the cervical spine provides good temporary relief of pain. Similar quality literature does not exist regarding the same procedure in the lumbar region. Lumbar facet

neurotomies reportedly produce mixed results. Facet neurotomies should be performed only after appropriate investigation involving controlled differential dorsal ramus medial branch diagnostic blocks.

- Other miscellaneous therapies, such as magnet therapy, have been evaluated and found to be ineffective or minimally effective.
- Some studies support neuroreflexotherapy (the temporary implantation of epidermal devices in trigger points in the back and referred tender points in the ear), but the procedure is invasive, and some questions exist regarding its potential benefit versus risk and cost.
- Lumbar supports have not been shown to have any lasting benefit beyond the acute phase of symptom relief.
- Moderate evidence suggests that back schools have better short-term effects than other treatments for chronic low back pain, and that such schools are more effective in an occupational setting than in a non-occupational setting. No good evidence supports using back schools for prevention, as opposed to treatment.
- Behavioral therapy may be an effective treatment for patients with chronic low back pain, but it is still unknown what type of patient benefits most from what type of behavioral treatment. Some studies provide evidence that intensive multidisciplinary bio-psycho-social rehabilitation with a functional restoration approach improves pain and function.

Activity Alteration

Bed rest has been used as a treatment for acute low back pain; however, debilitation and irritation can result from prolonged bed rest. The most severe cases of low back pain can be treated with one to two days of bed rest, but bed rest is not advisable as routine treatment.

Activities causing an increase in low back symptoms should be reviewed with the patient and modifications advised. Driving, workstation positions, repetitive motions, and other activities (that may or may not be obvious to the patient) may require modification.

While the patient is recovering from low back symptoms, activities that do not aggravate symptoms can be maintained, and exercises to prevent debilitation due to inactivity can be advised. The patient should be informed that this may temporarily increase symptoms. Work activity modification is an important part of any treatment regimen. Advice on how to avoid aggravating activities includes a review of work duties to decide whether or not modifications can be accomplished without employer notification and to determine whether modified duty is available. Making every attempt to maintain the patient at maximal levels of activity, including work activities, is recommended. Aerobic exercise is beneficial as a conservative management technique, and exercising as little as 20 minutes twice a week can be effective in managing low back pain.

Work Activities

Table 12-6 provides recommendations on activity modification and duration of absence from work. These guidelines are intended for patients without comorbidity or complicating factors, including employment or legal issues. They are targets to provide a guide from the perspective of physiologic recovery. The clinician can make it clear to patients and employers that:

- Even moderately heavy lifting, carrying, or working in awkward positions may aggravate back symptoms from low back strain or lumbosacral nerve root irritation, for example; and

*Table 12-6. Guidelines for Modification of Work Activities and Disability Duration**

		Recommended Target for Disability Duration**		**NHIS Experience Data*****	
Disorder	**Activity Modifications and Accommodation**	**With Modified Duty**	**Without Modified Duty**	**Median (cases with lost time)**	**Percent (no lost time)**
Lumbar strain	Bed rest for 1-2 days if needed for severe symptoms Avoid aggravating activities (e.g., bending, lifting, stooping, prolonged standing, walking, sitting) until full activity possible	0-2 days	7-14 days	13 days	19%
Lumbar disk protrusion, with radiculopathy	Bed rest for 2 days if needed for severe symptoms Avoid aggravating activities (e.g., bending, lifting, stooping, prolonged standing, walking, sitting) until full activity possible	0-4 days	7-14 days	29 days	36%
Spinal stenosis (aggravation)	Changes in position to avoid symptoms	0-4 days	7-14 days	16 days	19%
Post-laminectomy syndrome	Same as for lumbar disk protrusion, with referral to surgeon if patient does not improve	0-4 days	7-14 days	29 days	39%
Sciatica	Bed rest for 1-2 days if needed for severe symptoms	0-4 days	7-14 days	8 days	45%
Regional low back pain	Bed rest for 1-2 days if needed for severe symptoms	0-2 days	7-10 days	5 days	39%

* These are general guidelines based on consensus or population sources and are never meant to be applied to an individual case without consideration of workplace factors, concurrent disease or other social or medical factors that can affect recovery.
** These parameters for disability duration are "consensus optimal" targets as determined by a panel of ACOEM members in 1996, and reaffirmed by a panel of ACOEM members in 2002. In most cases, persons with one non-severe injury can return to modified duty immediately.
*** Based on the CDC NHIS (National Health Interview Survey), as compiled and reported in the 8th annual edition of *Official Disability Guidelines (ODG)*, © 2002 Work Loss Data Institute, all rights reserved.

- Any restrictions are intended to allow for spontaneous recovery or for time to build activity tolerance through exercise.

Measures to assist the patient in avoiding aggravating activities include a review of work duties to decide whether modifications can be made without employer notification and to determine whether modified duty is available. Make every attempt to maintain the patient at maximal levels of activity, including work activities.

Follow-up Visits

Patients with potentially work-related low back complaints should have follow-up every three to five days by a midlevel practitioner or physical therapist who can counsel the patient about avoiding static positions, medication use, activity modification, and other concerns. Health practitioners should take care to answer questions and make these sessions interactive so that the patient is fully involved in his or her recovery. If the patient has returned to work, these interactions may be conducted on site or by telephone to avoid interfering with modified- or full-work activities.

Physician follow-up can occur when a release to modified-, increased-, or full-duty is needed, or after appreciable healing or recovery can be expected, on average. Physician follow-up might be expected every four to seven days if the patient is off work and seven to fourteen days if the patient is working.

Special Studies and Diagnostic and Treatment Considerations

Lumbar spine x rays should not be recommended in patients with low back pain in the absence of red flags for serious spinal pathology, even if the pain has persisted for at least six weeks. However, it may be appropriate when the physician believes it would aid in patient management.

Unequivocal objective findings that identify specific nerve compromise on the neurologic examination are sufficient evidence to warrant imaging in patients who do not respond to treatment and who would consider surgery an option. When the neurologic examination is less clear, however, further physiologic evidence of nerve dysfunction should be obtained before ordering an imaging study. Indiscriminant imaging will result in false-positive findings, such as disk bulges, that are not the source of painful symptoms and do not warrant surgery. If physiologic evidence indicates tissue insult or nerve impairment, the practitioner can discuss with a consultant the selection of an imaging test to define a potential cause (magnetic resonance imaging [MRI] for neural or other soft tissue, computer tomography [CT] for bony structures).

Electromyography (EMG), including H-reflex tests, may be useful to identify subtle, focal neurologic dysfunction in patients with low back symptoms lasting more than three or four weeks. Diskography is not recommended for assessing patients with acute low back symptoms.

Table 12-7 provides a general comparison of the abilities of different techniques to identify physiologic insult and define anatomic defects. An imaging study may be appropriate for a patient whose limitations due to consistent symptoms have persisted for one month or more to further evaluate the possibility of potentially serious pathology, such as a tumor.

Relying solely on imaging studies to evaluate the source of low back and related symptoms carries a significant risk of diagnostic confusion (false-positive test results) because of the possibility of identifying a finding that was present before symptoms began and therefore has no temporal association with the symptoms. Techniques vary in their abilities to define abnormalities (Table 12-7). Imaging studies should be reserved for cases in which surgery is considered or red-flag diagnoses are being evaluated. Because the overall false-positive rate is 30% for imaging studies in patients over age 30 who do not have symptoms, the risk of diagnostic confusion is great.

Magnetic resonance (MR) neurography may be useful in isolating diagnoses that do not lend themselves to back surgery, such as sciatica caused by piriformis syndrome in the hip. However, MR neurography is still new and needs to be validated by quality studies.

Recent studies on diskography do not support its use as a preoperative indication for either intradiskal electrothermal (IDET) annuloplasty or fusion. Diskography does not identify the symptomatic high-intensity zone, and concordance of symptoms with the disk injected is of limited diagnostic value (common in non-back issue patients, inaccurate if chronic or abnormal psy-

Table 12-7. Ability of Various Techniques to Identify and Define Low Back Pathology

Technique	LS Strain	Disk Protrusion	Cauda Equina Syndrome	Spinal Stenosis	Post-laminectomy Syndrome
History	+ +	+ +	+ +	+ + +	+ + +
Physical examination	+ +	+ + +	+ + + +	+ +	+ + +
Laboratory studies	0	0	0	0	0
Imaging studies					
Radiography[1]	0	+	+	+ +	+
Computerized tomography (CT)[1,2]	0	+ + +	+ + +	+ + +	+ +
Magnetic resonance imaging (MRI)[1,2]	0	+ + + +	+ + + +	+ + +	+ + + +
Electromyography (EMG), sensory evoked potentials (SEPs)	0	+ + +	+	+	+

[1] Risk of complications (e.g., infection, radiation) highest for myeloCT, second highest for myelography, and relatively less for bone scan, radiography, and CT.

[2] False-positive results in up to 30% of people over age 30 who do not have symptoms and up to 50% in those over age 40.

Note: Number of plus signs indicates relative ability of technique to identify or define pathology.

chosocial tests), and it can produce significant symptoms in controls more than a year later. Tears may not correlate anatomically or temporally with symptoms. Diskography may be used where fusion is a realistic consideration, and it may provide supplemental information prior to surgery. This area is rapidly evolving, and clinicians should consult the latest available studies. Despite the lack of strong medical evidence supporting it, diskography is fairly common, and when considered, it should be reserved only for patients who meet the following criteria:

- Back pain of at least three months duration.
- Failure of conservative treatment.
- Satisfactory results from detailed psychosocial assessment. (Diskography in subjects with emotional and chronic pain problems has been linked to reports of significant back pain for prolonged periods after injection, and therefore should be avoided.)
- Is a candidate for surgery.
- Has been briefed on potential risks and benefits from diskography and surgery.

Surgical Considerations

Within the first three months after onset of acute low back symptoms, surgery is considered only when serious spinal pathology or nerve root dysfunction not responsive to conservative therapy (and obviously due to a herniated disk) is detected. Disk herniation, characterized by protrusion of the central nucleus pulposus through a defect in the outer annulus fibrosis, may impinge on a nerve root, causing irritation, back and leg symptoms, and nerve root dysfunction. The presence of a herniated disk on an imaging study, however, does not necessarily imply nerve root dysfunction. Studies of asymptomatic adults commonly demonstrate intervertebral disk herniations that apparently do not cause symptoms. Some studies show spontaneous disk resorption without surgery, while others suggest that pain may be due to irritation of the dorsal root ganglion by inflammogens (metalloproteinases, nitric oxide, interleukin-6, prostaglandin E2) released from a damaged disk in the absence of anatomical evidence of direct contact between neural elements and disk material. Therefore, referral for surgical consultation is indicated for patients who have:

- Severe and disabling lower leg symptoms in a distribution consistent with abnormalities on imaging studies (radiculopathy), preferably with accompanying objective signs of neural compromise
- Activity limitations due to radiating leg pain for more than one month or extreme progression of lower leg symptoms
- Clear clinical, imaging, and electrophysiologic evidence of a lesion that has been shown to benefit in both the short and long term from surgical repair
- Failure of conservative treatment to resolve disabling radicular symptoms

If surgery is a consideration, counseling regarding likely outcomes, risks and benefits, and, especially, expectations is very important. Patients with acute low back pain alone, without findings of serious conditions or significant nerve root compromise, rarely benefit from either surgical consultation or surgery. If there is no clear indication for surgery, referring the patient to a physical medicine practitioner may help resolve the symptoms.

Before referral for surgery, clinicians should consider referral for psychological screening to improve surgical outcomes, possibly including standard tests such as the second edition of the Minnesota Multiphasic Personality Inventory (MMPI-2). In addition, clinicians may look for Waddell signs during the physical exam.

Many patients with strong clinical findings of nerve root dysfunction due to disk herniation recover activity tolerance within one month; there is no evidence that delaying surgery for this period worsens outcomes in the absence of progressive nerve root compromise. With or without surgery, more than 80% of patients with apparent surgical indications eventually recover. Although surgery appears to speed short- to mid-term recovery, surgical morbidity (recovery and rehabilitation time and effects) and complications must be considered. Surgery benefits fewer than 40% of patients with questionable physiologic findings. Moreover, surgery increases the need for future surgical procedures with higher complication rates. In good surgery centers, the overall incidence of complications from first-time disk surgery is less than 1%. However, for older patients and repeat procedures, the rate of complications is dramatically higher. Patients with comorbid conditions, such as cardiac or respiratory disease, diabetes, or mental illness, may be poor candidates for surgery. Comorbidity should be weighed and discussed carefully with the patient. Following surgery, exercise is much better than manipulation for rehabilitation.

A. Lumbosacral Nerve Root Decompression

Direct methods of nerve root decompression include laminotomy, standard diskectomy, and laminectomy. Chemonucleolysis with chymopapain is an example of an indirect method. Indirect chemical methods are less efficacious and have rare but serious complications (e.g., anaphylaxis, arachnoiditis). Percutaneous diskectomy is not recommended because proof of its effectiveness has not been demonstrated. Recent studies of chemonucleolysis have shown it to be more effective than placebo, and it is less invasive, but less effective, than surgical diskectomy; however, few providers are experienced in this procedure because it is not widely used anymore. Surgical diskectomy for carefully selected patients with nerve root compression due to lumbar disk prolapse provides faster relief from the acute attack than conservative management; but any positive or negative effects on the lifetime natural history of the underlying disk disease are still unclear. Given the extremely low level of evidence available for artificial disk replacement or percutaneous endoscopic laser diskectomy (PELD), it is recommended that these procedures be regarded as experimental at this time.

B. Intradiskal Electrothermal Annuloplasty

Intradiskal electrothermal annuloplasty may show some advantages over diskectomy, but IDET is operator dependent and not considered ready for wholesale use by the public. Early outcomes may exaggerate the efficacy of IDET because some who initially improve later deteriorate. In addition, studies of IDET have relied on diskography, a technique not well supported by the medical evidence.

C. Implantable Spinal Cord Stimulators

Implantable spinal cord stimulators are rarely used and should be reserved for patients with low back pain for more than six months duration who have not responded to the standard nonoperative or operative interventions.

D. Management of Spinal Stenosis

Spinal stenosis usually results from soft tissue and bony encroachment of the spinal canal and nerve roots. It has a gradual onset and usually manifests as a degenerative process after age 50. Evidence does not currently support a relationship with work. The surgical treatment for spinal stenosis is usually complete laminectomy. Elderly patients with spinal stenosis who tolerate their daily activities usually do not require surgery unless bowel or bladder dysfunction develops. Surgery is rarely considered in the first three months after onset of symptoms, and a decision to proceed with surgery should not be based solely on the results of imaging studies. Some evidence suggests that patients with moderate to severe symptoms may benefit more from surgery than from conservative treatment.

E. Spinal Fusion

Except for cases of trauma-related spinal fracture or dislocation, fusion of the spine is not usually considered during the first three months of symptoms. Patients with increased spinal instability (not work-related) after surgical decompression at the level of degenerative spondylolisthesis may be candidates for fusion. There is no scientific evidence about the long-term effectiveness of any form of surgical decompression or fusion for degenerative lumbar spondylosis compared with natural history, placebo, or conservative treatment. There is no good evidence from controlled trials that spinal fusion alone is effective for treating any type of acute low back problem, in the absence of spinal fracture, dislocation, or spondylolisthesis if there is instability and motion in the segment operated on. It is important to note that although it is being undertaken, lumbar fusion in patients with other types of low back pain very seldom cures the patient. A recent study has shown that only 29% assessed themselves as "much better" in the surgical group versus 14% "much better" in the nonfusion group (a 15% greater chance of being "much better") versus a 17% complication rate (including 9% life-threatening or reoperation).

Summary of Evidence and Recommendations

See Table 12-8.

Table 12-8. Summary of Recommendations for Evaluating and Managing Low Back Complaints

Clinical Measure	Recommended	Optional	Not Recommended
History and physical exam	Basic history (B) History of cancer or infection (B) Signs or symptoms of cauda equina syndrome (C) History of significant trauma (C) Psychosocial history (C) Straight- and crossed-leg raising tests (B) Focused neurologic exam (B)	Pain drawing and visual analog scale (D)	
Patient education	Patient education about low back symptoms (B) Back school in occupational settings (C)	Back school in nonoccupational settings (C)	
Medication (See Chapter 3)	Acetaminophen (C) NSAIDs (B)	Opioids, short course (C) Muscle relaxants (C) Phenylbutazone (C)	Using opioids for more than 2 weeks (C) Oral corticosteroids (C) Colchicine (B) Antidepressants (C)
Physical treatment methods	Manipulation of low back during first month of symptoms without radiculopathy (C)	Manipulation for patients with radiculopathy (C) Relaxation techniques (D) At-home applications of local heat or cold to low back (D) Shoe insoles (C) In occupational setting, corset for prevention (C)	Manipulation for patients with undiagnosed neurologic deficits (D) Prolonged course of manipulation (longer than 4 weeks) (D) Traction (B) TENS (C) Biofeedback (C) Shoe lifts (D) Corset for treatment (D)

Table 12-8. (continued)

Clinical Measure	*Recommended*	*Optional*	*Not Recommended*
Injections		Epidural corticosteroid injections for radicular pain, to avoid surgery (C) Needle acupuncture (D)	Epidural injections for back pain without radiculopathy (D) Trigger-point injections (C) Ligamentous injections (C) Facet-joint injections (C)
Bed rest		Bed rest for 2 days for severe radiculopathy (D)	Bed rest for more than 2 days (B)
Activities and exercise	Temporary avoidance of activities that increase mechanical stress on spine (D) Gradual return to normal activities (B) Low-stress aerobic exercise (C) Conditioning exercises for trunk muscles after 2 weeks (C)		Back-specific exercise machines (D) Therapeutic stretching of back muscles (D)
Detection of physiologic abnormalities	If no improvement after 1 month, consider: Bone scan (C) Needle EMG and H-reflex tests to clarify nerve root dysfunction (C) SEPs to assess spinal stenosis (C)		EMG for clinically obvious radiculopathy (D) Surface EMG and F-wave tests (C) Thermography (C)
Radiographs of lumbosacral spine	When red flags for fracture are present (C) When red flags for cancer or infection are present (C)		Routine use during first month of symptoms in absence of red flags (B) Routine oblique views (B)
Imaging	CT or MRI when cauda equina, tumor, infection, or fracture are strongly suspected and plain film radiographs are negative (C) MRI test of choice for patients with prior back surgery (D) Assure quality criteria for imaging tests (B)	Myelography or CT myelography for preoperative planning if MRI is unavailable (D) MR neurography (D)	Using imaging test before 1 month in absence of red flags (B) Diskography or CT diskography (C)

Table 12-8. (continued)

Clinical Measure	Recommended	Optional	Not Recommended
Surgical considerations	Discuss surgical options with patients with persistent and severe sciatica and clinical evidence of nerve root compromise if symptoms persist after 4-6 weeks of conservative therapy (B) Standard diskectomy or microdiskectomy for herniated disk (procedures have similar efficacy) (B)	Chymopapain, used after ruling out allergic sensitivity, acceptable but less efficacious than diskectomy to treat herniated disk (C)	Disk surgery in patients with back pain alone, no red flags, and no nerve root compression (D) Surgery for spinal stenosis within the first 3 months of symptoms (D) Surgery for spinal stenosis when justified by imaging test rather than patient's functional status (D) Spinal fusion in the absence of fracture, dislocation, complications of tumor, or infection (C)
Psychosocial factors	Social, economic, and psychological factors can alter patient's response to symptoms and treatment (B)	Referral for evaluation prior to surgical intervention (C)	Referral for extensive evaluation and treatment prior to exploring patient expectations or psychosocial factors (D)

A = Strong research-based evidence (multiple relevant, high-quality scientific studies).
B = Moderate research-based evidence (one relevant, high-quality scientific study or multiple adequate scientific studies).
C = Limited research-based evidence (at least one adequate scientific study of patients with low back complaints).
D = Panel interpretation of information not meeting inclusion criteria for research-based evidence.

Algorithm 12-1. *Initial Evaluation of Occupational Low Back Complaints*

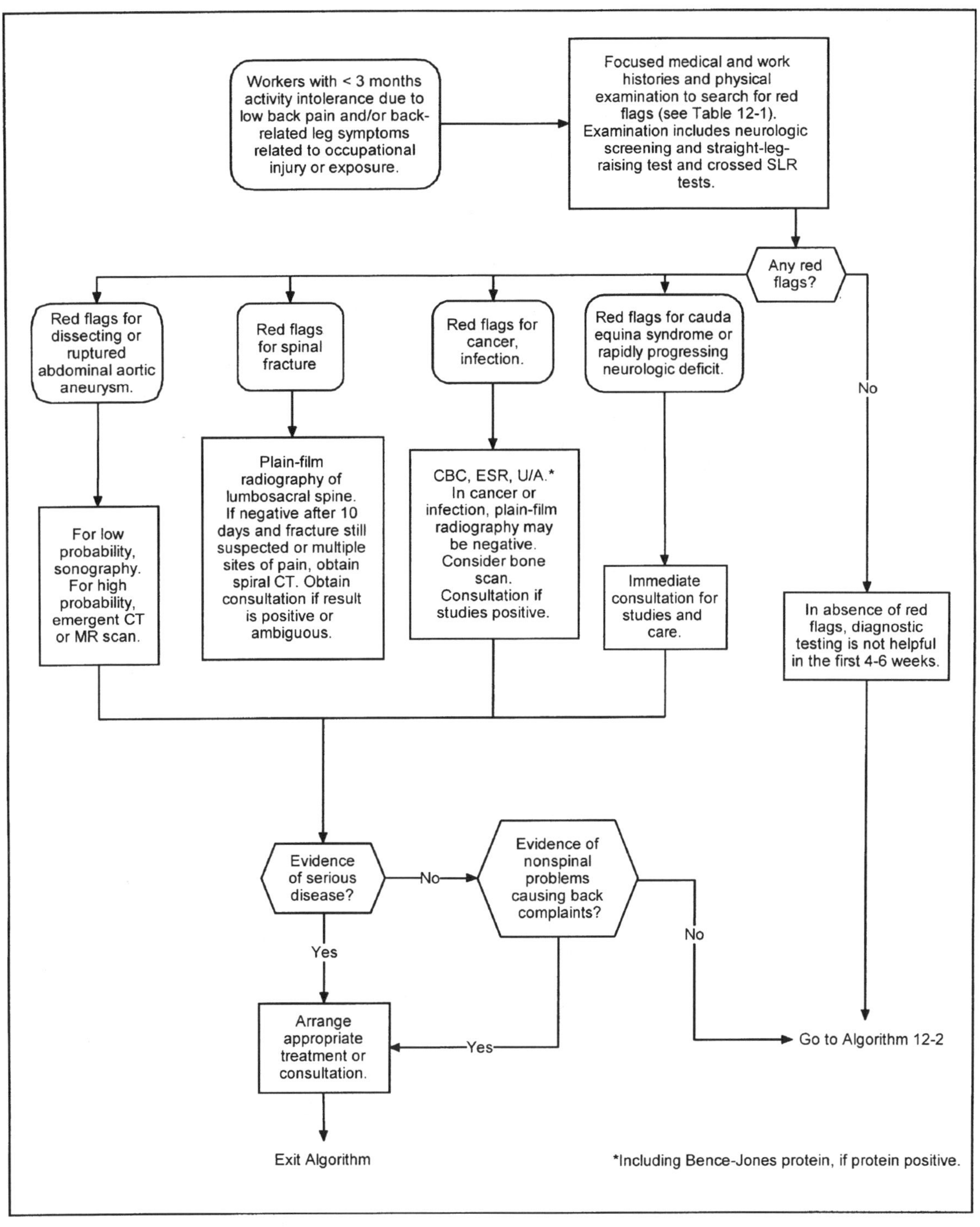

Algorithm 12-2. *Initial and Follow-up Management of Occupational Low Back Complaints*

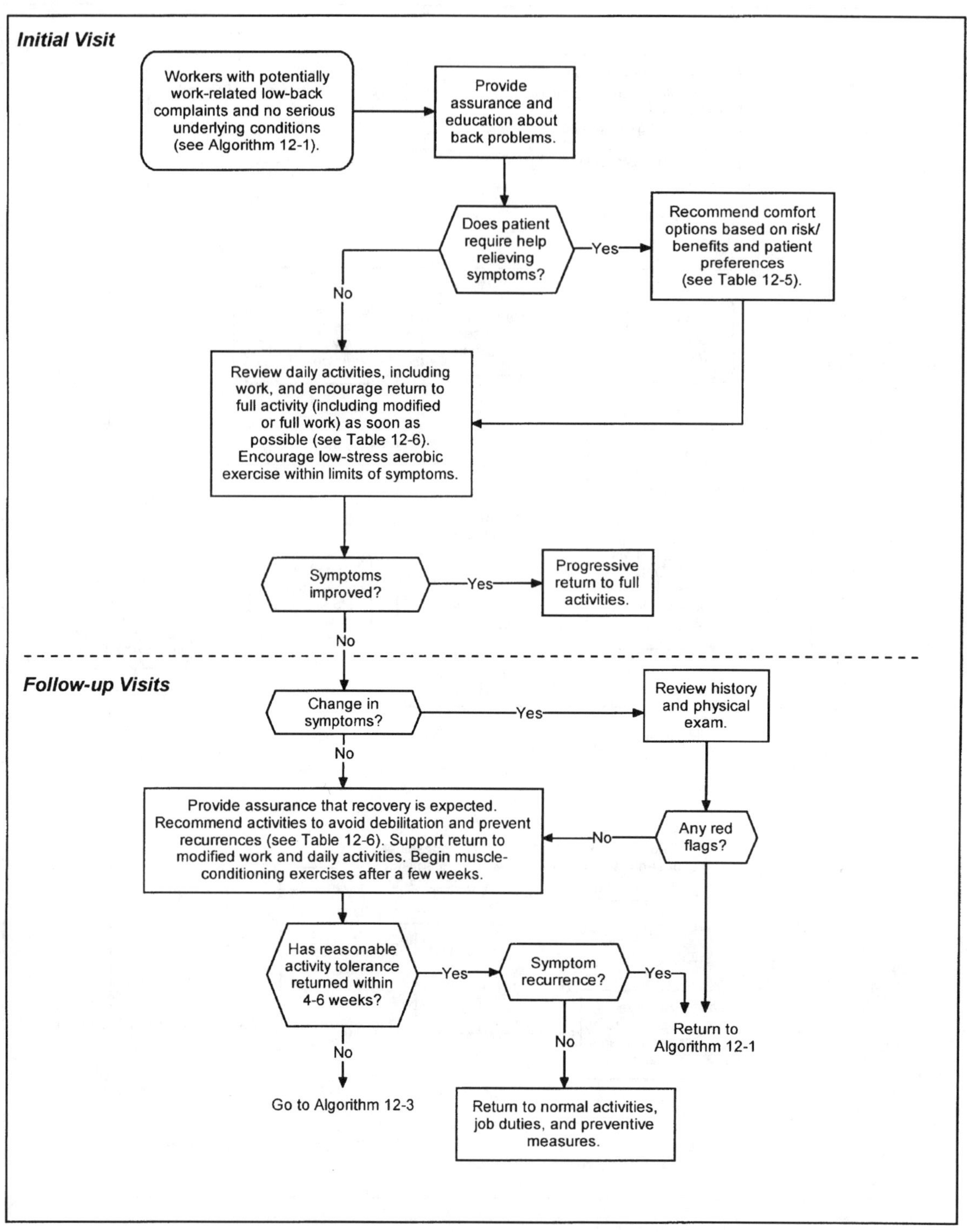

Algorithm 12-3. *Evaluation of Slow-to-recover Patients with Occupational Low Back Complaints (Symptoms > 4 Weeks)*

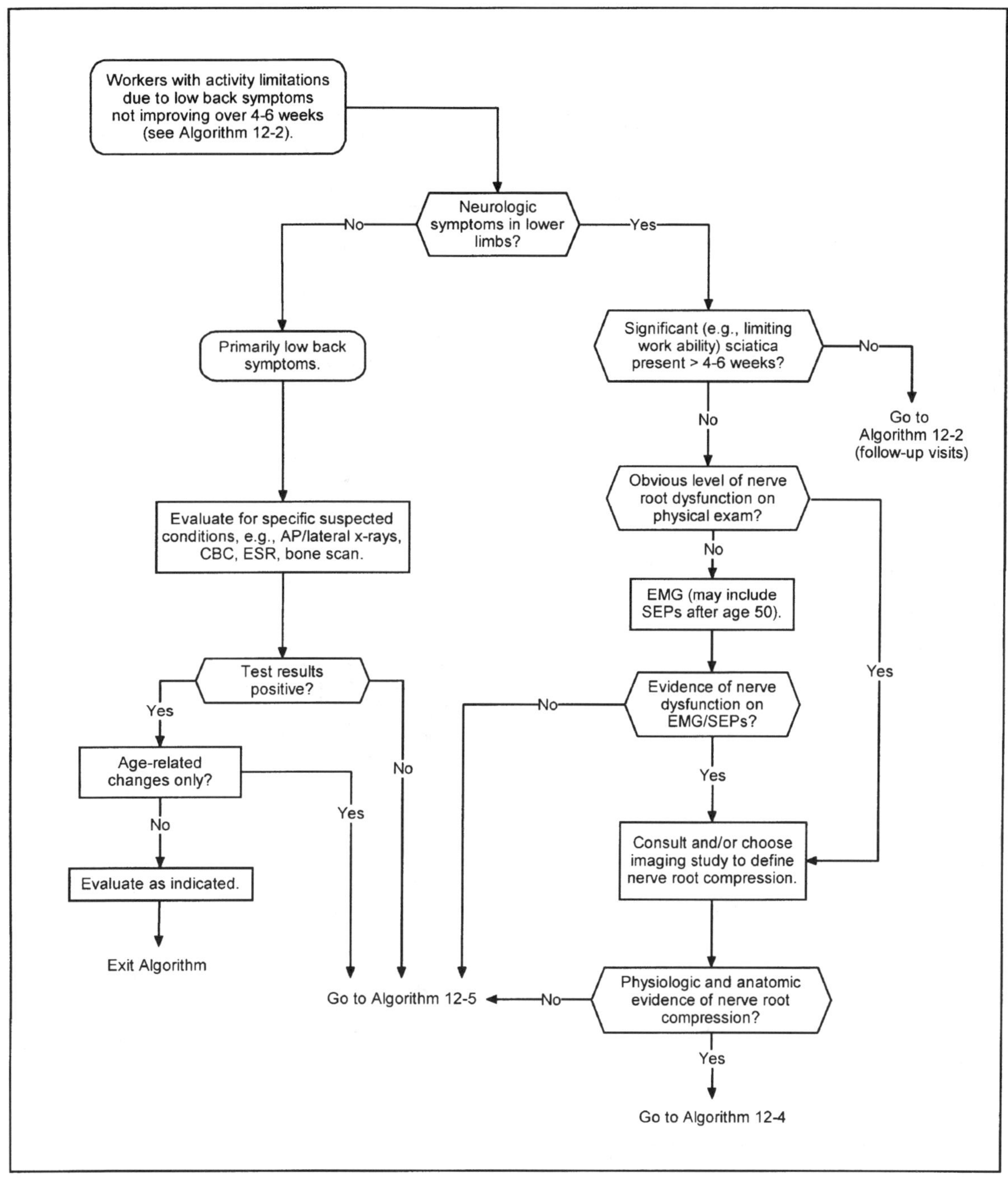

Algorithm 12-4. *Surgical Considerations for Patients with Anatomic and Physiologic Evidence of Nerve Root Compression and Persistent Low Back Symptoms*

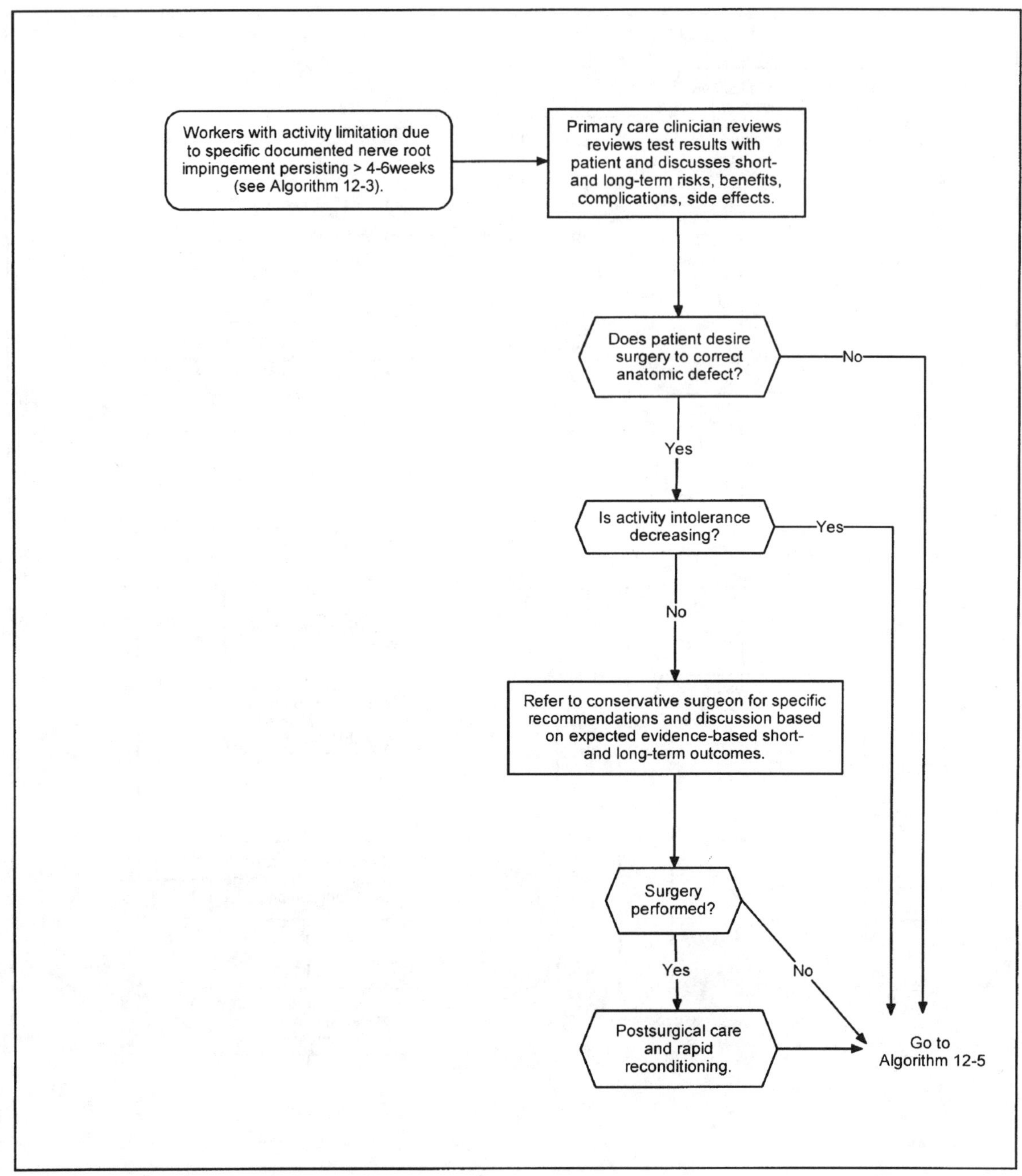

Algorithm 12-5. *Further Management of Occupational Low Back Complaints*

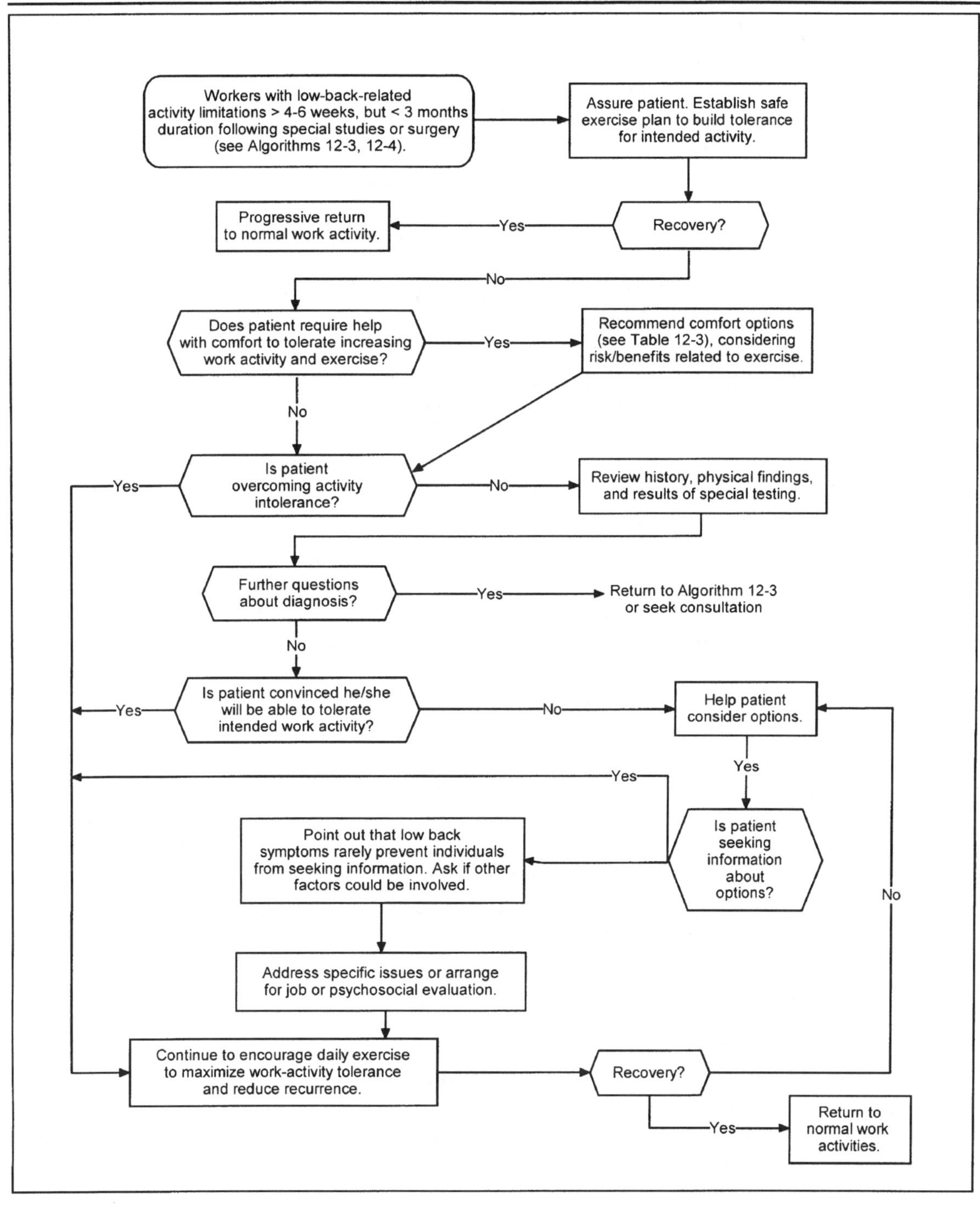

Note: The following references are additions to the 373 references cited in *Acute Low Back Problems in Adults.* (Bigos SJ, Bowyer O, Braen G, et al. *Acute Low Back Problems in Adults, Clinical Practice Guideline No. 14*, Rockville, Md: U.S. Department of Health and Human Services, Public Health Service, Agency for Health Care Policy and Research, AHCPR Pub. No. 95-0642, 1994.) Those references have been reviewed and are incorporated herein.

HISTORY AND PHYSICAL EXAMINATION

Bickerstaff ER. *Neurological Examination in Clinical Practice.* Oxford: Blackwell Scientific; 1975.

Devinsky O, Feldmann E. *Examination of the Cranial and Peripheral Nerves.* New York, NY: Churchill Livingstone; 1988.

Hestbaek L, Leboeuf-Yde C. Are chiropractic tests for the lumbo-pelvic spine reliable and valid? A systematic critical literature review. *J Manipulative Physiol Ther.* 2000;23:258-75.

Hoppenfeld S. *Orthopaedic Neurology: A Diagnostic Guide to Neurologic Levels.* Philadelphia, Pa: Lippincott; 1977.

Hsieh CY, Hong CZ, Adams AH, et al. Interexaminer reliability of the palpation of trigger points in the trunk and lower limb muscles. *Arch Phys Med Rehabil.* 2000;81:258-64.

Johanning E. Evaluation and management of occupational low back disorders. *Am J Ind Med.* 2000;37(1):94-111.

Joynt RJ, ed. *Clinical Neurology.* Vol. 3. Philadelphia, Pa: Lippincott-Raven; 1995.

Kilpikoski S, Airaksinen O, Kankaanpaa M, Leminen P, Videman T, Alen M. Interexaminer reliability of low back pain assessment using the McKenzie method. *Spine.* 2002;27:E207-14.

Smith RL. Therapists' ability to identify safe maximum lifting in low back pain patients during functional capacity evaluation. *J Orthop Sports Phys Ther.* 1994;19:277-81.

PATIENT EDUCATION

Burton AK, Waddell G, Tillotson KM, Summerton N. Information and advice to patients with back pain can have a positive effect. A randomized controlled trial of a novel educational booklet in primary care. *Spine.* 1999;24:2484-91.

Cherkin DC, Deyo RA, Battie M, Street J, Barlow W. A comparison of physical therapy, chiropractic manipulation, and provision of an educational booklet for the treatment of patients with low back pain. *N Engl J Med.* 1998;339:1021-9.

Cohen JE, Goel V, Frank JW, et al. Group education interventions for people with low back pain: an overview of the literature. *Spine.* 1994;19:214-22.

Derebery VJ, Giang GM, Saracino G, Fogarty WT. Evaluation of the impact of a low back pain educational intervention on physicians' practice patterns and patients' outcomes. *J Occup Environ Med.* 2002;44:977-84.

Elders LA, van der Beek AJ, Burdorf A. Return to work after sickness absence due to back disorders—a systematic review on intervention strategies. *Int Arch Occup Environ Health.* 2000;73:339-48.

Triano JJ, McGregor M, Hondras MA, Brennan PC. Manipulative therapy versus education programs in chronic low back pain. *Spine.* 1995;20:948-55.

van Tulder MW, Ostelo R, Vlaeyen JW, Linton SJ, Morley SJ, Assendelft WJ. Behavioral treatment for chronic low back pain: a systematic review within the framework of the Cochrane Back Review Group. *Spine.* 2001;26:270-81.

MEDICATION

See Chapter 3 references.

Mahmud MA, Webster BS, Courtney TK, Matz S, Tacci JA, Christiani DC. Clinical management and the duration of disability for work-related low back pain. *J Occup Environ Med.* 2000;42(12):1178-87.

Schnitzer TJ, Gray WL, Paster RZ, Kamin M. Efficacy of tramadol in treatment of chronic low back pain. *J Rheumatol.* 2000;27(3):772-8.

van Tulder MW, Koes BW, Bouter LM. Conservative treatment of acute and chronic nonspecific low back pain. A systematic review of randomized controlled trials of the most common interventions. *Spine.* 1997;22:2128-56.

van Tulder MW, Scholten RJ, Koes BW, Deyo RA. Nonsteroidal anti-inflammatory drugs for low back pain: a systematic review within the framework of the Cochrane Collaboration Back Review Group. *Spine.* 2000;25:2501-13.

PHYSICAL TREATMENT METHODS

Andersson GBJ, Lucente T, Davis AM, Kappler RE, Lipton JA, Leurgans S. A comparison of osteopathic spinal manipulation with standard care for patients with low back pain. *N Engl J Med.* 1999;341:1426-31.

Beurskens AJ, de Vet HC, Koke AJ, et al. Efficacy of traction for nonspecific low back pain. 12-week and 6-month results of a randomized clinical trial. *Spine.* 1997;22:2756-62.

Bigos SJ, McKee JE, Holland JP, Holland CL, Hildebrandt J. Back pain, the uncomfortable truth—assurance and activity problem. *Schmerz.* 2001;15:430-4.

Cates JR, Young DN, Guerriero DJ, et al. Evaluating the quality of clinical practice guidelines. *J Manipulative Physiol Ther.* 2001;24:170-6.

Cherkin DC, Eisenberg D, Sherman KJ, et al. Randomized trial comparing traditional Chinese medical acupuncture, therapeutic massage, and self-care education for chronic low back pain. *Arch Intern Med.* 2001;161:1081-8.

Cherkin DC, Deyo RA, Battie M, Street J, Barlow W. A comparison of physical therapy, chiropractic manipulation, and provision of an educational booklet for the treatment of patients with low back pain. *N Engl J Med.* 1998;339:1021-9.

Collacott EA, Zimmerman JT, White DW, Rindone JP. Bipolar permanent magnets for the treatment of chronic low back pain. *JAMA.* 2000;283:1322-5.

Flor H, Birbaumer N. Comparison of the efficacy of electromyographic biofeedback, cognitive-behavioral therapy, and conservative medical interventions in the treatment of chronic musculoskeletal pain. *J Consult Clin Psychol.* 1993;61:653-8.

Furlan AD, Brosseau L, Imamura M, Irvin E. Massage for low back pain. *Cochrane Database Syst Rev.* 2002;(2):CD001929.

Ghoname EA, Craig WF, White PF, et al. Percutaneous electrical nerve stimulation for low back pain: a randomized crossover study. *JAMA.* 1999;281:818-23.

Gose EE, Naguszewski WK, Naguszewski RK. Vertebral axial decompression therapy for pain associated with herniated or degenerated disks or facet syndrome: an outcome study. *Neurol Res.* 1998;20:186-90.

Hsieh CY, Adams AH, Tobis J, et al. Effectiveness of four conservative treatments for subacute low back pain: a randomized clinical trial. *Spine.* 2002;27:1142-8.

Kovacs FM, Llobera J, Abraira V, Lazaro P, Pozo F, Kleinbaum D. The KAP Group, effectiveness and cost-effectiveness analysis of neuroreflexotherapy for subacute and chronic low back pain in routine general practice: a cluster randomized, controlled trial. *Spine.* 2002;27:1149-59.

Jellema P, van Tulder MW, van Poppel MN, Nachemson AL, Bouter LM. Lumbar supports for prevention and treatment of low back pain: a systematic review within the framework of the Cochrane Back Review Group. *Spine.* 2001;26:377-86.

Kang JD, Georgescu HI, McIntyre-Larkin L, Stefanovic-Racic M, Donaldson WF III, Evans CH. Herniated lumbar intervertebral disks spontaneously produce matrix metalloproteinases, nitric oxide, interleukin-6, and prostaglandin E2. *Spine.* 1996;21:271-7.

Karasek M, Bogduk N. Twelve-month follow-up of a controlled trial of intradiskal thermal annuloplasty for back pain due to internal disk disruption. *Spine.* 2000;25:2601-7.

Linz DH, Shepherd CD, Ford LF, Ringley LL, Klekamp J, Duncan JM. Effectiveness of occupational medicine center-based physical therapy. *J Occup Environ Med.* 2002;44:48-53.

Milne S, Welch V, Brosseau L, et al. Transcutaneous electrical nerve stimulation (TENS) for chronic low back pain. *Cochrane Database Syst Rev.* 2001;(2):CD003008.

Mohseni-Bandpei MA, Stephenson R, Richardson B. Spinal manipulation in the treatment of low back pain: a review of the literature with particular emphasis on randomized controlled clinical trials. *Phys Ther Rev.* 1998;3: 185-94.

Saal JS, Saal JA. Management of chronic diskogenic low back pain with a thermal intradiskal catheter. A preliminary report. *Spine.* 2000;25:382-8.

Saal JA, Saal JS. Intradiskal electrothermal treatment for chronic diskogenic low back pain: a prospective outcome study with minimum 1-year follow-up. *Spine.* 2000;25:2622-7.

Saal JA, Saal JS. Intradiskal electrothermal treatment for chronic diskogenic low back pain: prospective outcome study with a minimum 2-year follow-up. *Spine.* 2002;27:966-73; discussion 973-4.

Scheer SJ, Radack KL, O'Brien DR Jr. Randomized controlled trials in industrial low back pain relating to return to work. Part 1. Acute interventions. *Arch Phys Med Rehabil.* 1995;76:966-73.

Scheer SJ, Radack KL, O'Brien DR Jr. Randomized controlled trials in industrial low back pain relating to return to work. Part 2. Diskogenic low back pain. *Arch Phys Med Rehabil.* 1996;77:1189-97.

Schiller L. Effectiveness of spinal manipulative therapy in the treatment of mechanical thoracic spine pain: a pilot randomized clinical trial. *J Manipulative Physiol Ther.* 2001;24(6):394-401.

Sherry E, Kitchener P, Smart R. A prospective randomized controlled study of VAX-D and TENS for the treatment of chronic low back pain. *Neurol Res.* 2001;23:780-4.

Stern PJ, Cote P, Cassidy JD. A series of consecutive cases of low back pain with radiating leg pain treated by chiropractors. *J Manipulative Physiol Ther.* 1995;18:335-42.

Tacci JA, Webster BS, Hashemi L, Christiani DC. Clinical practices in the management of new-onset, uncomplicated, low back workers' compensation disability claims. *J Occup Envir Med.* 1999;41:397-404.

Timm KE. A randomized-control study of active and passive treatments for chronic low back pain following L5 laminectomy. *J Orthop Sports Phys Ther.* 1994;20:276-86.

Triano JJ, McGregor M, Hondras MA, Brennan PC. Manipulative therapy versus education programs in chronic low back pain. *Spine.* 1995;20:948-55.

Urrutia G, Bonfill X, Del Pozo P, Fernandez A. Neuroreflexotherapy for non-specific low back pain (Protocol for a Cochrane Review). In: *The Cochrane Library.* Issue 3; 2002.

van Tulder MW, Cherkin DC, Berman B, Lao L, Koes BW. The effectiveness of acupuncture in the management of acute and chronic low back pain. A systematic review within the framework of the Cochrane Collaboration Back Review Group. *Spine.* 1999;24:1113-23.

van Tulder MW, Koes BW, Bouter LM. Conservative treatment of acute and chronic nonspecific low back pain. A systematic review of randomized controlled trials of the most common interventions. *Spine.* 1997;22:2128-56.

van Tulder MW, Blomberg SEI, de Vet HCW, van der Heijden G, Bronfort G, Bouter LM. Traction for low back pain with or without radiating symptoms (Protocol for a Cochrane Review). In: *The Cochrane Library.* Issue 3; 2003.

van Tulder MW, Cherkin DC, Berman B, Lao L, Koes BW. Acupuncture for low back pain. *Cochrane Database Syst Rev.* 2000;(2):CD001351.

van der Heijden GJ, Beurskens AJ, Koes BW, Assendelft WJ, de Vet HC, Bouter LM. The efficacy of traction for back and neck pain: a systematic, blinded review of randomized clinical trial methods. *Phys Ther.* 1995;75(2): 93-104.

Washington State Department of Labor and Industries. *Technology Assessment of the Dynatron STS.* Office of the Medical Director. April 30, 2002.

Werners R, Pynsent PB, Bulstrode CJ. Randomized trial comparing interferential therapy with motorized lumbar traction and massage in the management of low back pain in a primary care setting. *Spine.* 1999;24:1579-84.

West DT, Mathews RS, Miller MR, Kent GM. Effective management of spinal pain in one hundred seventy-seven patients evaluated for manipulation under anesthesia. *J Manipulative Physiol Ther.* 1999;22:299-308.

Zigenfus GC, Yin J, Giang GM, Fogarty WT. Effectiveness of early physical therapy in the treatment of acute low back musculoskeletal disorders. *J Occup Environ Med.* 2000;42:35-9.

INJECTIONS

Blomberg S, Svardsudd K, Tibblin G. A randomized study of manual therapy with steroid injections in low-back pain: telephone interview follow-up of pain, disability, recovery and drug consumption. *Eur Spine J.* 1994;3:246-54.

Bowman SJ, Wedderburn L, Whaley A, et al. Outcome assessment after epidural corticosteroid injection for low back pain and sciatica. *Spine.* 1993; 18:1345-50.

Carette S, Leclaire R, Marcoux S, et al. Epidural corticosteroid injections for sciatica due to herniated nucleus pulposus. *N Engl J Med.* 1997;336:1634-40.

Dechow E, Davies RK, Carr AJ, Thompson PW. A randomized, double-blind, placebo-controlled trial of sclerosing injections in patients with low back pain. *Rheumatol.* 1999;38:1255-9.

Esses SI, Moro JK. The value of facet joint blocks in patient selection for lumbar fusion. *Spine.* 1993;18:185-90.

Foster L, Clapp L, Erickson M, Jabbari B. Botulinum toxin A and chronic low back pain: a randomized, double-blind study. *Neurology.* 2001;56:1290-3.

Hopwood MB, Abram SE. Factors associated with failure of lumbar epidural steroids. *Reg Anesth.* 1993;18:238-43.

Klein RG, Eek BC, DeLong WB, et al. A randomized double-blind trial of dextrose-glycerine-phenol injections for chronic, low back pain. *J Spinal Disord.* 1993;6:23-33.

Kovacs FM, Abraira V, Pozo F, et al. Local and remote sustained trigger point therapy for exacerbations of chronic low back pain. A randomized, double-blind, controlled, multicenter trial. *Spine.* 1997;22:786-97.

Mam MK. Results of epidural injection of local anaesthetic and corticosteroid in patients with lumbosciatic pain. *J Indian Med Assoc.* 1995;93:17-8, 24.

Nelemans PJ, de Bie RA, de Vet HC, Sturmans F. Injection therapy for subacute and chronic benign low back pain. *Cochrane Database Syst Rev.* 2000;(2):CD001824.

Ongley MJ, Klein RG, Dorman TA, Eek BC, Hubert LJ. A new approach to the treatment of chronic low back pain. *Lancet.* 1987;2(8551):143-6.

Rozenberg S, Dubourg G, Khalifa P, Paolozzi L, Maheu E, Ravaud P. Efficacy of epidural steroids in low back pain and sciatica. A critical appraisal by a French Task Force of randomized trials. Critical Analysis Group of the French Society for Rheumatology. *Rev Rhum Engl Ed.* 1999;66(2):79-85.

BED REST

Allen C, Glasziou P, Del Mar C. Bed rest: a potentially harmful treatment needing more careful evaluation. *Lancet.* 1999;354(9186):1229-33.

Hagen KB, Hilde G, Jamtvedt G, Winnem M. Bed rest for acute low back pain and sciatica. *Cochrane Database Syst Rev.* 2000;(2):CD001254.

Hilde G, Hagen KB, Jamtvedt G, Winnem M. Advice to stay active as a single treatment for low back pain and sciatica. *Cochrane Database Syst Rev.* 2002;(2):CD003632.

Malmivaara A, Hakkinen U, Aro O, et al. The treatment of acute low back pain—bed rest, exercises, or ordinary activity? *N Engl J Med.* 1995;332: 351-5.

van Tulder MW, Koes BW, Assendelft WJ, Bouter LM, Daams J, van der Laan JR. Acute low back pain: activity, NSAIDs and muscle relaxants effective; bedrest and targeted exercise not effective; results of systematic reviews. *Ned Tijdschr Geneeskd.* 2000;144(31):1484-9.

Waddell G, Feder G, Lewis M. Systematic reviews of bed rest and advice to stay active for acute low back pain. *Br J Gen Pract.* 1997;47(423):647-52.

ACTIVITIES AND EXERCISE

Delitto A, Cibulka MT, Erhard RE, et al. Evidence for use of an extension-mobilization category in acute low back syndrome: a prescriptive validation pilot study. *Phys Ther.* 1993;73:216-22.

Faas A. Exercises: which ones are worth trying, for which patients, and when? *Spine.* 1996;21:2874-8; discussion 2878-9.

Hagen EM, Eriksen HR, Ursin H. Does early intervention with a light mobilization program reduce long-term sick leave for low back pain? *Spine.* 2000;1;25:1973-6.

Hall H, McIntosh G, Melles T, et al. Effect of discharge recommendations on outcome. *Spine.* 1994;19:2033-7.

Hansen FR, Bendix T, Skov P, et al. Intensive, dynamic back-muscle exercises, conventional physiotherapy, or placebo-control treatment of low-back pain: a randomized, observer-blind trail. *Spine.* 1993;18:98-108.

Indahl A, Velund L, Reikeraas O. Good prognosis for low back pain when left untampered. A randomized clinical trial. *Spine.* 1995;20:473-7.

Lindstrom I, Ohlund C, Eek C, et al. The effect of graded activity on patients with subacute low back pain: a randomized prospective clinical study with an operant-conditioning behavioral approach. *Phys Ther.* 1992;72:279-90; discussion 291-3.

Mellin G, Harkapaa K, Vanharanta H, et al. Outcome of a multimodal treatment including intensive physical training of patients with chronic low back pain. *Spine.* 1993;18:825-9.

Mellin G, Harkapaa K, Vanharanta H, et al. Outcome of a multimodal treatment including intensive physical training of patients with chronic low back pain. *Spine.* 1993;18:825-9.

Mitchell RI, Carmen GM. The functional restoration approach to the treatment of chronic pain in patients with soft tissue and back injuries. *Spine.* 1994;19:633-42.

Ostelo RW, de Vet HC, Waddell G, Kerckhoffs MR, Leffers P, van Tulder MW. Rehabilitation after lumbar disk surgery. *Cochrane Database Syst Rev.* 2002;(2):CD003007.

Scheer SJ, Watanabe TK, Radack KL. Randomized controlled trials in industrial low back pain. Part 3. Subacute/chronic pain interventions. *Arch Phys Med Rehabil.* 1997;78:414-23.

Schonstein E, Kenny DT, Keating J, Koes BW. Work conditioning, work hardening and functional restoration for workers with back and neck pain (Protocol for a Cochrane Review). In: *The Cochrane Library.* Issue 3; 2002.

van Tulder MW, Esmail R, Bombardier C, Koes BW. Back schools for non-specific low back pain. *Cochrane Database Syst Rev.* 2000;(2):CD000261.

van Tulder MW, Koes BW, Assendelft WJ, Bouter LM, Maljers LD, Driessen AP. Chronic low back pain: exercise therapy, multidisciplinary programs, NSAIDs, back schools and behavioral therapy effective; traction not effective; results of systematic reviews. *Ned Tijdschr Geneeskd.* 2000;144(31): 1489-94.

van Tulder MW, Malmivaara A, Esmail R, Koes B. Exercise therapy for low back pain: a systematic review within the framework of the Cochrane Collaboration Back Review Group. *Spine.* 2000;25:2784-96.

RADIOGRAPHY AND IMAGING

Carragee EJ, Chen Y, Tanner CM, Truong T, Lau E, Brito JL. Provocative diskography in patients after limited lumbar diskectomy: a controlled, randomized study of pain response in symptomatic and asymptomatic subjects. *Spine.* 2000;25:3065-71.

Carragee EJ, Paragioudakis SJ, Khurana S. 2000 Volvo Award winner in clinical studies: lumbar high-intensity zone and diskography in subjects without low back problems. *Spine.* 2000;25:2987-92.

Carragee EJ, Chen Y, Tanner CM, Hayward C, Rossi M, Hagle C. Can diskography cause long-term back symptoms in previously asymptomatic subjects? *Spine*. 2000;25:1803-8.

Carragee EJ, Tanner CM, Khurana S, et al. The rates of false-positive lumbar diskography in select patients without low back symptoms. *Spine*. 2000;25:1373-80; discussion 1381.

Donelson R, Aprill C, Medcalf R, Grant W. A prospective study of centralization of lumbar and referred pain. A predictor of symptomatic disks and annular competence. *Spine*. 1997;22:1115-22.

Filler AG, Kliot M, Howe FA, et al. Application of magnetic resonance neurography in the evaluation of patients with peripheral nerve pathology. *J Neurosurg*. 1996;85:299-309.

Kendrick D, Fielding K, Bentley E, Miller P, Kerslake R, Pringle M. The role of radiography in primary care patients with low back pain of at least 6 weeks duration: a randomised (unblinded) controlled trial. *Health Technol Assess*. 2001;5(30):1-69.

Kerry S, Hilton S, Patel S, Dundas D, Rink E, Lord J. Routine referral for radiography of patients presenting with low back pain: is patients' outcome influenced by GPs' referral for plain radiography? *Health Technol Assess*. 2000;4(20:i-iv, 1-119.

Littenberg B, Siegel A, Tosteson AN, Mead T. Clinical efficacy of SPECT bone imaging for low back pain. *J Nucl Med*. 1995;36:1707-13.

Mullin WJ, Heithoff KB, Gilbert TJ Jr, Renfrew DL. Magnetic resonance evaluation of recurrent disk herniation: is gadolinium necessary? *Spine*. 2000;25:1493-9.

SURGICAL CONSIDERATIONS

Agency for Health Care Research and Quality (AHRQ). Treatment of degenerative lumbar spinal stenosis. Rockville, Md: *Agency for Health Care Research and Quality (AHRQ)*. 1587630516. Evidence Report/Tech. 2001.

Boult M, Fraser RD, Jones N, et al. Percutaneous endoscopic laser diskectomy. *Aust N Z J Surg*. 2000;70:475-9.

Cinotti G, David T, Postacchini F. Results of disk prosthesis after a minimum follow-up period of 2 years. *Spine*. 1996;21:995-1000.

Franklin GM, Haug J, Heyer NJ, et al. Outcome of lumbar fusion in Washington State workers' compensation. *Spine*. 1994;19:1897-903; discussion 1904.

Fritzell P, Hagg O, Wessberg P, Nordwall A. Swedish Lumbar Spine Study Group, 2001 Volvo Award Winner in Clinical Studies: lumbar fusion versus nonsurgical treatment for chronic low back pain: a multicenter randomized controlled trial from the Swedish Lumbar Spine Study Group. *Spine*. 2001;26:2521-32; discussion 2532-4.

Gibson JN, Grant IC, Waddell G. Surgery for lumbar disk prolapse. *Cochrane Database Syst Rev*. 2000;(3):CD001350.

Gibson JN, Waddell G, Grant IC. Surgery for degenerative lumbar spondylosis. *Cochrane Database Syst Rev*. 2000;(3):CD001352.

Haro H, Crawford HC, Fingleton B, Shinomiya K, Spengler DM, Matrisian LM. Matrix metalloproteinase-7-dependent release of tumor necrosis factor-alpha in a model of herniated disk resorption. *J Clin Invest.* 2000; 105:143-50.

Jonsson B, Stromqvist B. Repeat decompression of lumbar nerve roots: a prospective two-year evaluation. *J Bone Joint Surg [Br].* 1993;75:894-7.

Katz JN, Lipson SJ, Lew RA, et al. Lumbar laminectomy alone or with instrumented or noninstrumented arthrodesis in degenerative lumbar spinal stenosis. Patient selection, costs, and surgical outcomes. *Spine.* 1997; 22:1123-31.

Klara PM, Ray CD. Artificial nucleus replacement: clinical experience. *Spine.* 2002;27:1374-7.

Lee CK, Vessa P, Lee JK. Chronic disabling low back pain syndrome caused by internal disk derangements: the results of disk excision and posterior lumbar interbody fusion. *Spine.* 1995;20:356-61.

Malter AD, Larson EB, Urban N, Deyo RA. Cost-effectiveness of lumbar diskectomy for the treatment of herniated intervertebral disk. *Spine.* 1996;21:1048-54; discussion 1055.

Mayer HM. Diskogenic low back pain and degenerative lumbar spinal stenosis—how appropriate is surgical treatment? *Schmerz.* 2001;15:484-91.

Stevens CD, Dubois RW, Larequi-Lauber T, Vader JP. Efficacy of lumbar diskectomy and percutaneous treatments for lumbar disk herniation. *Soz Praventivmed.* 1997;42:367-79.

Zeegers WS, Bohnen LM, Laaper M, Verhaegen MJ. Artificial disk replacement with the modular type SB Charite III: 2-year results in 50 prospectively studied patients. *Eur Spine J.* 1999;8(3):210-7.

PSYCHOSOCIAL FACTORS

Bush T, Cherkin D, Barlow W. The impact of physician attitudes on patient satisfaction with care for low back pain. *Arch Fam Med.* 1993;2:301.

Chapman SL, Pemberton JS. Prediction of treatment outcome from clinically derived MMPI clusters in rehabilitation for chronic low back pain. *Clin J Pain.* 1994;10:267-76.

Fritz JM, Wainner RS, Hicks GE. The use of nonorganic signs and symptoms as a screening tool for return-to-work in patients with acute low back pain. *Spine.* 2000;25(15):1925-31.

Gaines WG Jr, Hegmann KT. Effectiveness of Waddell's nonorganic signs in predicting a delayed return to regular work in patients experiencing acute occupational low back pain. *Spine.* 1999;24(4):396-400; discussion 401.

Gatchel RJ, Polatin PB, Kinney RK. Predicting outcome of chronic back pain using clinical predictors of psychopathology: a prospective analysis. *Health Psychol.* 1995;14(5):415-20.

Guzman J, Esmail R, Karjalainen K, Malmivaara A, Irvin E, Bombardier C. Multidisciplinary bio-psycho-social rehabilitation for chronic low back pain. *Cochrane Database Syst Rev.* 2002;(1):CD000963.

Hasenbring M, Marienfeld G, Kuhlendahl D, et al. Risk factors of chronicity in lumbar disk patients: a prospective investigation of biologic, psychologic, and social predictors of therapy outcome. *Spine.* 1994;19:2759-65.

Karjalainen K, Malmivaara A, van Tulder M, et al. Multidisciplinary biopsychosocial rehabilitation for subacute low back pain in working-age adults: a systematic review within the framework of the Cochrane Collaboration Back Review Group. *Spine.* 2001;26(3):262-9.

Klapow JC, Slater MA, Patterson TL, et al. An empirical evaluation of multidimensional clinical outcome in chronic low back pain patients. *Pain.* 1993;55:107-18.

Lanes TC, Gauron EF, Spratt KF, et al. Long-term follow-up of patients with chronic back pain treated in a multidisciplinary rehabilitation program. *Spine.* 1995;20:801-6.

Main CJ, Williams AC. Musculoskeletal pain. *BMJ.* 2002;325(7363):534-7.

McIntosh G, Frank J, Hogg-Johnson S, Bombardier C, Hall H. Prognostic factors for time receiving workers' compensation benefits in a cohort of patients with low back pain. *Spine.* 2000;25(2):147-57.

Paulsen JS, Altmaier EM. The effects of perceived versus enacted social support on the discriminative cue function of spouses for pain behaviors. *Pain.* 1995;60:103-10.

Polatin PB, Cox B, Gatchel RJ, Mayer TG. A prospective study of Waddell signs in patients with chronic low back pain. When they may not be predictive. *Spine.* 1997;22(14):1618-21.

Riley JL 3rd, Robinson ME, Geisser ME, Wittmer VT, Smith AG. Relationship between MMPI-2 cluster profiles and surgical outcome in low-back pain patients. *J Spinal Disord.* 1995;8(3):213-9.

Talo S, Puukka P, Rytokoski U, et al. Can treatment outcome of chronic low back pain be predicted? Psychological disease consequences clarifying the issue. *Clin J Pain.* 1994;10:107-21.

Tota-Faucette ME, Gil KM, Williams DA, et al. Predictors of response to pain management treatment: the role of family environment and changes in cognitive processes. *Clin J Pain.* 1993;9:115-23.

Trief PM, Carnrike CL Jr, Drudge O. Chronic pain and depression: is social support relevant? *Psychol Rep.* 1995;76:227-36.

Vendrig AA. Prognostic factors and treatment-related changes associated with return to work in the multimodal treatment of chronic back pain. *J Behav Med.* 1999;22(3):217-32.

Wetzel FT, McCracken L, Robbins RA, Lahey DM, Carnegie M, Phillips FM. Temporal stability of the Minnesota Multiphasic Personality Inventory (MMPI) in patients undergoing lumbar fusion: a poor predictor of surgical outcome. *Am J Orthop.* 2001;30(6):469-74.

GENERAL

Bigos SJ, Bowyer O, Braen G, et al. *Acute Low Back Problems in Adults. Clinical Practice Guideline No. 14.* Rockville, Md: U.S. Department of Health and Human Services, Public Health Service, Agency for Health Care Policy and Research. AHCPR Pub No. 95-0642, 1994.

PREVENTION

Daltroy LH, Iversen MD, Larson MG, et al. A controlled trial of an educational program to prevent low back injuries. *N Engl J Med.* 1997;337:322-8.

van Poppel MN, Koes BW, Smid T, Bouter LM. A systematic review of controlled clinical trials on the prevention of back pain in industry. *Occup Environ Med.* 1997;54:841-7.

Yassi A, Cooper JE, Tate RB, et al. A randomized controlled trial to prevent patient lift and transfer injuries of health care workers. *Spine.* 2001;26: 1739-46.

OTHER METHODS

Atcheson SG, Brunner RL, Greenwald EJ, Rivera VG, Cox JC, Bigos SJ. Paying doctors more: use of musculoskeletal specialists and increased physician pay to decrease workers' compensation costs. *Occup Environ Med.* 2001;43: 672-9.

Bigos SJ. Perils, Pitfalls, and accomplishments of guidelines for treatment of back problems. *Neurol Clin.* 1999;17:179-92.

Dreyfuss P, Halbrook B, Pauza K, Joshi A, McLarty J, Bogduk N. Efficacy and validity of radiofrequency neurotomy for chronic lumbar zygapophysal joint pain. *Spine.* 2000;25:1270-7.

Kang JD, Georgescu HI, McIntyre-Larkin L, Stefanovic-Racic M, Donaldson WF III, Evans CH. Herniated lumbar intervertebral disks spontaneously produce matrix metalloproteinases, nitric oxide, interleukin-6, and prostaglandin E2. *Spine.* 1996;21:271-7.

Leclaire R, Fortin L, Lambert R, Bergeron YM, Rossignol M. Radiofrequency facet joint denervation in the treatment of low back pain: a placebo-controlled clinical trial to assess efficacy. *Spine.* 2001;26:1411-6; discussion 1417.

Mam MK. Results of epidural injection of local anaesthetic and corticosteroid in patients with lumbosciatic pain. *J Indian Med Assoc.* 1995;93:17-8, 24.

Schroth WS, Schectman JM, Elinsky EG, et al. Utilization of medical services for the treatment of acute low back pain: conformance with clinical guidelines. *J Gen Intern Med.* 1992;7:486-91.

van Kleef M, Barendse GA, Kessels A, Voets HM, Weber WE, de Lange S. Randomized trial of radiofrequency lumbar facet denervation for chronic low back pain. *Spine.* 1999;24:1937-42.

Tacci JA, Webster BS, Hashemi L, Christiani DC. Clinical practices in the management of new-onset, uncomplicated, low back workers' compensation disability claims. *J Occup Envir Med.* 1999;41:397-404.

***Master Algorithm**. ACOEM Guidelines for Care of Acute and Subacute Occupational Knee Complaints*

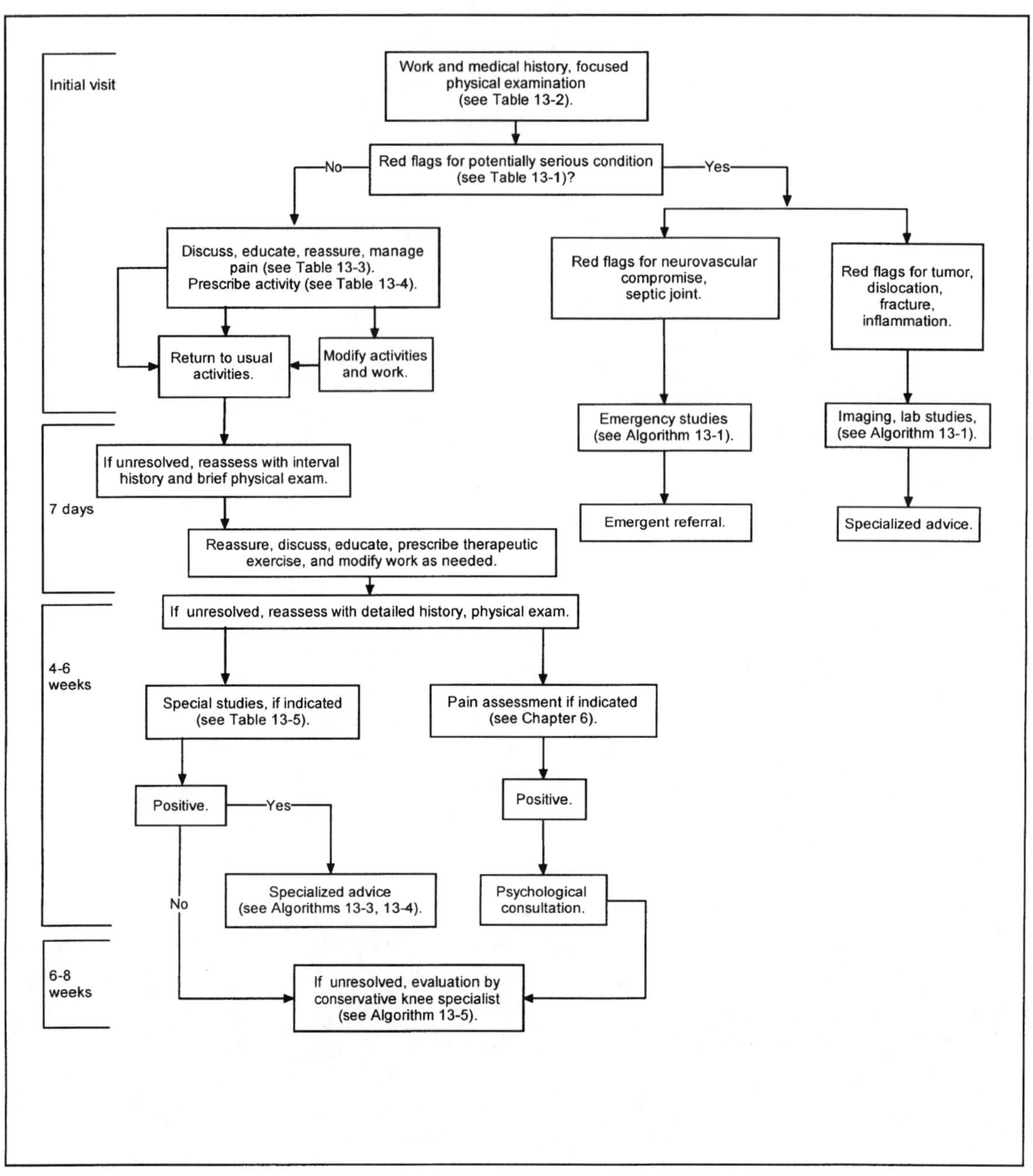

13 Knee Complaints

General Approach and Basic Principles

Knee complaints that are potentially related to work are common problems presenting to occupational and primary care providers—they are among the ten most common causes of reported occupational complaints and workers' compensation claims. Knee complaints account for 7-8% of total benefits paid for workers' compensation medical care and temporary disability, ranking them in the top ten for financial severity. However, about a quarter of the total expense is incurred for surgical procedures whose efficacy is not supported by available evidence, as summarized in this guideline.

Recommendations on assessing and treating adults with potentially work-related knee problems are presented in this clinical practice guideline. Topics include the initial assessment and diagnosis of patients with acute and subacute knee complaints that potentially are work related; identification of red flags that may indicate the presence of a serious underlying medical condition; initial management; diagnostic considerations and special studies for identifying clinical pathology; work-relatedness; modified duty and activity; return to work; and further management considerations, including the management of delayed recovery.

Algorithms for patient management are included. This chapter's master algorithm schematizes how primary care and occupational medicine practitioners generally can manage patients with acute and subacute knee complaints. The following text, tables, and numbered algorithms expand upon the master algorithm.

The principal recommendations for assessing and treating patients with knee complaints are as follows:

- The initial assessment of patients with acute and subacute knee problems focuses on detecting indications of potentially serious disease, termed red flags.
- In the absence of red flags, work-related knee complaints can be managed safely and effectively by occupational or primary care providers. The focus is on monitoring for complications, facilitating the

healing process, and facilitating return to work in modified- or full-duty.

- In the absence of red-flag signs or symptoms, evaluation and treatment can proceed in the acute phase for four to six weeks without performing special studies because the yield of treatment-altering findings is low and most patients' conditions improve within that period of time.
- Patients can be introduced to the concept of load and overload. Load is beneficial for the muscle, tendon, skeleton, and cartilage; overload is not beneficial. The adaptation of physical activities is crucial; total rest does more harm than good.
- Relieving discomfort can be accomplished most safely by temporary immobilization, reduction in weight bearing, and systemic nonprescription analgesics.
- Patients recovering from acute knee injury or infection should be encouraged to return to modified-duty work as soon as their condition permits.
- If symptoms persist beyond four weeks, referral for specialty care may be indicated.
- Nonphysical factors, such as psychosocial, workplace, or socioeconomic problems, may be investigated and addressed in cases of delayed recovery or return to work.

Initial Assessment

Thorough medical and work histories and a focused physical examination (see Chapter 2) are sufficient to assess the worker complaining of potentially work-related knee symptoms. The initial history and examination include evaluation for serious underlying conditions. This evaluation should consider the possibility of referred knee pain due to a disorder in another part of the body, particularly the low back or hip. Certain findings on the history and physical examination raise suspicion of serious underlying medical conditions known as red flags (see Table 13-1). Their absence rules out the need for special studies, referral, or inpatient care during the first four to six weeks, when spontaneous recovery is expected (provided any inciting workplace factors are mitigated). Knee complaints then can be classified into one of four working categories:

- **Potentially serious knee conditions:** fractures, dislocation, infection, neurovascular compromise, tumors, etc.
- **Mechanical disorders:** derangements of the knee related to acute trauma, such as ligament strain or meniscus or ligament tears
- **Degenerative disorders:** consequences of aging or repetitive use, or a combination thereof, such as patellofemoral syndrome (formerly commonly referred to as chondromalacia), bursitis, or tendinitis
- **Nonspecific disorders:** occurring in the knee and suggesting neither internal derangement nor referred pain

Table 13-1. Red Flags for Potentially Serious Knee Conditions

Disorder	Medical History	Physical Examination
Fractures	History of significant trauma	Bony crepitation Abnormal mobility Angulation of leg New deformity Point tenderness Inability to bear weight or walk
Dislocations	History of significant trauma Prior history of dislocation	Displaced patella Displaced tibia or fibula
Septic arthritis	Penetrating wound of the knee History of systemic infection Diabetes History of immunosuppression (e.g., transplant, chemotherapy, HIV)	Severe pain on motion Systemic signs of infection Local swelling and heat Abnormal complete blood count (CBC), erythrocyte sedimentation rate (ESR) Soft tissue swelling not consistent with effusion
Infected prepatellar bursitis	Minor trauma to prepatellar bursa area	No severe pain on motion Spreading local inflammation and cellulitis
Inflammation	History of autoimmune disease or gout Recurrent episodes Swollen joint Swelling in other joints	Local effusion, heat CBC, ESR may be abnormal Pain on motion
Tumor	History of primary tumor or metastatic disease	Local swelling Nontender mass
Compartment syndrome above or below the knee	History of fracture or other major trauma Very painful muscular compartment	Tense, very tender compartment Possibly distal signs of neurovascular compromise
Neurovascular compromise	History consistent with fracture or dislocation History of peripheral vascular disease History of diabetes Pain, pallor at or below the knee History of recent surgery, immobilization, or deep vein thrombosis	Decreased or absent pulse popliteal or pedal Pale, cold skin, distal to knee Paralysis of the distal lower extremity Painless swelling (Charcot's syndrome) Painful swelling in popliteal fossa or lower leg

Note: ICD-9 = *International Classification of Diseases,* 9th Edition.

Medical History

Asking the patient open-ended questions such as those listed below allows the clinician to gauge the need for further discussion or specific inquiries to obtain more detailed information (see also Chapter 2):

WHAT ARE YOUR SYMPTOMS?

- Do you have pain, weakness, limited motion, popping, clicking, locking, recurrent swelling, or giving way?
- For traumatic injury: Was the area deformed? Did you lose any blood or have an open wound?
- If swelling is reported: How long was it following the injury that your knee became swollen?
- Are the symptoms located primarily in the knee? Do you have pain or other symptoms elsewhere (e.g., low back, hip)?
- Is the pain constant or intermittent? What makes the problem worse or better?

DO THESE SYMPTOMS LIMIT YOUR ACTIVITIES? IF SO, HOW?

- Can you walk or carry weight? For how long?
- Can you lift? How much weight?
- Are your symptoms worse when climbing or going down stairs or hills?

WHEN DID YOUR CURRENT LIMITATIONS BEGIN? WAS THERE A SPECIFIC INCITING EVENT THAT LED TO THE SYMPTOMS?

- How did the limitations develop?
- How long have your activities been limited? More than four weeks?
- Have your symptoms changed? How?
- Have you had similar episodes previously?
- Have you had previous testing or treatment? With whom?
- What do you think caused the problem? How do you think it is related to work?
- What are your specific job duties? Do you use your knees? How? How often?

DO YOU HAVE OTHER MEDICAL PROBLEMS?

- Do you have any autoimmune or metabolic diseases, such as rheumatoid arthritis or gout?
- Do you have arthritis in any other joint?
- Have you had cancer?

WHAT DO YOU HOPE WE CAN ACCOMPLISH DURING THIS VISIT?

Knee complaints as described by the patient can sometimes be referred from other sources. Hip pathology can produce distal thigh symptoms and knee pain in the absence of knee pathology. Likewise, sciatic or femoral nerve irritation or hip disease can cause knee symptoms.

Physical Examination

Guided by the medical history, the physical examination includes:

- General observation of the patient
- Focused examination of the knee on the affected side
- Neurovascular screening

Care should be taken to document which knee—left or right—is the subject of the examination. Not infrequently, injured workers have prior workers' compensation claims that involve the opposite knee, or pain in the opposite knee that is unrelated to employment. Any ambiguity in documentation that identifies the knee being examined can lead to delay in acceptance of the patient's workers' compensation claim, delay in the authorization of time-loss benefits, delay in the authorization of payment of medical care, or even outright denial of the workers' compensation claim.

The physician should seek objective evidence of pathology that is consistent with the patient's subjective complaints. In many cases, careful examination will reveal one or more truly objective findings, such as swelling, deformity, atrophy, reflex changes or spasm. Any such findings should be thoroughly documented in the medical record both for reference during future visits, and for the value the information will have in the patient's workers' compensation claim. For some patients with knee complaints, however, there are no objective findings. Meticulous documentation of the patient's complaints at each visit is of the utmost importance in such cases.

Though it may seem a point too obvious to warrant mention, the physician should specifically note which knee—left or right—is the subject of the patient's complaints. Not infrequently, injured workers have prior workers' compensation claims that involve the opposite knee. Any ambiguity in documentation can lead to delay in acceptance of the patient's workers' compensation claim, delay in the authorization of time-loss benefits, delay in the authorization of payment of medical care, or even outright denial of the workers' compensation claim.

The physician should seek objective evidence of pathology that is consistent with the patient's subjective complaints. In many cases, careful examination will reveal one or more truly objective findings, such as swelling, deformity, atrophy, reflex changes, or spasm. Any such findings should be thoroughly documented in the medical record both for reference during future visits, and for the value the information will have in the patient's workers' compensation claim. For some patients with knee complaints, however, there are no objective findings. Meticulous documentation of the patient's complaints at each visit is of the utmost importance in such cases.

A. Focused Knee Examination

Knee examinations should be performed in a thorough and careful manner in order to identify any clinically significant pathology that may be present. A considerable number of patients may present with findings such as grinding, clicking, popping, and pain, yet do not necessarily have clinically significant intraarticular pathology or require more than conservative care. Patients presenting with sensations of instability or locking require further investigation.

Initially, the patient's gait and the appearance of the knees can be observed during stance. Difficulty walking, as well as deformity (e.g., excessive varus or valgus), swelling, redness, and inability to fully extend are all observable in this manner. In the supine position, smaller effusions, tenderness and its location (e.g., at joint lines), and range of motion can be determined. The posterior structures of the knee also can be inspected and palpated, including the popliteal fossa. Collateral ligament stability can be checked by applying varus and valgus stress (pressure) with the joint slightly flexed. Cruciate ligament competence is determined by pulling the tibia forward at 30 degrees (Lachman test) and 90 degrees (drawer test). The knee also can be examined at 0 degrees. The McMurray test is limited to testing defects of the posterior horn.

A history of anterior knee pain and popping and clicking may suggest patellofemoral syndrome (PFS, formerly known as chondromalacia patella). Patients with tenderness over the patellar tendon or its insertion may have patellar tendinitis or Osgood-Schlatter disease, a congenital condition. Knee catching, locking, or swelling may be secondary to meniscus tears, patellofemoral instability or ligamentous injury. Patellar instability often presents as a constant dull pain.

B. Neurovascular Screening

The neurologic and vascular status of the knee and distal lower extremity can be routinely assessed. Evidence of lumbar disk disease, with radiculopathy and radiation to the knee, also may be sought because neurologic changes may be present in the lower extremity.

C. Assessing Red Flags

Signs of neurovascular compromise, unreduced dislocation, infection, or tumor that correlate with the patient's medical history and test results may indicate a need for immediate consultation. A medical history suggestive of pathology originating somewhere other than in the knee may warrant examination of the back, hip, or other areas.

Diagnostic Criteria

If the patient does not have red flags for serious conditions, the clinician can then determine which common musculoskeletal disorder is present. The criteria presented in Table 13-2 follow the clinical thought process, from the mechanism of illness or injury to unique symptoms and signs of a particular disorder and, finally, to test results, if any tests are needed to guide treatment at this stage.

Table 13-2. Diagnostic Criteria for Non-red-flag Knee Conditions that Can Be Managed by Primary Care Physicians

Probable Diagnosis or Injury	Mechanism	Unique Symptoms	Unique Signs	Tests and Results
Meniscus tear (ICD-9 826.0, 836.0, 836.1, 836.11—new med, lat.—717.1-.3—old med, lat)	Squatting Twisting with foot planted (in younger workers) Repeated minor trauma (in older workers)	Locking of knee with flexion	Catching or locking of knee Quadriceps wasting (rare in acute phase)	MRI confirms tear (test indicated only if surgery is contemplated)
Collateral ligament tear (ICD-9 844.0.1)	Twisting Direct lateral or medial blow to the knee	Pain at lateral or medial side of knee	Excessive abduction or adduction at knee (> 30°) vs. other side when varus and valgus stress (pressure) is applied Tenderness at joint line Tenderness at origin, insertion of ligament	Stress films (not recommended but may be available) show ≥7-mm gap vs. other knee MRI can also confirm tear
Anterior cruciate tear (ICD-9 844.21, 717.83)	Noncontact pivot or twist of knee Direct blow to planted leg	Popping sound at injury site Immediate swelling Increased laxity	Positive Lachman's or anterior drawer sign Positive pivot-shift sign Hemarthrosis	Arthrometer reading 3 mm > that for other knee MRI confirms tear
Posterior cruciate tear (ICD-9 844.22, 717.84)	Blow to front of knee Severe injury of other structure with knee dislocation	Pain in interior knee	Positive posterior drawer test Sag sign positive	Arthrometer reading 3 mm > that for other knee MRI confirms tear

Table 13-2. (continued)

Probable Diagnosis or Injury	Mechanism	Unique Symptoms	Unique Signs	Tests and Results
Collateral ligament strain (ICD-9 844.0, 844.1)	Direct medial or lateral blow	Pain in lateral or medial knee Pain worse with weight bearing or rotation	Tenderness at joint lines laterally or medially with abduction or adduction Tenderness at origin or insertion of ligament	None
Cruciate ligament strain (ICD-9 844.2)	Noncontact pivot or twist of knee Direct blow to planted leg	Pain in interior knee	Pain but not displacement elicited by drawer and/or Lachman test	None
Patellofemoral syndrome (chondromalacia) (ICD-9 717.7)	Chronic vibration, impact Direct blow to patella Overuse	Popping or snapping Pain under patella with motion Pain on stairs, hills, quadriceps contraction	Tenderness under patella Grating under patella on motion	Possible misalignment on Merchant's view, with lateral displacement (inicated only if surgery is contemplated)
Effusion, nonspecific (ICD-9 719.06)	No history of acute trauma	Effusion may be worse with exercise	Effusion	Possible crystals in aspirate Possible positive serology for rheumatic disease
Patellar tendinitis (ICD-9 726.64)	Repeated minor trauma	Pain over patellar tendon	Tenderness over patellar tendon Pain on resisted quadriceps contraction	MRI is confirmatory (but not necessary except when considering surgery)
Prepatellar bursitis (ICD-9726.65)	Repeated minor trauma from kneeling work	Swelling over patella Inability to kneel due to swelling	Prepatellar bursal effusion	Aspirate positive for bacteria, etc., if infected
Nonspecific pain (ICD-9 719.46, 719.56, 719.76, 719.96)	Nonspecific No acute trauma	None	None	None
Patellar instability	Nonspecific	Knee catching, semilocking, swelling, constant dull pain	Abnormal patellar motion	None

Note: ICD-9 = *International Classification of Diseases,* 9th Edition.

Work-Relatedness

A thorough work history is crucial to establishing work-relatedness. See Chapter 2 for components of the work history.

Repeated trauma, for example crawling or working in a crouched position under load, is currently thought to contribute to tendinitis and nonspecific knee pain, although the strength of the association is not great. Working on the knees is thought to contribute to prepatellar bursitis. Trauma from vibration, such as jackhammer use, is thought to contribute to patellofemoral syndrome. Repetitive motion under load may contribute to meniscus damage in older workers. Acute trauma at work may cause acute meniscus tears, ligament strains, and ligament ruptures.

Patellar tendinitis and osteoarthritis usually do not have causative associations with acute trauma (see Chapter 1). However, aggravations of these conditions may have connection with work activities. Heavy workload, previous knee injury, and/or an overweight patient are all predictors of aggravation of osteoarthritis and can be addressed. The medical history becomes crucial in determining this relationship; nonwork as well as work activities have to be evaluated. If a history of past injury is associated with the onset of symptoms and the present complaint has the identical presentation, a relationship to the past injury may exist. It is important to establish the level of function that existed before the current health complaint. This is because the goal of treatment will be to return the patient at least to that state; because the underlying problem may well be chronic, its elimination may be unrealistic. The patient can be asked to identify when this level has been reached, because treatment beyond that point will likely be reduced to the level of maintenance and observation.

Initial Care

Comfort is often a patient's first concern. Nonprescription analgesics will provide sufficient pain relief for most patients with acute and subacute symptoms. If treatment response is inadequate (i.e., if symptoms and activity limitations continue), prescribed pharmaceuticals or physical methods can be added. Comorbid conditions, side effects, cost, and provider and patient preferences guide the clinician's choice of recommendations. Table 13-3 summarizes comfort options.

A number of treatment options are available to the clinician treating acute and subacute knee pain. These options include:

- Instruction in home exercise. Except in cases of significant injury, patients with knee problems can be advised to do early straight-leg-raising and active range-of-motion exercises, especially bicycling, as tolerated. The emphasis is on closed-chain exercises[1] and muscle re-

[1]Closed-chain exercises are those in which the feet remain in contact with the floor throughout the exercise. Squats are an example of closed-chain exercises. Conversely, open-chain exercises are those in which the feet do not maintain floor contact. Straight-leg extensions are open-chain exercises.

Table 13-3. Methods of Symptom Control for Knee Complaints

RECOMMENDED

Nonprescription Medications

Acetaminophen (safest)
Nonsteroidal anti-inflammatory drugs (NSAIDs) (aspirin, ibuprofen)

Nonprescribed Physical Methods

Adjustment or modification of workstation, job tasks, or work hours and methods
Stretching
Specific knee exercises for range of motion and strengthening (avoid leg extensions for PFSs but not SLRs)
At-home local applications of cold packs in first few days of acute complaints; thereafter, applications of heat packs
Aerobic exercise

Prescribed Pharmaceutical Methods

Other NSAIDs

Prescribed Physical Methods

Initial and follow-up visits for education, counseling, and evaluation of home exercise

OPTIONS

Meniscus Tears	Collateral Ligament Strain	Collateral Ligament Tear
Brief partial weight bearing as needed Immobilizer only if needed Quadriceps strengthening	Partial weight bearing (crutches) for 1 week Immobilizer if needed Quadriceps strengthening	Partial weight bearing (crutches) for 2 weeks
Cruciate Ligament Strain	**Cruciate Ligament Tear**	**Patellofemoral Syndrome**
Weight bearing as tolerated Quadriceps strengthening	Partial weight bearing (crutches) for 2 weeks Immobilizer only if needed Quadriceps and hamstring strengthening	Knee sleeve Avoid activities involving knee flexion Quadriceps strengthening
Effusion	**Patellar Tendinitis**	**Prepatellar Bursitis**
Possible aspiration	Quadriceps strengthening	Possibly aspiration of bursa
Nonspecific Knee Pain		
Ice		

training. Instruction in proper exercise technique is important and a few visits to a physical therapist can serve to educate the patient about an effective exercise program. The clinician or therapist should teach the patient rehabilitation programs for knee problems.

- Patient's at-home applications of heat or cold packs may be used before or after exercises and are as effective as those performed by a therapist.

- Some studies have shown that transcutaneous electrical neurostimulation (TENS) units and acupuncture may be beneficial in patients with chronic knee pain, but there is insufficient evidence of benefit in acute knee problems.
- Sophisticated rehabilitation programs involving equipment should be reserved for significant knee problems as an alternative to surgery or for postoperative rehabilitation. Properly conducted, these programs minimize the active participation of the therapist and direct the patient to take an active role in the program by simply using the equipment after instruction and then graduating to a home program.
- Physical modalities, such as massage, diathermy, cutaneous laser treatment, ultrasound, and biofeedback have no scientifically proven efficacy in treating acute knee symptoms.
- Invasive techniques, such as needle aspiration of effusions or prepatellar bursal fluid and cortisone injections, are not routinely indicated. Knee aspirations carry inherent risks of subsequent intraarticular infection.
  - A reddened, hot, swollen area may be a sign of cellulitis or infected prepatellar bursitis; thus, aspirating the joint through such an area is not recommended because microorganisms may be introduced into a previously sterile joint space.
  - If a patient has severe pain with motion, septic effusion of the knee joint is a possibility, and referral for aspiration, Gram stain, culture, sensitivity, and possibly lavage may be indicated. Initial atraumatic effusions without signs of infection may be aspirated for diagnostic purposes.
  - There is a high rate of recurrence of effusions after aspiration, but the procedure may be worthwhile in cases of large effusions or if there is a question of infection in the bursa.
  - Patients with recurrent effusions who have a history of gout or pseudogout may need aspiration to rule out infection, but more likely will need it only for comfort, if at all. Osteoarthritis can present with effusions, but findings of crepitus, palpable osteophytes, and history of chronic symptoms are usually sufficient to make the differential diagnosis.
  - Swelling and sponginess anterior to the patella is consistent with a diagnosis of prepatellar bursitis.
- Other miscellaneous therapies have been evaluated and found to be ineffective. In particular, iontophoresis and phonophoresis have no proven efficacy.
- Manipulation does not appear to be effective in alleviating knee pain.

Activity Alteration

The principle of maximizing activities while recovering from a physical problem applies to knee problems as well as problems involving other parts of the body.

Non-weight-bearing exercises, such as swimming or floor exercises, can be carried out while allowing the affected knee to rest before undergoing specific exercises to rehabilitate the area at a later date. Weight-bearing exercises, as tolerated, can begin as soon as possible provided no exacerbation of structural damage will occur. Weight bearing helps avoid the adverse effects of non-weight-bearing, such as loss of muscle mass, loss of strength, and diffuse osteopenia. The knee disorders under discussion almost always can bear weight, as tolerated. For example, treatment could include a partial weight-bearing gait using crutches with the affected leg on the floor and with the weight distributed between crutches and leg by adjusting the amount of force applied with arms on the crutches. Even at the acute stage, however, patients can usually perform appropriate lower extremity exercises, and can remove the immobilizer for active range-of-motion exercises, at least twice a day. Using load-bearing exercises and movement is far more beneficial to the muscle, tendon, skeleton, and cartilage than is total rest, but it also is crucial to avoid overloading the knee.

Activities and postures that increase stress on a structurally damaged knee tend to aggravate symptoms. Patients with acute ligament tears, strains, or meniscus damage of the knee can often perform only limited squatting and working under load during the first few weeks after return to work. Patients with prepatellar bursitis should avoid kneeling. Patients with any type of knee injury or disorder will find prolonged standing and walking to be difficult, but return to modified-duty work is extremely desirable to maintain activities and prevent debilitation. A brace can be used for patellar instability, anterior cruciate ligament (ACL) tear, or medical collateral ligament (MCL) instability although its benefits may be more emotional (i.e., increasing the patient's confidence) than medical. Usually a brace is necessary only if the patient is going to be stressing the knee under load, such as climbing ladders or carrying boxes. For the average patient, using a brace is usually unnecessary. In all cases, braces need to be properly fitted and combined with a rehabilitation program.

Work Activities

Occupational clinicians often are called on to make specific recommendations about activities at work for patients with acute limitations due to knee problems. Work-activity modification can be discussed at the initial and subsequent encounters with patients. Education about avoiding painful positions may help the patient maintain partial activities and thus avoid debilitation. The patient's age, general health and condition, and perceptions of safe limits for walking, standing, stooping, twisting, and kneeling (noted on initial history) help in formulating recommendations on reasonable starting points for activity.

The clinician can make it clear to patients and employers that:

- Even moderately heavy, unassisted carrying, stooping, crouching, etc. may aggravate knee symptoms caused by any of the diagnoses under discussion.

- Any restrictions are intended to allow for spontaneous recovery or for the time necessary for the development of activity tolerance through exercise.

Table 13-4 provides a guide for recommendations on activity modification, and data on disability duration. These are intended to apply to patients without comorbidity or complicating factors, including legal or employment issues. The activity modification table is intended to provide activity-related guidance that will maximize the chances for a prompt recovery. The disability-duration data are presented to provide assistance in determining when the length of recovery has reached the point that reconsideration should be given to the diagnosed condition, the treatment plan, or the injured worker's degree of participation in that plan.

Follow-up Visits

Patients with knee complaints should have follow-up every three to five days, whether in person or with brief telephone or e-mail contact, by a midlevel practitioner or physical therapist who can counsel the patient about avoiding static positions, medication use, activity modification, and other concerns. The practitioner can answer questions and make these sessions interactive so that the patient is fully involved in his or her recovery. If the patient has returned to work, these interactions may be done on site or by telephone to avoid interfering with modified- or full-work activities.

Physician follow-up is appropriate when a release to modified, increased, or full duty is needed, or after appreciable healing or recovery can be expected, on average. Physician follow-up might be expected every four to seven days if the patient is off work and every seven to fourteen days if the patient is working.

Special Studies and Diagnostic and Treatment Considerations

Special studies are not needed to evaluate most knee complaints until after a period of conservative care and observation. The position of the American College of Radiology (ACR) in its most recent appropriateness criteria list the following clinical parameters as predicting absence of significant fracture and may be used to support the decision *not* to obtain a radiograph following knee trauma:

- Patient is able to walk without a limp
- Patient had a twisting injury and there is no effusion

The clinical parameters for ordering knee radiographs following trauma in this population are:

- Joint effusion within 24 hours of direct blow or fall
- Palpable tenderness over fibular head or patella

*Table 13-4. Guidelines for Modification of Work Activities and Disability Duration**

Disorder	Activity Modifications and Accommodation	Recommended Target for Disability Duration**		NHIS Experience Data***	
		With Modified Duty	Without Modified Duty	Median (cases with lost time)	Percent (no lost time)
Meniscus tear	Weight-bearing as tolerated; no prolonged squatting, standing or walking. No stooping, crouching, or carrying	0-2 days	4-14 days	18 days	14%
Collateral ligament strain	Same as for meniscus tear	0-1 day	7-14 days	14 days	19%
Collateral ligament tear	Same as for meniscus tear	0-2 days	14-21 days	14 days	19%
Cruciate ligament strain	Same as for meniscus tear	0-1 day	7-10 days	14 days	19%
Cruciate ligament tear	Same as for meniscus tear	0-2 days	14-21 days	14 days	19%
Patellofemoral syndrome	Avoid activities involving knee flexation, e.g., frequent stair-climbing, hill-climbing, and prolonged walking	0 days	1-2 days	15 days	48%
Patellar tendinitis	Same as meniscus tear	0 days	2-7 days	15 days	48%
Prepatellar bursitis	Avoid kneeling, stooping, and crouching	0 days	2-14 days	15 days	48%
Effusion	Avoid prolonged standing, walking, stooping, crouching, and heavy carrying	0 days	2-5 days	11 days	31%
Regional knee pain	Same as for effusion	0 days	2-4 days	4 days	50%

* These are general guidelines based on consensus or population sources and are never meant to be applied to an individual case without consideration of workplace factors, concurrent disease or other social or medical factors that can affect recovery.

** These parameters for disability duration are "consensus-optimal" targets as determined by a panel of ACOEM members in 1996, and reaffirmed by a panel of ACOEM members in 2002. In most cases persons with one non-severe extremity injury can return to modified duty immediately. Restrictions should take into consideration the opposite extremity also to prevent strain injuries to the uninjured extremity.

*** Based on the CDC NHIS (National Health Interview Survey), as compiled and reported in the 8th annual edition of *Official Disability Guidelines (ODG)*, © 2002 Work Loss Data Institute, all rights reserved.

Table 13-5. Ability of Various Techniques to Identify and Define Knee Pathology

Technique	Meniscus Tear	Ligament Strain	Ligament Tear	Patello-femoral Syndrome	Tendinitis	Prepatellar Bursitis	Regional Pain
History	++	++	++	++++	+++	++	++
Physical examination	++++	++++	++++	++	++++	++++	++
Laboratory studies	0	0	0	0	0	0	0
Electromyography/nerve conduction velocity (EMG/NCV) studies	0	0	0	0	0	0	0
Imaging studies							
Radiography[1]	0	0	0	+	0	0	0
Bone scan[1]	0	0	0	+	0	0	0
Arthrography[1]	+++	0	+	0	0	0	0
Computed tomography (CT)[1]	0	0	0	0	0	0	0
Magnetic resonance imaging (MRI)[1]	++++	+++	++++	+++	+++	+++	0

[1] Risk of complications (e.g., infection, radiation) highest for arthrography, less for radiography and computer tomography (CT), and lowest for bone scan and MRI.

- Inability to walk (four steps) or bear weight immediately or within a week of the trauma
- Inability to flex knee to 90 degrees

Most knee problems improve quickly once any red-flag issues are ruled out. For patients with significant hemarthrosis and a history of acute trauma, radiography is indicated to evaluate for fracture.

Reliance only on imaging studies to evaluate the source of knee symptoms may carry a significant risk of diagnostic confusion (false-positive test results) because of the possibility of identifying a problem that was present before symptoms began, and therefore has no temporal association with the current symptoms. Even so, remember that while experienced examiners usually can diagnose an ACL tear in the nonacute stage based on history and physical examination, these injuries are commonly missed or overdiagnosed by inexperienced examiners, making MRIs valuable in such cases. Also note that MRIs are superior to arthrography for both diagnosis and safety reasons. Table 13-5 provides a general comparison of the abilities of different techniques to identify physiologic insult and define anatomic defects.

Surgical Considerations

Referral for surgical consultation may be indicated for patients who have:

- Activity limitation for more than one month; and
- Failure of exercise programs to increase range of motion and strength of the musculature around the knee.

Earlier, emergency consultation is reserved for patients who may require drainage of acute effusions or hematomas. Referral for early repair of ligament or meniscus tears is still a matter for study because many patients can have satisfactory results with physical rehabilitation and avoid surgical risk.

A. Anterior Cruciate Ligament (ACL) Tears

Anterior cruciate ligament reconstruction generally is warranted only for patients who have significant symptoms of instability caused by ACL incompetence. Anterior cruciate ligament tears often are followed by an immediate effusion of the knee. A history of frequent giving-way episodes, or falls during activities that involve knee rotation, is consistent with the condition. A physical examination in an acute setting may be unrevealing because of the effusion and immobilization of the knee. In addition, the physical examination may reveal clear signs of instability as shown by positive Lachman, drawer, and pivot-shift tests. It is important to confirm the clinical findings with MRI evidence of a complete tear in the ligament. Especially in cases involving partial ACL tears, substantial improvement in symptoms may occur with rehabilitation alone. In complete tears, consideration should be given to the patient's age, normal activity level, and the degree of knee instability caused by the tear. Surgical reconstruction of the ACL may provide substantial benefit to active patients, especially those under 50 years old. For the patient whose work or life does not require significant loading of the knee and other stressful conditions, ACL repair may not be necessary.

Complications of wound infection and untoward anesthetic events are possible but rare. Anterior cruciate ligament reconstruction is noted in the literature to have various rates of failure, and it is appropriate to warn the patient of this possibility. After the procedure, the rehabilitation period involves six months of intense concentration and work by the patient; the patient's willingness to undergo the rehabilitative process must be determined by the practitioner and may be discussed with the patient. Besides providing the patient with educational literature, the practitioner may want to have the patient meet with someone who is going through the rehabilitation process. Such a meeting might help the patient determine whether he or she will be able to follow through with the intense process. Older patients may be less motivated to go through rehabilitation, and the work environment can be examined before deciding upon the need for ACL repair.

B. Meniscus Tears

Arthroscopic partial meniscectomy usually has a high success rate for cases in which there is clear evidence of a meniscus tear—symptoms other than simply pain (locking, popping, giving way, recurrent effusion); clear signs of a bucket-handle tear on examination (tenderness over the suspected tear but not over the entire joint line, and perhaps lack of full passive flexion); and consistent findings on MRI. However, patients suspected of having meniscal tears, but without progressive or severe activity limitation, can be encouraged to live with symptoms to retain the protective effect of the meniscus. If symptoms are lessening, conservative methods can maximize healing. In patients younger than 35, arthroscopic meniscal repair can preserve meniscal function, although the recovery time is longer compared to partial meniscectomy. Arthroscopy and meniscus surgery may not be equally beneficial for those patients who are exhibiting signs of degenerative changes.

C. Collateral Ligament Tears

Isolated collateral ligament tears have been shown to heal with excellent results without surgical intervention. When accompanying cruciate or meniscus injuries are ruled out, the patient can be treated non-operatively. Rehabilitative exercises will be needed.

D. Patellofemoral Syndrome

Although arthroscopic patellar shaving has been performed frequently for PFS, long-term improvement has not been proved and its efficacy is questionable. Severe patellar degeneration presents a problem not easily treated by surgery. Patellectomy and patellar replacements in reasonably active patients yield inconsistent results, and the procedures have a reasonable place only in treating patients with severe rheumatoid arthritis or another rheumatoid condition. Lateral arthroscopic release may be indicated in cases of recurrent subluxation of the patella, but surgical realignment of the extensor mechanism may be indicated in some patients.

E. Osteochondral Defects

Cartilage grafts and/or transplantations for osteochondral defects are still somewhat controversial despite some scientific evidence of their effectiveness. These procedures are technically difficult and require specific physician expertise. They may be effective in patients less than 40 years old with active lifestyles, exhibiting a singular, traumatically caused grade III or IV femoral condyle deficit. The diameter of the deficit should not exceed 20 mm for osteochondral autograft transplant system (OATS) procedures. The OATS technique could be a suitable and cost-effective therapy, possibly preventing, or, at least, delaying the development of osteoarthrosis. Grafts and transplants are not recommended for individuals with obesity, inflammatory conditions or osteoarthritis, other chondral defects, associated ligamentous or meniscus pathology, or who are greater than 55 years of age.

Summary of Recommendations and Evidence

See Table 13-6.

Table 13-6. Summary of Recommendations for Evaluating and Managing Knee Complaints

Clinical Measure	Recommended	Optional	Not Recommended
History	Basic history, with careful search for mechanism of injury (C, D)		
Physical exam	Focused physical exam, including ligament testing and careful search for any swelling (C, D)		
Patient education	Patient education Full disclosure of diagnostic accuracy, prognosis, and expectations of treatment (D)		
Medication (See Chapter 3)	Acetaminophen Aspirin (C, D)	Opioids for severe pain NSAIDs (C, D)	Use of opioids for more than 2 weeks (C, D)
Physical treatment methods	Nonoperative rehabilitation for medial collateral ligament injuries (C, D) Short postoperative rehabilitation for ACL repair prior to home exercise program (D) Conservative treatment for selected ruptures of the ACL (D) Exercises for cases of anterior knee pain or ligament strain(D)		Passive modalities without exercise program (D) Manipulation (D)
Aspirations and injections	Aspiration of tense acute effusions (D) Aspiration of tense prepatellar bursa (D)	Repeated aspirations or corticosteroid injections (D)	Aspiration through infected area (D)
Rest and immobilization	Short period of immobilization after an acute injury to relieve symptoms (C)	Functional bracing as part of a rehabilitation program (D)	Prophylactic braces (D) Prolonged bracing for ACL deficient knee (D)

Table 13-6. (continued)

Clinical Measure	Recommended	Optional	Not Recommended
Activity and exercise	Stretching Aerobic exercise Maximal activity of other body parts while recovering from knee injury (D)		Excessive rest (may lead to generalized debilitation) (D)
Detection of neurologic abnormalities			Electrical studies (contraindicated for nearly all knee injury diagnoses) (D)
Radiography	Plain-film radiographs for suspected red flags (C)	Plain-film radiographs for tense hemarthroses (C)	Routine radiographic film for most knee complaints or injuries (C)
Imaging	MRI study to determine extent of ACL tear preoperatively (C)		MRI for ligament collateral tears (C)
Surgical considerations	Arthroscopic meniscectomy or repair for severe mechanical symptoms and signs or serious activity limitations if MRI findings are consistent for meniscal tear (C, D) ACL repair for symptomatic instability (i.e., serious activity limitation) if results of Lachman and pivot-shift tests and MRI are positive (C, D)	ACL reconstruction before rehabilitation has been attempted (C, D)	Surgical repair of isolated MCL ruptures (D) Immediate surgical reconstruction of all ACL tears on basis of MRI findings without physical findings confirming diagnosis or worker life demands requiring high knee performance (D)

A = Strong research-based evidence (multiple relevant, high-quality scientific studies).
B = Moderate research-based evidence (one relevant, high-quality scientific study or multiple adequate scientific studies).
C = Limited research-based evidence (at least one adequate scientific study of patients with knee complaints).
D = Panel interpretation of information not meeting inclusion criteria for research-based evidence.

Algorithm 13-1. *Initial Evaluation of Occupational Knee Complaints*

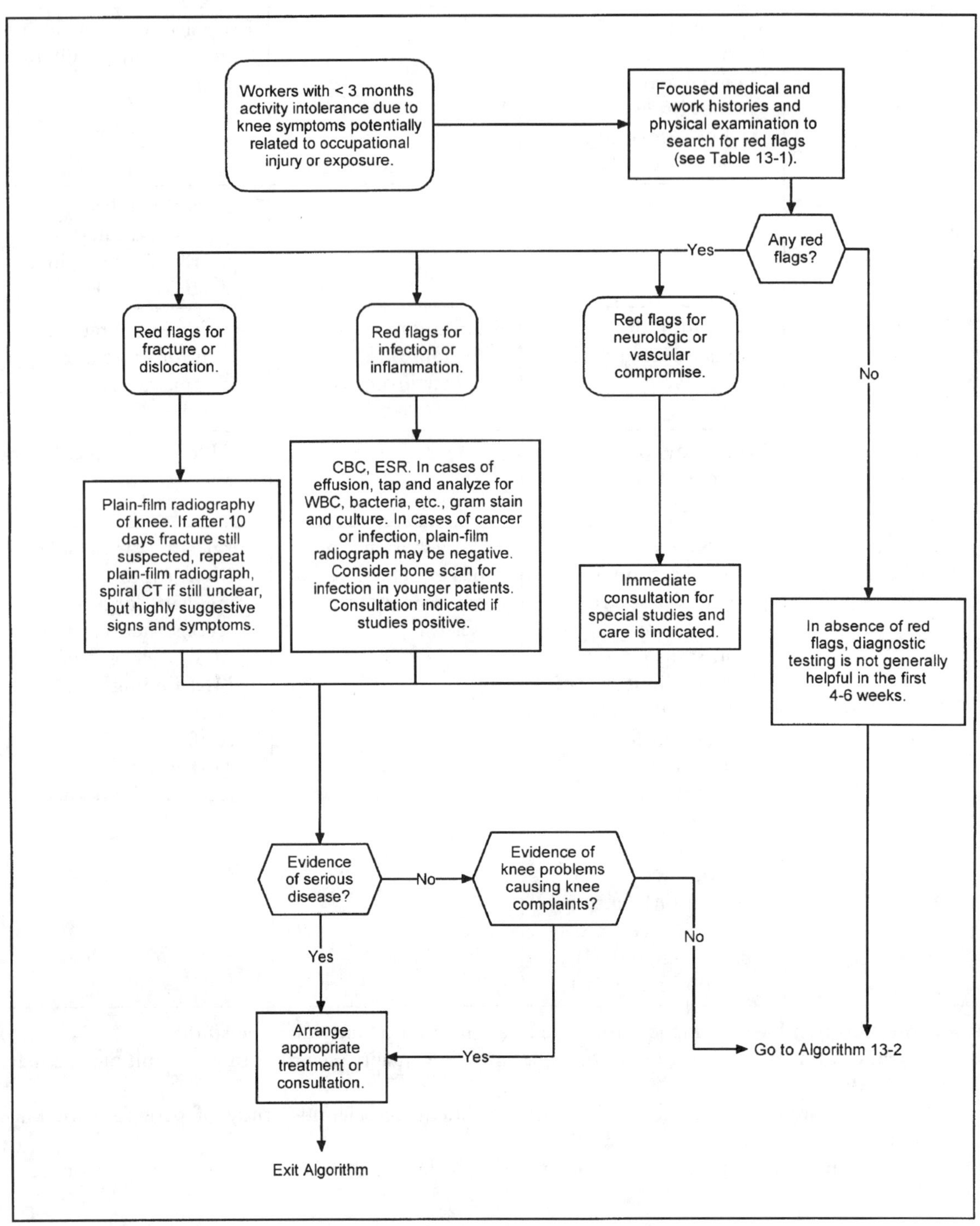

Algorithm 13-2. *Initial and Follow-up Management of Occupational Knee Complaints*

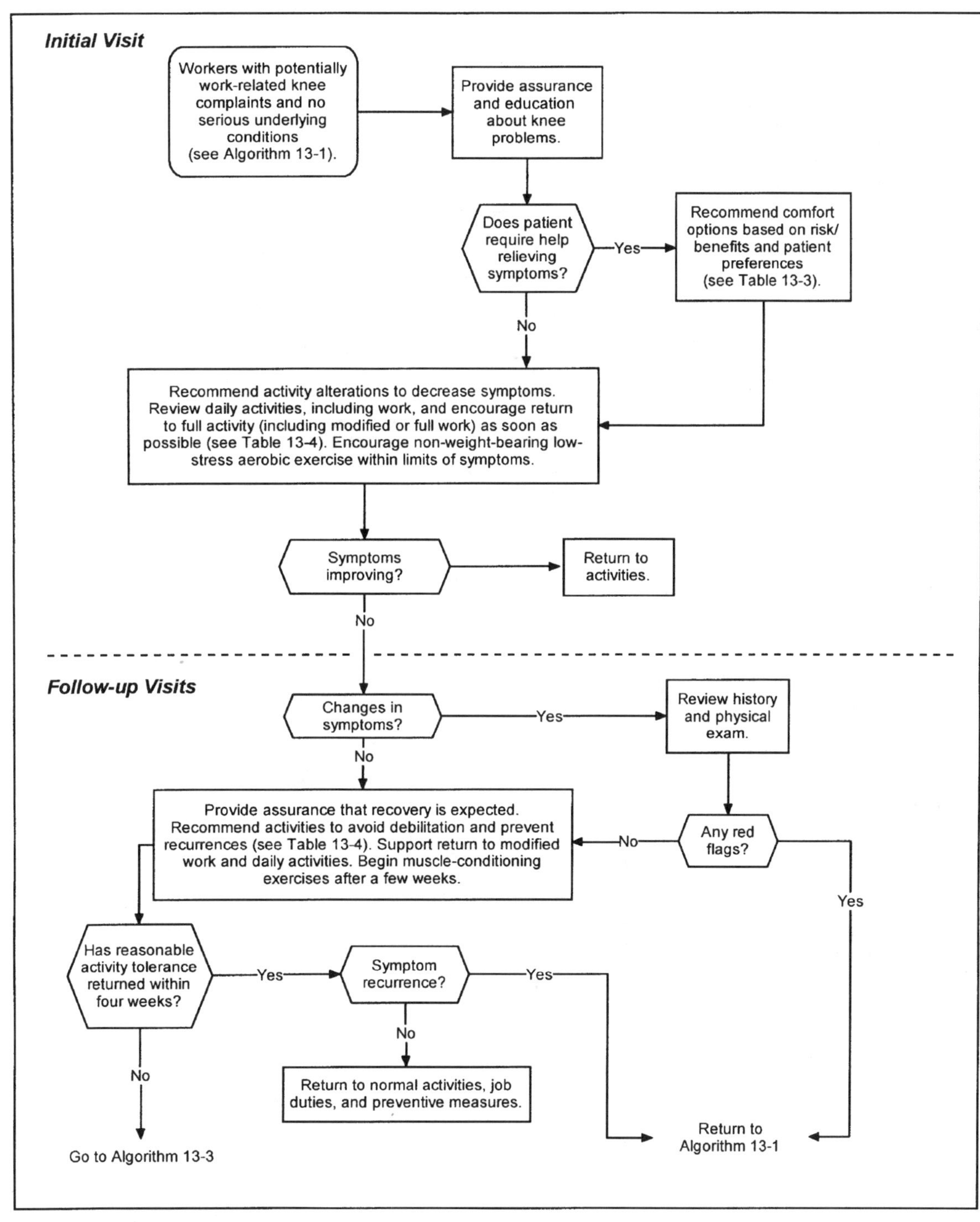

Algorithm 13-3. *Evaluation of Slow-to-recover Patients with Occupational Knee Complaints (Symptoms > 4 Weeks)*

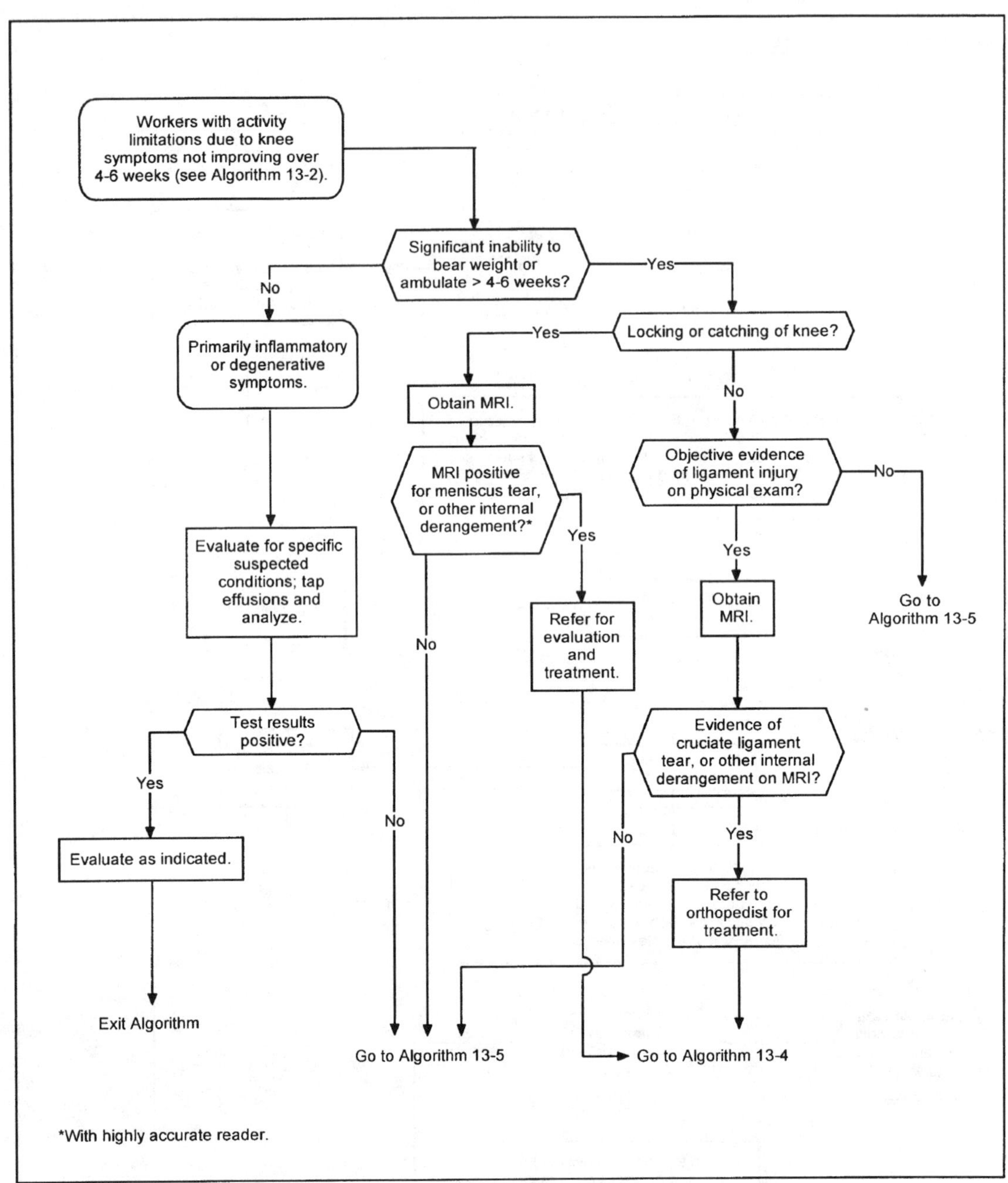

Algorithm 13-4. *Surgical Considerations for Patients with Anatomic Evidence of Torn Meniscus or Ligament and Persistent Knee Symptoms*

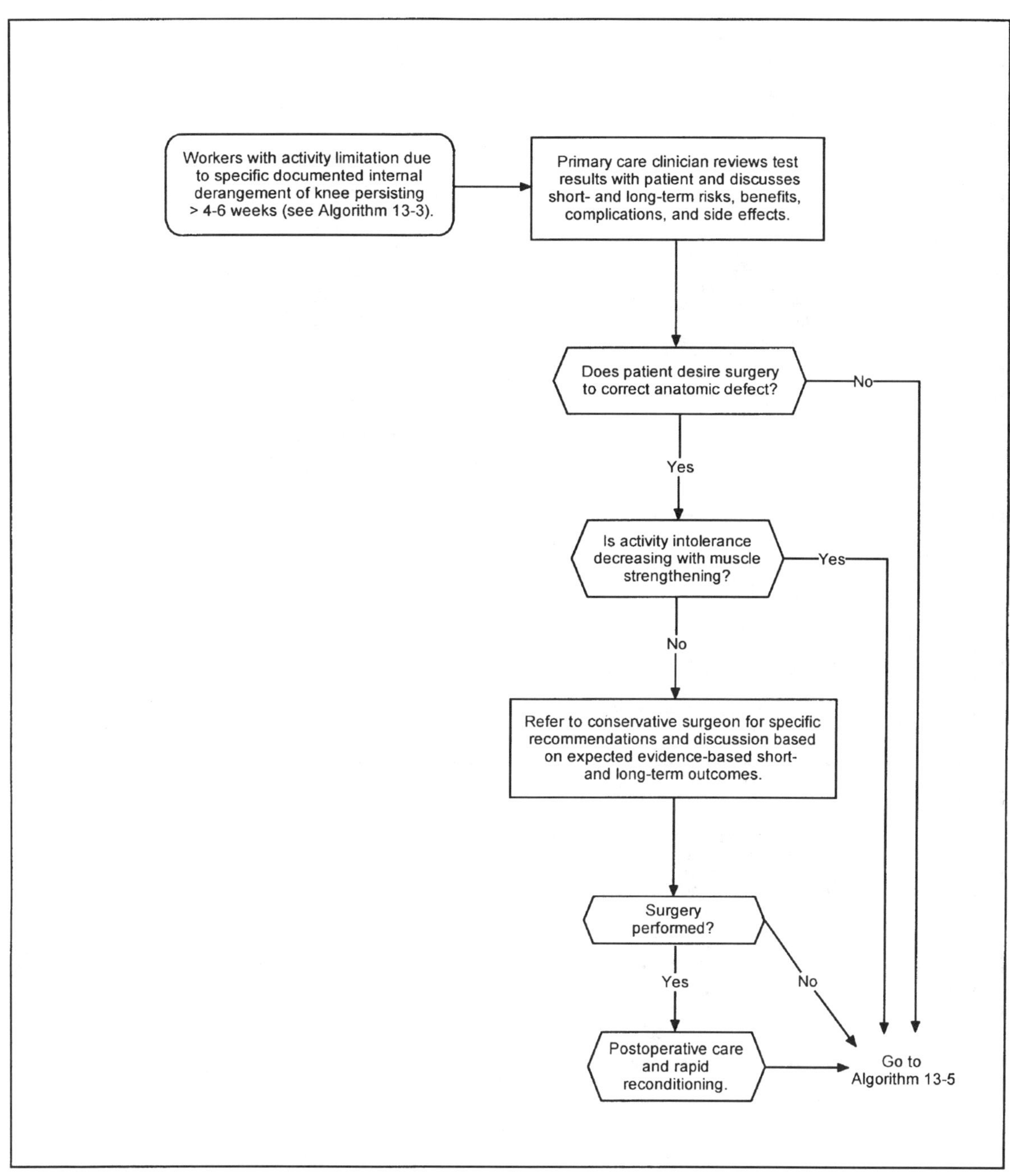

Algorithm 13-5. *Further Management of Occupational Knee Complaints*

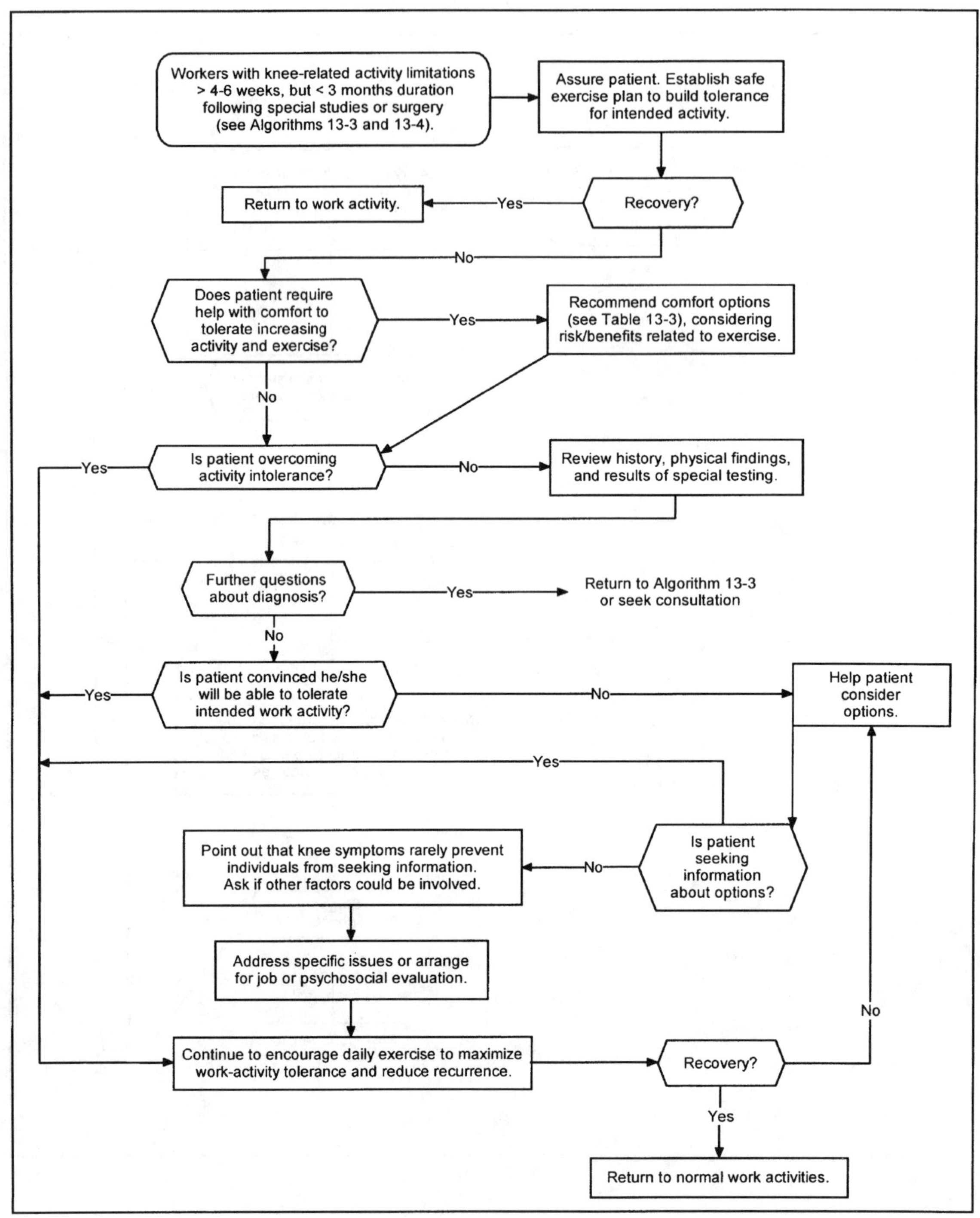

References

HISTORY

Hoher J, Munster A, Klein J, et al. Validation and application of a subject knee questionnaire. *Knee Surg Sports Traumatol Arthrosc.* 1995;3:26-33.

Kujala UM, Jaakkola LH, Koskinen SK, Taimela S, Hurme M, Nelimarka O. Scoring of patellofemoral disorders. *Arthroscopy.* 1993;9:159-63.

Smith JP III, Barrett GR. Medial and lateral meniscal tear patterns in anterior cruciate ligament-deficient knees. A prospective analysis of 575 tears. *Am J Sports Med.* 2001;29(4):415-9.

PHYSICAL EXAMINATION

Cooperman JM, Riddle DL, Rothstein JM. Reliability and validity of judgments of the integrity of the anterior cruciate ligament of the knee using the Lachman's test. *Phys Ther.* 1990;70:225-33.

Curtin W, O'Farrell D, McGoldrick F, et al. The correlation between clinical diagnosis of knee pathology and findings at arthroscopy. *Ir J Med Sci.* 1992;161:135-6.

Donaldson WF III, Warren RF, Wickiewicz T. A comparison of acute anterior cruciate ligament examinations. Initial versus examination under anesthesia. *Am J Sports Med.* 1985;13:5-10.

Evans PJ, Bell GD, Frank C. Prospective evaluation of the McMurray test. *Am J Sports Med.* 1993;21:604-8.

Fowler PJ, Lubliner JA. The predictive value of five clinical signs in the evaluation of meniscal pathology. *Arthroscopy.* 1989;5:184-6.

Gurtler RA, Stine R, Torg JS. Lachman test evaluated. Quantification of a clinical observation. *Clin Orthop.* 1987;216:141-50.

Johnson DL, Warner JJ. Diagnosis for anterior cruciate ligament surgery. *Clin Sports Med.* 1993;12:671-84.

Katz JW, Fingeroth RJ. The diagnostic accuracy of ruptures of the anterior cruciate ligament comparing the Lachman test, the anterior drawer sign, and the pivot shift test in acute and chronic knee injuries. *Am J Sports Med.* 1986;14:88-91.

Lucie RS, Wiedel JD, Messner DG. The acute pivot shift: clinical correlation. *Am J Sports Med.* 1984;12:189-91.

Oberlander MA, Shalvoy RM, Hughston JC. The accuracy of the clinical knee examination documented by arthroscopy: a prospective study. *Am J Sports Med.* 1993;221:773-8.

Roos EM, Roos HP, Ekdahl C, Lohmander LS. Knee injury and Osteoarthritis Outcome Score (KOOS)—validation of a Swedish version. *Scand J Med Sci Sports.* 1998;8(6):439-48.

Sandberg R, Balkfors B, Henricson A, et al. Stability tests in knee ligament injuries. *Arch Orthop Traum Surg.* 1986;106:5-7.

Schweitzer ME, Tran D, Deely DM, et al. Medial collateral ligament injuries: evaluation of multiple signs, prevalence and location of associated bone bruises, and assessment with MR imaging. *Radiology.* 1995;194:825-9.

Simonsen O, Jensen J, Mouritsen P, et al. The accuracy of clinical examination of injury of the knee joint. *Injury.* 1984;16:96-101.

Strand T, Solheim E. Clinical tests versus KT-1000 instrumented laxity test in acute anterior cruciate ligament tears. *Int J Sports Med.* 1995;16:51-3.

Thomee R, Augustsson J, Karlsson J. Patellofemoral pain syndrome: a review of current issues. *Sports Med.* 1999;28(4):245-62.

Watson CJ, Leddy HM, Dynjan TD, Parham JL. Reliability of the lateral pull test and tilt test to assess patellar alignment in subjects with symptomatic knees: student raters. *J Orthop Sports Phys Ther.* 2001;31(7):368-74.

ALTERNATIVE MEDICINE

Ezzo J, Hadhazy V, Birch S, et al. Acupuncture for osteoarthritis of the knee: a systematic review. *Arthritis Rheum.* 2001;44(4):819-2521.

Jensen R, Gothesen O, Liseth K, Baerheim A. Acupuncture treatment of patellofemoral pain syndrome. *J Altern Complement Med.* 1999;5(6):521-7.

Tillu A, Tillu S, Vowler S. Effect of acupuncture on knee function in advanced osteoarthritis of the knee: a prospective, non-randomised controlled study. *Acupunct Med.* 2002;20(1):19-21.

MEDICATIONS

See Chapter 3 references.

PHYSICAL TREATMENT METHODS

Beynnon BD, Fleming BC, Johnson RJ, et al. Anterior cruciate ligament strain behavior during rehabilitation exercises in vivo. *Am J Sports Med.* 1995;23:24-34.

Brody LT, Thein JM. Nonoperative treatment for patellofemoral pain. *J Orthop Sports Phys Ther.* 1998;28(5):336-44.

Brosseau L, Casimiro L, Milne S, et al. Deep transverse friction massage for treating tendinitis (Cochrane Review). In: *The Cochrane Library.* Issue 2; 2002. Oxford: Update Software.

Brosseau L, Casimiro L, Robinson V, et al. Therapeutic ultrasound for treating patellofemoral pain syndrome (Cochrane Review). In: *The Cochrane Library.* Issue 2; 2002. Oxford: Update Software.

Ciccotti MG, Lombardo SJ, Nonweiler B, et al. Non-operative treatment of ruptures of the anterior cruciate ligament in middle-aged patients. Results after long-term follow-up. *J Bone Joint Surg Am.* 1994;76(9):1315-21.

Colorado Division of Workers' Compensation. *Medical Treatment Guidelines, Lower Extremity Injury.* December 1, 2001.

Crossley K, Bennell K, Green S, McConnell J. A systematic review of physical interventions for patellofemoral pain syndrome. *Clin J Sport Med.* 2001;11(2):103-10.

D'hondt NE, Struijs PAA, Kerkhoffs GM, et al. Orthotic devices for treating patellofemoral pain syndrome (Cochrane Review). In: *The Cochrane Library.* Issue 2; 2002. Oxford: Update Software.

Juhn MS. Patellofemoral pain syndrome: a review and guidelines for treatment. *Am Fam Physician.* 1999;60(7):2012-22.

Miller MD, Hinkin DT, Wisnowski JW. The efficacy of orthotics for anterior knee pain in military trainees. A preliminary report. *Am J Knee Surg.* 1997;10(1):10-13.

Odensten M, Hamberg P, Nordin M, et al. Surgical or conservative treatment of the acutely torn anterior cruciate ligament. A randomized study with short-term follow-up observations. *Clinical Orthop.* 1985;198:87-93.

Osiri M, Welch V, Brosseau L, et al. Transcutaneous electrical nerve stimulation for knee osteoarthritis. *Cochrane Database Syst Rev.* 2000;(4):CD002823.

Philadelphia Panel. Philadelphia Panel evidence-based clinical practice guidelines on selected rehabilitation interventions for knee pain. *Phys Ther.* 2001;81(10):1675-700.

Rudzki SJ. Injuries in Australian army recruits. Part I: Decreased incidence and severity of injury seen with reduced running distance. Part II: Location and cause of injuries seen in recruits. *Military Med.* 1997;162(7):472-6.

Sandberg R, Balkfors B, Nilsson B, et al. Operative versus non-operative treatment of recent injuries to the ligaments of the knee. *J Bone Joint Surg [Am].* 1987;69:1120-6.

Schneider F, Labs K, Wagner S. Chronic patellofemoral pain syndrome: alternatives for cases of therapy resistance. *Knee Surg Sports Traumatol Arthrosc.* 2001;9(5):290-5.

Thomee R. A comprehensive treatment approach for patellofemoral pain syndrome in young women. *Phys Ther.* 1997;77(12):1690-703.

Thomson LC, Handoll HHG, Cunningham A, Shaw PC. Physiotherapist-led programmes and interventions for rehabilitation of anterior cruciate ligament, medial collateral ligament and meniscal injuries of the knee in adults (Cochrane Review). In: *The Cochrane Library.* Issue 2; 2002. Oxford: Update Software.

Welch V, Brosseau L, Peterson J, Shea B, Tugwell P, Wells G. Therapeutic ultrasound for osteoarthritis of the knee. *Cochrane Database Syst Rev.* 2001;(3):CD003132.

Zatterstrom R, Friden T, Lindstrand A, et al. Muscle training in chronic anterior cruciate ligament insufficiency—a comparative study. *Scand J Rehabil Med.* 1992;24:91-7.

Zatterstrom R, Friden T, Lindstrand A, Moritz U. Early rehabilitation of acute anterior cruciate ligament injury—a randomized clinical trial. *Scand J Med Sci Sports.* 1998;8(3):154-9.

Zatterstrom R, Friden T, Lindstrand A, Moritz U. Rehabilitation following acute anterior cruciate ligament injury—a 12-month follow-up of a randomized clinical trial. *Scand J Med Sci Sports.* 2000;10(3):156-63.

PREVENTION

BenGal S, Lowe J, Mann G, Finsterbush A, Matan Y. The role of the knee brace in the prevention of anterior knee pain syndrome. *Am J Sports Med.* 1997;25(1):118-22.

Felson DT, Zhang Y, Anthony JM, Naimark A, Anderson JJ. Weight loss reduces the risk for symptomatic knee osteoarthritis in women. The Framingham Study. *Ann Intern Med.* 1992;116(7):535-9.

Hartig DE, Henderson JM. Increasing hamstring flexibility decreases lower extremity overuse injuries in military basic trainees. *Am J Sports Med.* 1999;27(2):173-6.

Pope R, Herbert R, Kirwan J. Effects of ankle dorsiflexion range and pre-exercise calf muscle on injury risk in Army recruits. *Aust J Physiotherapy.* 1998;44(3):165-72.

Pope RP, Herbert RK, Kirwan JD, Graham BJ. A randomized trial of preexercise stretching for prevention of lower limb injury. *Med Sci Sports Exerc.* 2000;32(2):271-7.

Yeung EW, Yeung SS. Interventions for preventing lower limb soft-tissue injuries in runners (Cochrane Review). In: *The Cochrane Library.* Issue 2; 2002. Oxford: Update Software.

REST AND IMMOBILIZATION

Deppen RJ, Landfried MJ. Efficacy of prophylactic knee bracing in high school football players. *J Orthop Sports Phys Ther.* 1994;20:243-6.

Finestone A, Radin EL, Lev B, et al. Treatment of overuse patellofemoral pain: prospective randomized controlled clinical trial in a military setting. *Clin Orthop.* 1993;293:208-10.

Vailas JC, Pink M. Biomechanical effects of functional knee bracing: practical implications. *Sports Med.* 1993;15:210-8.

RADIOGRAPHY

Felson DT, Zhang Y, Hannan MT, et al. Risk factors for incident radiographic knee osteoarthritis in the elderly: the Framingham Study. *Arthritis Rheum.* 1997;40(4):728-33.

Ferguson J, Knottenbelt JD. Lipohaemarthrosis in knee trauma: an experience of 907 cases. *Injury.* 1994;25:311-2.

Hess T, Rupp S, Hopf T, et al. Lateral tibial avulsion fractures and disruptions to the anterior cruciate ligament: a clinical study of their incidence and correlation. *Clin Orthop.* 1994;303:193-7.

Roos H, Lindberg H, Gardsell P, et al. The prevalence of gonarthrosis and its relation to meniscectomy in former soccer players. *Am J Sports Med.* 1994:219-22.

Seaberg DC, Jackson R. Clinical decision rule for knee radiographs. *Am J Emerg Med.* 1994;12:541-3.

Stiell IG, Greenburg GH, Wells GA, et al. Derivation of a decision rule for the use of radiography in acute knee injuries. *Ann Emerg Med.* 1995; 26:405-13.

Stiell IG, Greenberg GH, Wells GA, et al. Prospective validation of a decision rule for the use of radiography in acute knee injuries. *JAMA.* 1996; 275:611-15.

Weber JE, Jackson RE, Peacock WF, Swor RA, Carley R, Larkin GL. Clinical decision rules discriminate between fractures and nonfractures in acute isolated knee trauma. *Ann Emerg Med.* 1995;26:429-33.

OTHER IMAGING PROCEDURES

Ross G, Chapman AW, Newberg AR, Sheller AD. Magnetic resonance imaging for the evaluation of acute posterolateral complex injuries of the knee. *Am J Sports Med.* 1997;25:444-8.

Schweitzer ME, Tran D, Deely DM, et al. Medial collateral ligament injuries: evaluation of multiple signs, prevalence and location of associated bone bruises, and assessment with MR imaging. *Radiology.* 1995;194:825-9.

Yao L, Dungan D, Seeger LL. MR imaging of tibial collateral ligament injury: comparison with clinical examination. *Skeletal Radiol.* 1994;23:521-4.

SURGERY

Agneskirchner JD, Brucker P, Burkart A, Imhoff AB. Large osteochondral defects of the femoral condyle: press-fit transplantation of the posterior femoral condyle (MEGA-OATS). *Knee Surg Sports Traumatol Arthrosc.* 2002;10(3):160-8.

Andersson C, Odensten M, Good L, et al. Surgical or non-surgical treatment of acute rupture of the anterior cruciate ligament: a randomized study with long-term follow-up. *J Bone Joint Surg [Am].* 1989;71:965-74.

Bobic V. Arthroscopic osteochondral autograft transplantation in anterior cruciate ligament reconstruction: a preliminary clinical study. *Knee Surg Sports Traumatol Arthrosc.* 1996;3(4):262-4.

Christen B, Jakob RP. Fractures associated with patellar ligament grafts in cruciate ligament surgery. *J Bone Joint Surg [Br].* 1992;74:617-9.

Cimino PM. The incidence of meniscal tears associated with acute anterior cruciate ligament disruption secondary to snow skiing accidents. *Arthroscopy.* 1994;10:198-200.

Engebretsen L, Benum P, Fasting O, et al. A prospective, randomized study of three surgical techniques for treatment of acute ruptures of the anterior cruciate ligament. *Am J Sports Med.* 1990;18:585-90.

Englund M, Roos EM, Roos HP, Lohmander LS. Patient-relevant outcomes fourteen years after meniscectomy: influence of type of meniscal tear and size of resection. *Rheumatology (Oxford).* 2001;40(6):631-9.

Gudad R. Autologous osteochondral transplantation (mosaicplasty) in the treatment of femoral condyle defects. *Medicina (Kaunas).* 2002;38(1):52-7.

Hazel WA Jr, Rand JA, Morrey BF. Results of meniscectomy in the knee with anterior cruciate ligament deficiency. *Clin Orthop.* 1993;292:232-8.

Howell JR, Handoll HHG. Surgical treatment for meniscal injuries of the knee in adults (Cochrane Review). In: *The Cochrane Library.* Issue 2; 2002. Oxford: Update Software.

Jager A, Starker M, Herresthal J. Can meniscus refixation prevent early development of arthrosis in the knee joint? Long-term results. *Zentralbl Chir.* 2000;125(6):532-5.

Jarvinen M, Natri A, Lehto M, et al. Reconstruction of chronic anterior cruciate ligament insufficiency in athletes using a bone-patellar tendon-bone autograft. A two-year follow up study. *Int Orthop.* 1995;19:1-6.

Jaureguito JW, Elliot JS, Lietner T, et al. The effects of arthroscopic partial lateral meniscectomy in an otherwise normal knee: a retrospective review of functional, clinical, and radiographic results. *Arthroscopy.* 1995;11:29-36.

Jensen NC, Riis J, Robertsen K, et al. Arthroscopic repair of the ruptured meniscus: one to 6.3 years follow up. *Arthroscopy.* 1994;10:211-4.

Jomha NM, Borton DC, Clingeleffer AJ, Pinczewski LA. Long-term osteoarthritic changes in anterior cruciate ligament reconstructed knees. *Clin Orthop.* 1999;(358):188-93.

Marcus A. Popular surgery for knee arthritis falls short; study finds arthroscopic procedure doesn't work. *Health Scout News.* July 10, 2002.

Morelli M, Nagamori J, Miniaci A. Management of chondral injuries of the knee by osteochondral autogenous transfer (mosaicplasty). *J Knee Surg.* 2002;15(3):185-90.

Moseley JB, O'Malley K, Petersen NJ, et al. A controlled trial of arthroscopic surgery for osteoarthritis of the knee. *N Engl J Med.* 2002;347(2):81-8.

Navarro R, Cohen M, Filho MC, da Silva RT. The arthroscopic treatment of osteochondritis dissecans of the knee with autologous bone sticks. *Arthroscopy.* 2002;18(8):840-4.

Odensten M, Hamberg P, Nordin M, et al. Surgical or conservative treatment of the acutely torn anterior cruciate ligament. A randomized study with short-term follow-up observations. *Clin Orthop Related Research.* 1985;198:87-93.

Sandberg R, Balkfors B, Nilsson B, et al. Operative versus non-operative treatment of recent injuries to the ligaments of the knee: a prospective randomized study. *J Bone Joint Surg [Am].* 1987;69:1120-6.

Wasiak J, Villanueva E. Autologous cartilage implantation for full thickness articular cartilage defects of the knee (Cochrane Review). In: *The Cochrane Library.* Issue 4; 2002. Oxford: Update Software.

***Master Algorithm**. ACOEM Guidelines for Care of Acute and Subacute Occupational Ankle and Foot Complaints*

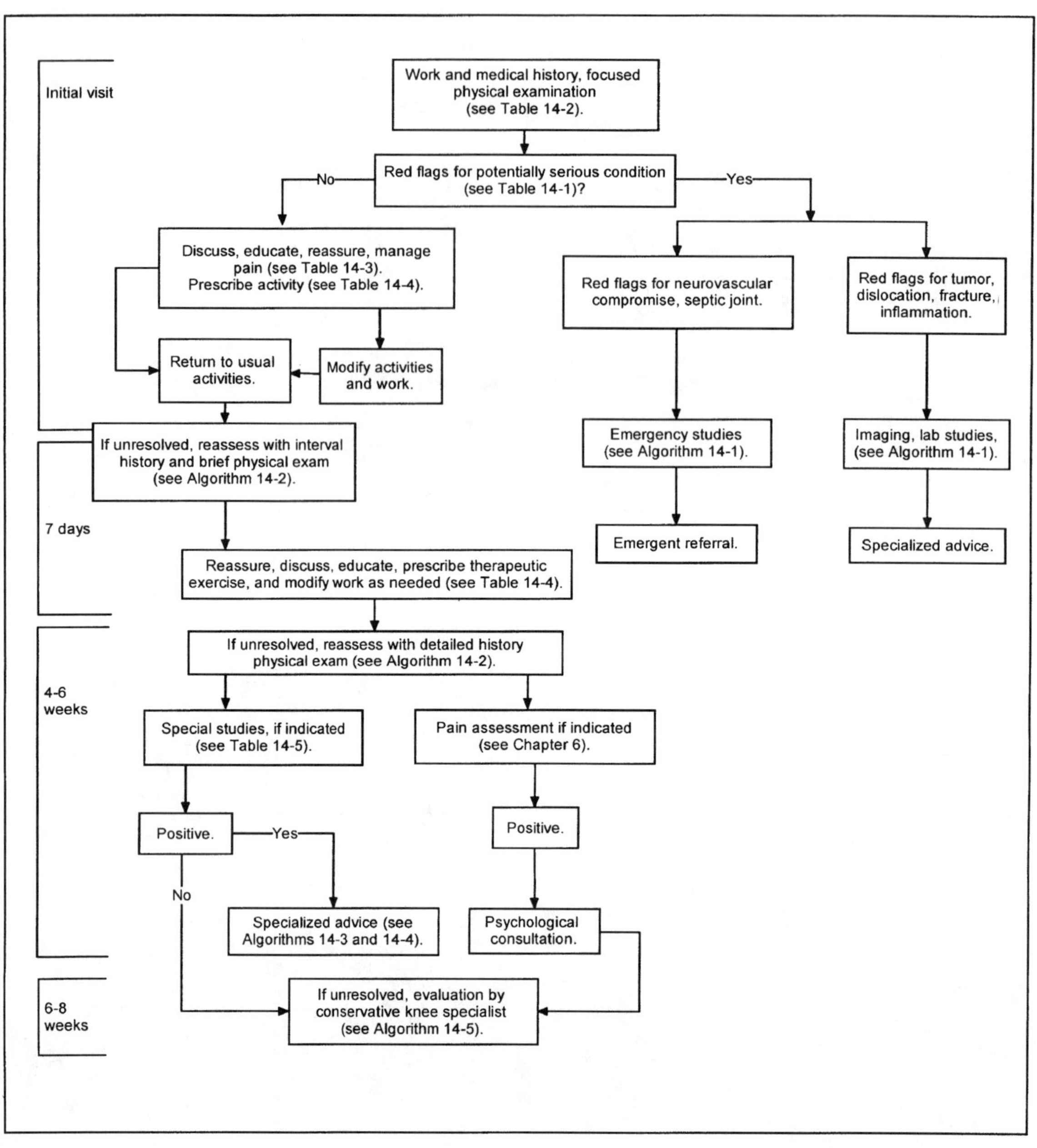

14 Ankle and Foot Complaints

General Approach and Basic Principles

Foot and ankle complaints that are potentially work related are common problems presenting to occupational and primary care providers; they are among the ten most common causes of reported work-related health complaints and workers' compensation claims. These complaints account for about 15% of claims, 7% of costs, and 6 to 7% of total lost workdays in workers' compensation, ranking them in the top ten for financial severity as well.

Recommendations for assessing and treating adults with potentially work-related ankle and foot problems are presented in this clinical practice guideline. Topics include the initial assessment and diagnosis of patients with acute and subacute ankle or foot complaints that may be work related, identification of red flags that may indicate the presence of a serious underlying medical condition, initial management, diagnostic considerations and special studies for identification of clinical pathology, work-relatedness, modified duty and activity, return to work, and further considerations, including the management of delayed recovery.

Algorithms for patient management are included. This chapter's master algorithm schematizes the recommended way primary care and occupational medicine practitioners should manage patients with acute or subacute ankle and foot complaints. The following text, tables, and numbered algorithms amplify the guidelines of the master algorithm.

The principal recommendations for assessing and treating patients with ankle and foot complaints are as follows:

- The initial appropriate assessment of patients with ankle and foot problems focuses on detecting red-flag indicators of potentially serious injury or disease.
- In the absence of red flags, work-related foot and ankle complaints can be safely and effectively managed by occupational or primary care providers. The focus is on monitoring for complications, facilitating activity and the healing process, and facilitating return to work in a modified- or full-duty capacity.

- Relieving discomfort can be accomplished most safely by temporary immobilization, elevation, use of heat and cold, restricted weight bearing, and systemic nonprescription analgesics.
- Patients recovering from acute foot and ankle injury or infection should be encouraged to return to modified work as soon as their condition permits.
- If symptoms persist more than four weeks, referral for specialty care may be indicated.
- Nonphysical factors, such as psychosocial, workplace, or socioeconomic problems and non-anatomic pain, should be addressed in an effort to resolve delayed recovery.

Initial Assessment

Thorough medical and work histories and a focused physical examination (see Chapter 2) are sufficient for the initial assessment of a patient complaining of potentially work-related foot or ankle symptoms. The initial medical history and examination involves evaluating for serious underlying conditions, including sources of foot and ankle pain in other parts of the body. Certain findings in this assessment raise suspicion of serious underlying medical conditions, which are referred to as red flags (see Table 14-1). Their absence rules out the need for special studies, referral, or inpatient care during the first four weeks, during which time spontaneous recovery is expected (provided any contributing workplace factors are mitigated). Foot and ankle complaints can then be classified into one of four working categories:

- **Potentially serious foot and ankle conditions:** fractures, acute dislocation, neurovascular compromise, tendon rupture, or infection
- Acute **mechanical disorders:** derangements of the foot or ankle related to acute trauma, such as ligament strain
- **Chronic mechanical or degenerative disorders:** possible consequences of aging or repetitive use, or a combination thereof, such as degenerative arthritis and chronic tendinitis, tenosynovitis, or tendinosis
- Referred pain or paresthesias
- **Nonspecific disorders:** occurring in the foot or ankle and suggesting neither internal derangement nor referred pain

Medical History

Asking the patient open-ended questions, such as those listed below, allows the clinician to gauge the need for further discussion or specific inquiries to obtain more detailed information (see also Chapter 2):

Table 14-1. Red Flags for Potentially Serious Ankle and Foot Conditions

Disorder	Medical History	Physical Examination
Fracture	History of significant trauma History of abnormal mobility History of deformity with or without spontaneous or self-reduction Painful swelling of ankle or foot	Significant swelling Significant bruising or hematoma Deformity of ankle or foot Abnormal mobility Bony crepitus
Dislocation	History of significant ankle or foot trauma History of ankle or foot deformity with or without spontaneous reduction or self-reduction	Swelling Possible deformity of ankle or foot
Infection	History of swelling of ankle or foot with increasingly red, hot area on the ankle or foot History of fever or chills History of diabetes or immunosuppression (e.g., transplant, chemotherapy, HIV)	Palpable mass Local heat, swelling, erythema Systemic signs of sepsis
Inflammation	History of inflammatory arthritis or autoimmune disease	Swelling and effusion of ankle or foot
Rapidly progressive neurologic compromise	History of neuropathy, decreased or absent sensation History of neurologic disease History of diabetes History of dislocation or fracture	Decreased sensation in feet and ankles Loss of vibratory or positional sense Dermatomal distribution Absent ankle jerk Motor loss in specific distribution Painless swelling (Charcot's joint)
Rapidly progressive vascular compromise	History of diabetes History of peripheral vascular disease or bypass grafts History of dislocation or fracture	Decreased or absent foot and ankle pulses Decreased capillary filling Cold, pale extremity
Acute gout	History of sudden recurring attacks of joint pain in the toes	Swelling Red, tender, warm first metatarsal joint
Achilles rupture	History of trauma Sharp pain to the Achilles tendon, may be accompanied by loud pop	Swelling and bruising Inability to point foot downward and stand or walk comfortably

WHAT ARE YOUR PROBLEMS WITH YOUR FOOT OR ANKLE?

- When did they begin?
- Did a specific inciting event cause the symptoms?
- Are your problems pain, weakness, and/or limited motion in your ankle or foot?
- For traumatic injuries: Was the area deformed or bent? Did you lose any blood or have an open wound?
- Are the problems located primarily in the foot or ankle? Do you have pain or other problems elsewhere (e.g., low back, knee)?
- Are your problems constant or intermittent?
- What makes the problem worse?
- What makes the problem better?
- What can't you do, and/or what do you have difficulty doing as a result of these problems?
- Can you walk or bear weight? For how long?
- How long have your activities been limited? More than four weeks?
- Have your problems changed?
- Have you had similar episodes previously?
- Have you had previous testing or treatment? With whom?
- What do you think caused the problem? How do you think it is related to work?
- What are your specific job duties?
- What activities cause problems for you?
- How long do you spend performing each duty on a daily basis?
- What other activities (hobbies, workouts, sports) do you engage in at home or elsewhere? Is this problem limiting you in those activities? If so, how? How often?
- What would you like to be able to do that you cannot do now?
- Do you have other medical problems?
- What do you hope we can accomplish during this visit?

A medical history suggesting pathology originating somewhere other than in the foot or ankle may warrant examination of the back, knee on the affected side, or other areas.

Physical Examination

Guided by the medical history, the preferred method of physical examination includes:

- General observation of the patient
- Regional examination of the feet and ankles
- Neurologic screening

In most cases, the examination is subjective because patient response or interpretation is required for findings on the examination. Some patients with foot or ankle problems have no objective findings. Some will present with painful or excessive range of motion and areas of tenderness or stiffness (loss of mobility). Atrophy is an objective finding and may be present in long-standing cases. A "frozen" area (marked loss of motion) may be present, as may signs of infection or deformity due to fracture or dislocation, although these cases are much less common than nonspecific pain.

Though it may seem a point too obvious to warrant mention, the physician should specifically note which ankle or foot—left or right—is the subject of the patient's complaints. Not infrequently, injured workers have prior workers' compensation claims that involve the opposite ankle or foot. Any ambiguity in documentation can lead to delay in acceptance of the patient's workers' compensation claim, delay in the authorization of time-loss benefits, delay in the authorization of payment of medical care, or even outright denial of the workers' compensation claim.

The physician should seek objective evidence of pathology that is consistent with the patient's subjective complaints. In many cases, careful examination will reveal one or more truly objective findings, such as swelling, deformity, atrophy, reflex changes, or spasm. Any such findings should be thoroughtly documented in the medical record both for reference during future visits, and for the value the information will have in the patient's workers' compensation claim. For some patients with ankle or foot complaints, however, there are no objective findings. Meticulous documentation of the patient's complaints at each visit is of the utmost importance in such cases.

A. Regional Foot and Ankle Examination

In the recommended focused foot and ankle examination, the clinician observes the foot for heel position and arch shape as the patient bears weight. Inspecting the medial and lateral aspects of the foot and ankle can help determine the most likely site of injury because swelling and ecchymosis often occur over the site of injury. Deformities due to fractures or dislocations may be visible abnormalities. Signs of infection (e.g., redness, heat, swelling) also may be visible.

Carefully palpate the foot for tender areas, and assess the lateral and medial ligamentous structures of the ankle. The distal fibula, distal tibia, proximal fibula, and proximal fifth metatarsal should be palpated because they are the areas most often injured in avulsion fractures. Inspecting and palpating the tendinous insertions of the leg muscles also may aid in the diagnosing the injury and rule out a more serious condition, such as an Achilles tendon rupture. The range of motion of the foot and ankle should be determined both actively and passively, for instance, by asking the patient to move the foot and ankle within the limits of symptoms and then engaging in gentle range of motion of the joints (rear foot, midfoot, forefoot, toes) passively for comparison. Resisted range of motion may be used to assess strength and the presence of injury in associated muscles. Atrophy of calf muscles is an objective finding, but one that arises only after weeks to months of problems.

Ligamentous testing can be performed to assess the presence of ankle instability. It includes the anterior drawer test, talar tilt test, and squeeze test. Observe adjacent ankle structures, such as the tendons. The anterior drawer test is performed with the foot in neutral position. Hold the foot firmly at the heel while applying a backward, posterior force to the tibia. If significant anterior displacement of the foot relative to the distal tibia can be felt, it indicates a significant injury to the anterior talofibular ligament. The talar tilt test gently applies inversion force to the affected ankle; due to immediate post-injury pain, this examination may best be performed after pain has subsided. A positive test indicates lateral ligamentous laxity. Findings from both the anterior drawer test and talar tilt test can be compared with the unaffected, contralateral ankle. The squeeze test may be used if medial injury or severe lateral injury has taken place. Place the hands about six inches distal to the knee with thumbs on the fibula and fingers on the medial tibia. Then squeeze the leg to bring the fibula and tibia together. Pain during this test indicates syndesmotic injury, and prolonged recovery is likely.

Observe weight-bearing skeletal alignment of the foot and ankle in relation to the whole body for local skeletal malalignment and correlated and compensatory motions and postures. Observe foot and ankle motion during gait; during other work-related tasks and other home-related tasks. Is pain the limiter of the task? Observe:

- Strength
- Pain location, intensity, link with activity
- Stiffness
- Balance
- Ligamentous laxity
- Joint accessory motion

B. Neurovascular Screening

Assessment of the neurologic and vascular status of the foot and ankle (including skin temperature, peripheral pulses, and the motor, reflex, and sensory status of the foot and ankle as well as the more proximal surrounding structures) is recommended. Observe the skin for trophic changes. Examination of lumbosacral nerve root function also is in order because L5 radiculopathy can affect the foot and toe extensors and S1 radiculopathy can affect plantar flexion (see Chapter 12). Patients with peripheral neuropathy (e.g., diabetics) may have decreased sensation in the foot or ankle and neuropathic joints presenting as acute swelling or inflammation. Peripheral nerve entrapment may be manifested as foot drop if the peroneal nerve at the knee is involved or, rarely, as a tarsal tunnel syndrome, presenting as numbness of the plantar surface of the foot and toes. Foot drop also can be seen in L5 neuropathy due to an L4-5 disc protrusion.

C. Assessing Red Flags

Physical examination evidence of neurovascular compromise that correlates with the medical history and test results may indicate a need for immediate consultation. The examination may further reinforce or reduce suspicions of tumor, infection, tendon rupture, metabolic disorder, fracture, or dislocation.

Diagnostic Criteria

If the patient does not have red flags for serious conditions, the clinician can then determine which common musculoskeletal disorder is present. The criteria presented in Table 14-2 follow the clinical thought process, from the mechanism of illness or injury to unique symptoms and signs of a particular disorder and finally to test results, if any tests are needed to make a correct diagnosis.

Table 14-2. Diagnostic Criteria for Non-red-flag Conditions that Can Be Managed by Primary Care Physicians

Probable Diagnosis or Injury	Mechanism	Unique Symptoms	Unique Signs	Tests and Results
Ankle sprain (ICD-9 845.0; medial 845.01, lateral 845.02)	Inversion of ankle Eversion of ankle	Pain at or below lateral or medial malleolus Swelling over or near malleolus	Swelling at or below malleolus Tenderness over medial or lateral ankle ligament With severe sprain, positive drawer sign for instability	None (radiograph negative if obtained)
Forefoot sprain (ICD-9 845.10)	Plantar flexion, extension, or inversion beyond range	Dorsal foot pain Swelling of dorsal foot	Swelling in dorsum of foot Tenderness over dorsum of foot	None (radiograph negative if obtained)
Ankle or foot tendonitis (ICD-9 726.71)	Acute overuse Repetitive trauma	Heel cord pain Pain over specific tendon unit with flexion or extension	Pain over muscle/tendon unit on motion or resisted motion of tendon unit Tenderness of involved tendon	None

Table 14-2. (continued)

Probable Diagnosis or Injury	Mechanism	Unique Symptoms	Unique Signs	Tests and Results
Neuroma (ICD-9 355.6)	Prolonged weight bearing Idiopathic	Gradual onset of pain and paresthesias on both sides of web space	Reproduction of symptoms by pressing metatarsals together or pressing the web space	None
Metatarsalgia (ICD-9 726.70)	Prolonged weight bearing Degenerative changes Idiopathic	Gradual onset of pain under metatarsal heads with weight bearing	Reproduction of metatarsal pain on compression Decreased tissue padding under metatarsal heads	None
Bunion, hallux valgus (ICD-9 727.1, 735.0)	Prolonged weight bearing Degenerative change	Lateral deviation of first toe Pain in first toe from overlap with tight footwear	Lateral angulation of great toe	Metatarsal angle of > 14 degrees
Plantar fasciitis (ICD-9 728.71)	Weight bearing (on hard surfaces) Idiopathic	Pain across sole of foot Pain with 1st step upon rising in the morning	Tenderness on compression of plantar fascia	None
Heel spur (ICD-9 726.73)	Prolonged weight bearing Degenerative change Idiopathic	Pain at heel with weight bearing First steps upon rising in A.M. very painful in heel	Point tenderness over plantar calcaneus	Ragiograph positive for plantar calcaneal spur (if obtained)
Metatarsal stress fracture (ICD-9 825.25)	Repetitive load	Pain in the dorsal forefoot on weight bearing	Point tenderness over metatarsal shaft	Radiograph positive later in course of disorder Bone scan or spiral CT positive
Toe fracture (ICD-9 826.1)	Direct trauma	Pain at fracture site (possibly)	Point tenderness Deformity Hematoma	Positive radiograph
Nonspecific foot or ankle pain (ICD-9 719.47, 719.57)	Unknown	Nonspecific pain in foot or ankle	None	None

Note: ICD-9 = *International Classification of Diseases*, 9th Edition.

Work-Relatedness

A thorough work history is crucial to establishing work-relatedness. See Chapter 2 for components of the work history.

Determining whether a complaint of a foot or ankle disorder is work related requires careful analysis and weighing all associated or apparently causal factors operative at the time (see Chapter 4). A predominance of work factors suggests that worksite intervention is appropriate. A cluster of cases in a work group suggests a greater probability of associated work-design or management factors.

Prolonged weight bearing may aggravate Morton's neuroma, metatarsalgia, hallux valgus, and plantar fasciitis, although the strength of the association is not great. Acute trauma at work can be associated with tendinitis, tenosynovitis, and ligament strains. Stress fractures can be related to a recent increase in walking or weight-bearing activities. The relation of "chronic strain" or degenerative joint disease to work in the absence of specific traumatic exposures has not been documented in well-designed studies.

Initial Care

Comfort is often a patient's first concern. Nonprescription analgesics, short-term non-weight bearing, cold application and elevation will provide sufficient pain relief for most patients with acute and subacute symptoms. If treatment response is inadequate (e.g., if symptoms and activity limitations continue), prescribed pharmaceuticals or physical methods can be added. Comorbid conditions, side effects, cost, and provider and patient preferences guide the clinician's choice of recommendations. Table 14-3 summarizes initial treatment options.

Physical Methods

- Instruction in home exercise may be considered. Except for cases of fractures, acute dislocations, or infection, patients may be advised to do early passive range-of-motion exercises at home. Instruction in proper exercise technique is important, and instruction by a physical therapist can educate the patient about an effective exercise program.
- Patients may use applications of heat or cold at home before or after exercises; these are as effective as those performed by a therapist. Applying cold regularly for 36 to 48 hours following acute injury and swelling is beneficial.
- Elevation and a brief period of non-weight bearing may be effective for pain management and resolution of swelling.
- Manipulation has not been shown to be effective in alleviating foot or ankle pain.

Table 14-3. Methods of Symptom Control for Ankle and Foot Complaints

RECOMMENDED
Nonprescription Medications
Acetaminophen (safest) NSAIDs (aspirin, ibuprofen, naproxen)
Physical Methods
Adjust or modify workstation, job tasks, or work hours and methods Stretching Specific foot and ankle exercises for range of motion and strengthening At-home applications of cold during first few days of acute complaint; thereafter, applications of heat or cold as patient prefers, unless swelling persists—then use cold Initial and follow-up visits for education, counseling, and evaluation of home exercise Aerobic exercise
Prescribed Pharmaceutical Methods
Other NSAIDs

OPTIONS

Ankle Sprain	Tendinitis/Tenosynovitis	Forefoot Sprain
Cold and elevation of foot Splint or immobilization in severe cases Gradual, early resumption of weight bearing as tolerated	Splint, temporary cast or surgical shoe if needed	Splint or surgical shoe if needed Encourage partial weight bearing
Neuroma	**Metatarsalgia**	**Hallux Valgus**
Toe separator at affected web space Wide shoes	Metatarsal arch bars Arch supports Rigid orthotics	Soft, wide shoes
Plantar Fasciitis	**Heel Spur**	**Nonspecific Ankle or Foot Pain**
Heel donut Soft, supportive shoes Rigid orthotics	Heel donut Air sole shoes	Activity as tolerated
Toe Fracture		
Buddy taping Splint or temporary cast if needed		

- Physical modalities, such as massage, diathermy, cutaneous laser treatment, ultrasound, transcutaneous electrical neurostimulation (TENS) units, and biofeedback have no scientifically proven efficacy in treating acute ankle or foot symptoms, although some are used commonly in conjunction with an active therapy program, such as therapeutic exercise. Insufficient high quality scientific evidence exists to determine clearly the effectiveness of these therapies.
- Limited evidence exists regarding extracorporeal shock wave therapy (ESWT) in treating plantar fasciitis to reduce pain and improve function. While it appears to be safe, there is disagreement as to its efficacy. Insufficient high quality scientific evidence exists to determine clearly the effectiveness of this therapy.
- Invasive techniques (e.g., needle acupuncture and injection procedures) have no proven value, with the exception of corticosteroid injection into the affected web space in patients with Morton's neuroma or into the affected area in patients with plantar fasciitis or heel spur if four to six weeks of conservative therapy is ineffective.
- Other miscellaneous therapies have been evaluated and found to be ineffective or minimally effective. In particular, iontophoresis and phonophoresis have little or no proven efficacy in treating foot and ankle complaints.
- Rigid orthotics (full-shoe-length inserts made to realign within the foot and from foot to leg) may reduce pain experienced during walking and may reduce more global measures of pain and disability for patients with plantar fasciitis and metatarsalgia.
- Night splints, as part of a treatment regimen that may include stretching, range-of-motion (ROM) exercises and nonsteroidal anti-inflammatory drugs (NSAIDs), may be effective in treating plantar fasciitis, though evidence is limited.
- There is limited evidence for the effectiveness of impulse compression or coupled electrical stimulation treatment to accelerate delayed fracture union.

Activity Alteration

Careful advice regarding maximizing activities within the limits of symptoms is imperative once red flags have been ruled out. Putting joints at rest in a brace or splint should be for as short a time as possible. Gentle exercise at the initial phase of recovery is desirable. For instance, partial weight bearing involves placing the affected foot or ankle on the ground with crutches on either side and having the patient place as much weight as possible on the foot, with the rest of the weight on the crutches. This practice is preferable to complete non-weight bearing. If the nature of the injury does not prohibit them, gentle range-of-motion exercises several times a day within limits of pain is better than complete immobilization. Toes exposed in a splint should be exercised; knee range-of-motion exercises should be performed; and straight-leg raising exercises should be done to maintain quadriceps strength.

Activities and postures that increase stress on a structurally damaged ankle or foot tend to aggravate symptoms. Correct undesirable correlated and compensatory motions and postures if possible. Weight bearing may be limited during the first few weeks, with gradual return to full weight bearing. Weight bearing with orthotics often returns function toward normal very quickly.

Work Activities

Table 14-4 provides a guide for activity modification and duration of absence from work. These recommendations apply to patients without comorbidity or complicating factors, including employment or legal issues. They are targets to provide a guide from the perspective of physiologic recovery. Key factors to consider in disability duration are age and type of job, especially if the regular work includes activities likely to worsen the condition. It is important for the clinician to clarify with patients and employers that:

- Even moderately heavy weight bearing and carrying may aggravate foot and ankle symptoms caused by tendinitis, plantar fasciitis, heel spurs, metatarsalgia, and some other conditions.
- Any restrictions are intended to allow for spontaneous recovery or time to build activity tolerance through exercise.

Follow-up Visits

Patients with ankle and foot complaints may have initial follow-up every three to five days by a midlevel practitioner or physical therapist who can provide counseling about avoiding static positions, medication use, activity modification, and other concerns. Care should be taken to answer questions and make these sessions interactive so that the patient is fully involved in his or her recovery. If the patient has returned to work, these interactions may be done on site or by telephone to avoid interfering with modified- or full-work activities.

Physician follow-up is appropriate when a release to modified-, increased-, or full-duty work is needed, or after appreciable healing or recovery is expected. Later physician follow-up might be expected every four to seven days if the patient is off work and every seven to fourteen days if the patient is working.

Special Studies and Diagnostic and Treatment Considerations

For most cases presenting with true foot and ankle disorders, special studies are usually not needed until after a period of conservative care and observation. Most ankle and foot problems improve quickly once any red-flag issues are ruled out. Routine testing, i.e., laboratory tests, plain-film radiographs of the foot or ankle, and special imaging studies are not recommended during the

*Table 14-4. Guidelines for Modification of Work Activities and Disability Duration**

Disorder	Activity Modifications and Accommodation	Recommended Target for Disability Duration**		NHIS Experience Data***	
		With Modified Duty	Without Modified Duty	Median (cases with lost time)	Percent (no lost time)
Ankle sprain	Partial to full weight-bearing	0-2 days	7-21 days	7 days	21%
Forefoot sprain	Partial to full weight-bearing	0-2 days	7-21 days	7 days	21%
Ankle or foot tendinitis	Weight-bearing as tolerated, but prolonged standing and walking should be avoided	0-1 day	7-21 days	41 days	63%
Neuroma (aggravation)	Same as for ankle or foot tendinitis	0-5 days	Indefinite	20 days	38%
Metatarsalgia	Same as for ankle or foot tendinitis	0-2 days	5 days	41 days	63%
Hallux valgus (aggravation) Hallux limitus	Same as for ankle or foot tendinitis	0-3 days	10-14 days	13 days	79%
Plantar fasciitis	Same as for ankle and foot tendinitis	0-2 days	10-14 days	3 days	61%
Heal spur (aggravation)	Same as for ankle and foot tendinitis	0-2 days	7-14 days	41 days	63%
Metatarsal stress fracture	Splint or case and partial weight-bearing	0-1 day	6 weeks	20 days	12%
Toe fracture	Buddy tape and open shoes Exposure to further trauma should be carefully avoided	0 days	1-2 weeks	13 days	21%
Regional foot and ankle pain	Allow all activities as tolerated Avoid activities that aggravate symptoms but start range-of-motion and conditioning exercises	0-2 days	5 days	4 days	49%

* These are general guidelines based on consensus or population sources and are never meant to be applied to an individual case without consideration of workplace factors, concurrent disease or other social or medical factors that can affect recovery.
** These parameters for disability duration are "consensus-optimal" targets as determined by a panel of ACOEM members in 1995, and reaffirmed by a panel of ACOEM members in 2002. In most cases persons with one non-severe extremity injury can return to modified duty immediately. Restrictions should take into consideration the opposite extremity also to prevent strain injuries to the uninjured extremity.
*** Based on the CDC NHIS (National Health Interview Survey), as compiled and reported in the 8th annual edition of *Official Disability Guidelines (ODG)*, © 2002 Work Loss Data Institute, all rights reserved.

first month of activity limitation, except when a red flag noted on history or examination raises suspicion of a dangerous foot or ankle condition or of referred pain.

In particular, patients who have suffered ankle injuries caused by a mechanism that could result in fracture can have radiographs if the Ottawa Criteria are met. This will markedly increase the diagnostic yield for plain radiography. The Ottawa Criteria are rules for foot and ankle radiographic series. An ankle radiographic series is indicated if the patient is experiencing any pain in the:

- Malleolar area, and any of the following findings apply: a) tenderness at the posterior edge or tip of the lateral malleolus; b) tenderness at the posterior edge or tip of the medial malleolus; or c) inability to bear weight both immediately and in the emergency department.
- Midfoot area, and any of the following findings apply: a) tenderness at the base of the fifth metatarsal; b) tenderness at the navicular bone; or c) inability to bear weight both immediately and in the emergency department.

Radiographic evaluation may also be performed if there is rapid onset of swelling and bruising; if patient's age exceeds 55 years; if the injury is high-velocity; in the case of multiple injury or obvious dislocation/subluxation; or if the patient cannot bear weight for more than four steps.

For patients with continued limitations of activity after four weeks of symptoms and unexplained physical findings such as effusion or localized pain, especially following exercise, imaging may be indicated to clarify the diagnosis and assist reconditioning. Stress fractures may have a benign appearance, but point tenderness over the bone is indicative of the diagnosis and a radiograph or a bone scan may be ordered. Imaging findings should be correlated with physical findings.

Disorders of soft tissue (such as tendinitis, metatarsalgia, fasciitis, and neuroma) yield negative radiographs and do not warrant other studies, e.g., magnetic resonance imaging (MRI). Magnetic resonance imaging may be helpful to clarify a diagnosis such as osteochondritis dissecans in cases of delayed recovery.

Cases of hallux valgus that fail conservative treatment merit standing plain films to plan surgery, and consultation with the potential surgeon is recommended. Sprains are frequently seen after emergency room treatment in which radiographs are obtained to rule out fractures. Minimal sprains can be treated symptomatically without films. Table 14-5 provides a general comparison of the abilities of different techniques to identify physiologic insult and define anatomic defects.

Surgical Considerations

Referral for surgical consultation may be indicated for patients who have:

- Activity limitation for more than one month without signs of functional improvement
- Failure of exercise programs to increase range of motion and strength of the musculature around the ankle and foot
- Clear clinical and imaging evidence of a lesion that has been shown to benefit in both the short and long term from surgical repair

Earlier, emergency consultation is reserved for patients who may require drainage of acute effusions or hematomas. Referral for early repair of ligament tears is controversial and not common practice. Repairs are generally reserved

Table 14-5. Ability of Various Techniques to Identify and Define Ankle and Foot Pathology

Technique	Sprain	Ligament Tear	Tendinitis	Neuroma	Metarsalgia	Hatallux Valgus	Fasciitis	Heel Spur	Metatarsal Fracture	Toe Fracture
History	++	++	++	++++	+++	+++	++	++	++	++++
Physical examination	++++	++++	++++	++++	++++	++++	++++	++++	+++	+++
Laboratory studies	0	0	0	0	0	0	0	0	0	0
Imaging studies										
Radiography	0	0	0	0	0	++	0	++	++	+++
Computed tomography (CT)	0	0	0	0	0	0	0	0	+++	+++
Magnetic resonance imaging (MRI)	0	++	++	++	0	0	0	0	0	0
Bone scan	0	0	0	0	0	0	0	0	++++	+++

Note: Number of plus signs indicates relative ability to identify or define pathology.

for chronic instability. Most patients have satisfactory results with physical rehabilitation and thus avoid the risks of surgery. If there is no clear indication for surgery, referring the patient to a physical medicine practitioner may help resolve the symptoms.

A. Neuroma

If a patient with a neuroma has persistent pain in a web space despite using toe separators, along with temporary relief from local cortisone injections, surgical removal of the neuroma may be indicated. Besides the usual counseling about possible wound complications and complications of anesthesia, the patient can be informed that the operation is not always effective because the surgeon may be unable to find the neuroma and excise it. Always counsel the patient about expectations for surgery so that he or she can make an informed decision about whether or not to proceed with surgery.

B. Hallux Valgus

Failure of conservative treatment (e.g., using wider shoes and/or arch supports, or aspiration of an overlying bursa) may lead to consideration of surgery. However, surgery should not be performed for cosmetic purposes because surgical complications such as infection can worsen appearance and a good functional result is the goal of treatment. Counseling patients about the postoperative course and recovery period is required because they may otherwise underestimate the length of time for recovery and the postoperative pain involved.

Summary of Recommendations and Evidence

See Table 14-6.

Table 14-6. Summary of Recommendations for Evaluating and Managing Ankle and Foot Complaints

Clinical Measure	Recommended	Optional	Not Recommended
History and physical exam	Basic history and physical exam, including evaluation of ability to bear weight, tenderness, and ligament stability (C)		
Patient education	Patient education regarding diagnosis, prognosis, and expectations of treatment (D)		
Medication (See Chapter 3)	Acetaminophen (C) NSAIDs (B)	Opioids, short course (C) NSAID creams (D)	Use of opioids for more than 2 weeks (C)
Injections	For patients with point tenderness in the area of a heel spur, plantar fasciitis, or Morton's neuroma, local injection of lidocaine and cortisone solution (D)		Repeated or frequent injections (D)
Physical treatment methods	For acute injuries, at-home ice applications, range-of-motion and strengthening exercises, as taught by primary provider (D)	Pneumatic or pulse devices to reduce swelling (C) ESWT for plantar fasciitis (C) Coupled electrical stimulation or impulse compression for fracture (C)	Passive physical therapy modalities, except as initial aid prior to home exercises (D) Laser treatment (B)
Rest and immobilization (e.g., braces, supports)	For acute injuries, immobilization and weight bearing as tolerated; taping or bracing later to avoid exacerbation or for prevention (C) For acute swelling, rest and elevation (D) For appropriate diagnoses, rigid orthotics, metatarsal bars, heel donut, toe separator (C)	Tension night splints for plantar fasciitis (B)	Prolonged supports or bracing without exercise (due to risk of debilitation) (D)

Table 14-6. (continued)

Clinical Measure	Recommended	Optional	Not Recommended
Activity and exercise	Stretching Aerobic exercise Maintenance of general activity to avoid debilitation (C) Early mobilization of patients with ankle sprain (C)		Full activity in presence of swelling and other signs of acute trauma (D)
Detection of physiologic abnormalities			Electrical studies for routine foot and ankle problems without clinical evidence of tarsal tunnel syndrome or other entrapment neuropathies (D)
Radiography	Plain-film radiographs only for patients with acute ankle injuries who have signs identified in Ottawa Criteria ankle rules (B) Further evaluation if radiographic films show ankle effusion > 13 mm anteriorly (C)		Routine plain-film radiographs for ankle injuries (B) Routine radiographic films for soft tissue diagnoses (D)
Surgical considerations	Bunionectomy if conservative treatment fails and radiographs are positive for > 14-degree intermetatarsal angle (D) Excision of neuroma if conservative treatment (injections, toe separator) fails (D) Reconstruction of lateral ankle ligament for symptomatic patients with ankle laxity demonstrated on physical exam and positive stress films (C)		Diagnostic arthroscopy of ankle if diagnosis obtainable by other non-invasive method (D) Arthroscopy of ankle for synovial impingement before conservative care, including injections, is tried (D)

A = Strong research-based evidence (multiple relevant, high-quality scientific studies).
B = Moderate research-based evidence (one relevant, high-quality scientific study or multiple adequate scientific studies).
C = Limited research-based evidence (at least one adequate scientific study of patients with foot or ankle complaints).
D = Panel interpretation of evidence not meeting inclusion criteria for research-based evidence.

Algorithm 14-1. *Initial Evaluation of Occupational Ankle and Foot Complaints*

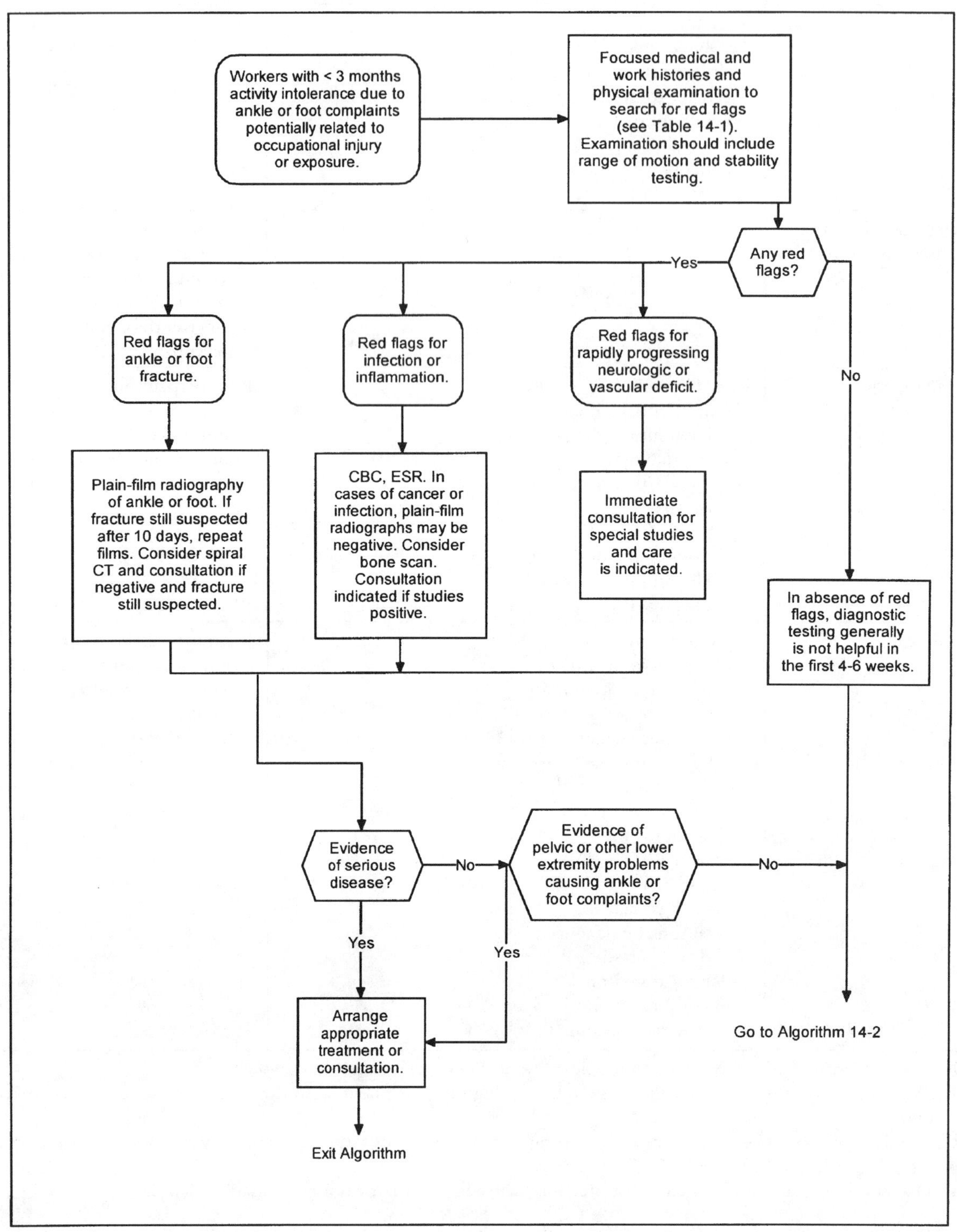

Algorithm 14-2. *Initial and Follow-up Management of Occupational Ankle and Foot Complaints*

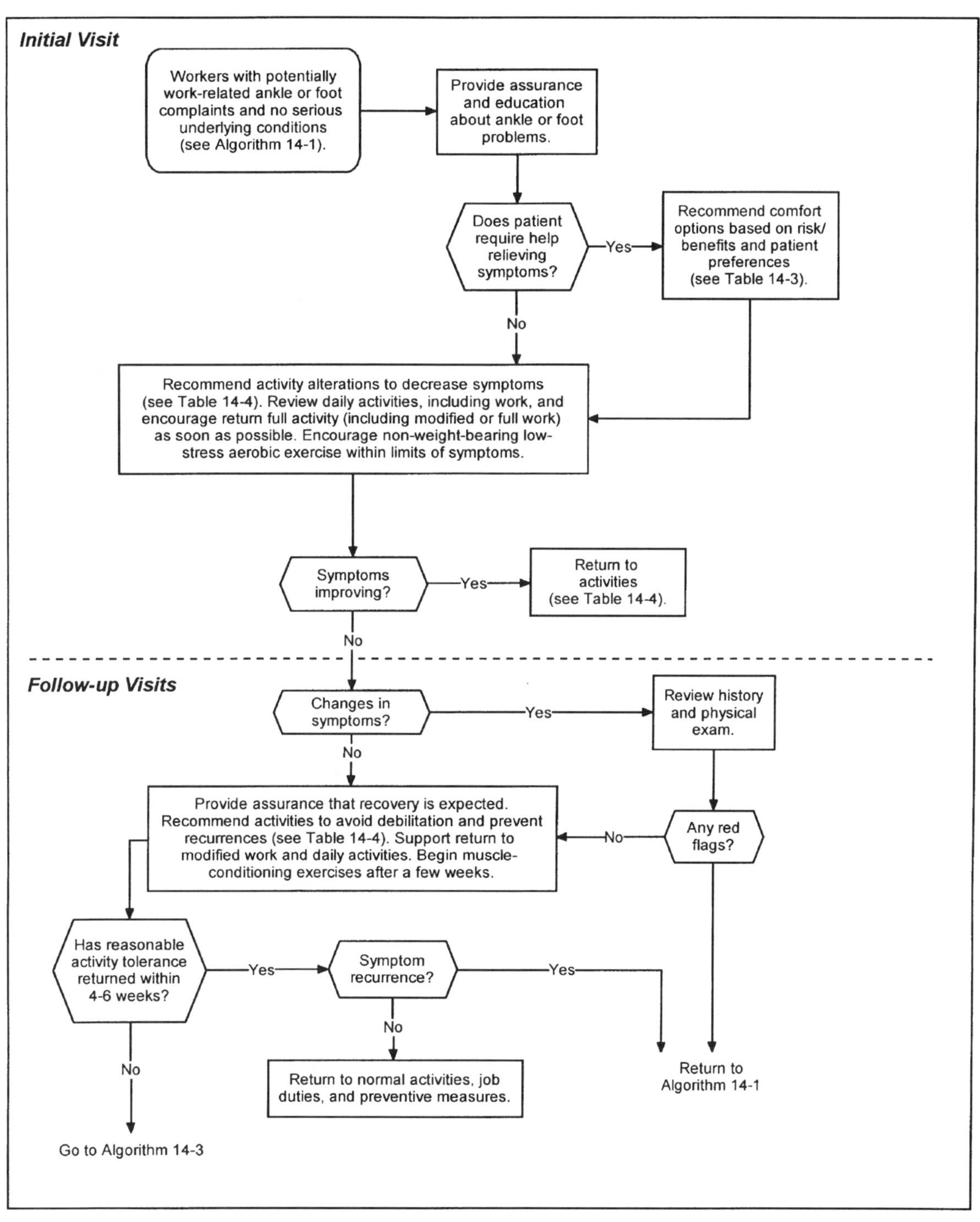

Algorithm 14-3. *Evaluation of Slow-to-recover Patients with Occupational Ankle and Foot Complaints (Symptoms > 4 Weeks)*

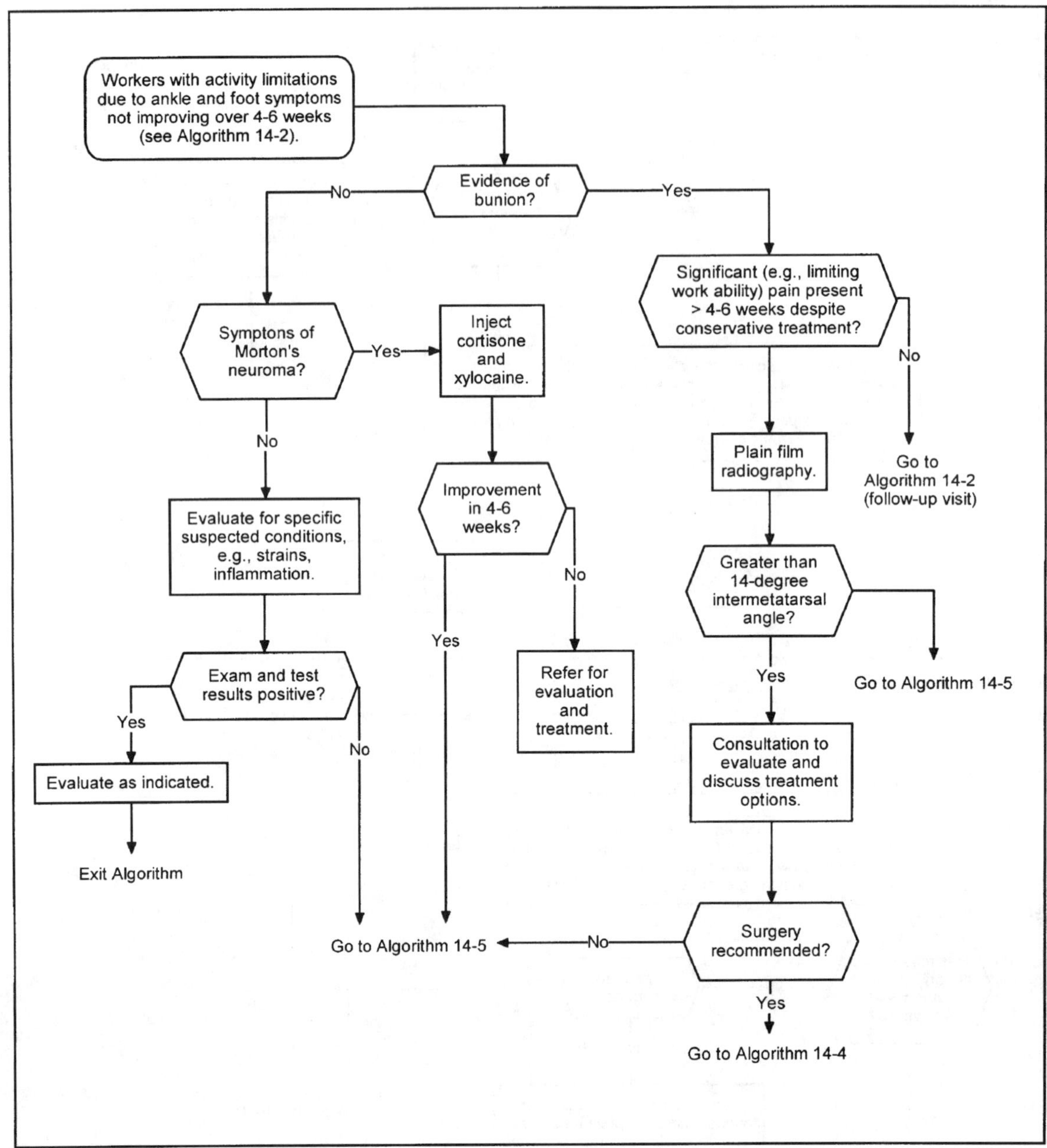

Algorithm 14-4. *Surgical Considerations for Patients with Anatomic and Physiologic Evidence of Bunion, or Morton's Neuroma, and Persistent Symptoms*

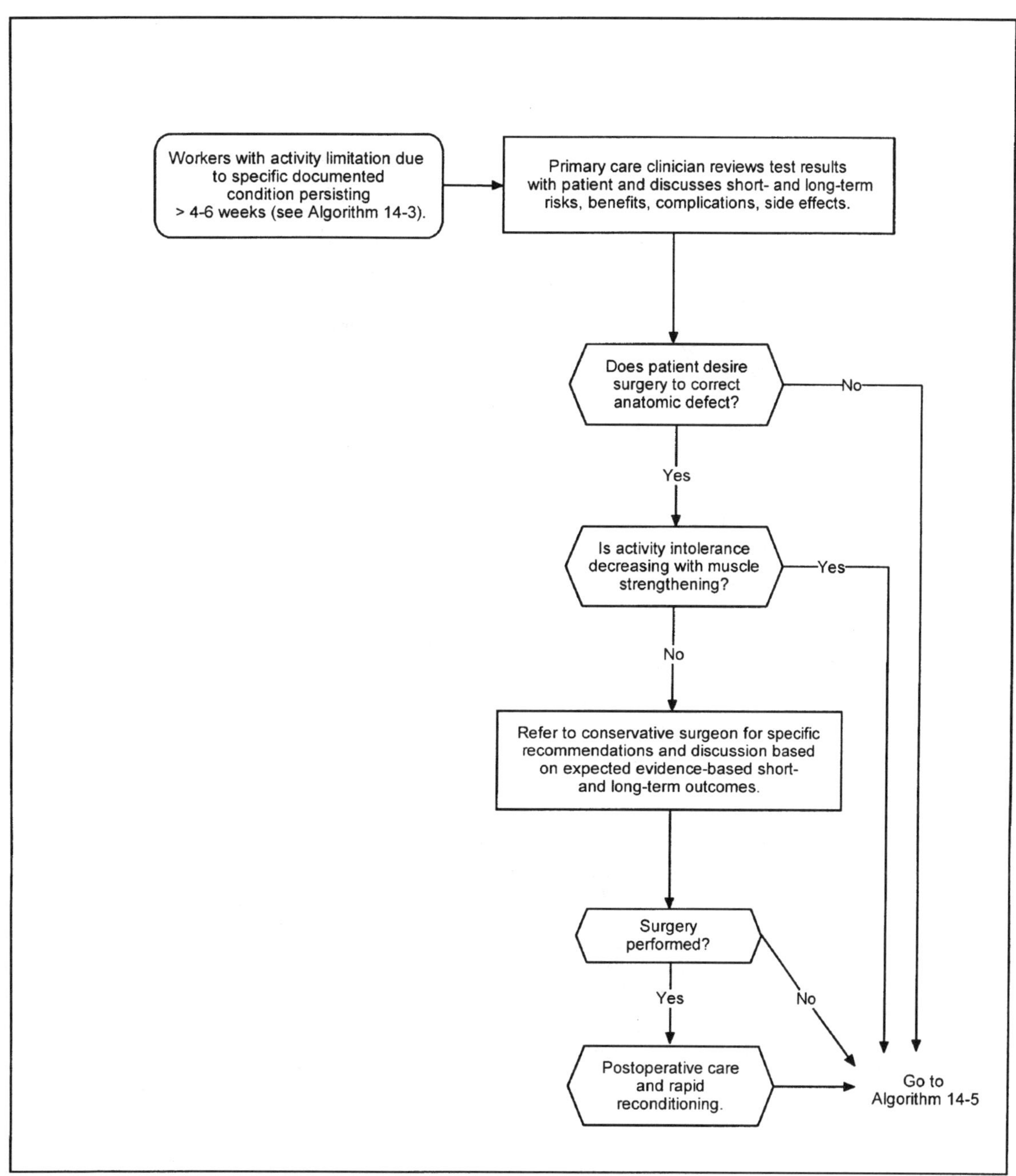

Algorithm 14-5. *Further Management of Occupational Ankle and Foot Complaints*

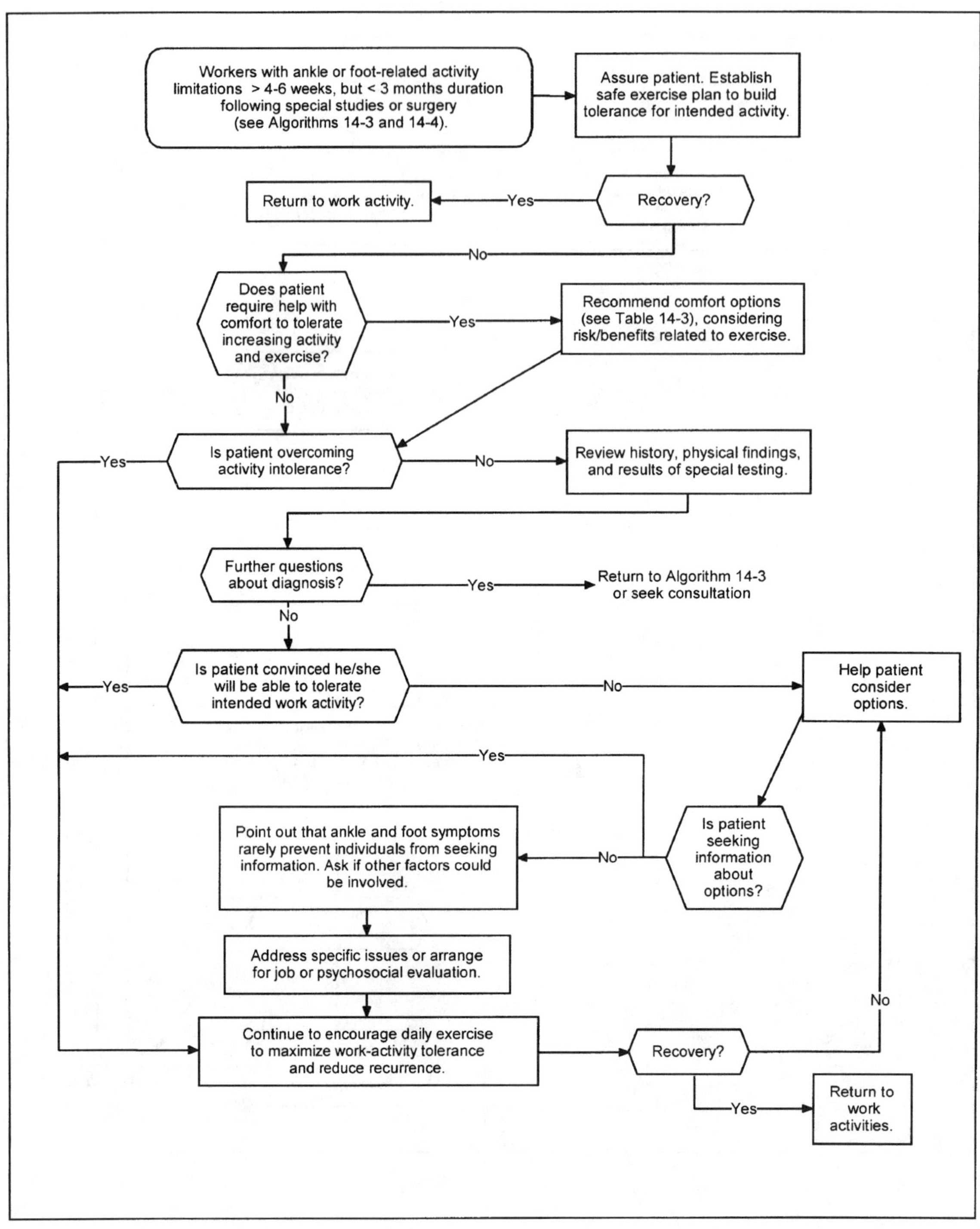

References

HISTORY AND PHYSICAL EXAMINATION

Kaikkonen AP, Jarvinen M. A performance test protocol and scoring scale for the evaluation of ankle injuries. *Am J Sports Med.* 1994;22:462-9.

Riegger-Krugh C, Keysor JJ. Skeletal malalignments of the lower quarter: correlated and compensatory motions and postures. *J Orthop Sports Phys Ther.* 1996;23(2):164-70.

Stiell IG, McKnight RD, Greenberg GH, et al. Interobserver agreement in the examination of acute ankle injury patients. *Am J Emerg Med.* 1992;10: 14-7.

Swain RA, Holt WS. Ankle injuries. *Postgrad Med.* 1993;93(3):91-100.

DISABILITY MANAGEMENT

Denniston PL, ed. *OSHA Durations Report: Return-to-Work by State, Industry & Age (plus Diagnosis, Body Part, Event, Gender and Length of Service).* Corpus Christi, Texas: Work Loss Data Institute; 2002.

MEDICATION

See Chapter 3 references.

PHYSICAL TREATMENT METHODS

Basford JR, Malanga GA, Krause DA, Harmsen WS. A randomized controlled evaluation of low-intensity laser therapy: plantar fasciitis. *Arch Phys Med Rehabil.* 1998;79(3):249-54.

Buchbinder R, Ptasznik R, Gordon J, Buchanan J, Prabaharan V, Forbes A. Ultrasound-guided extracorporeal shock wave therapy for plantar fasciitis: a randomized controlled trial. *JAMA.* 2002;288(11):1364-72.

Cosentino R, Falsetti P, Manca S, et al. Efficacy of extracorporeal shock wave treatment in calcaneal enthesophytosis. *Ann Rheum Dis.* 2001;60(11): 1064-7.

Crawford F, Atkins D, Edwards J. Interventions for treating plantar heel pain (Cochrane Review). In: *The Cochrane Library.* Issue 3; 2002.

Hammer DS, Rupp S, Kreutz A, Pape D, Kohn D, Seil R. Extracorporeal shockwave therapy (ESWT) in patients with chronic proximal plantar fasciitis. *Foot Ankle Int.* 2002;23(4):309-13.

Lynch DM, Goforth WP, Martin JE, Odom RD, Preece CK, Kotter MW. Conservative treatment of plantar fasciitis. A prospective study. *J Am Podiatr Med Assoc.* 1998;88(8):375-80.

McLauchlan GJ, Handoll HHG. Interventions for treating acute and chronic Achilles tendinitis (Cochrane Review). In: *The Cochrane Library.* Issue 3; 2002.

Myerson MS, Henderson MR. Clinical applications of a pneumatic intermittent impulse compression device after trauma and major surgery to the foot and ankle. *Foot Ankle.* 1993;14:198-203.

Ogden JA, Alvarez R, Levitt R, Cross GL, Marlow M. Shock wave therapy for chronic proximal plantar fasciitis. *Clin Orthop.* 2001;(387):47-59.

Ogden JA, Alvarez RG, Marlow M. Shockwave therapy for chronic proximal plantar fasciitis: a meta-analysis. *Foot Ankle Int.* 2002;23(4):301-8.

Rompe JD, Schoellner C, Nafe B. Evaluation of low-energy extracorporeal shock-wave application for treatment of chronic plantar fasciitis. *J Bone Joint Surg Am.* 2002;84-A(3):335-41.

Rompe JD, Hopf C, Nafe B, Burger R. Low-energy extracorporeal shock wave therapy for painful heel: a prospective controlled single-blind study. *Arch Orthop Trauma Surg.* 1996;115(2):75-9.

Van der Windt DA, Van der Heijden GJ, Van den Berg SG, Ter Riet G, De Winter AF, Bouter LM. Ultrasound therapy for acute ankle sprains (Cochrane Review). In: *The Cochrane Library.* Issue 3; 2002.

Weil LS Jr, Roukis TS, Weil LS, Borrelli AH. Extracorporeal shock wave therapy for the treatment of chronic plantar fasciitis: indications, protocol, intermediate results, and a comparison of results to fasciotomy. *J Foot Ankle Surg.* 2002;41(3):166-72.

REST AND IMMOBILIZATION, BRACES, SUPPORTS, AND OTHER SUPPORTIVE METHODS

Batt ME, Tanji JL, Skattum N. Plantar fasciitis: a prospective randomized clinical trial of the tension night splint. *Clin J Sport Med.* 1996;6(3):158-62.

Gross MT, Byers JM, Krafft JL, Lackey EJ, Melton KM. The impact of custom semirigid foot orthotics on pain and disability for individuals with plantar fasciitis. *J Orthop Sports Phys Ther.* 2002;32(4):149-57.

Johannes EJ, Sukul DM, Spruit JP, et al. Controlled trial of a semi-rigid bandage ('Scotchrap') in patients with ankle ligament lesions. *Curr Med Res Opin.* 1993;13:154-62.

Kerkhoffs GM, Rowe BH, Assendelft WJ, Kelly K, Struijs PA, van Dijk CN. Immobilisation and functional treatment for acute lateral ankle ligament injuries in adults (Cochrane Review). In: *The Cochrane Library.* Issue 3; 2002.

Powell M, Post WR, Keener J, Wearden S. Effective treatment of chronic plantar fasciitis with dorsiflexion night splints: a crossover prospective randomized outcome study. *Foot Ankle Int.* 1998;19(1):10-8.

Sitler M, Ryan J, Wheeler B, et al. The efficacy of a semirigid ankle stabilizer to reduce acute ankle injuries in basketball. A randomized clinical study at West Point. *Am J Sports Med.* 1994;22:454-61.

Yamamoto H, Ishibashi T, Muneta T, et al. Nonsurgical treatment of lateral ligament injury of the ankle joint. *Foot Ankle.* 1993;14(9):500-4.

Zwipp H, Schievink B. Primary orthotic treatment of ruptured ankle ligaments: a recommended procedure. *Prosthet Orthot Int.* 1992;16:49-56.

ACTIVITY AND EXERCISE

Dettori JR, Basmania CJ. Early ankle mobilization, part II: a one-year follow-up of acute, lateral ankle sprains (a randomized clinical trial). *Mil Med.* 1994;159:20-4.

Dettori JR, Pearson BD, Basmania CJ, et al. Early ankle mobilization, part I: the immediate effect on acute, lateral ankle sprains (a randomized clinical trial). *Mil Med.* 1994;159:15-20.

Eiff MP, Smith AT, Smith GE. Early mobilization versus immobilization in the treatment of lateral ankle sprains. *Am J Sports Med.* 1994;22:83-8.

Kerkhoffs GM, Struijs PA, Marti RK, Assendelft WJ, Blankevoort L, van Dijk CN. Different functional treatment strategies for acute lateral ankle ligament injuries in adults (Cochrane Review). In: *The Cochrane Library.* Issue 3; 2002.

RADIOGRAPHY

Clark TW, Janzen DL, Ho K, Grunfeld A, Connell DG. Detection of radiographically occult ankle fractures following acute trauma: positive predictive value of an ankle effusion. *AmJ Roentgenol.* 1995;164(5):1185-9.

Kelly AM, Richards D, Kerr L, et al. Failed validation of a clinical decision rule for the use of radiography in acute ankle injury. *N Z Med J.* 1994;107:294-5.

Packer GJ, Goring CC, Gayner AD, et al. Audit of ankle injuries in an accident and emergency department. *Br Med J.* 1991;302:885-7.

Pigman EC, Klug RK, Sanford S, Jolly BT. Evaluation of the Ottawa clinical decision rules for the use of radiography in acute ankle and midfoot injuries in the emergency department: an independent site assessment. *Ann Emerg Med.* 1994;24:41-5.

Pijnenburg AC, Glas AS, De Roos MA, et al. Radiography in acute ankle injuries: the Ottawa Ankle Rules versus local diagnostic decision rules. *Ann Emerg Med.* 2002;39(6):599-604.

Smith GF, Madlon-Kay DJ, Hunt V. Clinical evaluation of ankle inversion injuries in family practice offices. *J Fam Pract.* 1993;37:345-8.

Stiell IG, McKnight RD, Greenberg GH, et al. Implementation of the Ottawa Ankle Rules. *JAMA.* 1994;271:8270-332.

Vangsness CT Jr, Carter V, Hunt T, et al. Radiographic diagnosis of ankle fractures: are three views necessary? *Foot Ankle Int.* 1994;15:172-4.

Verma S, Hamilton K, Hawkins HH, et al. Clinical application of the Ottawa ankle rules for the use of radiography in acute ankle injuries: an independent site assessment. *Am J Roentgenol.* 1997;169(3):825-7.

SURGICAL CONSIDERATIONS

Ferrari J, Higgins JPT, Williams RL. Interventions for treating hallux valgus (abductovalgus) and bunions (Cochrane Review). In: *The Cochrane Library,* Issue 3; 2002.

Hall RL, Shereff MJ, Stone J, et al. Ankle arthroscopy in industrial injuries of the ankle. *Arthroscopy.* 1995;11:127-33.

Kashuk KB, Landsman AS, Werd MB, et al. Arthroscopic lateral ankle stabilization. *Clin Podiatr Med Surg.* 1994;11:407-23.

Kerkhoffs GM, Handoll HH, de Bie R, Rowe BH, Struijs PA. Surgical versus conservative treatment for acute injuries of the lateral ligament complex of the ankle in adults (Cochrane Review). In: *The Cochrane Library.* Issue 3; 2002.

Saxena A. Return to athletic activity after foot and ankle surgery: a preliminary report on select procedures. *J Foot Ankle Surg.* 2000;39(2):114-9.

Torkki M, Malmivaara A, Seitsalo S, Hoikka V, Laippala P, Paavolainen P. Surgery vs orthosis vs watchful waiting for hallux valgus: a randomized controlled trial. *JAMA.* 2001;285(19):2474-80.

Verhagen RA, de Keizer G, van Kijk CN. Long-term follow-up of inversion trauma of the ankle. *Arch Orthop Trauma Surg.* 1995;114:92-6.

15 Stress-related Conditions

This guideline is intended to help occupational physicians and primary care practitioners manage employed patients with acute stress-related conditions of relatively short duration. This guideline recognizes that factors inherent in the workplace can contribute to the development of stress. Topics covered in this chapter include the initial assessment and management of patients with acute stress-related conditions, identification of red flags requiring urgent mental health-care referral, work relatedness, and modified duty and return to work.

General Approach and Basic Principles

Stressors may be any life event or circumstance that exerts a physical, emotional, or cognitive demand on the individual. The lifetime prevalence of major stressful life events is 100%, so associated stress-related symptoms may be considered a normal condition of human existence.

- Stress is not a diagnosis, disease, or syndrome. It is a nonspecific set of emotions or physical symptoms that may or may not be associated with a disease or syndrome. Whether or not stress contributes to a disease or syndrome depends on the vulnerability of the individual; the intensity, duration, and meaning of the stress; and the nature and availability of modifying resources.
- The initial assessment of patients with acute stress-related conditions focuses on detecting potentially serious psychopathology, or red flag conditions, requiring urgent specialty referral. The majority of patients with stress-related conditions will not have red flags and can be safely and effectively managed by occupational or primary care physicians.
- Relief of stress depends on its precipitants, which are often multifactorial. Psychosocial, workplace, or socioeconomic issues can be explored with the patient to facilitate early identification of precipitating factors and appropriate interventions that may prevent delayed recovery or

relapse. An open, honest discussion of the underlying factors often results in an increase in the patient's insight and coping skills, which itself helps alleviate many stress-related symptoms.

- Worksite interventions may be helpful in mitigating or eliminating inciting stressors, depending on the source of the complaints.
- Medications generally have a limited role. Limit use of anti-anxiety agents to short periods of time, i.e., periods when overwhelming anxiety limits the patient's ability to work or effectively perform the activities of daily living. Antidepressant or antipsychotic medication may be prescribed for major depression or psychosis; however, this is best done in conjunction with specialty referral.
- Patients are encouraged to enhance their individual coping skills and to decrease or discontinue maladaptive coping mechanisms such as excessive use of alcohol, tobacco, or other drugs, or excessive food intake. Patients are counseled to redirect their energy to regular aerobic exercise, relaxation techniques, and cognitive coping mechanisms.
- For uncomplicated cases, absence from work should not exceed one work week. Referral for mental health professional assessment may be considered for patients whose anticipated absence from work will exceed one week.
- If symptoms become disabling despite primary care interventions or persist beyond three months, referral to a mental health professional is indicated.

Symptoms attributable to stress are common problems for patients presenting to occupational and primary care physicians. Up to 60% of patient visits are due to somatic manifestations of emotional states, and workers with job-related stress, anxiety, and depression miss an average of 16 days per year. The National Institute for Occupational Safety and Health (NIOSH) ranks psychological problems as one of the ten most important health problems affecting workers. Complaints of stress may be nonspecific physical or emotional manifestations or may be a clue to underlying psychiatric disorders. This guideline will help clinicians identify patients who need urgent referral for psychiatric care and provide a framework for treating the majority of patients who do not.

Models and Definitions

The word stress has been used extensively in lay and scientific literature to describe any or all parts of a complex and dynamic interaction of intrapersonal, interpersonal, organizational, community, and social factors or outcomes. It follows that "stress research" can focus on any of these levels. It is well beyond the scope of this guideline to review in detail the many models, constructs, and methodologic issues in the vast stress research literature, which includes cognitive and occupational psychology, health promotion, organizational dynamics, physiology, occupational medicine, psychiatry, and other medical specialties.

Common to most stress models is that the individual perceives distress when a mismatch between perceived demands and resources occurs. This model offers a practical framework physicians and patients can use to explore the patient's symptoms and develop a treatment plan.

Perceived demands can include any external or internal stressors, either work related or personal. One perceives demands through a "personal filter"—attitudes, values, and beliefs—that modify actual demands. Cognitive therapy techniques are designed to act at this level. Resources can be further defined as personal factors (e.g., coping skills, physical health), and external supports (e.g., family and other social supports, skills/knowledge, financial resources). Gender, ethnicity, and religion can act at all levels of this model.

The acuity of the stressor and the physical or psychological reaction can vary. An acute occupational stressor, such as reorganization, may have either an acute effect (e.g., increased heartburn or sleep disturbances) or exacerbate a chronic medical condition (e.g., difficulty with blood pressure control in hypertensive patients or relapse in individuals with duodenal ulcer) or both. Chronic stress, such as poor relations with a supervisor or an aging parent, may increase one's susceptibility to transient health effects (e.g., catching more colds) or affect chronic conditions (e.g., increase in frequency of migraine headaches) or both. Furthermore, stress indirectly can affect existing medical conditions. For example, an individual may postpone seeking personal medical care or be less likely to take medications regularly if he or she feels stressed. Not everyone who is stressed becomes ill, and not everyone who is ill seeks help. Emotional stress and mental health problems are associated with higher accidents and injury rates for workers.

A. Physiological Reactions

Autonomic and neuroendocrine responses to physical and psychological stressors have been extensively studied. The fight or flight response, first described by Cannon in 1914, refers to a short-lived physical reaction to an acute perceived threat. The cerebral cortex perceives a threat, and via the hypothalamus, activates the autonomic nervous system and stimulates the adrenal medulla to secrete epinephrine and norepinephrine, resulting in the classic fight or flight reaction. The General Adaptation Syndrome, described by Hans Selye in 1936, describes a more complex physiologic reaction to sustained stress, involving three phases:

- The alarm phase is essentially the fight or flight adrenergic response.
- The resistance phase is characterized by a remission of the adrenergic response and a concomitant increase in cortisol secretion, as the cerebral cortex also stimulates the pituitary to release adrenocorticotropic hormone (ACTH). Metabolism and muscle strength are heightened

during this phase to allow maximal physical resistance to the threat, but at the expense of physical resources.

- The exhaustion phase occurs when prolonged cortisol secretion no longer results in physical resistance, but rather depletes physical resources such as decreased immunity.

These early models have proved too simplistic and mechanistic to explain the negative and positive effects of stress in everyday life or to determine the effect of mediators such as meaning and individual factors on the outcome of stress in people. As research in psychoneurology has increased, more sophisticated models of psychophysiologic reactions to stress have been described.

Medical conditions reported to be affected by stress include asthma, autoimmune diseases, dermatitis, duodenal and peptic ulcer disease, eczema, heart disease (angina, myocardial infarction), irritable bowel disease, migraine and tension headache, mucous colitis, paroxysmal tachycardia, systemic lupus erythematosus, ulcerative colitis, and urticaria. Psychosocial variables also are correlated with musculoskeletal disorders and delayed recovery.

B. Role of Social Factors

Key elements of one's psychosocial milieu have been found to be associated with health parameters and outcomes. Holmes and Rahe demonstrated an association between both positive and negative major life events and health outcomes. The positive impact of social supports on mental health and chronic disease was demonstrated in large-population cachement studies. Marital status, family integrity, community involvement, and self-perceptions of social support are studied most often, but aspects of religious life also have been found to be positively associated with health outcomes.

C. Role of the Workplace in Stress

A Swedish sawmill study was the first to show a difference in a health parameter (an increase in norepinephrine levels) associated with the degree of control over a job among workers in the same mill. Subsequent research demonstrated that the psychosocial work environment is a risk factor for certain health outcomes and modifies certain medical conditions.

The three main models of occupational stress focus on the duration of stress and the resulting chronic effects. These are the person-environment fit, demand-control, and effort-reward models.

- The person-environment fit model posits that poor job fit, or perceived incongruence between skills and job demands or between career goals and actual opportunities, results in emotional distress.
- Demand-control has been, by far, the most extensively studied occupational stress model since the early 1980s. This model proposes that

high job demands and low decision latitude (or ability to exert control over job demands) interact to result in job strain. Job strain consistently has been linked with cardiovascular mortality and heart disease as well as with effects on intermediate parameters proximal to health outcomes, such as hypertension and left ventricular mass. Recent modifications of the demand-control model allow for the influence of personal traits and learning from psychosocial job experience accrued over a lifetime.

- The effort-reward model integrates social and biologic factors with psychological factors. This model posits that high effort without social rewards elicits strong recurrent feelings of anger, depression, and demoralization, which results in sustained autonomic arousal and consequent adverse health outcomes, such as hypertension and myocardial infarction.

Table 15-1 summarizes specific risk factors identified from the large body of research evaluating specific factors inherent in the job or work organization and associated with employees' health outcomes and mental health. It is important to recognize that specific occupations in the service sector or others with unique demands may carry inherent risk for work-related stress disorders (e.g., nurses, caregivers, teachers, firefighters, law enforcement officers).

Initial Assessment

The initial assessment of patients presenting with stress-related complaints seeks to screen for potentially serious psychiatric disorders, to assess the patient's physical and psychosocial situation, and to establish an effective treatment plan. It is important to adequately evaluate and document the presenting complaint, any prior medical or psychiatric illness, and immediate safety concerns. Attributing symptoms to stress often indicates a diagnosis of exclusion and requires a more thorough assessment, which can be achieved through a short-term plan that includes initial counseling and education and a plan for reassessment. Good communication skills as well as observing confidentiality and boundaries of privacy are vitally important, and are essential to obtain the information for correct diagnosis and establish a basis for treatment. Privacy means considering other sources of help and information with the patient's knowledge and understanding. The patient must also understand who initiated the assessment and who will be privy to any or all of the results.

The initial assessment is a critical tool for detecting potential emotional problems that require the attention of a psychiatrist or other mental health professional to assure safe and optimal treatment. The initial screening should be focused more on recognizing indications for urgent mental health referral (red flags) than on specific psychiatric diagnosis (see Table 15-2). Red-flag indicators include impairment of mental functions, overwhelming symptoms, or signs of substance abuse. The practitioner performing the assessment is advised to keep a high index of suspicion for depression, which is a prevalent

Table 15-1. Potential Stressors

Personal	Interpersonal	Job	Organizational	Societal
Chronic illness	Relationship with peers, supervisor, or subordinates	High demands and low control	Lack of advancement opportunities	Unemployment
Inadequate skills or training	Marital discord, divorce, or other relationship issues	Work overload or underload	Threat of downsizing or mergers	Crime (or fear of)
Bereavement	Emotional labor	Role ambiguity Role conflict	Survivor guilt	Poor economy
Child or elder care issues	Violence (or threat of)	Lack of recognition or reward	Fear of redundancy	War, civil unrest
Personality factors (Type A, hostility, cynicism)	Sexual or other harassment	Insufficieint or excessive supervision		
Stage-of-life issues	Litigation	Shiftwork issues		
Stage-of-career issues	Lack of social support	Work pace		
Job satisfaction		Physical hazards		
Personal values and goals				

and underdiagnosed condition. Absence of red-flag indicators rules out the need for urgent referral or inpatient care.

Medical History

The medical history is fundamental to assessment, triage, and counseling patients with stress-related conditions. Presenting complaints often include multi-system, diffuse, or vague symptom complexes; however, many of the symptoms associated with stress also may be symptoms of other physical or major psychiatric disorders. The history includes physical and emotional symptoms, perceived causes of stress and their meaning to the patient, coping mechanisms, and perceived level of functioning.

Active listening skills are of paramount importance to help the patient identify symptoms, psychosocial stressors, coping mechanisms, and other re-

Table 15-2. Red Flags for Potentially Serious Psychiatric Conditions

Disorder	Medical History	Physical and Mental Status Examination
Thought disorder	Paranoia Hallucinations Bizarre beliefs Delusions	Thought disorder Delusions Impaired reality testing
Affective disorder	Loss of interest in life Sleep, appetite disturbance Change in libido Low self-esteem Suicidal ideation Impaired functioning	Depressed affect Psychomotor retardation
Post-traumatic stress syndrome	History of traumatic event Flashbacks	Increased arousal after re-experience
Possible harm to self or others	Suicidal or homicidal ideation Threats of violence to self or others Has a plan and the means Child or spouse abuse	Thoughts or feelings of violence Feelings of being out of control
Cognitive disorganization or dysfunction	Cognitive impairment Impaired impulse control Impaired social judgment Impaired functioning	Disoriented to time or place Inability to comprehend or follow directions Acute cognitive changes
Substance abuse	Increased alcohol or drug intake Preoccupation with obtaining and using substance Impairment of social or work role Disruptive behavior History of withdrawal Desire for detoxification	Intoxication Tolerance Withdrawal symptoms Elevated liver function studies Agitation Hallucinations Diaphoresis
Overwhelming emotional state	Overwhelming emotions Inability to make decisions Impaired functioning (activities of daily living)	Emotional affect Withdrawal behavior

sources. Open-ended questions are helpful in constructing a semi-structured interview. By asking open-ended direct questions and remaining nonjudgmental, the practitioner helps engender trust, which is critical to the patient's revealing important information. Often, the patient may be embarrassed to divulge the most disturbing symptoms and stressors. Asking direct, detailed questions about difficult situations (e.g., thoughts of suicide, domestic abuse) and specific areas of functioning indicates the practitioner's comfort with the subject, gives the patient permission to reveal this information, and helps him or her trust that it will be received in a nonjudgmental way.

A. Symptoms

The medical history includes the patient's description of current symptoms, their duration, and perceived stressors as well as a recounting of any previous episodes. The patient's estimate of functional impairment is a means to assess the severity of the problem and may guide treatment and the timing of other individual or organizational interventions. When a patient presents with a complaint of stress, it is important to evaluate his or her needs, risks, and strengths before dealing with external factors. Not all stressed individuals will seek help even if they are having trouble with work or difficulty adapting or are physically and/or emotionally ill. It is always important to know why, or at whose direction, the patient is seeking help. The patient may initiate the request or may be referred by a supervisor, human resources manager, medical personnel, union, or a representative of the employer's employee assistance program (EAP). The physician may need to enlist the help of these individuals to gather information and develop a treatment plan after evaluating the patient.

B. Stressors

Effective counseling rests on clearly eliciting biopsychosocial stressors and understanding what they mean to the patient. Patients rarely describe irrelevant events or factors. Frequently, however, patients do not describe the most disturbing stressors and symptoms unless specific direct questions are asked. For this reason, initial assessment of stress-related problems may include a standardized interview format and an informal mental status examination that provides the basic observations needed to evaluate impairment of mental functioning. Only by attempting to identify all principal areas of stress and dysfunction can the clinician make specific diagnoses and treatment recommendations. While it is important to recognize and acknowledge organizational and situational factors, it is not always possible to quickly or easily modify or eliminate an external stressor.

Physicians need to be attuned to symptoms of burnout which, like stress, is not a specific diagnosis or disease. It is characterized by depersonalization, emotional exhaustion, and a reduced sense of personal accomplishment. Burnout may be expressed in nonspecific physical or emotional symptoms or may lead to psychiatric illness or impairment, such as depression or dissociation.

C. Coping Mechanisms

Before a clinician can help the patient enhance his or her coping skills, it is important to understand how he or she has characteristically coped with stressful situations. Again, asking direct questions about the patient's means of coping with stressful situations will be revealing. Coping mechanisms can be active or passive. Examples of active coping skills include proactively confronting issues and requesting assistance from supervisors, coworkers, or others (e.g., EAP personnel). Passive coping mechanisms are escape behaviors, such as denying or avoiding issues or focusing on escape mechanisms (e.g., weekends, retirement), or engaging in behaviors that provide symptom relief but do not directly address the stressor. Remember, however, that changing one's focus may be an escape or a way to develop new adaptations. Good judgment and careful self-evaluation are part of making any change to deal effectively with a problem. Alcohol and drugs are dysfunctional ways to reduce stress and may contribute to unrealistic self-evaluation; therefore, it is very important to ask specifically about the frequency and amount of alcohol, tobacco, or other drug use. The CAGE questions ("have you ever tried to cut down," "ever been angry when confronted," "ever felt guilty about your drinking," or "needed an eye-opener") can be useful in screening for alcohol dependency. With women patients in particular, it is important to ask about eating habits; weight changes; and changes in eating, cooking, and shopping behaviors because these also may reveal maladaptive coping mechanisms.

D. Other Resources

Asking the patient direct questions is helpful in identifying resources. Asking the patient to assess what other resources are available for support is often helpful. Some patients may effectively manage their problems alone, while others may not, particularly those who avoid asking others for help because they distort the meaning of help or are too embarrassed to ask others. The process of identifying to whom or where the patient may turn for additional support, and what that means to the patient, will help develop a treatment plan. This is also likely to increase the patient's sense of control and compliance with the plan and ultimately improve the outcome. Support may include family, a trusted friend, resources in the religious community, or formal support groups.

Physical Examination

The focus of the physical examination will be based on the presenting symptoms. However, it always includes a general assessment of the patient's current mental and physical state. The clinician needs to maintain a high index of suspicion for underlying depression and for other underlying medical disorders that might present with psychosomatic symptoms, including substance abuse, withdrawal, and evidence of domestic violence.

A standardized mental status examination allows the clinician to detect clues to an underlying psychiatric disorder, assess the impact of stress, and document a baseline of functioning. All aspects of a mental status examination can be routinely incorporated into an informal interview rather than having a set list of questions. It is especially important to address inconsistencies between the patient's presenting complaints or answers to questions and observed behaviors, and to address those inconsistencies in a curious, positive

Table 15-3. Mental Status Examination

General observations	Appearance and demeanor Behavioral activity	Eye contact Motor behavior (psychomotor retardation or excitement)
Mood and affect	Depression, anxiety, anger Anhedonia, loneliness, euphoria Mood swings	Range of affect Inappropriate affect Emotional liability
Thought processes	Quality and/or fluency of speech Coherence and relevance Evasiveness	Loose associations Concrete thinking Neologisms, echolalia, etc.
Thought content	Delusions (and type) Phobias Guilt, self-reproach	Obsessive ideas Thoughts of suicide or death
Somatic functioning	Appetite Energy levels Sleep functioning	Libido Sensory impairment Somatic concerns
Perceptions	Hallucination (and type) Illusions	Depersonalization Derealization
Sensorium	Orientation to person, place, time Clarity of consciousness	Dissociation
Cognitive functions	Disturbance of memory or attention	Intelligence
Judgment	Estimate judgment in areas of family and other social relations, work situation, and future plans	
Insight	Estimate degree of awareness of self, contribution to problems, and solutions	
Potential for harm	Ask about thoughts and plans for self-injury, suicide, violence toward others	

manner. Table 15-3 presents the major areas to cover in the mental status examination.

Diagnostic Testing

A. General Approach

Always exercise sound medical judgment and evaluate for potentially life-threatening or other serious diseases that the history and physical examination may suggest, including ischemic cardiac disease, dysrhythmias, thyroid or other endocrine disorders, asthma, and depression. On the other hand, avoid the temptation to perform exhaustive testing to exclude the entire differential diagnosis of the patient's physical symptoms because such searches are generally unrewarding. Testing for use of illicit drugs or steroids can be considered if the presentation is suggestive and the remainder of the history and physical examination does not offer other possibilities. Consider specialty referral if persistent symptoms are not consistent with clinical findings. In general, neuropsychological testing is not indicated early in the diagnostic evaluation. Rather, it is most useful in assessing functional status or determining workplace accommodations in individuals with stable cognitive deficits.

B. Diagnosis and Coding

If the primary reason for the patient's health care visit is a somatic manifestation, the practitioner can code the presenting symptom or the medical condition exacerbated by stress. The *International Classification of Diseases,* 9th Edition (ICD-9) also allows for V-codes to indicate psychosocial stressors. Examples include bereavement (V62.82), academic problems (V62.3), occupational problems (V62.2), acculturation problems (V62.4), and phase-of-life problems (V62.89). Unfortunately, reimbursement policies often dictate coding practices, and this type of information may be lost.

If the primary reason for the patient's visit is emotional manifestations of stress, it may be coded according to the criteria set forth in the *Diagnostic and Statistical Manual of Mental Disorders,* 4th Edition (DSM-IV), provided the symptoms and signs meet the full criteria for diagnosis. The following require that specific criteria be met:

- Anxiety disorder NOS, 300.00
- Acute stress disorder, 308.3
- Somatoform disorder, 300.81
- Adjustment disorder, 309
- Physiologic malfunction arising from mental factors and (coded by organ system), 306

If specific criteria are not met, it may be best to code the event as an adjustment disorder or simply as a V-code in order to assure a realistic treatment approach and avoid labeling of the patient, which may be detrimental.

DSM-IV allows for coding of psychosocial and environmental stressors on Axis 4. Axis 1 is reserved for coding clinical disorders; Axis 2 is reserved for personality disorders and mental retardation. Comorbid medical conditions are coded on Axis 3, and the global assessment of functioning (GAF) score is coded on Axis 5. In reality, the GAF often is not coded accurately. This score is composed of both symptom and functional dimensions, but often the examiner assigns a code only on the basis of the patient's presentation of symptoms and perceived distress.

The diagnosis, pattern, and severity of symptoms and the need for referral will determine treatment. All of the following can be explored as initial treatment, as helpful adjuncts to psychotherapy, or as interim relief measures while the patient is waiting for the initial visit with a mental health care provider. For most patients without a concomitant psychiatric disorder, recovery is expected during the first few weeks provided that stressors are mitigated and/or resources and coping mechanisms are enhanced. Because there is no concrete way to determine how treatment is progressing, it is suggested that patients keep a written journal of their progress, including details on sleeping and eating habits, exercise schedule, and handling of workload. Other things worth mentioning are any identifiable barriers to progress and how they are approached.

A. Patient Education

Education is a cornerstone of effective treatment. Patients may find it therapeutic to understand the mechanism and natural history of the stress reaction and that it is a normal occurrence when their resources are overwhelmed. Education also provides the framework to encourage the patient to enhance his or her coping skills, both acutely and in a preventive manner by regularly using stress management techniques. Physicians, ancillary providers, support groups, and patient-appropriate literature are all education resources.

B. Referral

Specialty referral may be necessary when patients have significant psychopathology or serious medical comorbidities. Some mental illnesses are chronic conditions, so establishing a good working relationship with the patient may facilitate a referral or the return-to-work process. Treating specific psychiatric diagnoses are described in other practice guidelines and texts.

It is recognized that primary care physicians and other nonpsychological specialists commonly deal with and try to treat psychiatric conditions. It is recommended that serious conditions such as severe depression and schizophrenia be referred to a specialist, while common psychiatric conditions, such as mild depression, be referred to a specialist after symptoms continue for more than six to eight weeks. The practitioner should use his or her best professional judgment in determining the type of specialist. Issues regarding work stress and person-job fit may be handled effectively with talk therapy through a psychologist or other mental health professional. Patients with more serious conditions may need a referral to a psychiatrist for medicine therapy.

C. Management of Medical Conditions

All new medical conditions or exacerbations of chronic medical conditions should be evaluated and treated according to the best clinical practices.

D. Modification of Maladaptive Coping Mechanisms

Patients can be educated on the adverse effects of maladaptive coping mechanisms, their current symptoms, and their ability to develop new, adaptive coping mechanisms. Be aware that it is often counterproductive to encourage a patient to abandon a coping mechanism until new coping mechanisms are established. Nonetheless, counseling to reduce or discontinue tobacco, alcohol, or drugs does communicate appropriate concern.

Nicotine is an antidepressant that functions much like an MAO (monoamine oxidase) inhibitor; and its usage may be difficult to stop until the patient's health crisis has stabilized and/or a new coping mechanism has been learned. Alcohol and drugs, on the other hand, can actively interfere with learning new ways of coping. In some cases, abstinence is a necessary precondition to learning. Furthermore, alcohol and hypnotics themselves may produce an anxiety state that is difficult to distinguish from a psychiatric disorder for at least four to six weeks. Patients with these kinds of complex issues often require referral.

The physician can encourage adaptive coping mechanisms such as reducing intake of caffeine (a sympathomimetic), refined sugar, and high-fat foods and increasing their intake of complex carbohydrates. Patients also can be counseled on proper sleep and sleep hygiene.

E. Aerobic Exercise

The clinician can be of significant assistance by helping the patient design a graded exercise program appropriate to his/her fitness level. Exercise can be both curative and preventive because evidence suggests that conditioned individuals are better able to resist the physiologic consequences of stress. Aerobic exercise metabolizes glucose, fatty acids, and other metabolites of the stress hormones that are released as part of the neuroendocrine response. Such activity may act in another way by increasing endorphin levels, thus positively influencing mood.

F. Stress Management Techniques

The majority of stress research has focused on stress management techniques for individuals. The following techniques can be offered as a way to help reduce the symptoms of stress and give the patient control over stressful situations and offer a measurable and concrete result; they also may curb the patient's desire to increase use of tobacco, alcohol, or other drugs, or excessive eating. The choice of technique may be influenced by the patient's presenting symptoms. For example, relaxation techniques may be particularly effective for individuals manifesting muscle tension. The psychology literature contains much information about meditation, relaxation techniques, and biofeedback for stress and anxiety, with considerable debate on the theories and mechanism of action (e.g., placebo, operant conditioning). To complicate matters, some techniques are offered alone or in conjunction with other modalities (e.g., hypnosis) or are modifications of techniques.

1. RELAXATION TECHNIQUES

The goal of relaxation techniques is to teach the patient to voluntarily change his or her physiologic (autonomic and neuroendocrine) and cognitive functions in response to stressors. Using these techniques can be preventive or helpful for patients in chronically stressful conditions, or they even may be curative for individuals with specific physiologic responses to stress. Relaxation techniques include meditation, relaxation response, and progressive relaxation. These techniques are advantageous because they may modify the manifestations of daily, continuous stress. The main disadvantages are that formal training, at a cost, is usually necessary to master the technique, and the techniques may not be a suitable therapy for acute stress.

Transcendental meditation (TM) is the most widely practiced form of meditation in the West. Other forms of meditation are associated with Eastern religions or philosophies, which may limit their appeal in the West. Transcendental meditation has been studied extensively as an adjunct treatment for hypertension as well as a stress-reduction technique. It has been shown to result in sustained and improved scores on the Hamilton and Beck Anxiety and Depression inventories three years after initial training in a group of patients with anxiety disorders.

Autogenic training and biofeedback are other relaxation methods designed to empower individuals to self-regulate physiologic responses. Both require training and practice.

Other relaxation techniques focus on simple, every day destressors, such as going for a walk, playing with children or pets, spending time alone, or talking with a friend or counselor. Integrating these activities into a stressful time can help create the more stable life balance that is better suited for coping with demanding external stimuli.

2. BEHAVIORAL TECHNIQUES

Time management, conflict resolution, or assertiveness training may be appropriate, depending on the assessment of demands facing the patient as well as his or her coping mechanisms and skills. Often, these programs are offered as employee training by the employer at little or no cost.

3. COGNITIVE TECHNIQUES AND THERAPY

Fundamental to cognitive therapy is the premise that the individual plays an important role in how he or she perceives or modifies his or her situation. Cognitive therapy can be problem-focused, with strategies intended to help alter the perception of stress; or emotion-focused, with strategies intended to alter the individual's response to stress. Familiarity and fluency with the many cognitive theories, therapies, and techniques is beyond most physicians' set of skills without specialized training. Studies on the effectiveness of cognitive therapy performed by psychologists exist, but studies evaluating attenuated cognitive techniques have not been done.

Nevertheless, for patients who do not merit a mental health referral or who refuse it, reviewing some basic techniques may be helpful. Increasing self-awareness and helping the individual find a way to reframe the stimulus or respond differently is common to many cognitive techniques. One commonly employed practice in primary care is to encourage the patient to keep a diary of his or her symptoms and stressors. This may help the patient link stressors with symptoms and offers the added advantage of measuring the frequency of symptoms. Other techniques focus on the patient's identifying and re-characterizing situations, stopping distorted thinking, or choosing his or her response to stress. Clarifying values may be helpful for patients who feel torn between roles and responsibilities. In a brief relationship with a patient, it is usually more useful to help him or her consider alternative thinking, behaviors, and plans than to confront dysfunctional thinking.

4. STRESS INOCULATION THERAPY

Stress inoculation therapy is another cognitive technique that bears special mention because it may be useful on an individual level or for specific occupational groups. This technique involves identifying sources of predictable stress, then preparing and practicing a plan to deal with the stressors. The results of limited studies performed in occupational groups (law enforcement, caregivers to mentally retarded clients) have been encouraging.

G. External Resources and Referrals

Employee assistance programs (EAPs) are comprehensive worksite-based programs designed to assist in the early identification and resolution of productivity problems associated with employees who are impaired or likely to be impaired by behavioral problems. Employee assistance programs have evolved to provide counseling for many types of common problems.

Employee assistance programs generally are funded by the employer and may be in-house or external. Some EAPs have little or no understanding of the workplace. Their primary function is to provide referral to external resources. If an occupational health professional has employers as clients, it is very helpful to have some understanding of the scope of, and how to access, their EAPs as well as other mental health benefits.

Many EAPs offer a management referral as an intervention tool for the employer concerned about employee-performance issues. This allows the employer to formally request that a professional associated with the EAP evaluate an employee if that employee demonstrates problems with job performance that may result from a mental health, substance abuse, or psychosocial problem. The EAP will give the employer some feedback, ranging from confirmation that an appointment was kept to on-going feedback as to whether the employee is making a good-faith effort with therapy or other interventions. It is often helpful when the referring physician receives feedback from the EAP.

H. Pharmacotherapy

1. ANXIOLYTICS

Anxiolytics are not recommended as first-line therapy for stress-related conditions because they can lead to dependence and do not alter stressors or the individual's coping mechanisms. They may be appropriate for brief periods in cases of overwhelming symptoms that interfere with daily functioning or to achieve a brief alleviation of symptoms that allow the patient to recoup emotional or physical resources. If medication is requested or is needed for a longer time, physicians may consider psychiatric disorders and appropriate referral.

2. ANTIDEPRESSANTS

Brief courses of antidepressants may be helpful to alleviate symptoms of depression; but because they may take weeks to exert their maximal effect, their usefulness in acute situations may be limited. Antidepressants have many side effects and can result in decreased work performance or mania in some people. Incorrect diagnosis of depression is the most common reason antidepressants are ineffective. Long-standing character issues, not depression, may be the underlying issue. Given the complexity and increasing effectiveness of available agents, referral for medication evaluation may be worthwhile.

3. ANTIPSYCHOTICS

Continuing an established course of antipsychotics is important, but they can decrease motivation and effectiveness at work. If a referral is made, it is still important to plan how the patient using these drugs will manage at work or return to work even after being referred for specific psychiatric treatment.

I. Modified Work and Accommodations

Occupational physicians are expected to offer specific instructions about work ability or job accommodations to facilitate successful return to work. Patients with acute stress-related conditions may not be viewed as having disabilities under the Americans with Disabilities Act (ADA). Nonetheless, it may be appropriate to suggest workplace modifications if they will facilitate the patient's reentry and retention in the work environment. Examples of accommodations include: 1) working with the patient and his or her supervisor or human resources manager to clarify the patient's responsibilities and performance expectations; 2) clarifying the frequency and degree of feedback from supervisor; or 3) temporary reassignment of specific stressful tasks. All job modifications should be limited in duration. As the patient improves, the clinician can work with the patient and the supervisor on job redesign and/or task redistribution to increase efficiency and reduce stressors. Other examples of accommodations include flexible hours, job sharing, reassigning tasks between workers, reassigning the patient to a vacant position, physical changes in the work environment to reduce stimuli (noise, visual, people), providing laptop computers to allow the patient to work at home, increasing supervisory sessions, and offering additional training and skill building. Further assistance on designing accommodations can be obtained from the Job Accommodation Network at 800-ADA-WORK, and from other resources.

J. Organizational Interventions

Physicians who provide services to an employer are in a unique position to counsel the employer on all aspects of occupational health, including occupational stress. Crisis interventions can be helpful for acute events such as downsizing or a catastrophic workplace event. Assessments and interventions are also available to help organizations with chronically high-stress levels, as manifested by high turnover, absenteeism, and other indicators that employees are under stress, such as increased EAP use and increased medical claims.

The occupational physician can consider adding to worksite audit tools those psychosocial characteristics of the work environment linked with stress. This may be helpful in objectively framing work-related stress as a health issue to management or to human resources personnel and identifying risk factors.

Organizational stress assessment tools have been developed, validated, and used effectively worldwide. Examples include the Pressure Management Indicator (PMI), Occupational Stress Inventory (OSI), and Generic Job Stress Questionnaire developed by NIOSH. These are usually administered to a work group or an entire organization to assess sources of organizational stress, individual stressors, and individuals' coping mechanisms. Such tools often are followed with a group intervention, such as a focus group, to further explore the sources and potential remedies for the organizational stress. Potential remedies include increased employee participation, redesigning the work group or job, consultation on management and supervisory skills and styles, implementing flexible schedules, reorganization, information exchange, changing rewards, or changing organizational norms (e.g., change in corporate "culture"). Organizational development, a human resources specialty area that assesses and implements organizational change programs, traditionally has "ownership" of this area within large companies. Organizational psychologists and psychiatrists are potential resources for assessing and "treating" organizational stress.

K. Disability Duration

The ultimate goal of therapy is to preserve the patient's functioning at work and in social relationships. Patients can be encouraged to use time off from work appropriately (e.g., bereavement leave, vacation, personal days, time that may be available under the provisions of the Family and Medical Leave Act, etc.) to address stressors outside of work if they are otherwise medically able to work. Returning a patient to work without actively addressing the underlying problem and providing appropriate treatment may lead to increased stress with resultant depression, insecurity, and/or jeopardized employment.

The duration of disability for patients whose medical condition warrants an absence will vary with the diagnosis, severity of current symptoms, and any comorbid conditions. There is no gold standard for stress-related disability durations. According to the Occupational Safety and Health Administration (OSHA), 23 days is the median number of days away from work for acute reactions to stress precipitated by discrete catastrophic events (ICD-9 308). Observed disability for anxiety disorders (ICD-9 308.3, 308.4, 308.9) in national databases is zero to five days, which is consistent with recommended disability durations in major duration guidelines (*Official Disability Guidelines*, Reed). Referral for mental health assessment may be considered if anticipated absence from work is expected to be more than one week.

Work-Relatedness

From a purely medical and psychological standpoint, stress involves the complex dynamics of the many factors and modifiers. The workers' compensation process in the United States is largely a legal and not a medical process. Determining what role the workplace played in causing or exacerbating a stress-related complaint involves careful analysis, review of the scientific evidence, and considered professional judgment.

The workers' compensation system generally classifies injuries according to the nature of the injury and its proximal cause, as follows:

- **Mental-mental:** a psychological or psychosocial stressor causes psychological injury
- **Mental-physical:** a psychological or psychosocial stressor causes physical injury
- **Physical-mental:** a physical event (e.g., assault, trauma) causes psychological injury (e.g., post-traumatic stress disorder)
- **Physical-physical:** a physical stressor causes physical injury

Compensation for stress-related disorders varies by state. Some states stipulate that the stressful event or circumstances must be unusual. For example, California allows compensation for psychiatric injuries that can be shown to be predominately caused by employment. Similarly, North Dakota allows compensation for mental injuries that are causally related to employment with a medical degree of certainty. If stress aggravates physical illnesses, such as coronary artery disease, conduction disturbances, hypertension, asthma, and other diseases, it is compensable in some systems if the stress is medically determined to be significant. In some states, psychological or physical disorders can be regarded as stress-related or stress-induced if reasonably believed to have been incited by a stressor. The necessary proportion of contribution varies and is often determined by statute. In some cases, the proportions are different if physical violence is involved or a specific disease is at issue. Case law and statutory changes prove this area of workers' compensation is rapidly evolving and the local workers' compensation commission can provide the most recent guidance.

Follow-up Visits

Frequency of follow-up visits may be determined by the severity of symptoms, whether the patient was referred for further testing and/or psychotherapy, and whether the patient is missing work. These visits allow the physician and patient to reassess all aspects of the stress model (symptoms, demands, coping mechanisms, and other resources) and to reinforce the patient's supports and positive coping mechanisms. Generally, patients with stress-related complaints can be followed by a midlevel practitioner every few days for counseling about coping mechanisms, medication use, activity modifications, and other concerns. These interactions may be conducted either on site or by telephone to avoid interfering with modified- or full-duty work if the patient has returned to work. Follow-up by a physician can occur when a change in duty status is anticipated (modified, increased, or full duty) or at least once a week if the patient is missing work.

Failure to Improve

Failure to improve may be due to an incorrect diagnosis, unrecognized medical or psychological conditions, or unrecognized psychosocial stressors. Again, it bears repeating to maintain a high index of suspicion for the prevalent but underdiagnosed condition of depression. If a patient expresses chronic dissatisfaction with work or has experienced significant dissatisfaction for several months, referral for psychiatric assessment or vocational counseling may be appropriate.

References

GENERAL REFERENCES

Cummings N, Vanden Bos G. The twenty-year Kaiser-Permanente experience with psychotherapy and medical utilization: implications for national health policy and national health insurance. *Health Policy Q.* 1981;1:159-74.

Kahn JP, Langlieb AM, eds. *Mental Health in the Workplace: A Handbook for Organizations and Clinicians.* San Francisco, Calif: Jossey-Bass; 2003.

Olfson M, Broadhead E, Weissman M, et al. Subthreshold psychiatric symptoms in a primary care group practice. *Arch Gen Psychiatry.* 1996;53:880-6.

U.S. Department of Health and Human Services, Public Health Service, Agency for Health Care Policy and Research Publication. *Clinical Practice Guideline Number 5, Depression in Primary Care: Volume 1, Detection and Diagnosis; Volume 2, Treatment of Major Depression.* No. 93-0550 and -0551; April 1993.

U.S. Department of Health and Human Services, Public Health Service. *Healthy People 2000 Midcourse Review and 1995 Revisions.* Washington, DC; 1995.

DIAGNOSIS AND CODING

American Psychiatric Association. *Diagnostic and Statistical Manual of Mental Disorders.* 4th ed. Washington, DC. American Psychiatric Association; 1994.

World Health Organization. *The International Classification of Diseases.* 9th Revision. Geneva, Switzerland: World Health Organization; 1997.

DISABILITY AND WORKERS' COMPENSATION

Denniston PL Jr, Ranavaya MI, Kennedy CW, et al. Return-to-work best practice guidelines. In: Denniston PL Jr, ed. *Official Disability Guidelines 2003.* 8th ed. Encinitas, Calif: Work Loss Data Institute; 2002.

Mancuso L. *Case Studies on Reasonable Accommodations for Workers with Phychiatric Disabilities.* Washington, DC: The Washington Business Group on Health; 1992.

Reed, P. The *Medical Disability Advisor: Workplace Guidelines for Disability Durations.* 4th Ed. Boulder, Colo: Reed Group, Ltd; 2001.

Schulman B. Stress. In: Demeter S, Anderson G, Smith G, eds. *Disability Evaluation.* St. Louis, Mo: Mosby; 1996.

1996 Analysis of Workers' Compensation Laws. Washington, DC: U.S. Chamber of Commerce; 1996.

OCCUPATIONAL STRESS

Anderzen I, Arnetz BB. Psychophysiological reactions to international adjustment. Results from a controlled, longitudinal study. *Psychother Psychosom.* 1999;68(2):67-75.

Arnetz BB. Technological stress: psychophysiological aspects of working with modern information technology. *Scand J Work Environ Health.* 1997;23 Suppl 3:97-103.

Burton WN, Conti DJ, Chen C-Y, et al. The role of health risk factors and disease on worker productivity. *J Occup Environ Med.* 1999;41(10):863-77.

Holmes S. Work-related stress: a brief review. *J R Soc Health.* 2001;121(4):230-5.

Hurrell JJ Jr, Nelson DL, Simmons BL. Measuring job stressors and strains: where we have been, where we are, and where we need to go. *J Occup Health Psychol.* 1998;3(4):368-89.

Johnson JV, Johansson G, eds. *The Psychosocial Work Environment: Work Organization, Democratization and Health.* Amityville, NY: Baywood Publishing; 1991.

Kasl S. The influence of the work environment on cardiovascular health: a historical, conceptual, and methodological perspective. *J Occup Psychol.* 1996;1(1):42-56.

Karasek R, Theorell T. *Healthy Work: Stress, Productivity and the Reconstruction of Working Life.* New York, NY: Basic Books; 1990.

Kawakami N, Araki S, Kawashima M, Masumoto T, Hayashi T. Effects of work-related stress reduction on depressive symptoms among Japanese blue-collar workers. *Scand J Work Environ Health.* 1997;23(1):54-9.

Keita GP, Hurrell J, eds. *Job Stress in a Changing Workforce: Investigating Gender, Diversity, and Family Issues.* Washington, DC: American Psychological Association; 1994.

Kompier M, Cooper C, eds. *Preventing Stress, Improving Productivity: European Case Studies in the Workplace.* London and New York, NY: Routledge; 1999.

Nordstrom CK, Dwyer KM, Merz CN, Shircore A, Dwyer JH. Work-related stress and early atherosclerosis. *Epidemiology.* 2001;12(2):180-5.

Peterson M, Wilson JF. The culture-work-health model and work stress. *Am J Health Behav.* 2002;26(1):16-24.

Sauter S, Murphy L, eds. *Organization Risk Factors for Job Stress.* Washington, DC: American Psychological Association; 1995.

Smith A. The scale of perceived occupational stress. *Occup Med (Lond).* 2000;50(5):294-8.

Tennant C. Work-related stress and depressive disorders. *J Psychosom Res.* 2001;51(5):697-704.

Theorell T, Karasek R. Current issues relating to psychosocial job strain and cardiovascular disease research. *J Occup Psychol.* 1996;1(1):9-26.

Theorell T. How to deal with stress in organizations? A health perspective on theory and practice. *Scand J Work Environ Health.* 1999;25(6):616-24.

Seigrist J. Adverse health effects of high effort/low-reward conditions. *J Occup Psychol.* 1996;1(1):27-41.

Schwartz J, Pickering T, Landsbergis P. Work-related stress and blood pressure: current theoretical models and considerations from a behavioral medicine perspective. *J Occup Health Psychol.* 1996;1(3):287-310.

van der Klink JJ, Blonk RW, Schene AH, van Dijk FJ. The benefits of interventions for work-related stress. *Am J Public Health.* 2001;91(2):270-6.

DEPRESSION

ACOEM Occupational Mental Health Committee. A screening program for depression. *J Occup Environ Med.* 2003;45(4):346-8.

Dewa CS, Goering P, Lin E, Paterson M. Depression-related short-term disability in an employed population. *J Occup Environ Med.* 2002;44(7):628-33.

Druss BG, Schlesinger M, Allen HM. Depressive symptoms satisfaction with health care, and 2-year work outcomes in an employed population. *Am J Psychiatry.* 2001;158(5):731-4.

Moncrieff J, Wessely S, Hardy R. Active placebos versus antidepressants for depression (Cochrane Review). In: *The Cochrane Library.* Issue 2; 2002. Oxford: Update Software.

Pignone MP, Gaynes BN, Rushton JL, et al. Screening for depression in adults: a summary of the evidence for the US Preventive Services Task Force. *Ann Intern Med.* 2002;136(10):765-76.

US Preventive Services Task Force. Screening for Depression: Recommendations and Rationale. *Ann Intern Med.* 2002;136(10):760-4.

Westen D, Morrison K. A multidimensional meta-analysis of treatments for depression, panic, and generalized anxiety disorder: an empirical examination of the status of empirically supported therapies. *J Consult Clin Psychol.* 2001;69(6):875-99.

POST-TRAUMATIC STRESS DISORDER

Suzanna R, Bisson J, Wessely S. Psychological debriefing for preventing post traumatic stress disorder (PTSD) (Cochrane Review). In: *The Cochrane Library.* Issue 2; 2002. Oxford: Update Software.

TREATMENT

Cotton D. *Stress Management: An Integrated Approach to Therapy.* New York, NY: Brunner/Mazel; 1990.

Ezoe S, Morimoto K. Behavioral lifestyle and mental health status of Japanese factory workers. *Prev Med.* 1994;23(1):98-105.

Gorman JM. Treatment of generalized anxiety disorder. *J Clin Psychiatry.* 2002;63(Suppl)8:17-23.

Harris JS. Home study program. Stressors and stress in critical care. *Crit Care Nurse.* 1984;4(1):83-97.

Hawton K, Townsend E, Arensman E, et al. Psychosocial and pharmacological treatments for deliberate self harm (Cochrane Review). In: *The Cochrane Library.* Issue 2; 2002. Oxford: Update Software.

Ivanevich J, Matteson M, Freedman S, et al. Worksite stress management interventions. *Am J Psychol.* 1990;45(2):252-61.

Keyes J. Stress inoculation training for staff working with persons with mental retardation: a model program. In: Murphy L, Hurrell J, Sauter S, et al, eds. *Job Stress Interventions.* Washington, DC: American Psychological Association; 1995:45-56.

McCann I, Holmes D. Influence of aerobic exercise on depression. *J Pers Soc Psychol.* 1984;46(5):1142-7.

Miller JJ, Fletcher K, Kabat-Zinn J. Three-year follow-up and clinical implications of a mindfulness meditation-based stress-reduction intervention in the treatment of anxiety disorders. *Gen Hosp Psychiatr.* 1995;17(3):192-200.

Muchnick-Baku S, Traw K. *Employee Assistance Programs: An Evolving Human Resource Management Strategy.* Washington, DC: Washington Business Group on Health; 1992.

Murphy L, Hurrell J, Sauter S, et al, eds. *Job Stress Interventions.* Washington, DC: American Psychological Association; 1995.

Pittler MH, Ernst E. Kava extract for treating anxiety (Cochrane Review). In: *The Cochrane Library.* Issue 2; 2002. Oxford: Update Software.

Quick JC, Murphy L, Hurrell J, eds. *Stress and Well-Being at Work: Assessments and Interventions for Occupational Mental Health.* Washington, DC: American Psychological Association; 1992.

Roskies E, Seraganian P, Oseahon R, et al. The Montreal type A intervention project: major findings. *Health Psychol.* 1986;5(1):45-69.

Srisurapanont M, Jarusuraisin N. Opioid antagonists for alcohol dependence (Cochrane Review). In: *The Cochrane Library.* Issue 2; 2002. Oxford: Update Software.

Williams S. *Managing Pressure for Peak Performance: The Positive Approach to Stress.* London: Kogan Page; 1994.

ORGANIZATIONAL INTERVENTIONS

Cartwright S, Cooper C, Murphy L. Diagnosing a healthy organization: a proactive approach to stress in the workplace. In: Murphy L, Hurrell J, Sauter S, et al, eds. *Job Stress Interventions.* Washington, DC: American Psychological Association; 1995:217-34.

Cooper C, Sloan S, Williams S. *Occupational Stress Indicator (Pressure Management Indicator) Management Guide.* Windsor, England: NFER-Nelson; 1988.

Ganster D. Interventions for building healthy organizations: suggestions from the stress research literature. In: Murphy L, Hurrell J, Sauter S, et al, eds. *Job Stress Interventions.* Washington, DC: American Psychological Association; 1995:323-36.

Goetzel RZ, Ozminkowski RJ, Sederer LI, Mark TL. The business case for quality mental health services: why employers should care about the mental health and well-being of their employees. *J Occup Environ Med.* 2002;44(4):320-30.

Goetzel RZ, Anderson DR, Whitmer RW, et al. The relationship between modifiable health risks and health care expenditures: an analysis of the multi-employer HERO health risk and cost database. *J Occup Environ Med.* 1998;40(10):843-54.

Osipow S, Spokae A. *A Manual for Measure of Occupational Stress, Strain and Coping.* Odessa, Fla: Par, Inc; 1983.

SOCIAL SUPPORT AND HEALTH

Berkman L. Social networks, support and health: taking the next step forward. *Am J Epidemiol.* 1986;123:559-62.

Berkman L, Syme L. Social networks, host resistance, and mortality: a nine-year follow-up study of Alameda County residents. *Am J Epidemiol.* 1979;109:186-204.

Cassel J. The contribution of the social environment to host resistance. *Am J Epidemiol.* 1976;104:107-23.

Cromwell BA, George L, Blazer D, et al. Psychosocial risk factors and urban/rural differences in the prevalence of major depression. *Br J Psychiatry.* 1986;149:304-14.

Gardner J, Lyon J. Cancer in Utah Mormon men by lay priesthood level. *Am J Epidemiol.* 1982;116:243-57.

Gardner J, Lyon J. Cancer in Utah Mormon women by church activity level. *Am J Epidemiol.* 1982;116:258-65.

Holmes T, Rahe R. The social readjustment rating scale. *J Psychosom Research.* 1967;11:213-8.

House J, Landis K, Umberson D. Social relationships and health. *Science.* 1988;241:540-5.

Levin J, Vanderpool H. Is frequent religious attendance really conducive to better health? Toward an epidemiology of religion. *Soc Sci Med.* 1987; 24(7):589-600.

Levin J. Religion and health: is there an association, is it valid, and is it causal? *Soc Sci Med.* 1994;38(11):1475-82.

Vilhjalmosson R. Life stress, social support and clinical depression: a reanalysis of the literature. *Soc Sci Med.* 1993;37(3):331-42.

Wilson I, Cleary L. Linking clinical variables with health-related quality of life: a conceptual model of patient outcomes. *JAMA.* 1995;273:59-65.

STRESS AND MEDICAL CONDITIONS

Alfredsson L, Karasek R, Theorell T. Myocardial infarction risk and psychosocial work environment: an analysis of the male Swedish working force. *Soc Sci Med.* 1982;16:463-7.

Anda R, Williamson D, Escobedo L, et al. Self-perceived stress and the risk of peptic ulcer disease: a longitudinal study of U.S. adults. *Arch Intern Med.* 1992;152:829-33.

Armstrong D, Arnold R, Classen MA, et al. RUDER—A prospective, two-year multicenter study of risk factors for duodenal ulcer relapse during maintenance therapy with ranitidine. *Dig Dis Sci.* 1994;39(7):1425-33.

Bush DE, Ziegelstein RC, Tayback M, et al. Even minimal symptoms of depression increase mortality risk after acute myocardial infarction. *Am J Cardiol.* 2001;88:337-41.

Ellard K, Beaurepaire J, Jones M, et al. Acute and chronic stress in duodenal ulcer disease. *Gastroenterology.* 1990;99:1628-32.

Ferketich MA, Schwartzbaum JA, et al. Depression as an antecedent to heart disease among women and men in the NHANES I study. *Arch Intern Med.* 2000;160:1261-8.

Ford DE, Mead LA, Chang PP, Cooper-Patrick L, Wang NY, Klag MJ. Depression is a risk factor for coronary artery disease in men. *Arch Intern Med.* 1998;158:1422-6.

Frasure-Smith N, Lesperance F, Talajic M. Depression following myocardial infarction: impact on 6-month survival. *JAMA.* 1993;270:1819-25.

Holtman G, Armstrong D, Poppel E, et al. Influence of stress on the healing and relapse of duodenal ulcers: a prospective, multicenter trial of 2109 patients with recurrent duodenal ulceration treated with ranitidine. *Scand J Gastroenterol.* 1992;27:917-23.

Hui M, Shui P, Lok SF, et al. Life events and daily stress in duodenal ulcer disease: a prospective study of patients with active disease and in remission. *Digestion.* 1992;52:165-72.

Karasek R, Theorell T, Schwartz J, et al. Job characteristics in relation to the prevalence of myocardial infarction in the U.S. Health Examination Survey (HES) and the Health and Nutrition Examination Survey (HANES). *Am J Public Health.* 1988;78(8):910-8.

Karasek R, Baker D, Marxer F, et al. Job decision latitude, job demands, and cardiovascular disease: a prospective study of Swedish men. *Am J Public Health.* 1981;71:694-705.

Kawakami N, Haratani T, Araki S. Effects of perceived job stress on depressive symptoms in blue-collar workers of an electrical factory in Japan. *Scand J Work Environ Health.* 1992;18(3):195-9.

Knox S, Theorell T, Svensson J, et al. The relation of social support and working environment to medical variables associated with elevated blood pressure in young males: a structural model. *Soc Sci Med.* 1985;21(5):525-31.

Landsbergis P, Schnall P, Warren K, et al. Association between ambulatory blood pressure and alternative formulations of job strain. *Scand J Work Environ Health.* 1994;20:349-63.

Lerner D, Levine S, Malspeis S, et al. Job strain and health-related quality of life in a national sample. *Am J Public Health.* 1994;84:1580-5.

Lindquist TL, Beilin LJ, Knuiman M. Effects of lifestyle, coping and work-related stress on blood pressure in office workers. *Clin Exp Pharmacol Physiol.* 1995;22(8):580-2.

Maschewsky W. The relation between stress and myocardial infarction: a general analysis. *Soc Sci Med.* 1982;16:455-62.

Pieper C, LaCroix A, Karasek R. The relation of psychosocial dimensions of work with coronary heart disease risk factors: a meta-analysis of five United States data bases. *Am J Epidemiol.* 1989;129(3):483-94.

Richter JE. Stress and psychological and environmental factors in functional dyspepsia. *Scand J Gastroenterol.* 1991;26(S182):40-6.

Schnall P, Pieper C, Schwartz J, et al. The relationship between "job strain," workplace diastolic blood pressure, and left ventricular mass index: results of a case-control study. *JAMA.* 1990;263(14):1929-35.

Vanitallie TB. Stress: a risk factor for serious illness. *Metabolism.* 2002;51(6 Suppl 1):40-5.

OTHER

The following references, compiled by C. Donald Williams, MD, were kindly provided by the Academy of Organizational and Occupational Psychiatry for inclusion in this chapter.

Azima F. Group psychotherapy with personality disorders. In: Kaplan H, Sadock H, eds. *Comprehensive Group Psychotherapy.* 3rd ed. Baltimore, Md: Williams & Wilkins; 1993:393-406.

Bonnie RJ, Monahan, eds. *Mental Disorder, Work Disability, and the Law.* Chicago, Ill: University of Chicago Press; 1996.

Bruce ML, Seeman TE, Merrill SS, Blazer DG. The impact of depressive symptomatology on physical disability: MacArthur studies on successful aging. *Am J Public Health.* 1994;84:1796-9.

Druss BG, Rosenheck RA, Sledge WH. Health and disability costs of depressive illness in a major U.S. corporation. *Am J Psychiatry.* 2000;157(8):1274-8.

Dubovsky SL, Thomas M. Psychotic depression: advances in conceptualization and treatment. *Hosp Community Psychiatry.* 1992;43(12):1189-98.

Duckro PN, Chibnall JT, Tomazic TJ. Anger, depression, and disability: a path analysis of relationships in a sample of chronic posttraumatic headache patients. *Headache.* 1995;35:7-9.

Dworkin RH, Handlin DS, Richlin DM, Brand L, Vannucci C. Unraveling the effects of compensation, litigation, and employment on treatment response to chronic pain. *Pain.* 1985;23:49-59.

Eells TD. Can therapy affect physical health? *J Psychother Pract Res.* 2000;9(2)100-4.

Gallagher RM. Referral delay in back pain patients on worker's compensation. *Psychosomatics.* 1996;37:270-84.

Grant BL, Robbins DB. Disability, workers compensation, and fitness for duty. In: Kahn JP, ed. *Mental Health in the Workplace: A Practical Psychiatric Guide.* New York, NY: Van Nostrand Reinhold; 1993.

Hall HV, Pritchard DA. *Detecting Malingering and Deception.* New York: St. Lucie Press; 1996.

Hendler NL, Kozikowski JG. Patients involved in litigation. *Psychosomatics.* 1993;34:494-501.

Johnson P, Indvik J. The impact of unresolved trauma on career management. *Internl J Career Manag.* 1994;6(2):12-8.

Kouzis A, Eaton W. Psychopathology and the initiation of disability payments. *Psychiatric Services.* 2001;51:908-13.

Langer CS. Title I of the Americans with Disabilities Act. In: Snyder JW, Klees JE, eds. *Law and the Workplace: Occupational Medicine: State of the Art Reviews.* 1996;11:1-16.

Leig JP, Markowitz SB, Fahs M, Shin C, Landrigan PJ. Occupational injury and illness in the United States. *Arch Intern Med.* 1997;157:1557-68.

Minnesota Department of Labor and Industry. *State Workers' Compensation Anti-Fraud Activity: Survey Results*; 1995.

Mischoulon D. An approach to the patient seeking psychiatric disability benefits. *Acad Psych.* 1999;22:128-36.

Modlin HC. Compensation neurosis. *Bull Am Acad Psychiatry Law.* 1986;14(3):263-71.

Oldham JM, Skodol AE, Kellman HD, et al. Comorbidity of axis 1 and axis 2 disorders. *Am J Psychiatry.* 1995;152:571-8.

Porter K. Combined individual and group psychotherapy. In: Kaplan H, Sadock H, eds. *Comprehensive Group Psychotherapy.* 3rd ed. Baltimore, Md: Williams & Wilkins; 1993.

Rogers R, ed. *Clinical Assessment of Malingering and Deception.* New York, NY: The Guilford Press; 1988.

Schouten R. Pitfalls of clinical practice: the treating clinician as expert witness. *Harv Rev Psychiatry.* 1993;1:64-5.

Schouten R. Approach to the patient seeking disability. In: Stern TA, Herman JB, Slavin PL, eds. *The MGH Guide to Psychiatry in Primary Care.* New York, NY: McGraw Hill; 1998:121-6.

Schouten R, Williams CD. Psychiatric assessment and management of chronic disability syndromes. In: Stoudemire A, Fogel BS, Greenberg D, eds. *Psychiatric Care of the Medical Patient.* 2nd ed. New York, NY: Oxford University Press; 2000.

Sederer L, Clemens N. The business case for high-quality mental health care. *Psychiatric Serv.* 2001;53:143-5.

Strasburger LH, Gutheil TG, Brodsky A. On wearing two hats: role conflict in serving as both psychotherapist and expert witness. *Am J Psychiatry.* 1997;154:448-56.

Walker EA, Gelfand MD, Gelfand AN, Creed F, Katon WJ. The relationship of current psychiatric disorder to functional disability and distress in patients with inflammatory bowel disease. *Gen Hosp Psychiatry.* 1996;18:220-9.

Williams CD. Group psychotherapy in the treatment of injured workers. Paper presentation. APA Annual Meeting. 1997.

Zuckerman D. Reasonable accommodations for people with mental illness under the ADA. *Mental Physical Disability Law Reporter.* 1993;17:311-20.

Zwerling C, Whitten PS, Davis CS, Sprince NL. Occupational injuries among workers with disabilities. *JAMA.* 1997;278:2163-9.

***Master Algorithm**. ACOEM Guidelines for Care of Eye Complaints*

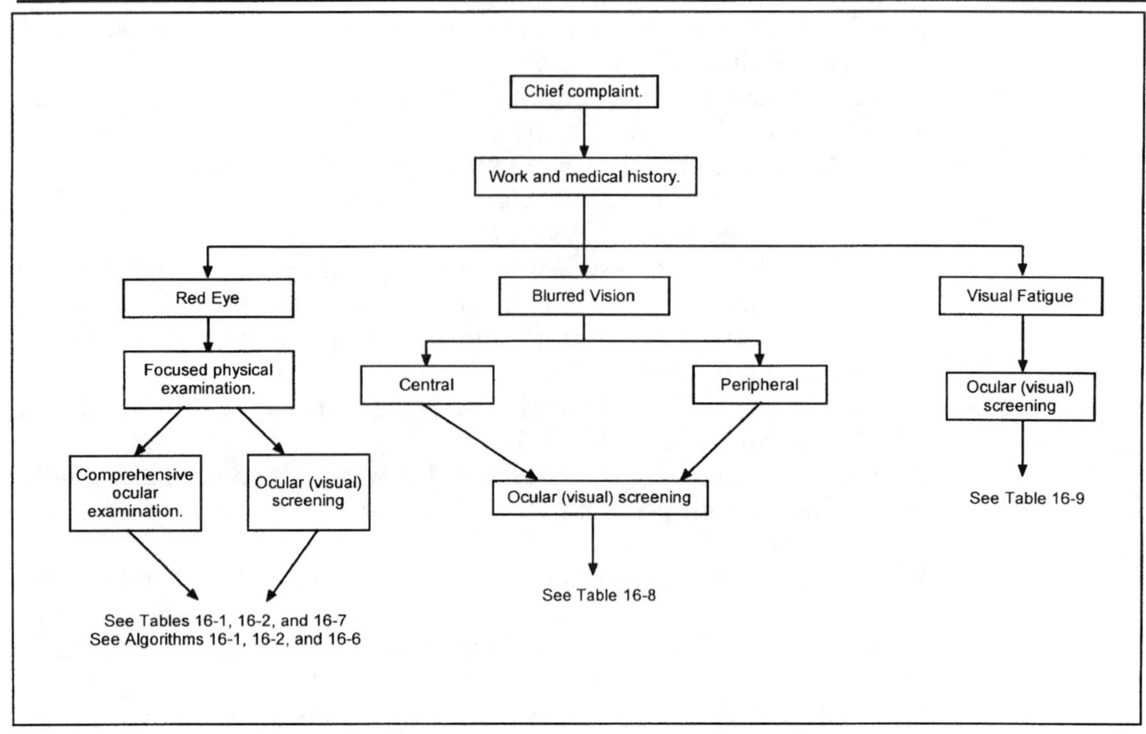

16 Eye

Unfortunately, occupational eye injuries are common and carry the potential for severe visual impairment and subsequent visual disability. The first responder's evaluation on whether the problem is a red flag or non-red-flag condition, and the action taken can make the difference between a subsequently healed normal eye and blindness. Some cannot wait for referral to an ophthalmologist and require immediate action. This chapter provides comprehensive guidelines and practical recommendations for treating the three major eye complaints seen most frequently in workers:

- Red eye
- Blurred vision
- Visual fatigue

This chapter contains straightforward guidelines on handling the problems and provides detailed information on treatment modalities that generally are not available to primary care personnel. Additional resources for further study are also provided.

General Approach and Basic Principles

Patients with work-related eye complaints are seen commonly by occupational and primary care providers. Eye complaints account for approximately 4% of workers' compensation claims and 1% of total payments.

An estimated 2.5 million people suffer eye injuries each year. Between 40,000 and 60,000 of these injuries are associated with severe vision loss, making careful monitoring, proper documentation, and timely referral paramount. Besides trauma cases, millions of patients visit emergency rooms each year for nontraumatic acute eye conditions such as conjunctivitis. Recommendations for assessing and treating adults with potentially work-related acute eye complaints (i.e., those of 48 hours duration or less) are presented in this clinical practice guideline. Topics include the initial assessment and diagnosis of patients with potentially work-related eye complaints, identification of red flags that may indicate the presence of a serious underlying medical condition, initial management, diagnostic considerations, and special studies for identifying clinical pathology, work-relatedness, return to work in a full- or modified-duty capacity, and further management considerations, including the management of delayed recovery.

The patient may present with the following symptoms:

- Red eye
- Blurred vision (central or peripheral)
- Visual fatigue (a phenomenon related to intensive use of the eyes)

Patient Management

Patient management is delineated in the algorithms. The master algorithm illustrates how primary care and occupational medicine practitioners generally should manage patients with eye complaints. The following text, tables, and numbered algorithms expand on the master algorithm.

The principal recommendations for assessing and treating patients with eye complaints are as follows:

- Initial assessment should focus on detecting indications of potentially serious ocular pathology, termed red flags, and determining an accurate diagnosis. For these purposes, red flags are defined as a sign or symptom of a potentially serious condition indicating that further consultation, support, or specialized treatment may be necessary.
- In the absence of red flags, occupational or primary care providers can safely and effectively handle work-related eye complaints. Conservative treatment can proceed for 48 to 72 hours for superficial foreign bodies, corneal abrasions, conjunctivitis, and ultraviolet radiation damage. Normally, tissues of the eye heal rapidly. If eye damage is not well on the way to resolution within 48 to 72 hours, referral to a specialist is indicated. Nonspecific eye complaints may be monitored for a longer period of time while ergonomic and other adjustments are made. The focus is on monitoring for complications, facilitating the healing process, and determining fitness for return to work in a modified- or full-duty capacity.
- Corneal discomfort can be relieved safely with a topically applied ophthalmic nonsteroidal anti-inflammatory drug (NSAID), a systemic nonprescription analgesic, or an intramuscular or intravenous narcotic in severe ocular/face injuries when symptoms or physical findings mandate. Patients requiring narcotic analgesics generally should be referred for ophthalmologic care. Avoid using topical anesthetics for purposes other than diagnosis or treatment because they may obscure worsening pathology and thus inadvertently cause further injury.

- Visual acuity should be assessed and documented carefully at each examination prior to other examinations or treatment, except for cases of chemical burns.
- Patients recovering from acute eye injury or infection should be encouraged to return to modified work as their condition permits.
- Nonphysical factors, such as psychosocial, workplace, or socioeconomic problems, should be addressed in an effort to resolve delayed recovery.

Presenting Symptoms

The patient may present with symptoms of red eye, blurred vision (central or peripheral), or visual fatigue (see Master Algorithm and Algorithm 16-1).

1. *Red eye* refers to hyperemia of the superficially visible vessels of the conjunctiva, episclera, or sclera. Hyperemia, or engorgement of the conjunctival blood vessels, also known as inflammation,[1] can be caused by disorders of these structures or of adjoining structures, including the cornea, iris, ciliary body, or ocular adnexa. Red eye can be characterized in three categories:
   a. Infections
   b. Sterile inflammation
   c. Trauma to the eyeball and/or periorbita
2. *Blurred vision* is a symptom of decreased visual acuity (central and peripheral). The central visual acuity is measured with an Early Treatment Diabetic Retinopathy Study (ETDRS) or Snellen chart at 20 feet (6 meters), at the working intermediate (i.e., computer operators 20 to 30 inches), and near (16 inches) distance. Peripheral vision (visual acuity) is measured by visual fields.
3. *Visual fatigue* describes a phenomenon related to intensive use of the eyes. It includes complaints of eye or periocular pain, itching, burning, tearing, oculomotor changes, focusing problems, performance degradation, and/or after-colors.

[1]In its broadest sense, the process of inflammation may be considered as the response of a tissue or tissues to a noxious stimulus. The tissue may be predominantly cellular (the retina), composed mainly of extracellular materials (the cornea), or a mixture of both (the uvea). The response may be localized or generalized and the noxious stimulus may be infectious or noninfectious. In general, inflammation is an immune (nonspecific or specific) response to a foreign stimulus or agent. Inflammation is not synonymous with infection. Inflammation may be caused by an infection, e.g., postoperative staphylococcal endophthalmitis, but it also may be caused by noninfectious agents such as thermal burns. Conversely, infection is not always accompanied by significant inflammation. For example, in certain diseases of the immune mechanism, widespread infection may be present, but the individuals are incapable of mounting an inflammatory response.

Management of Red Eye

Primary care physicians commonly see patients who complain of a red eye. This condition may result from a simple disorder such as a subconjunctival hemorrhage that will resolve spontaneously. The general physician may treat numerous other causes. Vision threatening disorders that cause a red eye require early recognition and prompt referral to an ophthalmologist for optimal management based on the results of the initial examination.

History

Information obtained from a careful history and examination directs the approach to management. The onset of a red eye, duration of the redness, and clinical course should be noted to help to distinguish the causative agents (see Table 16-1, Master Algorithm, and Algorithms 16-1, 16-2, and 16-3).

The patient's complaint may reveal the cause of the red eye. For example, itching may signify allergies. A scratchy or burning sensation suggests lid, conjunctival, or corneal disorders, including foreign bodies, in-turning eyelashes, and dry eyes. Localized lid pain or tenderness is a common presenting complaint of a stye or an acute chalazion of the lid. Table 16-1 relates the symptoms and the causes of these disorders.

Deep, intense, aching pain is not localized, but may reflect corneal laceration, iritis, or acute glaucoma, as well as sinusitis or tension headaches. Photophobia suggests problems arising from the anterior segment of the eye, such as corneal abrasions, iritis, and acute glaucoma. A halo effect around lights is a sign of corneal edema commonly seen in acute glaucoma. Individuals who have corneal edema associated with contact lens wear also may experience halo vision.

Table 16-1. Symptoms of Red Eye

Symptom	Referral Advisable if Present	Acute Glaucoma	Acute Iridocyclitis	Keratitis	Bacterial Conjunctivitis	Viral Conjunctivitis	Allergic Conjunctivitis
Blurred vision	Yes	3	1-2	3	0	0	0
Pain	Yes	2-3	2	2	0	0	0
Photo-phobia	Yes	1	3	3	0	0	0
Colored halos	Yes	2	0	0	0	0	0
Exudation	No	0	0	0-3	3	2	1
Itching	No	0	0	0	0	0	2-3

Note: The range of severity of the symptom is indicated by 0 (absent) to 3 (severe).
Source: Table modified from Bradford CA, ed. *Basic Ophthalmology.* 7th ed. San Francisco, Calif: American Academy of Ophthalmology; 1999.

Asking the patient open-ended questions such as those listed below allows the clinician to judge the need for further discussion or specific inquiries to obtain more detailed information.

- What are your symptoms?
  - Are you experiencing pain, sensitivity to light, blurring or loss of vision, or headache?
  - Is your problem located primarily in the eye or near the eye? Do you have pain or other symptoms elsewhere?
  - Are your symptoms constant or intermittent? What makes the problem worse or better?
- How do these symptoms limit you?
  - How long can you look at something?
  - Can you see clearly?
- When did your current limitations begin?
  - How long has your vision been limited? More than a day or two?
  - Have your symptoms changed? How?
- Have you had similar episodes previously?
- Have you had any previous testing or treatment? With whom?
- What do you think caused the problem?
- What are your specific job duties? How long do you spend performing each duty?
- Do you have other medical problems? Diabetes? High blood pressure? Glaucoma?
- What do you hope we can accomplish during this visit?

Observation of the Patient

When the patient enters the examination area, the physician can observe his or her ability to see the way in and to gauge depth. Photophobia or pain can be inferred if the affected eye is held shut. Tearing or discharge can be observed as well.

A history of chemical splash is an emergency, and examination may be delayed until after the eye is flushed to dilute the chemical.

Examination

The primary care physician should evaluate the red eye with a visual acuity chart, a penlight (slit lamp preferred), a tonometer, a sterile fluorescein dye strip, topical anesthetic drops, and an ophthalmoscope. Most clinics today have a Titmus or Stereo Optical visual screener or an Armed Forces Tester, a noncontact "puff" tonometer (Reichert Optical Company), and a slit lamp. A systematic approach to the examination should then be conducted, beginning by examining the face, orbital area, and lids and ending with a close view of the eyeball. The preferred method for examining the eyeball includes using the slit-lamp biomicroscope and the ophthalmoscope (see Master Alagorithm, and Algorithms 16-1, 16-2, and 16-3).

How to Examine the Red Eye

The American Academy of Ophthalmology specifies nine diagnostic steps to use when evaluating a patient with a red eye (Bradford):

1. Determine whether the visual acuity is normal or decreased using a Snellen chart or (preferred) ETDRS chart at 20 feet or six meters, or the 1 meter ETDRS chart if required.
2. Decide by inspection what pattern of redness is present and whether it is due to subconjunctival hemorrhage, conjunctival hyperemia, ciliary flush, or a combination of these.
3. Detect the presence of conjunctival discharge and categorize it as to amount—profuse or scant—and character—purulent, mucopurulent, serous, or hemorrhagic.
4. Detect opacities of the cornea, including large keratic precipitates, or irregularities of the corneal surface, such as corneal edema, corneal leukoma (a white opacity caused by scar tissue), and irregular corneal reflection. Conduct the examination using a biomicroscope, or penlight and transilluminator, at least. Biomicroscopy is the practice standard.
5. Search for disruption of the full thickness of the corneal epithelium by staining the cornea with fluorescein[2] and lack of corneal epithelium vitality by staining with rose bengal.

[2]Fluorescein, applied primarily as a 2% alkaline solution and with impregnated paper strips, is used to examine the integrity of the conjunctival and corneal epithelia. Defects in the corneal epithelium will appear green in ordinary light and bright yellow when a cobalt blue filter is used in the light path. Similar lesions of the conjunctiva appear bright orange or yellow in ordinary illumination. Fluorescein also has been used in the fitting of rigid contact lenses, although it cannot be used for soft lenses, which absorb the dye. Prepared sterile ophthalmic strips are used diagnostically for staining the anterior segment of the eye when (1) delineating a corneal injury, herpetic ulcer, or foreign body, (2) determining the site of an intraocular injury, (3) fitting contact lenses, (4) making the fluorescein test to ascertain postoperative closure of a sclerocorneal (also referred to as corneoscleral) wound in delayed anterior chamber re-formation, and (5) making the lacrimal drainage test. **Never use fluorescein sodium (Bioglo) while the patient is wearing soft contact lenses because the lenses may become stained.** Whenever fluorescein is used, flush the eyes with sterile normal saline solution and wait at least 1 hour before replacing the lenses. Soft Glo can be used.

Fluorescein sodium strips are manufactured as Fluor-I-Strips (sterile strips 9 mg each) by Bausch & Lomb Pharmaceuticals, Inc. (5500 Hidden River Parkway, Tampa, FL 32627), Bioglo (sterile strips 1 mg each) by Eye Care and Cure Corp. (1140 North Rosemont Blvd., Tucson, AZ 85712), Soft Glo (5 mg—it was established in 1972 and reverified in 1999 that this fluorescein does not stain soft contact lenses and may be used in soft lens wearers without the specific precautions noted for the other products listed; use of Soft Glo will save potential staining of soft contact lenses) by Eye Care and Cure Corp. (1140 North Rosemont Blvd., Tucson, AZ 85712), and Rose Bengal Ophthalmic Strips (1.3 mg of rose bengal, individually wrapped, sterile—these are particulary useful for demonstrating abnormal conjunctival or corneal epithelium; devitalized cells stain bright red, whereas normal cells show no change; the abnormal epithelial cells present in dry eye disorders are effectively revealed by this stain) by Akorn, Inc. (2500 Millbrook Drive, Buffalo Grove, IL 60089).

6. Use of a slit lamp (biomicroscope) allows one to estimate the depth of the anterior chamber as normal or shallow and to detect any microscopic blood or white blood cells, which would indicate either hyphema or hypopyon, respectively. (A hypopyon is indicated by the presence of protein and white blood cells in the anterior chamber, e.g., when a corneal ulcer is present, and a hyphema is indicated by protein and red blood cells in the anterior chamber.)
7. Detect irregularity of the pupils and determine whether one pupil is larger than the other. Observe the reactivity of the pupils to light to determine whether one pupil is more sluggish than the other or is nonreactive.
8. Determine whether the intraocular pressure is high, normal, or low by performing tonometry if indicated clinically, e.g., if acute angle-closure glaucoma is suspected. (Tonometry is contraindicated when external infection or lack of globe integrity is obvious.)
9. Detect the presence of proptosis, lid malfunction, or any limitations of eye movement.

A comprehensive examination is preferred in patients with ocular diseases or injuries. At a minimum, perform a visual acuity assessment prior to any treatment, except in chemical injuries, where immediate irrigation is mandated. Ocular (visual) screening is extremely useful and can fulfill the minimal examination requirements.

Methods of Testing

Visual Acuity: Quantitative Bilateral Tests. Acuity is measured at infinity (as a minimum) and near and intermediate distances (based on job description) and is performed with and without corrective devices (e.g., glasses or contact lenses) and without removing other corrective devices (e.g., intraocular lenses).

Slit-Lamp Biomicroscopy. Slit-lamp examination is the standard method of examining the eye. The slit lamp uses intense illumination and magnification.[3] Use of the slit-lamp biomicroscope has been established as a competency by the American College of Occupational and Environmental Medicine for occupational health physicians. The general findings noted in a slit-lamp exami-

[3]A slit lamp features an oblique (condensed) illumination and a magnifying system. With refinements, this system is used in current slit lamps. All detail is seen by the viewer by reflected light. Substances that do not reflect light are not visible; they are termed *optically empty,* such as normal tears and the aqueous humor. Structures that transmit light, but can be seen in the beam, are termed *reluctant,* such as the cornea, lens, and vitreous. Structures that do not transmit light are *opaque.* The examiner must use special techniques for illumination and focusing that enhance the examination. The methods include (1) diffuse illumination; (2) direct or focal illumination (the most useful and important type of slit-lamp illumination, whereby tissues such as the cornea are seen as an optical section or a block of tissue known as a *parallelepiped*); (3) retroillumination, where the area is being illuminated by reflected rays (e.g., a corneal foreign body or corneal ulcer); and (4) indirect illumination.

nation (biomicroscope) and their clinicopathologic correlations appear at the end of this chapter under "Additional Resources."

How to Interpret the Findings of Red Eye

The associated signs and symptoms (see Tables 16-1 and 16-2) of various disorders overlap to some extent. Although many conditions can cause a red eye, several signs and symptoms signal danger. The presence of one or more of these danger signals alerts the physician that the patient has a disorder requiring an ophthalmologist's attention (i.e., a red flag). Table 16-3 provides the differential diagnosis.

Table 16-2. Signs of Red Eye

Symptom	Referral Advisable if Present	Acute Glaucoma	Acute Iridocyclitis	Keratitis	Bacterial Conjunctivitis	Viral Conjunctivitis	Allergic Conjunctivitis
Ciliary flush	Yes	1	2	3	0	0	0
Conjunctival hyperemia	No	2	2	2	3	2	1
Corneal opacification	Yes	3	0	1-3	0	0-1	0
Corneal epithelial disruption	Yes	0	0	1-3	0	0-1	0
Pupillary abnormalities	Yes	Mid-dilated, nonreactive	Small; may be irregular	Normal or small	0	0	0
Shallow anterior chamber depth	Yes	3	0	0	0	0	0
Elevated intraocular pressure	Yes	3	−2 to +1	0	0	0	0
Proptosis	Yes	0	0	0	0	0	0
Discharge	No	0	0	Sometimes	2-3	2	1
Preauricular lymph-node enlargement	No	0	0	0	0	1	0

Note: The range of severity of the symptom is indicated by 0 (absent) to 3 (severe).
Source: Table modified from Bradford CA, ed. *Basic Ophthalmology.* 7th ed. San Francisco, Calif: American Academy of Ophthalmology; 1999.

Table 16-3. Differential Diagnosis—Red Eye

- *Acute angle-closure glaucoma.* An uncommon form of glaucoma due to sudden and complete occlusion of the anterior chamber angle by iris tissue—serious. The more common chronic open-angle glaucoma causes no redness of the eye.
- *Iritis or iridocyclitis.* An inflammation of the iris alone or of the iris and ciliary body; often manifested by ciliary flush—serious.
- *Herpes simplex keratitis.* An inflammation of the cornea caused by the herpes simplex virus; common—potentially serious; can lead to corneal ulceration.
- *Conjunctivitis.* Hyperemia of the conjunctival blood vessels; cause may be bacterial, viral, allergic, or irritative; common—often not serious.
- *Episcleritis.* An inflammation (often sectorial) of the episclera, the vascular layer between the conjunctiva and the sclera; uncommon, without discharge—not serious; possibly allergic, occasionally painful.

Source: Table modified from Berson FG. *Basic Ophthalmology for Medical Students and Primary Care Residents.* 6th ed. San Francisco, Calif: American Academy of Ophthalmology; 1993.

Diagnostic Criteria

If the patient does not have red flags for serious conditions, the clinician can then determine which other eye disorder is present. The criteria presented in Figure 16-1 follow the clinical thought process from the mechanism of illness or injury to unique symptoms and signs of a particular disorder and finally to test results, if any tests were needed to guide treatment at this stage.

The clinician must be aware that several symptoms and signs are common to a number of eye injuries or disorders (see Tables 16-1 and 16-2). Therefore, accurate diagnosis depends on linking the mechanism of injury or pathogenesis, symptoms, signs, and findings of the eye examination with findings on magnification and, if necessary, with fluorescein staining of the eye. In the following lists, an asterisk (*) after a symptom or sign indicates a danger signal.

Symptoms of Red Eye (see Table 16-1)

Blurred Vision. Blurred vision often indicates serious ocular disease. Blurred vision that improves with blinking suggests a discharge or mucus on the ocular surface.

Severe pain.* Pain may indicate keratitis, ulcer, iridocyclitis, or acute glaucoma. Patients with conjunctivitis may complain of a scratchiness or mild irritation, but do not have severe pain.

Photophobia.* Photophobia is an abnormal sensitivity to light that accompanies iritis. It may occur either alone or secondary to corneal inflammation. Patients with conjunctivitis have normal light sensitivity.

Colored halos.* Rainbow-like fringes or colored halos seen around a point of light are usually a symptom of corneal edema, often resulting from an abrupt rise in intraocular pressure. Therefore, colored halos are a danger symptom suggesting acute glaucoma as the cause of a red eye.

Exudation. Exudation, also called mattering, is a typical result of conjunctival or eyelid inflammation and does not occur with iridocyclitis or glaucoma. Patients often complain that their lids are "stuck together" on awakening. Corneal ulcer is a serious condition that may or may not be accompanied by exudate. Mucoid discharge generally is related to allergic conditions. Watery discharge may occur with viral conditions, and a purulent discharge is related to bacterial conditions.

Itching. Although a nonspecific symptom, itching usually indicates an allergic conjunctivitis.

Signs of Red Eye (see Table 16-2)

Reduced visual acuity.* Reduced visual acuity suggests a serious ocular disease, such as an inflamed cornea, iridocyclitis, glaucoma, or vitreous hemorrhage. It never occurs in simple conjunctivitis unless the associated cornea is involved.

Ciliary flush.* Ciliary flush is an injection of the deep conjunctival and episcleral vessels surrounding the cornea. It is seen most easily in daylight and appears as a faint violaceous ring in which individual vessels cannot be seen by the unaided eye. These engorged vessels, whose origin is the ciliary body, are a manifestation of inflammation of the ciliary body and the anterior segment of the eyeball. Ciliary flush is a danger sign often seen in eyes with corneal inflammations, iridocyclitis, or acute glaucoma. Usually ciliary flush is not present in conjunctivitis.

Conjunctival hyperemia. Conjunctival hyperemia is an engorgement of the larger and more superficial bulbar conjunctival vessels. A nonspecific sign, it may be seen in almost any of the conditions causing a red eye.

Corneal opacification.* In a patient with a red eye, corneal opacities always denote disease. These opacities may be detected by direct illumination with a penlight, or they may be seen with a direct ophthalmoscope (with a plus lens in the viewing aperture) outlined against the red fundus reflex. Several types of corneal opacities may occur, including:

- Keratic precipitates, or cellular deposits on the corneal endothelium, usually too small to be visible. Occasionally forming large clumps, these precipitates can result from iritis or chronic iridocyclitis.
- A diffuse haze obscuring the pupil and iris markings. This may be characteristic of corneal edema. It is frequently seen in acute glaucoma.
- Localized opacities. These may be due to keratitis or ulcer.

Corneal epithelial disruption.* Disruption of the corneal epithelium, which occurs in corneal inflammations and trauma, can be detected in two ways. The first method uses fluorescein vital stain, which detects disruption of the epithelium.

- The examiner should be positioned in such a way as to observe the reflection from the cornea of a single light source (e.g., window or penlight) as the patient moves his or her eye into various positions. Epithelial disruptions cause distortion and irregularity of the light reflected by the cornea.
- Apply fluorescein to the eye. Areas denuded of all layers of the epithelium will stain a bright green with a blue filter (see footnote 2, page 420).

The second method uses rose bengal vital stain, which detects degeneration or absence of one or more layers of the epithelium.

- Examiner positioned in the same manner as described above.
- Apply rose bengal vital stain. Diseased epithelium will stain a reddish purple color (see footnote 2, page 420).

Pupillary abnormalities.* The pupil in an eye with iridocyclitis typically is somewhat smaller than that of the other eye due to reflex spasm of the iris sphincter muscle. The pupil is also distorted occasionally by posterior synechiae, which are inflammatory adhesions between the lens and the iris. In acute glaucoma, the pupil is usually fixed, mid-dilated (about 5 to 6 mm), and slightly irregular. Conjunctivitis does not affect the pupil.

Shallow anterior chamber depth.* In a red eye, a shallow anterior chamber (especially related to acute ocular pain, nausea, and sometimes vomiting) always suggests the possibility of acute angle-closure glaucoma. Anterior chamber depth can be grossly estimated through side illumination with a penlight. The most exact technique and practice standard involves using a slit lamp with or without a diagnostic anterior segment contact lens. Intraocular pressure (IOP) is then measured.

Elevated IOP.* IOP is unaffected by common causes of red eye other than iridocyclitis and glaucoma. In any red eye without obvious infection, IOP can be measured to rule out glaucoma as clinically indicated (routinely at the time of all eye screening examinations generally after age 40); however, under some circumstances, routine screening for IOP should be part of the examination.

Proptosis.* Proptosis is a forward displacement of the globe. Proptosis of sudden onset suggests serious trauma, orbital infection, or tumor. The most common cause of chronic proptosis is thyroid disease. Orbital mass lesions also result in proptosis and should be considered. Proptosis may be accompanied by conjunctival hyperemia or limitation of eye movement. Small amounts of proptosis are detected most easily by standing behind a seated patient and looking downward to compare the positions of the two corneas. Acute orbital proptosis secondary to trauma is an ophthalmologic emergency because it may cause severe pressure on the eyeball, which can lead to central retinal artery occlusion.

Preauricular nodes. The type of discharge may be an important clue to the cause of conjunctivitis. Preauricular node enlargement can be a prominent feature of common viral as well as some unusual varieties of chronic granulomatous conjunctivitis, known collectively as Parinaud's oculoglandular syndrome. Usually, such enlargement does not occur in acute bacterial conjunctivitis. The adenovirus is found most commonly, especially in epidemic keratoconjunctivitis, which generally is spread by direct contact with secretions and often results from failure to wash hands after direct contact with infected patients.

Special Studies and Diagnostic Treatment Considerations

Special studies are not indicated during the first 2 to 3 days of treatment except for red flag conditions. Most patients with eye problems improve quickly once any red flag issues are ruled out. The clinical history and physical findings generally are adequate to diagnose the problem and provide treatment.

If the patient's limitations due to eye symptoms, other than nonspecific complaints, do not improve in 3 to 5 days, reassessment is recommended. After again reviewing the patient's limitations, history, and physical findings, the clinician may consider referral for further diagnostic studies and discuss these options with the patient. For patients with limitations after 3 to 5 days and unexplained physical findings, such as localized pain or visual disturbance, referral may be indicated to clarify the diagnosis and assist recovery.

Selection of Special Studies

Radiography of the globe may be indicated if the patient's history indicates the possibility of injury by a penetrating high-speed radiopaque foreign body. Ultrasonography can be used to locate non- and radiopaque foreign bodies. Computed tomographic (CT) scan of the orbit may be indicated in cases of significant blunt trauma and associated fractures at the time of initial evaluation and treatment. **Magnetic resonance imaging (MRI) is never indicated when there may be a possibility of a metallic foreign body**. Table 16-4 compares (generally) the abilities of different techniques to identify physiologic insult and define anatomic injury (see Algorithm 16-4).

Types of Red Eye

Occupational Eye Infections

Occupational hazards cause very few eye infections either directly or primarily. Rather, most occupational eye infections are attributable to workers who

Table 16-4. Ability of Various Techniques to Identify and Define Ocular Pathology

Technique	Identify Physiologic Insult	Identify Anatomic Defect
History	+ + +	+
Physical examination, including visual acuity testing and funduscopy	+ + + +	+ + + +
Fluorescein staining	0	+ + + +
Slit-lamp examination	0	+ + + +
Tonometry	+ + +	0
Imaging studies		
Plain-film radiography	0	+ [a]
Ultrasonography	0	+ + + + [b]
CT scan	0	+ + + + [a]
MRI	0	+ + + + [c]

Note: Specificity and repetitiveness from 0 (absent) to + + + + (maximum).
[a]For evaluating suspected periorbital and other depressed fractures.
[b]For evaluating suspected retinal detachment, chamber dimensions, and intraocular foreign bodies.
[c]For evaluating foreign body and intracranial pathology.

transfer the disease process. The significant eye infections include epidemic keratoconjunctivitis (EKC), infections caused by bloodborne pathogens, and tropical disease.

- *Epidemic keratoconjunctivitis (EKC)*. This is a classic condition originally described as shipyard conjunctivitis in 1934. In Western countries, EKC occurs mostly in industrial plants, where the disease periodically affects a considerable number of workers. Outbreaks appear from time to time in hospitals (Leopold), families (Dawson et al.), children (Dawson; Darwell, et al.), and ophthalmologic clinics, perhaps due to the use of unsterilized tonometers, eyedroppers, or finger-to-eye transmission (Pillat; Jawetz et al.; Dawson and Darwell; and others). Males are affected more frequently than females.
- *Bloodborne pathogens*. Infections also may be acquired by exposure to bloodborne pathogens, as in the acquired immune deficiency syndrome (AIDS), human immunodeficiency virus (HIV) infection, and hepatitis B virus (HBV) infection. Bloodborne pathogen exposure may be acquired by the spread of infectious products from afflicted individuals. Cross contamination may occur through the use of contaminated instruments, hands, etc. Bloodborne pathogen regulations (CFR 1910.1030) apply to occupational exposures from blood and other potentially infectious materials (e.g., semen, vaginal secretions, cerebrospinal fluid, synovial fluid, pleural fluid, pericardial fluid, peritoneal fluid, amniotic fluid, saliva in dental procedures, tears, body fluid visibly contaminated with blood, and all bodily fluids in situations where it is difficult or impossible to differentiate between bodily fluids,

as well as any unfixed tissue or organ other than intact skin from a living or dead human). An exposure is defined as a specific eye, mouth, or other mucous membrane, nonintact skin, or parenteral contact with blood or other potentially infectious materials resulting from the performance of an employee's duties. The term includes any pathogenic microorganisms present in human blood that can cause disease in persons who are exposed. These examples include hepatitis C, malaria, and syphilis. The intent of the regulation is to prevent the development of an exposure incident through appropriate administrative controls and personal protective equipment. An applanation tonometer, for example, must be thoroughly cleansed and sterilized after being used on an individual with HIV in the tears before using it on another individual because it may transmit the virus. Personal protective equipment appropriate to a procedure must be used.

- *Topical disease.* Some infectious diseases of the eye are not unique to the duties of individuals but rather are acquired from tropical conditions found in the area of employment. Examples include onchocerciasis, leishmaniasis, and trachoma.

PREVENTION AND CONTROL OF OCCUPATIONAL EYE INFECTIONS

Occupational eye infections spread by medical personnel through the use of inappropriate procedures are not uncommon. Various controls may be employed to help eliminate these infections:

- *Administrative controls.* These are designed to prevent dissemination of infectious agents to the eye. Members of medical departments are at risk for conditions such as EKC and AIDS. Tropical conditions can be readily referenced by geographic areas of the world and specific administrative controls should be implemented as recommended by the Centers for Disease Control and Prevention (CDC). Hands should always be washed between patient contacts.
- *Safe work practices.* The medical staff should help to prevent transmitting diseases person to person (i.e., EKC and AIDS). On some occasions, bodily secretions or blood products containing the AIDS virus may be cleaned up by nonmedical staff, and similar safe practices must be used.
- *Personal protective equipment for examiners.* In accordance with dictates of the Occupational Safety and Health Administration (OSHA, 29 CFR 1910.132), personal protective equipment must be worn by individuals who may be exposed to hazardous conditions. Using disposable gloves and eye and face protection is mandated in situations where medical personnel may be exposed to or may transmit infectious products from themselves to others. Such equipment includes type C spectacles with a full side shield, type D spectacles with a detachable side shield, type E spectacles with a nonremovable lens, and type H

cover goggles with indirect ventilations, as dictated by the American National Standards Institute (ANSI Z87.1-2003). In cases involving potential exposure to AIDS, personal protective equipment is mandated and directed in 29 CFR 1910.1030. Exposure from splattering or droplet generation would necessitate using the eye protection noted above and a mask or an ANSI Z87.1 type N face shield.

- *Employee education and training*. OSHA regulations (29 CFR 1910.132) mandate training about potential hazards and their prevention by using appropriate personal protective equipment. No individual who may be exposed to hazards should be allowed to work in such an environment without appropriate education and training.

Ocular Trauma

A new standardized classification of ocular trauma has been proposed and is known as the Birmingham Eye Trauma Terminology (BETT) (Figure 16-1 and Table 16-5).[4] Definitions in medical dictionaries are tailored to general medical use and cannot be applied effectively to ocular trauma. The new system always uses the entire globe as the tissue of reference; therefore, the type of the injury is described unambiguously without having to indicate the tissue involved. When a tissue is specified, it refers to wound location, not to injury type. A corneal penetrating injury thus involves an open globe injury with the wound being in the cornea. The system provides unambiguous definitions for each term and a complete classification of injury types.[5] **This new system should be used in all cases of ocular trauma**.

When the BETT system was published in 1996, it was reasonably expected that it eventually would become the standardized international language of ocular trauma. Ophthalmologists were urged to use this terminology in clinical practice and research. It is mandated by *Graefes' Archives, Klinische Monatsblätter*, and *Ophthalmology*.

[4]The new classification has been endorsed by the American Academy of Ophthalmology, the Board of Directors of the International Society of Ocular Trauma, the United States Eye Injury Registry, the Hungarian Eye Injury Registry, the Vitreous Society, the World Eye Injury Registry, and the Retina Society.

[5]In 1999, Pizzarello reported that a dramatic change in the type of eye injuries had occurred in the past 50 years. As the manufacturing sector eroded and the workplace changed, the nature of eye injuries also shifted. Liggett, Pince, and Barlow (1990) found that in inner city Los Angeles, only 8% of eye injuries occurred at work. The most common locations were in the home or on the street. Schein, Hibbard, and Shingleton, et al. (1988) found that 48% of injuries seen at an urban emergency room occurred at the workplace. This represents a wide discrepancy, and there is much discussion about the true extent of work-related eye injury. It is clear that many of the work-related injuries take place in auto repair and construction activities compared with the injuries in heavy industrial reported in prior years. Statistics from Prevent Blindness America estimate that there are approximately 2.4 million eye injuries each year, of which approximately 250,000, or about 10%, occur at the workplace. Increasingly, children are injured while at play or participating in sports. It is estimated that such injuries are in excess of 150,000 per year. The emphasis therefore has shifted to a more broad-based approach to eye safety. In addition, more private groups have become involved in injury prevention.

Figure 16-1. The New Standardized Classification of Eye Trauma

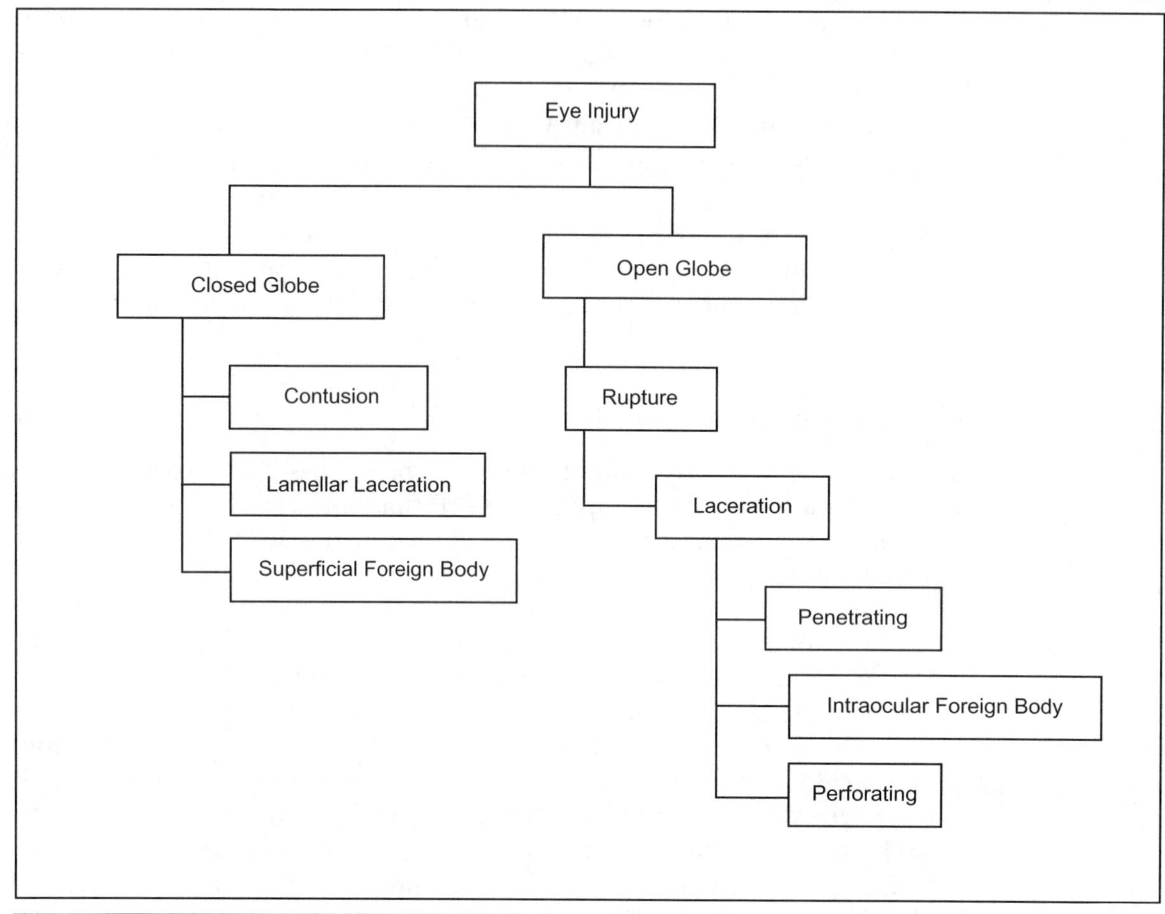

Source: Figure modified from Kuhn F, Morris R, Witherspoon CD, Heimann J, Jeffers JB, Treister G. A standardized classification of ocular trauma. *Graefes Arch Clin Ophthalmol.* 1966;234(6):399-403.

Elements of the History of Ocular Injury

While a detailed, accurate history is essential in all injuries, it is especially important to obtain a detailed history of an ocular injury because incorrect or misleading information may lead to blindness. Such information may be obtained from a variety of sources, including the patient, the first responder(s), and others involved in or associated with the accident (see Master Algorithm and Algorithms 16-1, 16-2, and 16-3).

Information for acute trauma should include the four *W*s:

- *Where:* Location of the accident
- *When:* Time and date
- *Who:* Other individuals involved

Table 16-5. BETT Glossary of Terms (Definitions and Explanations)	
Eyewall	Sclera and cornea

Although the eyewall technically has three coats posterior to the limbus, for clinical and practical purposes, violation of only the most external structure is taken into consideration.

Closed globe injury	No full-thickness wound of eyewall
Open globe injury	Full-thickness wound of eyewall
Contusion	No (full-thickness) wound

The injury is either due to direct energy delivery by the object (e.g., choroidal rupture) or to the changes in the shape of the globe (e.g., angle recession).

Lamellar laceration	Partial-thickness wound to the eyewall
Rupture	Full-thickness wound of the eyewall caused by blunt object

Because the eye is filled with incompressible liquid, the impact results in a momentary increase of the IOP. The eyewall yields at its weakest point (at the impact site or elsewhere; e.g., an old cataract wound dehisces even though the impact occurred elsewhere); the actual wound is produced by an inside-out mechanism.

Laceration	Full-thickness wound of the eyewall caused by a sharp object

The wound occurs at the impact site by an outside-in mechanism.

Penetrating injury	Entrance wound

Both wounds caused by the same agent.

Note: Some injuries remain difficult to classify. For instance, an intravitreal BB pellet is technically an intraocular foreign body (IOFB) injury. However, because this is a blunt object that requires a huge impact force if it enters, not just contuses, the eye, there is an element of rupture involved. In such situations, an ophthalmologist should either describe the injury as "mixed" (i.e., rupture with an IOFB) or select the most serious type of the mechanisms involved.

- *What:* A detailed description of the accident circumstances, including force and load

If chemical exposure was involved, seek available Material Safety Data Sheets (MSDSs) information. Critical data include:

- What chemical? MSDS information:[6]
  - *Type of chemical* (alkali, acid, solvent)

[6]Under federal law, 29 CFR 1910.1200, Hazard Communication, MSDS are to be furnished by the employer to the worker or his or her health care provider on request. Unfortunately, the quality of the information on MSDSs varies greatly because the information is supplied by the mnanufacturer of the product and there is no effective mechanism in place to ensure that it is accurate.

- *Type of exposure* (liquids, solids, fumes)
- *Dose of exposure*
- *pH* of the material
- *Concentration* of the material
- *Solubility* of the material
- *Contact* time

- Emergency medical care provided by first responder(s):
  - Product manufacturer
  - Availability of chemical data:
    - Material Safety Data Sheets (MSDSs)
    - Regional poison control center
    - Internet

OCULAR EXAMINATION FOR EYE INJURY

The examination of the injured eye should include:

- Visual acuity (each eye separately) with best correction or pinhole
- Inspection of the ocular structure. (If an open globe is suspected, no pressure should be exerted on the globe.)
- Position of the eyes and eye movements (six cardinal positions) if globe is intact
- Examination of the pupils for size and reaction to light
- Gross visual fields by confrontation
- Ophthalmoscopy
- Intraocular pressure (IOP) determination if acute glaucoma is suspected and the globe is intact

It is important for primary care physicians to make immediate referrals to the closest ophthalmologist or eye institute when eye injuries exceed their capability. Make the patient comfortable (with intravenous analgesics, if necessary), and protect the injured eye from further injury by applying a rigid Fox shield or equivalent. Depending on the type of injury, transport the patient on a stretcher.

Yardsticks that can be used to evaluate standard emergency care include:

1. The detail and accuracy of the history obtained at the time of or after admission
2. The thoroughness of the admission examination
3. The correlation of critical results with medication and/or other treatment provided to the patient

Initializing an Eye and Face Safety Program

Ninety-five percent of all eye injuries may be preventable. Eyes, as well as other parts of the body, may be exposed to a large variety of hazards in the home, due to hobbies, on the farm, in school, and at the work site.

PERSONAL PROTECTIVE EQUIPMENT

The goal of the Occupational Safety and Health Act of 1970 is to ensure safe and healthy working conditions for working men and women. It applies equally to areas outside the workplace where the hazards may be exactly the same. The Act's General Duty Clause requires that the "employer furnish to each of his employees employment . . . which is free from recognized hazards that are causing or are likely to cause death or serious harm." The preferred method of preventing exposure is by implementing engineering or administrative controls of the hazard(s) (see Chapter 1 for details).

If engineering controls of physical, chemical, or biologic hazards are not feasible, appropriate and effective personal protective equipment (PPE) should be used. Eye and face protectors are well-known examples of PPE. Protecting the eye from injury by physical, chemical, and radiologic agents is mandatory in any occupational safety program. To prevent an eye injury, it is essential to select the correct eye protective equipment after hazard(s) have been engineered out to the maximum amount possible.

While engineering controls are primary in the prevention of eye injuries, PPE is required under OSHA regulations (29 CFR 1910.132, Personal Protective Equipment; CFR 1910.133, Eye and Face Protection) and the American National Standards Institute (ANSI) Standard Z-87.1 (2003), incorporated by reference, and should be in use if engineering controls are not feasible. The new Z-87.1 standard now has testing criteria for both the frame and the lenses. Lenses now have two levels for performance—basic impact and high impact. Examples include:

- Safety spectacles with side shields when there is a hazard of flying objects—high impact
- Safety goggles or welding face shields with UV protection in welding and torch soldering—basic impact
- Face shields for severe exposure in chopping, grinding, masonry work, riveting, and sanding—high impact
- Goggles and face shields for chemicals—depends on other factors

Due to the fact that lenses have two levels of performance, the supplier/issuer needs to be informed of the result of the hazard analysis required in 29 CFR 1910.132.

Additional standards include ANSI Standard Z-136.1 (2000 or later) for safe use of lasers, and ANSI Standard Z-136.3 (1996 or later) for safe use of lasers in health care facilities, as required when lasers are operational.

Assessing Red Flags and Indications for Immediate Referral

Physical examination evidence of severe ocular compromise that correlates with the medical history and test results may indicate a need for immediate consultation. The examination may further reinforce or reduce suspicions of infection or major trauma (e.g., open globe, chemical exposure, or radiation damage). A medical history suggestive of pathology in an area other than the eye may warrant examination of the head, neck, or other areas.

TIMING OF REFERRALS OR SPECIAL STUDIES

Referrals for work-related eye complaints generally fall into two categories—immediate and following conservative treatment. Immediate referral to an ophthalmologist is necessary for many cases of eyelid disorders or injuries, open globe wounds or penetrating foreign bodies in the eye, thermal and chemical injuries (e.g., alkali, acid, solvent, or hydrofluoric acid burns), central retinal artery and/or vein occlusions, acute glaucoma, corneal ulcers, and retrobulbar hemorrhages.

Once these red flags have been ruled out, conservative treatment by the primary care physician can proceed for 48 to 72 hours for superficial foreign bodies, corneal abrasions, nonalkali chemical splashes, conjunctivitis, and non-ionizing radiation damage.

Normally, tissues of the eye heal rapidly. If eye damage is not well on the way to resolution within 48 to 72 hours, referral to an ophthalmologist (Eye MD) is indicated. Nonspecific eye complaints may be monitored for a longer period of time while making ergonomic and other adjustments.

As indicated below, some special studies, such as radiography and ultrasonography of the globe or orbit, may be indicated in the acute period to rule out fracture of the orbit or the presence of a foreign body, either intraocularly or in the orbit. Diagnose and begin treatment for conditions that need referral while stabilizing the patient and preparing him or her for transfer. A series of general and diagnostic modalities for the red flag and non-red-flag conditions are provided in Tables 16-6 and 16-7 (see also Algorithms 16-1, 16-2, 16-4, and 16-5).

Red Eye Differential Diagnosis

Red eye can be categorized generally in four classes—conjunctivitis, iritis, keratitis (corneal inflammation or foreign body), and acute glaucoma. The changes in vision, type of discharge, presence or absence of pain, pupillary size, presence of conjunctival injection, pupillary response to light, IOP, appearance of the cornea, and anterior chamber depth assist in making the diagnosis (see Table 16-3).

Table 16-6. Red Flags for Potentially Serious Eye Conditions Requiring Immediate Ophthalmologic Examination

Disorder	Medical History	Physical Examination
Ocular injury, open globe	Trauma due to high-velocity foreign-body injury Visual loss Bleeding Local pain	Visible foreign body in globe; deformity of the globe Loss of globe pressure Distorted pupil and/or iris Subconjunctival hemorrhage
Ocular injury, closed globe	Direct blow Visual loss Diplopia	Eyelid ecchymosis Subconjunctival hemorrhage Vitreous hemorrhage Lens dislocation Retinal edema and/or tear Decreased visual acuity Hyphema Retrobulbar hemorrhage Extraocular motion deviation
Thermal burns	Exposure of eyes to hot material/ extreme heat Superficial eye pain Photophobia	Burns of lids and/or surrounding structures Damage to cornea, conjunctiva, and/or sclera Decreased visual acuity
Radiation injury	Exposure of eyes to ultraviolet, laser, or bright light Delayed severe superficial eye pain (4-6 hours) Tearing Photophobia	Blepharospasm Tearing Corneal punctate staining and/or sloughing of epithelium Retinal damage
Chemical burns	Alkali, acid, solvent splash Painless visual loss	Corneal erosion Conjunctival chemosis Necrosis of anterior segment of tissues and vessels Decreased visual acuity Circumcorneal vascular ischemia Necrosis of cornea and/or conjunctiva Glaucoma
Hydrofluoric (HF) acid burns	HF acid splash Delayed damage	Necrosis of cornea and/or conjunctiva Decreased visual acuity
Corneal ulcer	Abrasion or infection Superficial pain Foreign-body sensation Photophobia Visual loss	Corneal infiltrates and ulcers Decreased visual acuity Ulceration on slit-lamp exam and fluorescein staining

Table 16-7. Diagnostic Criteria for Non-red-flag Eye Conditions That Can Be Managed by Primary Care Physicians

Probable Diagnosis or Injury	Mechanism	Unique Symptoms	Unique Signs	Tests and Results
Corneal abrasion (ICD-9 918.1), conjunctival abrasion (ICD-9 918.2)	Direct contact Contact lens Aerosol chemicals	Superficial pain Foreign-body sensation	Possibly visible abrasion on magnification	Fluorescein staining reveals abrasion with use of cobalt blue light Visual acuity test results abnormal
Nonionizing radiation exposure (ICD-9 990)	Ultraviolet (welding) light Bright light (sun) Laser	Severe photophobia Tearing Sandy sensation Possibly reduced visual acuity	Injection Blepharospasm Corneal erosion or sloughing Decreased visual acuity Central scotoma	Fluorescein staining reveals punctate lesions under cobalt blue light Amsler grid abnormality
Chemical splash (ICD-9 983.0 non; 983.1 acid; 983.2 alkali)	Chemical splash (nonacid, nonalkali; acid; alkali)	Chemical exposure Painful Visual loss	Corneal erosion Possibly diffuse inflammation of periorbita, lids and anterior segment Eye burn	Fluorescein staining reveals punctate lesions or abrasion under cobalt blue light
Foreign body (ICD-9 871.5 magnetic; ICD-9 871.6 nonmagnetic; ICD-9 930.0-9 on external eye)	Projectile material	Foreign-body sensation	Visible foreign body Possible corneal abrasion Possible rust ring	Fluorescein staining may reveal abrasion under cobalt blue light
Blepharitis (ICD-9 373.0 seborrheic; ICD-9 373.00 infectious; ICD-9 373.00 parasitic)	Infectious or eyelid gland dysfunction	Burning, itching of lids Wake up with eyelids stuck together	Dry or greasy scales of lid Loss of eyelashes in chronic state	None
Stye (ICD-9 373.12 internal hordeolum; ICD-9 373.11 external hordeolum)	Acute *Staphylococcus* infection of glands of Moll, Zeis, and Meibomian	Acute localized infection of eyelid in area of cilia or meibomian glands	Localized acute infection or abscess	None
Chalazion (ICD-9 373.2)	Chronic granulomatous inflammation of either of the gland Zeis, Moll, or Meibomian	Generally painless lid thickening, frequently following hordeolum	Palpable nodule associated with cilia of eyelid or meibomian glands	
Conjunctivitis (ICD-9 372.03 bacterial; ICD-9 077.4 viral)	Microbial infection Viral infection Parasitic infection	Blurred vision or eye stuck shut Discharge	Purulent, watery mucous discharge	Culture positive for bacteria

Table 16-7. (continued)

Probable Diagnosis or Injury	Mechanism	Unique Symptoms	Unique Signs	Tests and Results
Visual fatigue (ICD-9 368.13)	Ergonomic factor Refractive error Work habits Workplace illumination	Headache Colored afterimages Eye fatigue Diplopia Blurred vision, especially near vision	Possibly refractive error for working distance	Evaluate worksite for the visual ergonomic status
Subjunctival hemorrhage	May develop from rubbing the eyes, sneezing, Valsalva May be associated with bleeding disorders and hypertension	Asymptomatic	Generally a light amount of subjunctiva blood	None Rule out foreign body

Note: ICD-9 = *International Classification of Diseases,* 9th Edition.

Management or Referral

The conditions that a primary care physician may appropriately treat include blepharitis, stye and chalazion, and conjunctivitis. Patients requiring prolonged treatment or those in whom the expected response to treatment does not occur promptly may be referred to an ophthalmologist.

Red-Flag Conditions and Preferred Specific Treatment

Blunt Trauma

Ocular contusions are caused by blunt trauma to the eye or periorbital structures that may cause contusion of the globe and/or periorbita. There may be no symptoms; however, some patients complain of local pain, visual loss, diplopia, or a red eye. The clinician may observe any of the following—ecchymosis of the eyelid; corneal edema; subconjunctival hemorrhage; microscopic or gross hyphema; reduced visual acuity or abnormal visual fields; dislocation or subluxation of the lens; retinal tears, edema, or detachment; or restriction of ocular motion if extraocular muscles are trapped in a blowout fracture.

Retrobulbar Hemorrhage

A retrobulbar hemorrhage may increase the pressure on the globe such that the IOP may become greater than the perfusion pressure of the eye, leading to total ischemia of the retina. A relaxing incision at the lateral canthus must be completed within 10 minutes of the rise in IOP or the eye may be irreversibly damaged secondary to the high IOP.

Orbital Floor Fractures

Much discussion and controversy surround managing blowout fractures of the orbit. At various times, recommendations have included operating on all orbital floor fractures and operating on none of them. As the understanding of blowout fractures and their sequelae has evolved over time, so too has an understanding of when surgery is appropriate, and who benefits from such surgery. In the past, the focus often was on early versus late repair. At present, the focus is on understanding the mechanisms of diplopia and enophthalmos in orbital floor fractures, the best way to evaluate a patient, and the best way to restore maximal function and appearance (Harstein and Roper-Hall, 2000).

Diplopia caused by orbital floor blowout fractures is one of the major complications of orbital injuries. When vertical movement of the eye is impaired, surgery is indicated and is performed after complete resolution of orbital hemorrhage and edema. The maximal time before the first surgical procedure is 14 days (Taher, 1993).

Treatment indications for orbital floor fractures are evolving. Nonresolving oculocardiac reflex, the "white-eyed" blowout fracture, and early enophthalmos or hypoglobus are indications for immediate surgical repair. Surgery within 2 weeks is recommended in cases of symptomatic diplopia with positive forced ductions and evidence of orbital soft tissue entrapment on computed tomographic (CT) scan or large orbital floor fractures that may cause latent enophthalmos or hypo-ophthalmos (Burnstine, 2002).

Hyphema

Complications of traumatic hyphema include increased IOP, peripheral anterior synechiae, optic atrophy, corneal blood staining, secondary hemorrhage, and accommodative impairment. The reported incidence of secondary anterior chamber hemorrhage, i.e., rebleeding, in the setting of traumatic hyphema ranges from 0 to 38%. The risk of secondary hemorrhage may be higher among African Americans than among whites. Secondary hemorrhage is generally thought to convey a worse visual prognosis, although the outcome may depend more directly on the size of the hyphema and the severity of associated ocular injuries. Some issues involved in managing a patient with hyphema are using various medications (e.g., cycloplegics, systemic or topical steroids, antifibrinolytic agents analgesics, and antiglaucoma medications), the patient's activity level, use of a patch and shield, outpatient versus inpatient management, and medical versus surgical management. Special considerations are widely accepted in managing children, patients with hemoglobin S, and patients with hemophilia. It is important to identify and treat ocular injuries that often accompany traumatic hyphema. Consider each of these management issues and refer to the pertinent literature in formulating the following recommendations:

- Advise routine use of topical cycloplegics and corticosteroids, consider systemic antifibrinolytic agents or corticosteroids, and always use a rigid shield.
- Recommend activity restriction (quiet ambulation). If compliance (with medication use or activity restrictions), follow-up, or increased risk for complications (e.g., history of sickle cell disease or hemophilia) is a concern, inpatient management can be offered.
- Indications for surgical intervention include the presence of corneal blood staining or dangerously increased IOP despite maximum tolerated medical therapy, among others.

A study was performed to evaluate the clinical course of patients treated for traumatic microhyphema and the occurrence of elevated IOP and secondary hemorrhage. A total of 162 patients met the study criteria. All patients were treated initially as outpatients according to the protocol for traumatic microhyphema (i.e., atropinization, bed rest, shield, and restriction of antiplatelet medications). Three patients were subsequently hospitalized. The occurrence of IOP elevation (> 21 mmHg) and rebleeding was recorded. Of 150 patients with normal IOP at presentation, only 1 (0.7%) developed an elevated IOP at any point to warrant treatment (28 mmHg). Rebleeding was documented in three patients, one of whom developed a layered hyphema. Few complications result from traumatic microhyphema treated with standard measures. Closeness of follow-up may be determined by IOP on presentation. Secondary hemorrhage seems to be unaffected by the use of topical corticosteroids (Recchia, et al., 2002).

Burns

THERMAL BURNS OF THE EYE

Thermal burns of the eye are caused by exposure to hot gases, liquids, or solids. Unless there is local contact only with the eye, the periocular structures are typically damaged as well. Damage may range from superficial burns of the lids and surrounding structures to superficial destruction of the cornea, conjunctiva, or sclera, to greater destruction including exposure of the globe. If damage exceeds superficial burns of the lids and surrounding structures, prompt intervention by a specialist is imperative.

ELECTROMAGNETIC RADIATION INJURY TO THE EYE

Patients with electromagnetic radiation injury to the eye may have no initial symptoms. Severe cases may show a marked decrease in central visual acuity, but there may be severe delayed consequences. Depending on the exact electromagnetic spectrum, the symptoms or signs may be localized to the external segment, lens, retina, and choroid. This type of injury can cause scarring of the cornea or retina or cataracts. Visual field disorders also may result from damage to the retina or choroid. Burns from the blue end of the visible spectrum and ultraviolet A are discussed under nonionizing radiation exposure.

CHEMICAL BURNS

When they make contact with ultrasensitive eye tissues, toxic substances immediately begin to cause damage. Studies show that after the first 10 seconds of chemical contact, chances of full recovery become fleeting. Aside from general tissue damage, acids and alkalis can change the pH in the eye itself. From this detrimental change, severe eye damage, including blindness, may result. A history of chemical exposure is an emergency, and examination should be delayed until after the eye is flushed to dilute the chemical. It is imperative that emergency flushing begin immediately. To ensure the best chances for a minimal amount of eye damage, correct emergency equipment, proper placement, and knowledge of its use are necessary in the workplace. The requirements governing medical services and first aid is covered in OSHA 1910.151(a)(b), whereas ANSI Z-358.1, Emergency Eyewash and Shower Equipment, provides guidance. At the site, water is the initial dilution agent to flush the eye or body. Subsequently, an isotonic saline or balanced Ringer's solution is preferred and should be used, if available (otherwise, use sterile intravenous fluids), until a tear pH of about 7 is obtained after ceasing irrigation for 10 minutes. Proper flushing usually takes at least 15 minutes, but can take as long as 24 hours.

Irrigation technique. ANSI Z-358.1, Emergency Eyewash and Shower Equipment, sets forth the requirements for having the facilities to dilute a chemical within 10 seconds of undergoing an industrial eye chemical hazard. Once at the site of an industrial injury, emergency medical personnel or first responders should resolve pain and blepharospasm by applying a topical ophthalmic anesthesic (proparacaine hydrochloride). The interpalpebral fissure should be widened by means of a lid retractor (e.g., Demarres), the eye should be irrigated directly with isotonic saline, Ringer's lactate, or other ocular solutions, and a contact lens should be removed to facilitate irrigation of the eyeball. The irrigation is not completed until the upper lid is double everted so that all cul-de-sacs (recesses) of the conjunctiva are thoroughly irrigated and visualized. Irrigation should continue until the conjunctival secretions show a consistent pH of approximately 7 after ceasing irrigation for 10 minutes.

In the event of a chemical exposure, begin eye irrigation immediately, and remove contact lenses as soon as practical. Do not delay irrigation while waiting for contact lens removal because the lens may come out with the irrigation or can be removed when irrigation is complete.

Contact lenses adhere to the cornea and sometimes the paralimbal conjunctiva, depending on the type, and they have been shown to protect the cornea and/or conjunctiva beneath the lens. However, they do not fulfill the requirements of PPE. If a contact lens has not been washed out during the irrigation, emergency medical personnel may remove it following completion of irrigation.

Alkali burns. Alkali burns of the eye typically cause pain initially and may have disastrous consequences if not treated immediately. Alkali exposure can cause corneal ulceration or conjunctival, scleral, and/or anterior segment degeneration that is manifested as a blanched or "marbleized" appearance. The cornea may become opacified. The diagnosis is usually based on a history of exposure to alkaline chemicals, but occasionally testing the pH of tears or residual liquid is required.

Immediate referral to an ophthalmologist is recommended. Irrigation in most cases should be continued until the patient is seen by the ophthalmologist. A casual examination of the eye may reveal that the globe is white because there is severe ischemia of the conjunctiva or episcleral vessels, a finding that would be noted during a slit-lamp examination.

Acid burns. Acid burns of the eye, caused by acid splashes or vapors, can have the immediate effects of corneal erosion, corneal necrosis, and decreased visual acuity unless irrigation is accomplished immediately. In patients with acid burns, the eye looks inflamed immediately, unlike alkali burns, where the eye is white due to necrosis of the superficial ocular vessels. Delayed effects are unusual in patients with acid burns; hydrofluoric (HF) acid burns are the exception.

Hydrofluoric acid burns. Hydrofluoric acid causes delayed tissue destruction out of proportion to the apparent exposure. With an HF acid concentration of less than 20%, the onset of symptoms may be delayed up to 24 hours. With high concentrations, symptoms may begin relatively quickly. The patient's main complaint is severe eye pain out of proportion to the apparent exposure. HF acid penetrates tissue remarkably well and causes deep as well as superficial necrosis.

HF acid exposure must be treated immediately with copious irrigation with water or isotonic saline solution for 5 minutes and then by calcium gluconate 1% solution or Ringer's lactate solution providing Ca^{2+} and Mg^{+} atoms to the cell replacing the Ca^{2+} and Mg^{+} atoms that were incorporated into insoluble calcium and magnesium fluoride molecules. Immediate referral to an ophthalmologist after emergency care is recommended while calcium gluconate is irrigated into the eye.

Corneal Ulceration

Corneal ulcers, which can permanently damage vision, are an ophthalmologic emergency. They may be bacterial, viral, fungal, or parasitic in origin and may occur following corneal lacerations, abrasions, and intrusion of foreign bodies.

They may result from poorly fitted or inadequately cleaned contact lenses. Patients with corneal ulcers present with complaints of changes in visual acuity, photophobia and/or eye pain, tearing, and a sensation that a foreign body is in the eye. The presence of corneal ulcers can be determined by direct visualization, but magnified viewing with fluorescein staining is needed to completely rule out their presence.

Open Globe Eye Injury

Direct trauma to the eye from high-velocity objects can cause laceration or perforation of the globe. The trauma can be perforating or penetrating. Patients with damage to the integrity of the globe can present with decreased visual acuity, local pain, and bleeding. The cardinal sign is distortion of the globe with loss of tension or IOP; the pupil is not round, but rather is distorted and/or nonreactive. In addition, ecchymosis or other signs of damage to periorbital structures are evident. The clinician may observe subconjunctival hemorrhage, distortion of the iris or pupil, or herniation of the iris through the cornea. There also may be retinal damage. The injured eye should be protected with a metallic or plastic shield. Transfer by stretcher is recommended.

Non-red-flag Conditions (see Table 16-7)

Occupational health or other primary care physicians could treat the conditions listed in Table 16-7 after thorough evaluation and be within their scope of practice.

Abrasion of the Cornea or Conjunctiva

A corneal abrasion involves denuding of the five layers of corneal epithelium. Corneal abrasions may be divided into three classes based on healing time, degree of iridocyclitis, and potential infection complications. The three types are as follows (see Table 16-8 and Algorithm 16-3):

- *Simple.* Generally less than 3 mm in greatest diameter. Usually heals in 24 hours without treatment.
- *Complex.* Secondary to fingernails, thorns, tree branches, or oyster shells. These have a delayed and variable healing time, ocular pain and ciliary spasm, and a high rate of recurrent erosion. Use NSAIDs with ophthalmic antibiotics and, frequently, cycloplegics.
- *Potentially contaminated with bacteria.* Secondary to contact lenses, dirt, barnyard, or other traumatic materials. These have a higher potential rate of corneal infection or corneal ulcers from *Pseudomonas aerugi-*

Table 16-8. Types of Corneal/Conjunctival Abrasions

Technique	Simple (<3 mm in Greatest Diameter)	Complex Conjunctiva (Secondary to Fingernails, Thorns, Tree Branches, or Oyster Shells)	Potentially Contaminated (Contact Lenses, with Dirt, Barnyard, or Other Traumatic Materials)
Healing time	Within 24 hours	24-48 hours or longer	24-48 hours
Fluorescein staining	Yes	Yes	Yes
Complications:			
Recurrent erosion	No	Higher incidence	No
Keratitis/corneal ulcer	No	Higher incidence	Yes
Patching	No generally; some patients may be more comfortable, especially with corneal pain	May be needed to control corneal pain, including bandage contact lenses for recurrent erosions; may need surgery	Never
NSAID ophthalmic solution/topical	No generally; may be used as a substitute for patching	Use routinely	Routinely needed
Ophthalmic antibiotics/topical ointments Fluoroquinolones (e.g., ciprofloxacin, ofloxacin, norfloxacin)	No	Yes	Yes; routine use prophylactically and therapeutically for keratitis/corneal ulcer (e.g., *Pseudomonas aeruginosa*)
Cycloplegics:			
Short-acting mydriacyl 1%	No, only when incidence of ciliary spasm	No	No
Intermediate-acting cyclogyl 1% solutions	No	No	No
Longer-acting scopolamine 1%, homatropine 5% (large abrasions/iritis)	No	Yes	Yes
Topical steroids	No	No, only if prescribed by an ophthalmologist	No, only if prescribed by an ophthalmologist
Tetanus booster	No	No	Verify immunization state; tetanus toxoid as per prophylaxis protocols
Referral—generally	None	Ophthalmologist	Ophthalmologist

nosa. No patching is the rule because it encourages bacterial growth. Applying cycloplegics and ophthalmic antibiotics topically is indicated.

Recurrent Corneal Erosion

The patient has symptoms of recurrent attacks of acute ocular pain, photophobia, and tearing, often when awakening or during sleep when the eyelids are rubbed or opened. In addition, the patient often has a history of a prior corneal abrasion in the involved eye.

The signs are localized roughening of the corneal epithelium or a corneal abrasion (fluorescein dye may lightly stain and outline the area). Epithelial changes may resolve within hours of the onset of symptoms so that no abnormality is present when the patient is examined.

Damage to the corneal epithelium basement membrane from dystrophy of the cornea or previous corneal abrasions, especially of the complex type, is the most likely cause. The diagnosis is confirmed by a history of recent trauma, previous corneal abrasions, ocular surgery, family history (corneal dystrophy), and slit-lamp examination with fluorescein staining.

Treatment for an acute episode may be performed by a primary care physician, but subsequent episodes that do not resolve in 36 to 48 hours should be referred to an ophthalmologist. Apply a cycloplegic drop (e.g., cyclopentolate or homatropine) and use antibiotic ointment. If the defect is large, a pressure patch may be applied. After epithelial healing is complete, apply artificial tears (e.g., Refresh Plus, TheraTears, or Celluvisc) and artificial tear ointment (e.g., Refresh P.M.) or 5% sodium chloride drops four to eight times per day and 5% sodium chloride ointment at bedtime for at least 3 months.

If the corneal epithelium is loose and heaped and not healing, the ophthalmologist will consider debridement of the abnormal epithelium. The following treatments may be considered for erosions that are not responsive to the preceding treatment:

- An extended-wear bandage soft contact lens for several months
- Anterior stromal puncture (generally used in extremely symptomatic, refractory cases with erosions outside the visual axis)
- Epithelial debridement with diamond burr polishing of Bowman's membrane (effective for large areas of epithelial irregularity and lesions in the visual axis)
- Phototherapeutic keratectomy (PTK). Excimer laser ablation of the superficial stroma is successful in up to 90% of patients with recurrent erosions from corneal dystrophies. Follow-up may be required every 1 to 2 days until the epithelium has healed and then every 1 to 6 months depending on the severity and frequency of the episodes.

Nonionizing Radiation Exposure from Ultraviolet and Bright Visible Spectrum

This energy may arise from welders' torches, mercury vapor lamps, and the sun. The onset of symptoms, including photophobia, corneal pain, lacrimation, and blepharospasm, usually occurs 5 to 12 hours after exposure; healing usually occurs within 24 hours (see Tables 16-9 and 16-10).

Foreign Bodies of the Cornea or Conjunctiva

These may be superficial and may be removed less than 6 hours after the injury. Superficial foreign bodies generally may be removed with a moist swab soon after injury and should be handled like a simple abrasion (see Table

Table 16-9. Nonionizing Radiation Burns

Technique	**Ultraviolet Burns (Welders, mercury vapor lamps, sun) Clinical Findings**
Healing time	Onset symptoms of photophobia, pain, lacrimation, blepharospasm, 5-12 hours after exposure; healing < 24 hours
Fluorescein staining	Yes
Complications:	
Recurrent erosion	No
Keratitis/corneal ulcer	No, unless the patient is using topical anesthetics routinely
Patching	No generally; some patients may be more comfortable with patching
NSAID ophthalmic solution/topical	Yes
Ophthalmic antibiotics/topical ointments:	
Erythromycin, polymyxin B	No
Gentamycin, tobramycin (gram-positive and gram-negative bacteria, especially *P. aeruginosa*)	No
Cycloplegics:	
Short-acting Mydriacyl 1%, Cyclogyl 1% solutions	Yes, if ciliary spasm is present
Longer-acting scopolamine .25%, homatropine 5% (large abrasions/iritis)	No
Topical steroids	No
Tetanus booster	No
Referral—generally	None, unless healing is not complete in 24 hours

Table 16-10. Types of Foreign Bodies of the Cornea or Conjunctiva

Technique	Simple (Foreign Body < 6 hours)	Complex (Foreign Body with Metallic Pigmentation, Swelling of Tissues)
Healing time	Within 24 hours	24-72 hours or longer depending on amount of metallic residue and length of time foreign body has been in contact with the tissues
Fluorescein staining	Yes	Yes
Complications:		
Recurrent erosion	No	No
Keratitis/corneal ulcer	No	Higher incidence of keratitis/ corneal ulcer
Patching	No	No
NSAID ophthalmic solution/ topical	No, usually only mild superficial corneal pain	Yes, based on corneal pain present
Ophthalmic antibiotics/topical ointments:		
Fluoroquinoles (e.g., ciprofloxacin, ofloxacin, norfloxacin)	No	Yes; routine use prophylactically and therapeutically for keratitis/corneal ulcer and endophthalmitis
Cycloplegics:		
Short-acting mydriacyl 1%	No, only when incidence of ciliary spasm	Yes, if iritis/iridocyclitis present.
Intermediate cyclogyl 1% solutions	No	The type and concentration depends on the degree of ititis/iridocyclitis and how long you desire cycloplegia.
Longer-acting scopolamine .25%, homatropine 5% (large abrasions/iritis)	No	
Topical steroids	No	No; only if prescribed by an ophthalmologist
Tetanus booster	No	Based on type of foreign body; verify immunization state; tetanus toxoid as per prophylaxis protocols
Referral—generally	None	Ophthalmologist

16-8). Foreign bodies can be divided into two types (Table 16-10 presents details for treating various types of foreign bodies):

- *Simple.* A superficial foreign body removed within hours generally will heal within 24 hours and have a low rate of inflammation of the cornea or conjunctiva and no iritis.
- *Complex.* A foreign body of the cornea and conjunctiva in which the trauma has taken place generally will heal in 24 to 48 hours. A metallic foreign body may be surrounded by swollen necrotic tissue and metallic pigmentation.

Chemical Splashes

Chemical splashes from a solvent, acid, or alkali agent generally are red flag conditions, but preliminary treatment by a primary care physician can be provided before referring the patient to an ophthalmologist. Primary treatment is irrigation of the eye with water and/or isotonic saline until the pH returns to approximately 7, measured by pH paper, 10 minutes after stopping irrigation.

Subconjunctival Hemorrhage

In the absence of blunt trauma, hemorrhage beneath the subconjunctiva (the potential space between the conjunctiva and the sclera) requires no treatment and, unless recurrent, no evaluation. Causes may include a sudden increase in ocular venous pressure, such as occurs with coughing, sneezing, vomiting, or vigorous rubbing of the eye. Many subconjunctival hemorrhages occur during sleep when no prodomal conditions exist. If recurrent, an underlying bleeding disorder should be ruled out.

Blepharitis

Response to the treatment of blepharitis, or inflammation of the eyelid, is often frustratingly slow, and relapses are common. The mainstays of treatment are as follows:

- Apply a warm compress over the closed eyelids for 10 to 15 minutes with the cloth rewarmed (by running through hot water) as it cools. The compress helps to increase the fluidity of the meibomian glands and loosen the debris from the bases of the lashes.
- To remove the secretions, follow compresses with lid scrubs, such as baby shampoo diluted with water (one drop of shampoo in cup of water) on a cotton ball or clean cloth, which is preferable to a cotton-tipped applicator. These measures may be performed two to four times daily.

- Apply a topical antibiotic (erythromycin or bacitracin) following lid scrubs twice daily. Tetracycline (orally, daily) or doxycycline (orally, daily) is added for patients with rosacea or chronic blepharitis who are not responding to conservative measures. For pregnant or breast-feeding women and children younger than 12 years of age, substitute erythromycin.
- Give patients with punctate epithelial keratitis (PEK) artificial tears five to six times daily.

Chalazion

Chalazion is a chronic granulomatous inflammation of a meibomian gland that may develop spontaneously or may follow a hordeolum, acute meibomitis, or stye. Chalazia are chronic granulomata of fat bodies and they may require excision. Because most chalazia are sterile, antibiotic therapy is of no value, but hot compresses may be useful for early lesions. Incision with curettage is indicated when lesions do not resolve spontaneously or with other medical therapy. A persistent or recurring lid mass should undergo biopsy because it may be a rare meibomian gland carcinoma or a squamous cell carcinoma of the conjunctiva rather than a benign chalazion.

Bacterial Conjunctivitis

Bacterial conjunctivitis is treated with frequent antibiotic eye drops as well as antibiotic ointment applied at bedtime. Cool compresses may give some relief. There is no specific medical treatment for viral conjunctivitis, but patients should be instructed in proper precautions to prevent contagion. Corticosteroids have no place in treating infectious conjunctivitis. Eye drops containing a combination of antibiotics and corticosteroids are not indicated for the treatment of ocular inflammation by the primary care or occupational medicine physician.

Stye or Hordeolum

A stye or hordeolum is an acute inflammation of the eyelid that may be characterized as an external swelling (involving the hair follicle or associated glands of Zeis or Moll) or an internal swelling (involving the meibomian glands). An external hordeolum occurs on the surface of the skin at the edge of the lid. An internal hordeolum presents on the conjunctival surface of the lid. Styes, generally localized abscess, are treated initially with hot compresses and topical antibiotics. An internal or external hordeolum (stye) may be a sequela of acute blepharitis (meibomitis) and require incision and drainage of the abscess. Incision with curettage is indicated when lesions do not resolve spontaneously or with medical therapy.

Initial and Definitive Care of Red Flag and Non-red-flag Conditions

Patient Comfort

Comfort is often a patient's first concern. Nonprescription analgesics provide sufficient pain relief for most patients with acute eye symptoms. Persistence of eye pain is a red flag. If treatment response is inadequate (i.e., symptoms and limitations continue), prescription pharmaceuticals can be tried, but only briefly, before referring the patient to an ophthalmologist. Comorbid conditions, side effects, cost, and provider and patient preferences guide the clinician's choice of recommended agents. Table 16-11 summarizes comfort options.

Generally, three sources of pain are secondary to a red eye:

- Periorbital pain
- Cornea, conjunctival, or eyelid pain
- Ciliary and iris spasm

Conditions that require referral must be diagnosed and treated initially, and the patient must be stabilized while making preparations for transfer. A series of general and diagnostic treatment modalities for red flag and non-red flag conditions are provided.

Anesthetic Agents

Topical anesthetics of short onset and duration with a low potential for causing hypersensitivity (e.g., proparacaine hydrochloride 0.5%) are used commonly during the eye examination and treatment only to facilitate removal of superficial foreign bodies or rust rings or to facilitate the examination when blepharospasm or severe local pain prevents adequate visualization of the eye (e.g., in patients with flash burns or severe corneal abrasions).

The agents listed in Table 16-11 allow the clinician to perform ocular

Table 16-11. Topical Anesthetic Agents

USP or National Formulatory Name	Trade Name	Concentration (%)
Cocaine hydrochloride	—	1-4
Proparacaine hydrochloride	AK-Taine Alcaine Ophthetic	0.5 0.5 0.5
Tetracaine hydrochloride	AK-T-Caine Pontocaine hydrochloride	0.5 0.5

Source: From *Physicians Desk Reference for Ophthalmic Medicine.* 3rd ed. 2002; Table 11.

procedures such as tonometry, removing foreign bodies from the surface of the eye, and lacrimal canalicular manipulation and irrigation. Cocaine, the prototypical topical anesthetic, is a natural compound; the others are synthetic. Cocaine is now used rarely as an anesthetic agent. Topical anesthetics should not be used on an open globe. The practitioner should inquire about allergy to local anesthetics before using them. Proparacaine hydrochloride has the shortest onset, duration, and hypersensitivity. Chronic use by welders, for example, may lead to keratitis. Take adequate precautions to prevent pilfering of the clinic's bottles of anesthetic. A new delivery system for topical ophthalmic anesthetics in the form of a strip is now in the final predistribution stage.

Analgesics

SYSTEMIC

The safest and most effective analgesic medication for acute eye problems appears to be acetaminophen. Opioids may be no more effective than acetaminophen but should be avoided if possible or used only until an emergent referral to an ophthalmologist is made. Details regarding major orbital or periorbital trauma appear in Chapter 3.

OPHTHALMIC TOPICAL

Four topical nonsteroidal anti-inflammatory drugs (NSAIDs) are available for ophthalmic application that function as local anesthetics and analgesics. They are diclofenac, flurbiprofen, ketorolac, and suprofen[7] (see Table 16-14).

Studies that evaluated the effectiveness of an ophthalmic NSAID in treating noninfected, non-contact lens-related, traumatic corneal abrasions without a pressure patch have been completed (Kaiser, 1995). After randomization, patients receiving ketorolac tromethamine 0.5% ophthalmic solution noted significantly decreased levels of pain, photophobia, and foreign-body sensation compared with the control vehicle group. In addition, the time before resuming normal activities was shorter in the group that received ketorolac tromethamine 0.5% ophthalmic solution. There was no statistical difference in the amount of tearing, healing time, acuity changes, or complication rates between

[7] Flurbiprofen and suprofen, which are indicated only to inhibit intraoperative miosis, are very similar in activity, and some hospitals use them interchangeably. Diclofenac has an official indication for the postoperative prophylaxis and treatment of ocular inflammation. Ketorolac is indicated for treating postoperative inflammation and relieving ocular itching due to seasonal allergic conjunctivitis. It also has shown some success in alleviating the pain associated with keratotomy. Both diclofenac and ketorolac also have been used successfully to prevent and treat cystoid macular edema. NSAIDs cause little, if any, rise in IOP. The Ocular PF ophthalmic solution of ketorolac without preservative does not cause such transient stinging and burning on instillation (20% of patients in a clinical trial) whereas the solution with preservative does (40%). Diclofenac (Voltaren ophthalmic) caused stinging and burning in 15% of patients, but keratitis was reported in 28% of patients undergoing cataract surgery. Ocular PF ophthalmic would appear to be best tolerated by patients with fewer side effects.

the two groups. Ketorolac tromethamine 0.5% ophthalmic solution provides increased patient comfort without clinically adverse effects when used as adjunctive therapy in treating noninfected, non-contact lens-related traumatic corneal abrasions (Kaiser, 1995).

Pressure Patching

The cornea is richly supplied by sensory nerves whose endings ramify in the epithelium. These nerves are among the most sensitive in the body. A corneal epithelial defect produces immediate pain, tearing, photophobia, and foreign-body sensation that often motivates the patient to seek medical attention. A corneal abrasion is limited to the superficial corneal epithelium and usually results from trauma secondary to fingers, branches, paper, or metal. The defects generally heal within 2 to 3 days without any long-term complications. Corneal abrasions are very common and account for up to 10% of new admissions to eye emergency units (Kaiser, 1995).

Antibiotic ointment, with or without a topical mydriatic and a pressure patch, has been the traditional treatment of traumatic, non-contact lens-related corneal abrasions. Unfortunately, using a pressure patch is not a benign treatment because it removes binocular vision, can be uncomfortable for the patient, and may retard healing. Several studies have questioned the effectiveness of patching corneal abrasions. To date, no large-scale study has been performed to evaluate the effectiveness of pressure patching to treat traumatic corneal abrasions and after removing corneal foreign bodies.

Kaiser (1995) reported that patients with traumatic corneal abrasions healed significantly faster, had less pain, and had fewer reports of blurred vision when they were not wearing a patch. There was no difference in the amount of photophobia, tearing, foreign-body sensation, or blurred vision. Finally, compliance in the no-patch group was better. In Hulbert's study (1991) of both pain and healing after foreign-body removal, it appears that both parameters were influenced favorably by not patching.

Potential disadvantages of patching can be noted. Pseudomonas ulcers have been documented after eye patching of corneal abrasions caused by contact lenses. Also, patching has been noted to decrease the natural irrigation effect of tears and to decrease corneal oxygen tension while increasing corneal temperature. Adverse effects on depth perception and visual fields are well known.

In cases of open globe and/or major injury to the orbit, the injured eye should be covered with a metallic or plastic shield for protection.

Mydriatics and Cycloplegics (see Table 16-12)

The autonomic drugs that produce mydriasis (pupillary dilatation) and cycloplegia (paralysis of accommodation and iris constriction muscles) are among the most frequently used topical medications in ophthalmic practice. The most commonly used mydriatic is the direct-acting adrenergic agent phenylephrine

Table 16-12. Mydriatics and Cycloplegics

Generic Name	Trade Name	Concentration (%)	Onset/Duration of Action
Phenylephrine hydrochloride	AK-Dilate Mydfrin Neo-Synephrine Available generically	Solution 2.5%, 10% Solution 2.5% Solution 2.5%, 10% Solution 2.5%, 10%	30-60 minutes/3-5 hours
Hydroxyamphetamine hydrobromide*	Paremyd	Solution 1%	15-60 minutes/3-4 hours
Atropine sulfate	Atropisol Atropine-Care Isopto Atropine Available generically	Solution 1% Solution 1% Solution 1% Solution 1% Ointment 1%	45-120 minutes/7-14 days
Cyclopentolate hydrochloride	AK-Pentolate Cyclogyl Pentolair Available generically	Solution 1% Solution 0.5%, 1%, 2% Solution 1% Solution 1%	30-60 minutes/6-24 hours
Homatropine hydrobromide	Isopto Homatropine Available generically	Solution 2%, 5% Solution 2%, 5%	30-60 minutes/3 days
Scopolamine hydrobromide	Isopto Hyoscine	Solution 0.25%	30-60 minutes/4-7 days
Tropicamide	Mydriacyl AK-Tropicacyl Available generically	Solution 0.5%, 1% Solution 0.5%, 1% Solution 0.5%, 1%	20-40 minutes/4-6 hours

*In combination with tropicamide 0.25%.
Note: Dapiprazole hydrochloride (Rev-Eyes) ophthalmic solution 0.5% sterile (Bausch & Lomb Pharmaceutical, Inc.).
Source: From *Physicians Desk Reference for Ophthalmic Medicine.* 3rd ed. 2002; Table 2.

hydrochloride, usually in a 2.5% concentration. The other mydriatic, an indirectly acting adrenergic hydroxyamphetamine, is available only in combination with tropicamide.

Phenylephrine is used alone or, more commonly, in combination with a cycloplegic agent for refraction or for pupillary dilatation. The 2.5% concentration is favored for these cases. The possibility of severe adverse systemic effects arises from using the 10% solution.

Anticholinergic agents have both cycloplegic and mydriatic activity. They usually are used for refraction, pupillary dilatation, relief of inflammation, and relief from iris and ciliary spasm. It is important to remember that the effect of these medications depends on many factors, including age, race, and eye color. For example, the mydriatics and cycloplegics tend to be less effective in dark-eyed than in blue-eyed individuals.

The drug dapiprazole hydrochoride can be used to reverse the effects of phenyephrine and, to a lesser extent, tropicamide. Activity against phenylephrine is excellent: 88% reversal is seen at the end of 1 hour. Against tropicamide, results are significantly lower: 38% at the end of 2 hours. When using both drugs, it therefore remains important to instruct the patient to use sunglasses and to avoid driving or operating dangerous machinery.

There is no significant alteration in IOP in normotensive (intraocular tension with normal pressure under glaucoma treatment) glaucomatous eyes.

Antimicrobial Therapy (see Table 16-13)

Antibiotics are used routinely in ophthalmology for both treatment and prophylaxis. They are used prophylactically to manage foreign bodies and corneal abrasions and in pre- and postoperative care, where they are administered as an ophthalmic solution or ointment. Because these antibiotics are prescription drugs, no known over-the-counter antibiotics are available to be used.

Corneal abrasions associated with contact lens wear are commonly evaluated and treated in acute care clinics and emergency departments by nonophthalmologists. The risk of progression to suppurative keratitis in this setting requires management distinct from that of other mechanical (e.g., fingernail scratch) corneal abrasions. The antibiotic chosen should reflect the need for prophylaxis against Pseudomonas. Conditions favoring bacterial growth, specifically occlusive patching and/or use of steroid-containing compounds, must be avoided, and a 24-hour follow-up examination is recommended (Schein, 1993).

Again, ensure that the patient is not allergic to the proposed antibiotic prior to its use. Patients with more serious conditions, such as bacterial corneal ulcers (red flag), or those whose foreign-body abrasion is not healed in 24 hours or is showing no evidence of healing should be referred to an ophthalmologist for further treatment. Patients with potentially contaminated corneal abrasions or foreign bodies may have their tetanus immunization evaluated and may be treated in accordance with the tetanus immunization protocol.

Table 16-13. Commercially Available Ophthalmic Antibacterial Agents

Generic Name	Trade Name	Concentration of Ophthalmic Solution (1%)	Concentration of Ophthalmic Ointment
	Individual Agents		
Bacitracin	AK-Tracin	Not available	500 units/g
Chloramphenicol[a]	AK-Chlor	0.5%	Not available
	Chloromycetin	0.16-0.5%	1%
	Chloroptic	0.5%	1%
	Available generically	0.5%	Not available

Table 16-13. (continued)

Generic Name	Trade Name	Concentration of Ophthalmic Solution (1%)	Concentration of Ophthalmic Ointment
Ciprofloxacin hydrochloride	Ciloxan	0.3%	0.3%
Erythromycin	Llotycin Available generically	Not available Not available	0.5% 0.5%
Gentamicin sulfate	Garamycin Genoptic Gentacidin Gentak Available generically	0.3% 0.3% 0.3% 0.3% 0.3%	0.3% 0.3% 0.3% 0.3% 0.3%
Levofloxacin	Quixin	0.5%	Not available
Norfloxacin	Chibroxin	0.3%	Not available
Ofloxacin	Ocuflox	0.3%	Not available
Sulfacetamide sodium	AK-Sulf Bleph-10 Cetamide Isopto Cetamide Sulamyd Sodium Sulf-10 Available generically	10% 10% Not available 15% 10%, 30% 10% 10%, 15%, 30%	10% 10% 10% Not available 10% Not available 10%
Tobramycin sulfate	Tobrex Tobralcon Available generically	0.3% 0.3% 0.3%	0.3% 0.3% Not available
Mixtures			
Polymyxin B/bacitracin zinc	AK-Poly-Bac Polysporin Available generically	Not available	10,000 units 500 units/g
Polymyxin B/ neomycin/bacitracin	AK-Spore Neosporin Available generically	Not available	10,000 units 3.5 mg 400 units/g
Polymyxin B/ neomycin/gramicidin	AK-Spore Neosporin Available generically	10,000 units 1.75 mg 0.025 mg/ml	Not available
Polymyxin B/ oxytetracycline	Terramycin TERAK	Not available	10,000 units 5 mg/g
Polymyxin B/ trimethoprim	Polytrim Available generically	10,000 units 1 mg/ml	Not available

[a]Although noted, used very rarely.
Source: Table from *Physician's Desk Reference for Ophthalmic Medicine*. 3rd ed. 2002; Table 2.

Ocular Anti-inflammatory Agents (Steroids)

The wide variety of medications available to treat ocular inflammation are listed in Table 16-14. Corticosteroids (steroids) are used most commonly, and

Table 16-14. Topical Anti-inflammatory Agents

Name and Dosage Form	Trade Name	Concentration
Topical Steroids		
Dexamethasone	Maxidex Ophthalmic Suspension	0.1%
Dexamethasone sodium phosphate ophthalmic ointment	AK-Dex Decadron Available generically	0.05% 0.05% 0.05%
Dexamethasone sodium phosphate ophthalmic solution	AK-Dex Decadron Available generically	0.1% 01% 01%
Fluorometholone ophthalmic ointment	FML S.O.P.	0.1%
Fluorometholone ophthalmic suspension	Fluor-Op FML FML Forte Available generically	0.1% 0.1% 0.25% 0.1%
Fluorometholone acetate ophthalmic suspension	Flarex Eflone	0.1% 0.1%
Loteprednol etabonate	Lotemax	0.5%
Medrysone ophthalmic suspension	HMS	1%
Prednisolone acetate ophthalmic suspension	Pred Mild Econopred Econopred Plus Pred Forte Available generically	0.12% 0.125% 1% 1% 1%
Prednisolone sodium phosphate ophthalmic solution	AK-Pred Inflamase Available generically AK-Pred Inflamase Forte Available generically	0.125% 0.125% 0.125% 1% 1% 1%
Rimexolone ophthalmic suspension	Vexol	1%
Nonsteroidal Anti-inflammatory Drugs		
Diclofenac ophthalmic solution	Voltaren	0.1%
Ketorolac ophthalmic solution	Acular	0.5%

Source: Table from *Physician's Desk Reference for Ophthalmic Medicine*. 3rd ed. 2002; Table 8.

many are available in combination with antibiotics and/or other medications. Ocular anti-inflammatory drugs (steroids) should not be initiated by the primary care physician but may be followed after initiation by an ophthalmologist. Herpes simplex keratitis may be difficult to diagnose by a nonophthalmologist and can be extremely progressive when steroids are used without the presence of an appropriate antiviral agent.

Corticosteroids once were thought to be contraindicated in infectious disease states. However, it is now appreciated that steroids, when used in conjunction with appropriate antimicrobial, antifungal, or antiviral agents, may help to prevent more serious ocular damage. The correct diagnosis and appropriate agent are critical. Steroids may be administered by four different routes when treating ocular inflammation. Table 16-15 lists the preferred route for various conditions.

Topical corticosteroids can elevate IOP and, in susceptible individuals, can induce glaucoma. Some corticosteroids, such as fluorometholone acetate, medrysone, and loteprednol, cause less elevation of IOP than others. Corticosteroids also may cause cataract formation, a complication more likely with high systemic use.

Management of Blurred Vision

Blurred vision is a symptom of a decrease in visual acuity that may be central or peripheral. The patient presenting with symptoms or signs of blurred vision

Table 16-15. Usual Route of Steroid Administration in Ocular Inflammation

Condition	Route
Blepharitis	Topical
Conjunctivitis	Topical
Episcleritis	Topical
Scleritis	Topical and/or systemic
Keratitis	Topical
Anterior uveitis	Topical and/or periocular
Posterior uveitis	Systemic and/or periocular
Endophthalmitis	Systemic/periocular, intravitreal
Optic neuritis	Systemic or periocular
Cranial arteritis	Systemic
Sympathetic ophthalmia	Systemic and topical

Source: Table from *Physician's Desk Reference for Ophthalmic Medicine*. 3rd ed. 2002; Table 9.

may be referred to an ophthalmologist or, based on results of visual (ocular) screening, an optometrist (see Algorithm 16-8).

Central[8]

1. A central decrease in visual acuity may be transient or last longer than 24 hours. Transient visual loss (vision returns to normal within 24 hours, usually within 1 hour).
   a. Few seconds (usually bilateral): Papilledema
   b. Few minutes: Amaurosis fugax [transient ischemic attack (TIA), unilateral], vertebrobasilar artery insufficiency (bilateral)
   c. Between 10 and 60 minutes: Migraine (with or without subsequent headache)
2. Visual loss lasting longer than 24 hours.
   a. Sudden painless loss: Retinal artery or vein occlusion, ischemic optic neuropathy, vitreous hemorrhage, retinal detachment, optic neuritis (usually pain with eye movements)
   b. Gradual, painless loss (over weeks, months, or years): Cataract, open-angle glaucoma, chronic retinal disease [e.g., age-related macular degeneration (ARMD), diabetic retinopathy]
   c. Painful loss: Acute angle-closure glaucoma, optic neuritis (pain with eye movements), uveitis, corneal hydrops (keratoconus)
3. Gradual change in refractive error (over months, years).
   a. Myopia—nearsightedness
   b. Hyperopia—farsightedness
   c. Presbyopia—lack of accommodation for reading or performing tasks at near (approximately 9 inches or 22 centimeters)

Peripheral[9]

The peripheral vision (visual acuity) can be measured by means of a visual field examination. Visual field types of defects (identified below) will help to determine the anatomic defects and the most likely diagnosis.

Altitudinal defect. Ischemic optic neuropathy.
Arcuate scotoma. Glaucoma.
Binasal field defect. Glaucoma, bitemporal retinal disease (e.g., retinitis pigmentosa).

[8]Information modified from Rhee DJ, Pyfer MF, Rhee DM, eds. *The Wills Eye Manual: Office and Emergency Room Diagnosis and Treatment of Eye Diseases.* 3rd ed. Philadelphia, Pa: Lippincott, Williams & Wilkins; 1999. Chapter 1, p. 1-2.

[9]Information modified from Rhee DJ, Pyfer MF, Rhee DM, eds. *The Wills Eye Manual: Office and Emergency Room Diagnosis and Treatment of Eye Diseases.* 3rd ed. Philadelphia, Pa: Lippincott, Williams & Wilkins; 1999. Chapter 2, p. 16.

Bitemporal hemianopia. Chiasmal lesion (e.g., pituitary adenoma, meningioma, craniopharyngioma, aneurysm, glioma)

Blind spot enlargement. Papilledema, glaucoma, optic nerve drusen, optic nerve coloboma, medulated nerve fibers off the disc, drugs, myopic disc with a crescent, others.

Central scotoma. Macular disease, optic neuritis, ischemic optic neuropathy (more typically produces an altitudinal field defect), optic atrophy (e.g., from tumor compressing the nerve, toxic/metabolic disease).

Homonymous hemianopsia. Optic tract or lateral geniculate body lesion; temporal, parietal, or occipital lobe lesion of the brain (stroke and tumor more common; aneurysm and trauma less common).

Migraine. May cause a transient homonymous hemianopsia.

Constriction of the peripheral fields leaving only a small residual central field. Glaucoma, retinitis pigmentosa, or some other peripheral retinal disorder, chronic papilledema, after panretinal photocoagulation, central retinal artery occlusion with cilioretinal artery sparing, bilateral occipital lobe infarction with macular sparing, nonphysiologic visual loss, carcinoma-associated retinopathy.

Management of Visual Fatigue

Visual fatigue is a term used to describe phenomena related to intensive use of the eyes. It can include complaints of eye or periocular pain, itching or burning, tearing, oculomotor changes, focal problems, performance degradation, after-colors, and other phenomena. Patients presenting with signs or symptoms of visual fatigue may be referred to an ophthalmologist or optometrist (see Algorithm 16-9).

The ability to perform most tasks depends on many visual and nonvisual variables, and the factors that influence the visual performance include:

- The patient's visual capability
- The visibility of the task
- Psychological and general physiologic factors

Studies indicate that the visual complaints occur in 50 to 90% of video display terminal (VDT) workers. The vision problems result from visual inefficiencies and eye-related symptoms. They are caused by a combination of individual visual system problems and poor visual ergonomics. The problems occur whenever the task's visual demands exceed the patient's visual abilities. The visual symptoms can be resolved, for the most part, with good visual ergonomics, by properly managing the environment, and by providing proper visual care. Ergonomics is the science of designing machines and work tasks with the capabilities and limitations of the human being in mind.[10]

[10]Information modified from Blais BR. Basic principles of occupational ophthalmology. In: Tassman W, Jaeger EA, eds. *Duane's Clinical Ophthalmology.* Vol. 5, Chap. 47. Philadelphia, Pa: Lippincott, Williams & Wilkins; 2002.

Visibility of Tasks

The ability to perform a task safely, efficiently, and comfortably depends on its visibility, as well as on the worker's visual capabilities. Naturally, the better the visibility, the easier it is to perform the task, and the factors influencing a task's visibility include:

- Size
- Distance
- Illumination
- Glare
- Contrast
- Color
- Time available to view task
- Movement of the task
- Atmospheric conditions

Ergonomic research supports the following regarding VDTs:

- Place frequently used displays in the primary visual display area. The top of the display should be opposite the operator's eyes, which face forward, extending down to a point at which the operator is looking down at a 30-degree angle. Devices viewed as they are operated, such as buttons, keyboards, and controls, should be seen in this area, at the work surface, and in the plane of the operator's eyes.
- The optimal viewing distance for visual displays is about 50 centimeters (20 inches). Workers with refractive error or presbyopia can wear corrective lenses designed specifically for the job. Lenses of this type also can be incorporated into multifocal eyeglasses (progressive add lenses) with overviews (add on segment at the top of the lens).
- Proper illumination is important and may be evaluated for each task. Visual performance can be impaired by whole-body vibration in the range of 10 to 25 cycles per second (hertz). Such vibration, which may be generated by power saws, cranes, conveyors, and other machinery should be damped or separated from the worker.

Vision Screening for the Worker

In order to determine the exact loss of function in patients with blurred vision and visual fatigue, a visual (ocular) function screening should be completed (see Algorithms 16-7, 16-8, and 16-9).

Elements of Visual (Ocular) Function

Visual (ocular) function requirements are important to the safety, health, and efficiency of industrial workers in nearly all occupations. Vision is most important for identifying distant objects and for detailed perception of shape and color. Visual senses allow workers to judge distance and gauge movements in the visual field.

Visual screening was defined by a joint proposal from the American Academy of Pediatrics, the American Academy of Ophthalmology, the American College of Occupational and Environmental Medicine, and the American Academy of Pediatric Ophthalmology and Strabismology. The definition is based on the following:

- The key element is determination of screening visual acuity, both quantitative and bilateral.
- Graduated visual acuity stimuli should be employed to allow quantitative determination of visual acuity (e.g., Snellen chart).
- Screening may include determination of contrast sensitivity, ocular alignment, color vision, and visual fields.

Current Testing Methods

Most required visual tests may be provided by using visual screeners (see "Additional Resources").

Work-Relatedness

A thorough work history is crucial to establishing work-relatedness (see Chapters 2 and 4 for components of the work history). Determining whether an eye complaint is related to work requires careful analysis and weighing of all associated or apparently causal factors operative at the time. In most traumatic eye complaints, the etiology is relatively clear. However, identifying the source of cataracts, for example, may be more difficult. In cases of nonspecific eye complaints, such as "eye strain" or headache, a predominance of work factors suggests that worksite intervention to prevent recurrences and hasten recovery is appropriate. A cluster of cases in a work group suggests a greater probability of associated work-design or management factors. The following discussion applies primarily to these clusters but also may be useful in other cases.

Eye complaints can be associated with workstation design or positioning; thus an accurate and thorough history, including a review of work- and non-work-related activities, is required. Questioning about ergonomics of the worksite, including tasks, use of a headset, computer screen placement, and many other factors, is important.

Work Activities

THE PROSPECTIVE WORKER

In order to apply the postoffer examination findings, detailed knowledge of the job is required. Such information is derived from a visual analysis of the occupation. These data, or visual skills demanded of the worker, are written into the job requirements and meet with eventual tabulation (see Algorithm 16-7).

This visual survey must be accomplished so that the occupational health professional can enter the shops, learn the jobs and shop language, and be completely familiar with the workers' daily environment. From this point on, the occupational health professional can be of great help to the medical director and the personnel director, who are trying to place new workers in jobs where they can attain their full work capacity. From material gained at the time of the visual analysis, the worker receives eye protection for the job requirements and is offered protection against impact through the use of case-hardened glass or plastic. Using such a device provides a twofold result—good working vision and eye protection. Knowing the job's requirements is necessary to prescribe proper lenses because occupational glasses offer visual potential based on the working distance and a safety defense determined by the job's characteristic hazards.

Each individual applying for a position should undergo a complete physical appraisal, which should include a vision (ocular) screening procedure. In more progressive plants, the visual screening could include a battery of tests supplied by a single ocular screening or rating instrument.

In a well-integrated program, the results from these procedures can then be matched against the job's visual requirements. Failure to meet the guidelines established for that particular job places the worker and company management at risk both from a safety and production standpoint. The occupational health practitioner can play a key role by using these tests to interpret the job applicant's visual skills. In large plants, the practitioner interprets the findings of testing done by nontechnical employees (e.g., ophthalmic personnel or occupational health nurse). Small organizations will conduct the examination themselves or have it done by an off-site primary care physician.

Medical and personnel directors can then use the test and examination data to place the prospective worker in a job best suited to his or her visual function.

Preventive Medicine Guidelines

Preventive medicine guidelines are published in the American Medical Association (AMA) current procedural terminology (CPT) code guidelines and include the following activities:

1. *Visual screening history.* A general overview of the individual's visual history is required. See Table 16-16 for a proposed applicant questionnaire.

Table 16-16. Visual History Questionnaire

Visual History Questionnaire

Name ____________________ Date ________

Address ____________________

Occupation ____________________ Age ________

Eye History

Do you have a history of eye problem(s)? ☐Yes ☐No

If so, what is the diagnosis?

☐myopia (nearsightedness) ☐hyperopia (farsightedness) ☐astigmatism

☐presbyopia ☐lazy eye ☐ color vision (red/green deficiency) ☐color vision (blue/yellow deficiency)

☐cataract ☐macular degeneration ☐night blindness

☐congenital/acquired eye disease (specify) ____________________

☐eye injury (specify) ____________________

☐other eye condition ____________________

Family History

Does your father's family have an inherited eye condition? ☐Yes ☐No

If yes, specify ____________________

____

Does your mother's family have an inherited eye condition? ☐Yes ☐No

If yes, specify ____________________

____

General History

Do you have ☐diabetes ☐hypertension ☐glaucoma

Do you wear glasses? ☐ Yes ☐No

Do you own more than one pair of prescription glasses? ☐ Yes ☐No

If so, for what do you use your second pair?

☐sunglasses ☐reading ☐ occupational ☐ sports

Do you use safety or protective goggles? ☐ Yes ☐No

If so, do you wear them over spectacles or contact lenses? ☐ Yes ☐No

Do you use garden tools, such as weed whackers or lawn mowers? ☐ Yes ☐No

Do you have a home workshop or power tools? ☐ Yes ☐No

Do you use dangerous liquids such as alkalies or acids? ☐ Yes ☐No

Do you have safety prescription glasses for use in your workshop, hobbies or home activities? ☐ Yes ☐No

What are your hobbies? ____________________

Do you participate in any sports? ☐ Yes ☐No

If so, which ones? ____________________

Do you wear protective sports goggles? ☐ Yes ☐No

Have you ever heard of polycarbonate lenses? ☐ Yes ☐No

Visual History Questionnaire developed by Bernard R. Blais, MD, and reproduced with permission from Titmus Optical, Inc., Petersburg, Va.

2. Complete visual (ocular) screening examinations.
   a. Visual acuity quantitative bilateral tests measured at infinity (as a minimum) and at near and intermediate distances (based on job description) contrast sensitivity done periodically, and all performed with and without corrective devices (e.g., glasses, contact lenses) and without removing other visual corrective devices (e.g., intraocular lenses)
   b. Color vision—at a minimum, red and green hues, but preferable also to include blue and yellow
   c. Gross visual fields by confrontation at a minimum
   d. Heterophoria (horizontal and vertical) and depth perception stereopsis
   e. Intraocular tensions (e.g., puff tonometer when the globe is intact and the eye is not infected).
3. *Counseling participatory guidelines—risk factor reductions.* Interpretation of findings against standards (Purdue University, Federal Aviation Administration, U.S. Department of Transportation, U.S. Department of Energy, etc.), counseling, anticipatory guidance/risk factor reduction interventions.
4. Ordering appropriate laboratory and diagnostic procedures, followed by referral to an appropriate eye specialist depending on the defect, when an individual fails to meet standards, and preparing a written report.

ADA Issues: Performing Essential Functions with or without Accommodation

The Americans with Disabilities Act of 1990 (ADA), as implemented by most facilities in July of 1992, under Title 1 on employability, requires that individuals must be able to perform the essential functions of the position with or without reasonable accommodation without significant risk or direct threat to themselves and to others. Many federal agencies have published visual industrial standards. Physicians must carefully consider any contradictions between regulatory requirements and the ADA guidelines.

On the initial history, noting the patient's age, general health and condition, and perceptions of safe actions, considering current visual limitations, helps to provide criteria for recommended work activities. The availability of modified duty is an essential part of managing a patient with a work-related eye injury or disorder. Modified duty can be a job requiring less than perfect vision or the patient's original job adapted to his or her abilities. The clinician should make clear to patients and employers that monocular vision can pose a safety hazard by decreasing the field of vision and stereopsis unless job modifications or accommodations (or both) are provided.

Table 16-17 provides a guide for activity modification and duration of absence from work. These recommendations are intended for patients without comorbidity or complicating factors, including employment or legal issues. They are targets to provide a guide from the perspective of physiologic recovery.

*Table 16-17. Guidelines for Modification of Work Activities and Disability Duration**

Disorder	Activity Modifications and Accommodation	Recommended Target for Disability Duration†		NHIS Experience Data‡	
		With Modified Duty	**Without Modified Duty**	**Median (Cases with Lost Time)**	**Percent (no lost time)**
Corneal abrasion	If not patched, generally none. Modification for loss of binocular visual acuity, stereopsis, fields of vision if patched	0-3 days	0-5 days	2 days	46
Chemical splash (mild) (alkaline and acid)	Modification for loss of visual acuity	1-3 days	1-5 days	3 days	53
Foreign body on external eye	Modification for loss of binocular visual acuity, stereopsis, fields of vision if patched, otherwise generally none	0 days	0-5 days	2 days	67
Conjunctivitis	Provision for hygiene to prevent spread of infection by direct contact or shared articles	0 days	0 days	2 days	52
UV radiation	Modification for loss of visual acuity, stereopsis, fields of vision if patched	1 day	1 day	3 days	53
From radiation therapy				15 days	53
Nonspecific eye symptoms (visual disturbances)	Workstation adjustment	0 days	0 days	5 days	96

*These are general guidelines based on consensus or population sources and are never meant to be applied to an individual case without consideration of workplace factors, concurrent disease, and other social or medical factors that can affect recovery.

†These parameters for disability duration are "consensus optimal" targets as determined by a panel of ACOEM members in 1996 and reaffirmed by a panel of ACOEM members in 2002. In most cases, persons with one nonsevere injury can return to modified duty immediately.

‡Based on the CDC NHIS (National Health Interview Survey), as compiled and reported in the eighth annual edition of *Official Disability Guidelines (ODG)*, copyright © 2002, Work Loss Data Institute, all rights reserved.

***Algorithm 16-1**. Care of Red Eye Complaints*

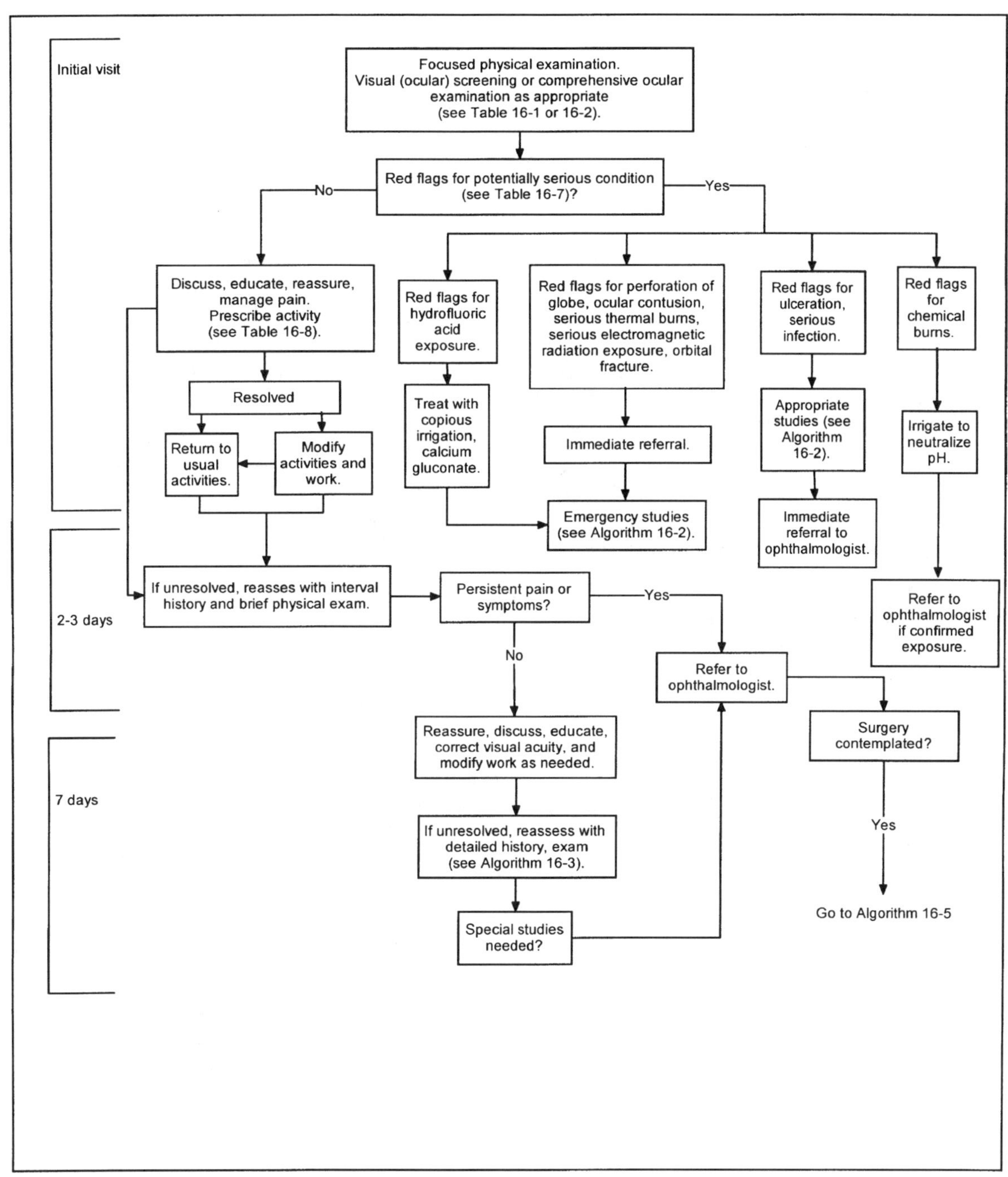

Algorithm 16-2. *Initial Evaluation of Occupational Red Eye Complaints*

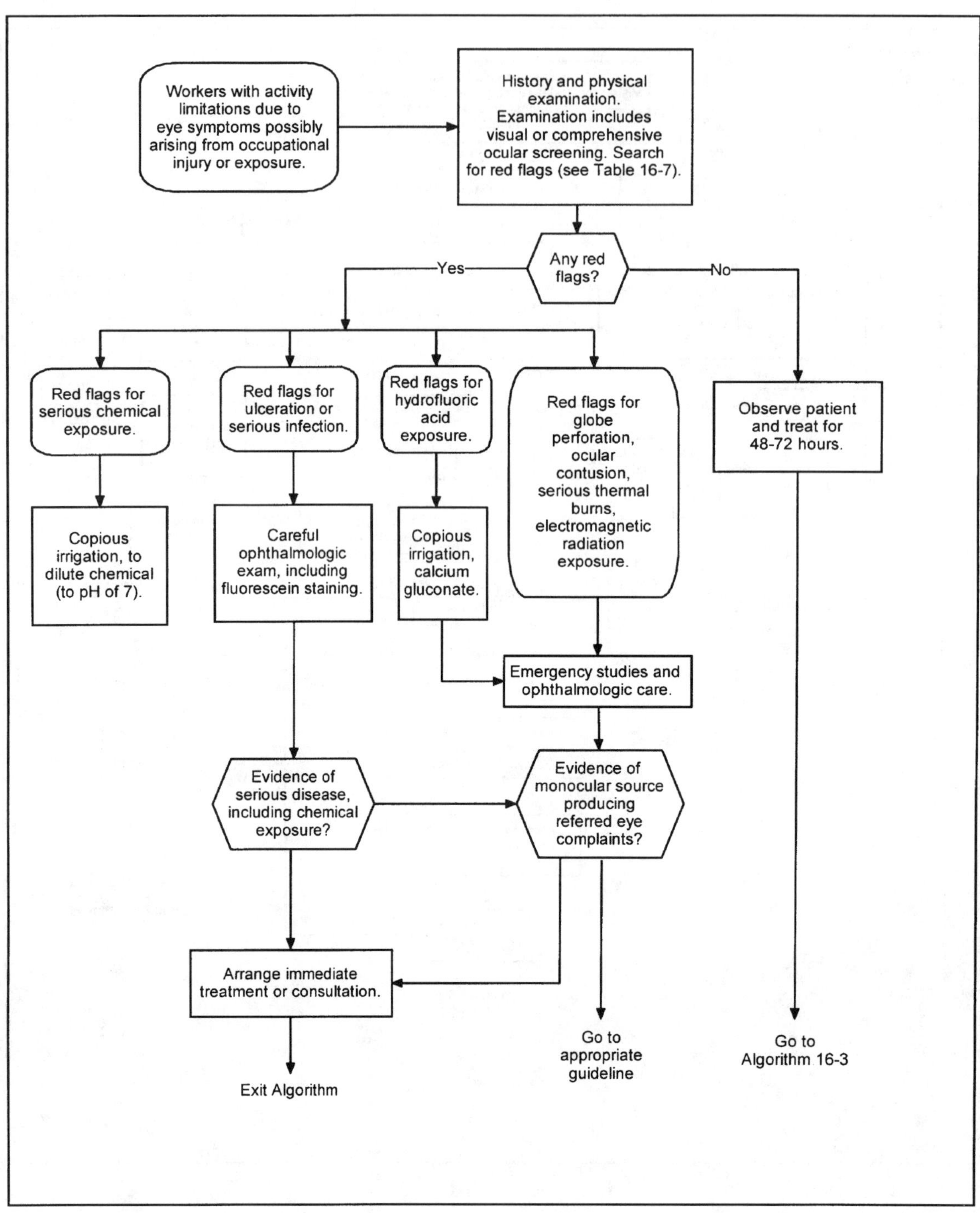

Algorithm 16-3. *Initial and Follow-up Management of Non-red Flag Occupational Eye Complaints*

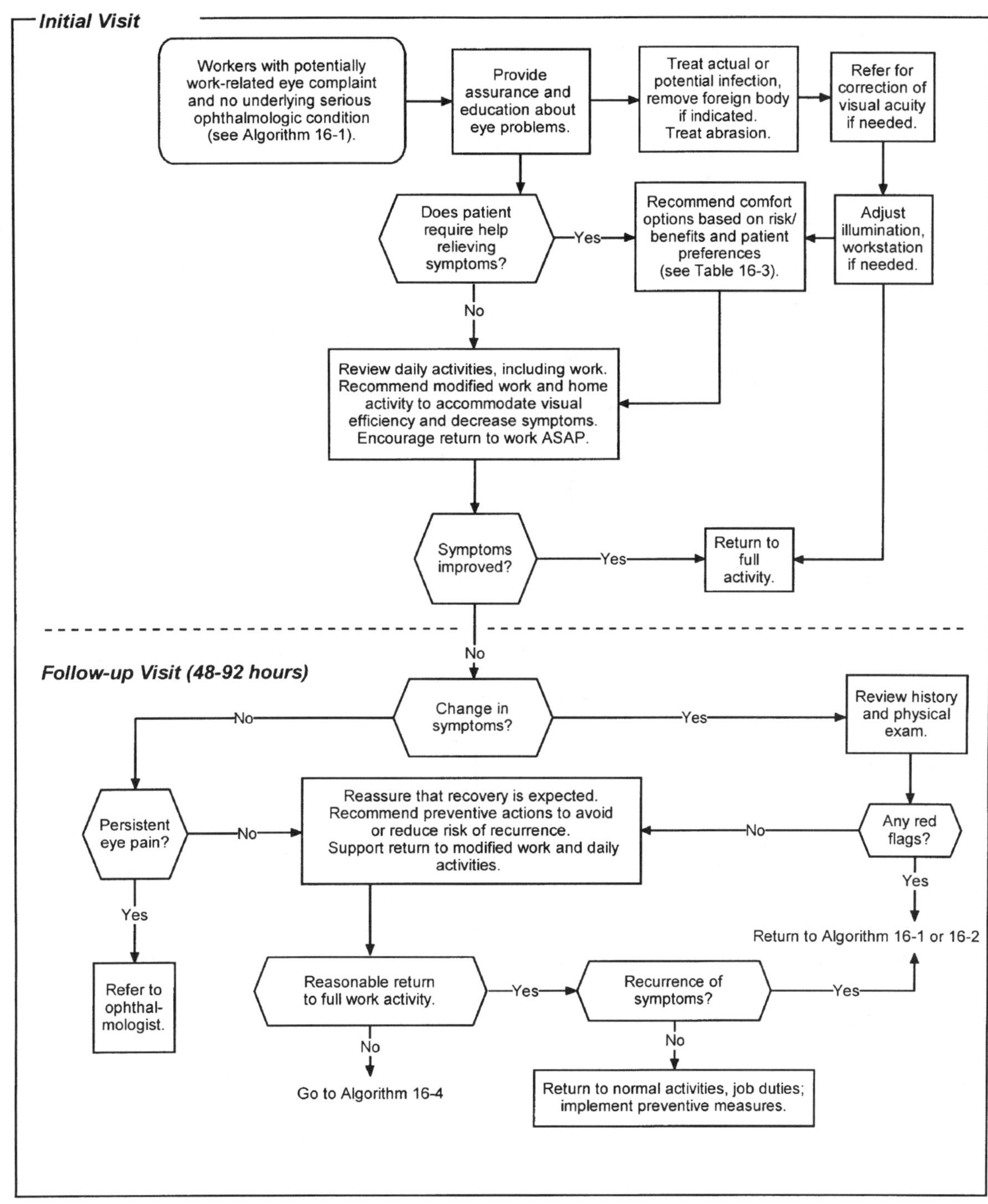

Algorithm 16-4. *Evaluation of Slow-to-recover Patients with Occupational Eye Complaints (Symptoms >7 Days)*

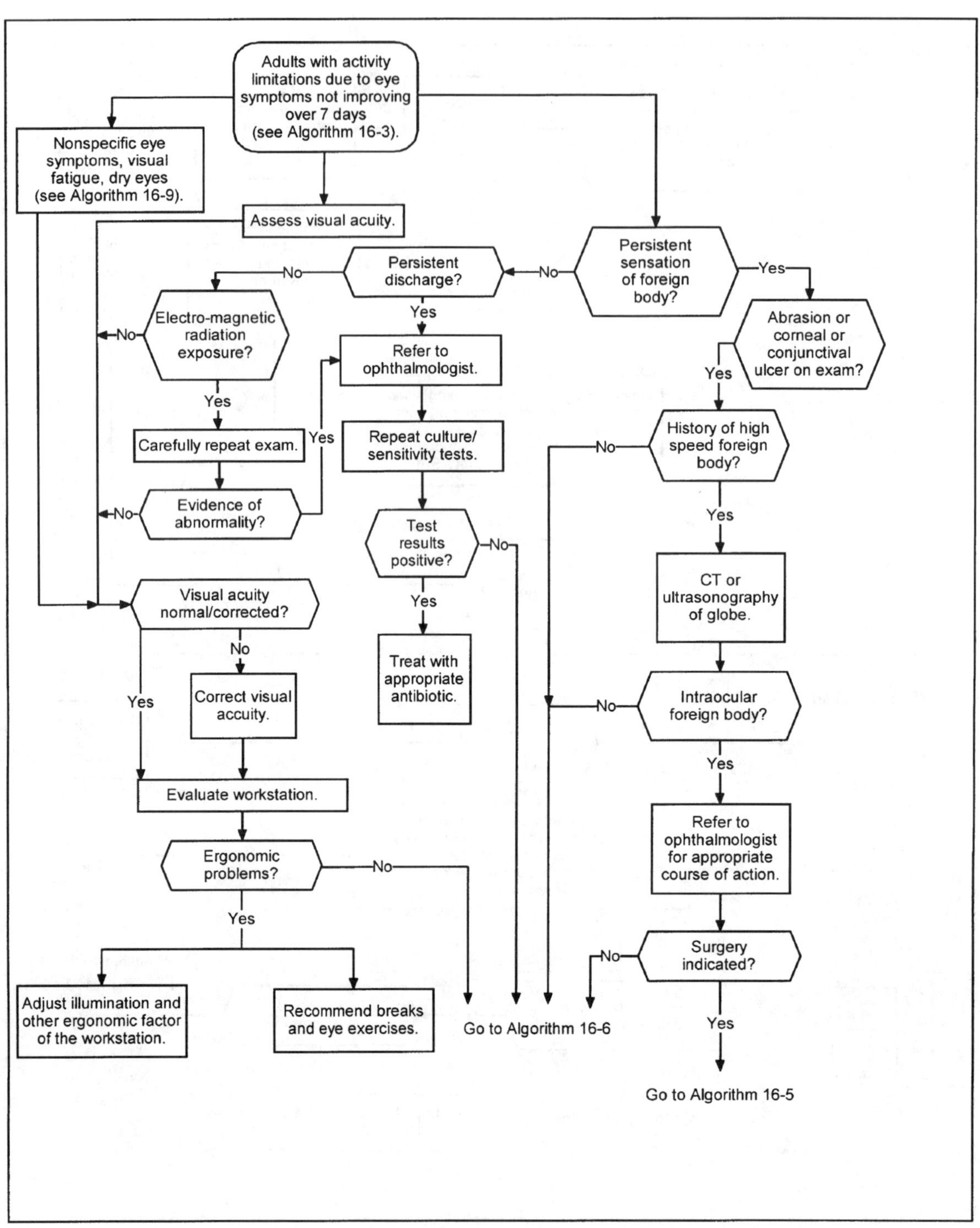

Algorithm 16-5. *Surgical Considerations for Patients with Persistent Visual Symptoms*

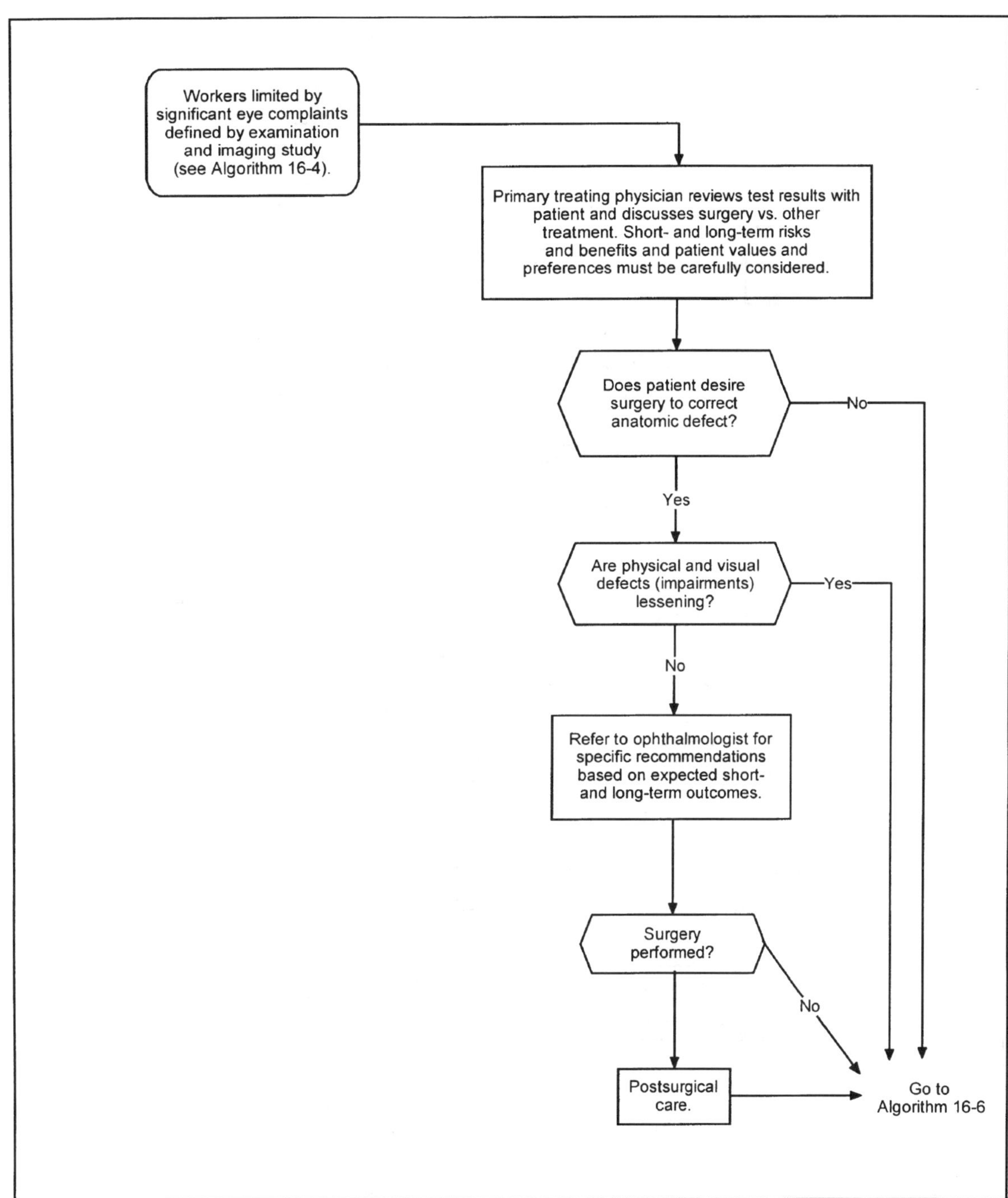

Algorithm 16-6. *Further Management of Occupational Eye Complaints*

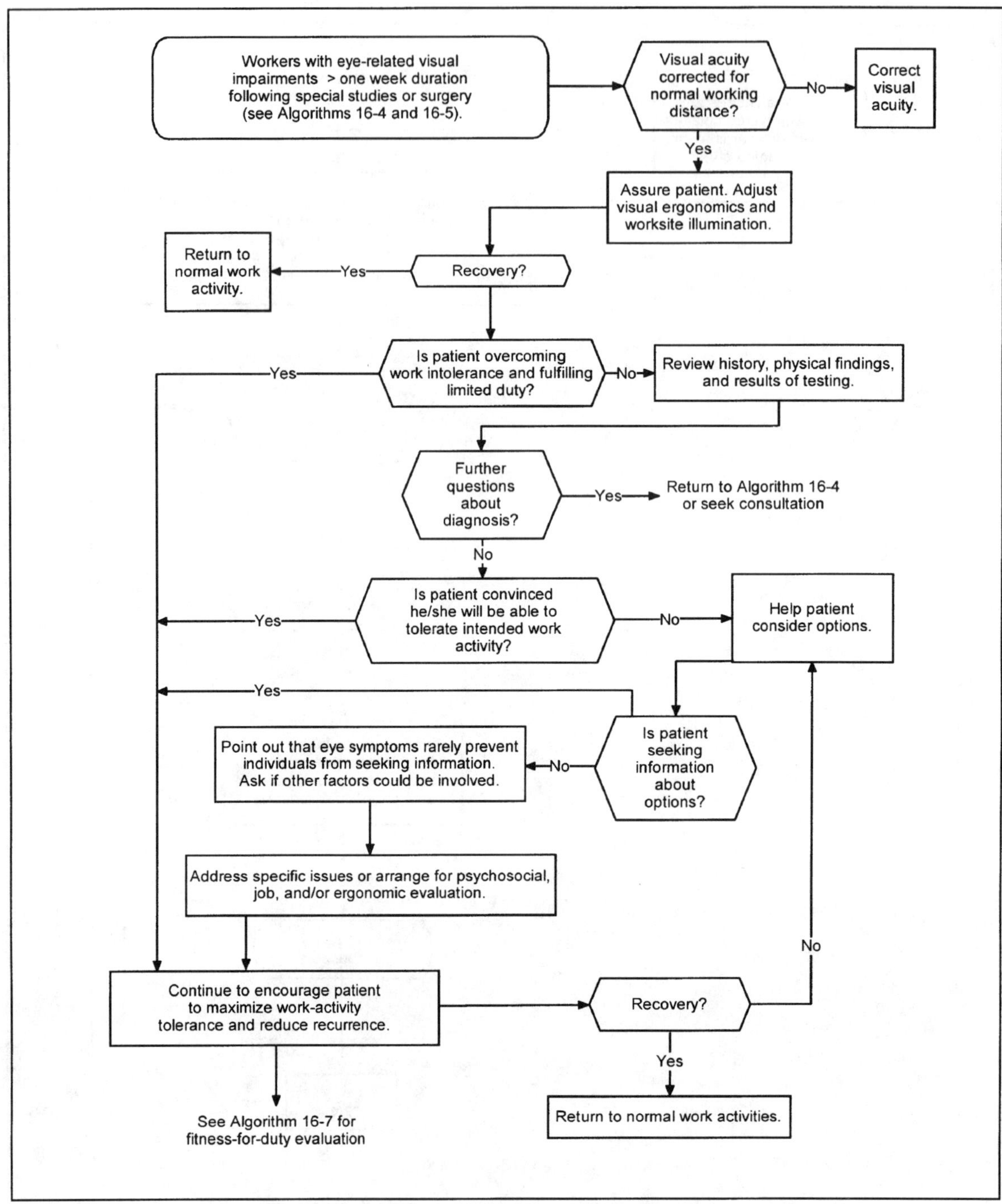

Algorithm 16-7. *Visual Screening (Fitness-for-duty Evaluation)*

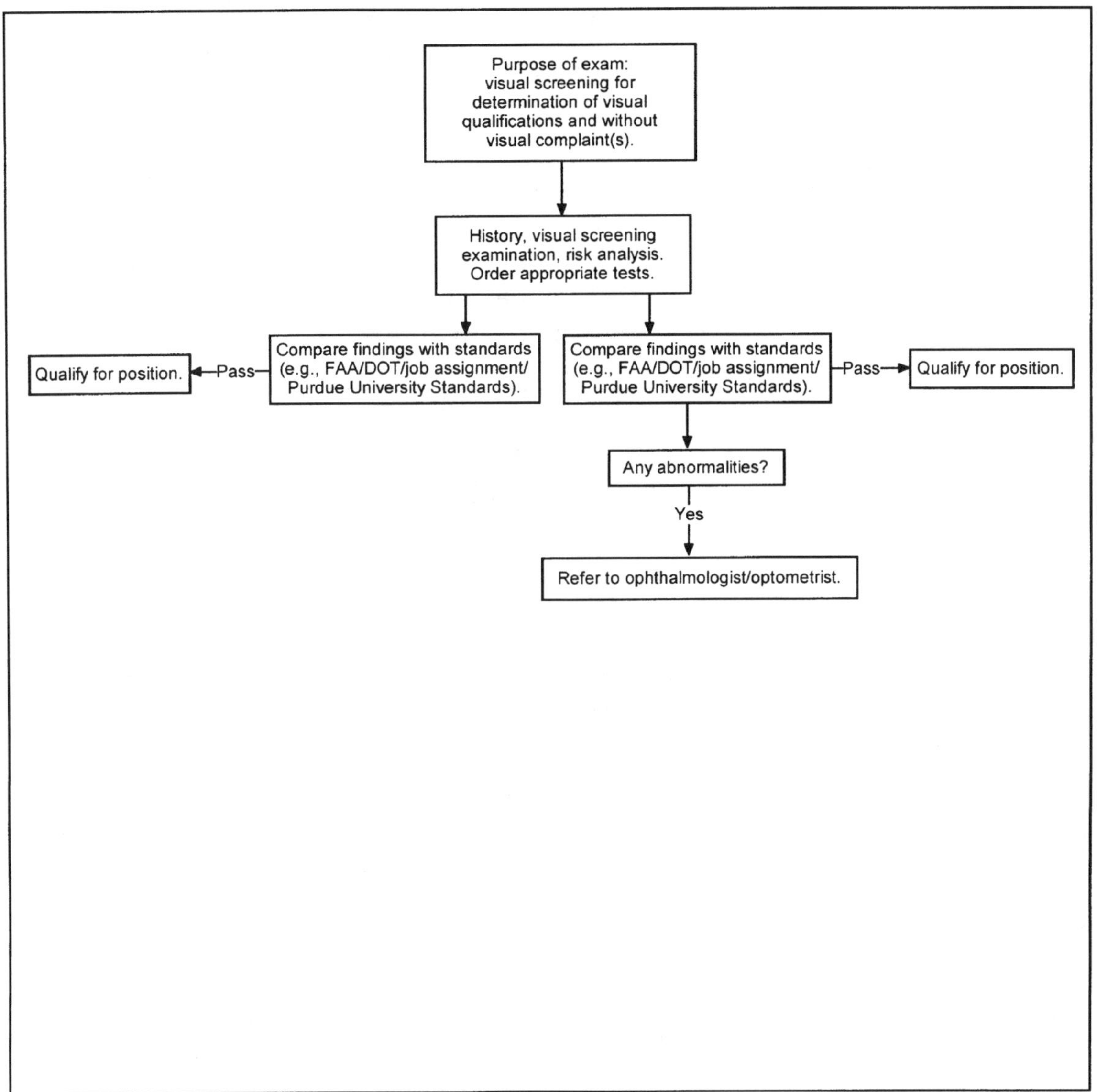

Algorithm 16-8. *Care of Eye Complaints – Blurred Vision*

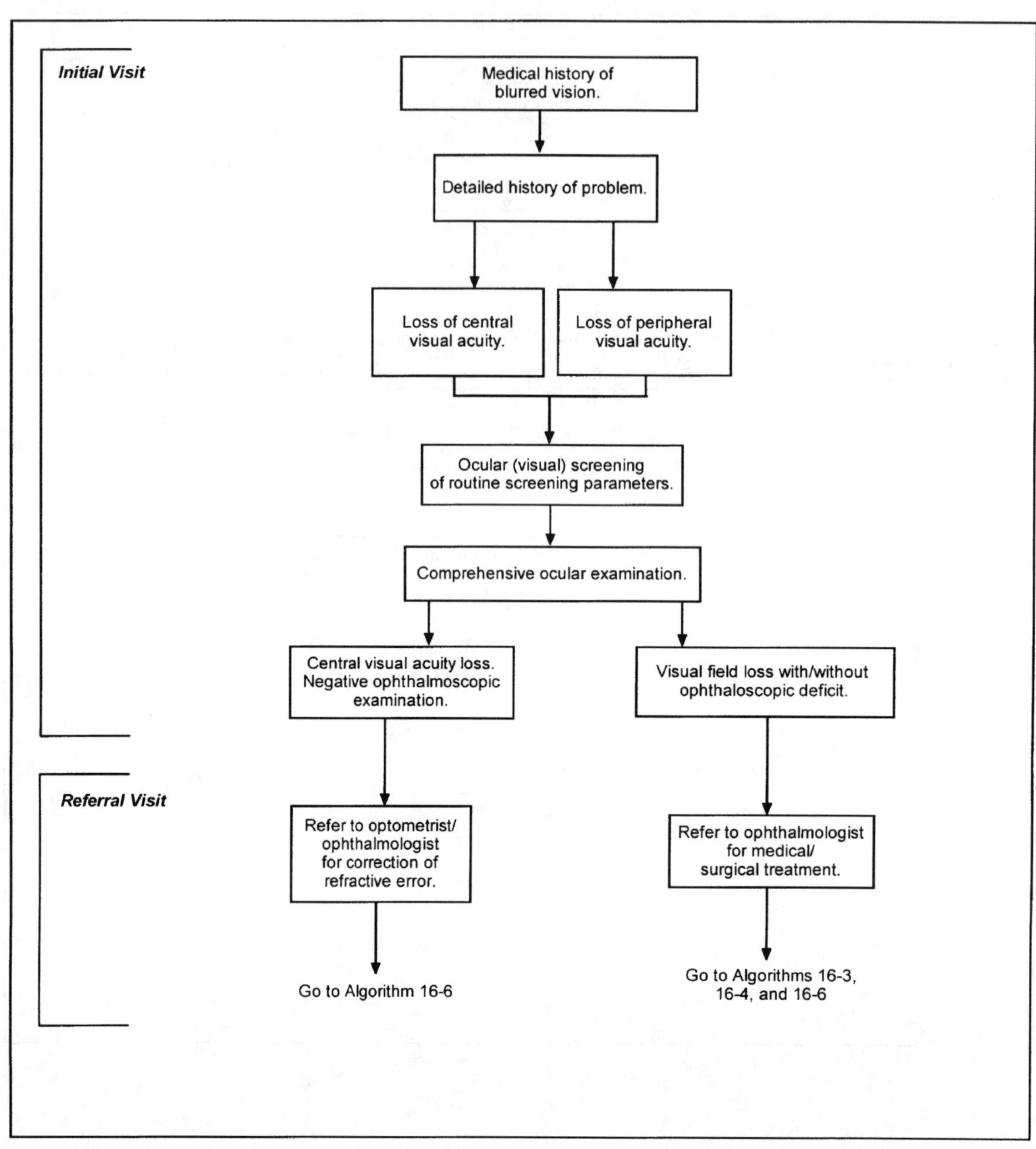

Algorithm 16-9. *Care of Eye Complaints – Visual Fatigue*

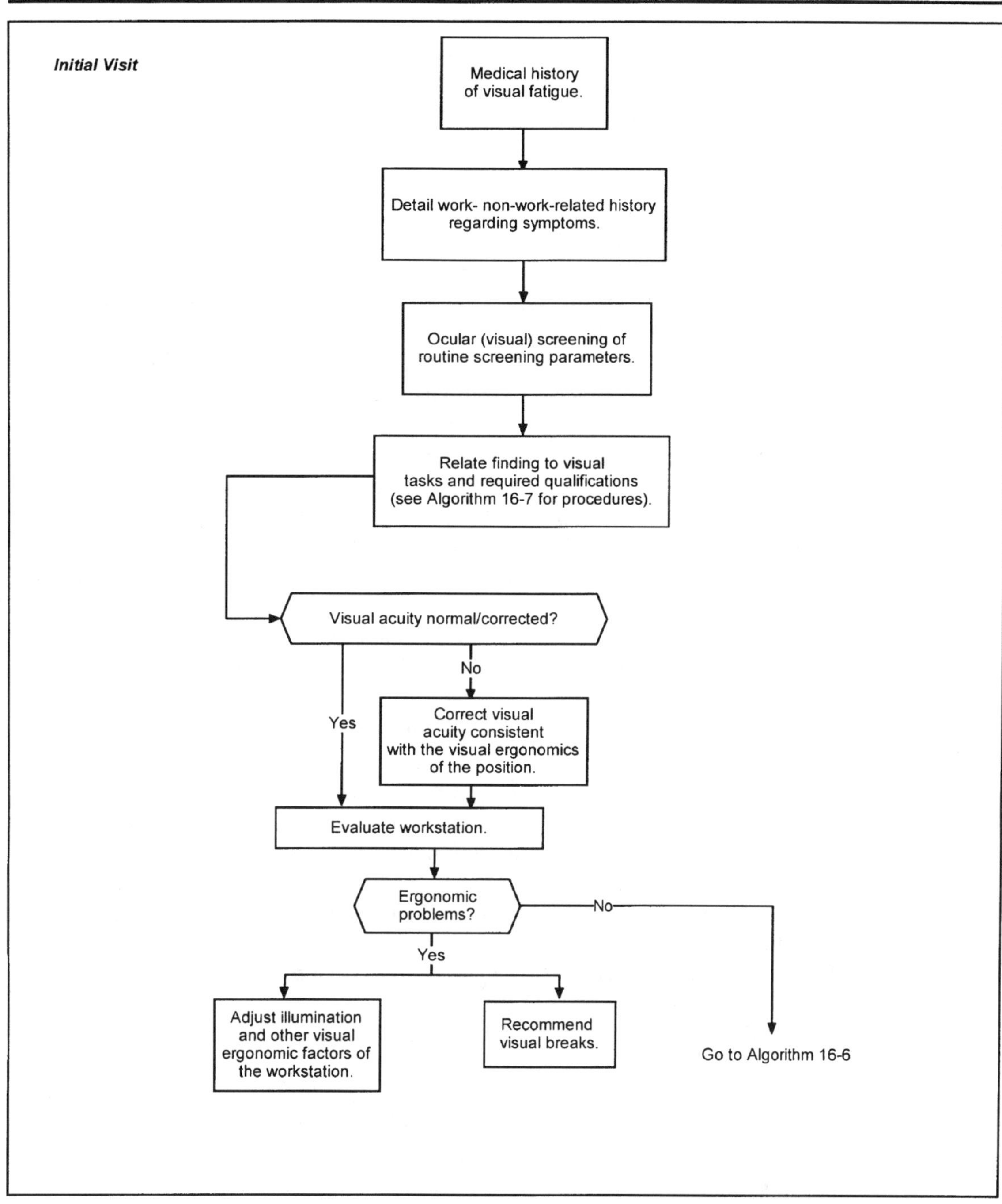

References

GENERAL APPROACH AND BASIC PRINCIPLES

Basic and Clinical Science Course, Section 8: *External Disease in Cornea.* San Francisco, Calif: American Academy of Ophthalmology (updated annually).

Berson FG. *Basic Ophthalmology for Medical Students and Primary Care Residents.* 6th ed. San Francisco, Calif: American Academy of Ophthalmology; 1993.

Blais BR. Basic principles of industrial ophthalmology. *Ophthalmol Clin of North Am.* 2000;12(3).

Blais BR. The new AMA ratings. *Occup Health Saf.* 2000;69(9):28-39.

Blais BR, Tredici TS, Williams J. Occupational ophthalmology. In: McCunney R, ed. *A Practical Approach to Occupational and Environmental Medicine.* 3rd ed. Chap. 34. Philadelphia, Pa: Lippincott Williams & Wilkins; 2003.

Blais BR. Basic principles of occupational ophthalmology. In: Tasman W, Jaeger EA, eds. *Duane's Clinical Ophthalmology.* Vol. 5, Chap. 47. Philadelphia, Pa: Lippincott Williams & Wilkins; 2002.

Blais BR. Visual impairment and disability assessment. In: Brigham CR, Ensalada LH, Talmadge JB, eds. *Clinics of Occupational and Environmental Medicine.* Philadelphia, Pa: Saunders; 2001.

Bradford CA. *Basic Ophthalmology.* 7th ed. San Francisco, Calif: American Academy of Ophthalmology; 1999.

Margo CE, Harman LE, Mulla ZD. Public health and the eye. The reliability of clinical methods in ophthalmology *Surv Ophthalomol.* 2002;47(4):375-86.

Newell FW. *Ophthalmology Principles and Concepts.* 8th ed. St. Louis, Mo: Mosby; 1996.

Pizzarello L. Eye safety and the economic impact of eye injuries during the last century in the United States. In Pizzarello L, Easterbrook M, eds. *Sports and Industrial Ophthalmology: Ophthalmology Clinics of North America.* 1999;12(3).

Prevent Blindness America. *Summary Materials.* Schaumburg, Ill: Prevent Blindness America; 1996.

Trobe JD. *Physicians Guide to Eyecare.* San Francisco, Calif: American Academy of Ophthalmology; 1993.

Trobe JD. *Physicians Guide to Eyecare.* 2nd ed. San Francisco, Calif: American Academy of Ophthalmology; 2001.

Tasman W, Jaeger EA, eds. *Duane's Clinical Ophthalmology.* Vol. 4, Chaps. 4-9A and 39-43. Philadelphia, Pa: Lippincott; 1991.

Wilson FM. *Practical Ophthalmology.* San Francisco, Calif: American Academy of Ophthalmology; 1996.

MANAGEMENT OF RED EYE

Bertolini J, Pelucio M. The red eye. *Emerg Med Clin North Am.* 1995;13(3): 561-79.

Gold EH, Lewis RA. *Clinical Eye Atlas.* Chicago, Ill: AMA Press; 2002.

OSHA. Rules and regulations. *Fed Reg.* 2001;66(13):5915-6135.

Reed EJ, Pyfer MF. *Wills' Eye Manual: Office and Emergency Room Treatment and Diagnosis of Eye Disease.* 3rd ed. Baltimore, Md: Williams & Wilkins; 1999.

Silverman H, Nunez L, Feller DB. Treatment of common eye emergencies. *Am Fam Phys.* 1992;45(5):2279-87.

OBSERVATION OF PATIENT AND EYE EXAMINATION

McNicholas MM, Brophy DP, Power WJ, et al. Ocular trauma: evaluation with US. *Radiology.* 1995;195(2):423-7.

SPECIAL STUDIES AND DIAGNOSTIC TREATMENT CONSIDERATIONS

Cascone G, Filippello M, Ferri R, Scimone G, Zagami A. B-scan echographic measurement of endobular foreign bodies. *Ophthalmologica.* 1994;208(4): 192-4.

Kramer M, Hart L, Miller JW. Ultrasonography in the management of penetrating ocular trauma. *Int Ophthalmol Clin.* 1995;35(1):181-92.

Kwong JS, Munk PL, Lin DT, Vellet AD, Levin M, Buckley AR. Real-time sonography in ocular trauma. *AJR.* 1992;158(1):179-82.

Maguire AM, Enger C, Eliott D, et al. Computed tomography in the evaluation of penetrating ocular injuries. *Retina.* 1991;11(4):405-11.

Rubsamen PE, Cousins SW, Winward KE, Byrne SF. Diagnostic ultrasound and pars plana vitrectomy in penetrating ocular trauma. *Ophthalmology.* 1994;101(5):809-14.

Shellock FG, Kanal E. Re: Metallic foreign bodies in the orbits of patients undergoing MR imaging: prevalence and value of radiography and CT before MR. *Am J Roentgenol.* 1994;162(4):985-6.

Weissman JL, Beatty RL, Hirsch WL, et al. Enlarged anterior chamber: CT finding of ruptured globe. *Am J Neuroradiol.* 1995;16(4 Suppl):936-8.

Williamson MR, Espinosa MC, Boutin RD, Orrison WW Jr, Hart BL, Kelsey CA. Metallic foreign bodies in the orbits of patients undergoing MR imaging: prevalence and value of radiography and CT before MR. *Am J Roentgenol.* 1994;162(4):981-3.

TYPES OF RED EYE

Alfaro DV, Roth D, Liggett PE. Post-traumatic endophthalmitis: Causative organisms, treatment, and prevention. *Retina.* 1994;14(3):206-11.

Ariyasu RG, Kumar S, LaBree LD, et al. Microorganisms cultured from the anterior chamber of ruptured globes at the time of repair. *Am J Ophthalmol.* 1995;119(2):181-8.

OCCUPATIONAL EYE INFECTIONS

Dawson C, Darrell R. Infections due to adenovirus type 8 in the United States. I. An outbreak of epidemic keratoconjuctivitis originating in a physician's office. *N Engl J Med.* 1963;268:1031.

Dawson C, Darrell R. Hanna L, Jawetz E. Infections due to adenovirus type 8 in the United States II. Community-wide infection with adenovirus type 8. *N Engl J Med.* 1963;268:1034-7.

Dawson C, Jawetz E, Hanna L, Winn WE, Thompson C. A family outbreak of adenovirus 8 infection (epidemic keratoconjunctivitis). *Am J Hyg.* 1960;72:279-83.

Duke Elder, SS, ed. *System of Ophthalmology.* Vol. VIII, Part 1. London: Henry Kimpton; 1965:353.

Holmes WJ. Epidemic infectious conjunctivitis. *Hawaii Med J.* 1941;1(2):11.

Jawetz E, Kimura SJ, Hanna L, Coleman VR, Thygeson P, Nicholas A. Studies on the etiology of epidemic keratoconjunctivitis. *Am J Ophthalmol.* 1953;40(5 Part 2):200-9; discussion 209-11.

Jawetz E, Thygson P, Hanna L, Nicholas A, Kimura SJ. The etiology of epidemic keratoconjunctivititis. *Am J Ophthalmol.* 1957;43(4 Part 2):79-83.

Leopold IH. Characteristics of hospital epidemics of epidemic keratoconjunctivitis. *Am J Ophthalmol.* 1957;43(4 Part 2):93-7.

Olson RJ, White GL Jr, Kreisler KR. Occupational eye disorders. In: Rom WN, ed. *Environmental and Occupational Medicine.* Boston, Mass: Little, Brown and Company; 1992:601-6.

OSHA. 29 CFR 1910.1030. *Fed Reg.* 1991;56(235):64-175.

OSHA. Instruction CPL, 2-2.44 C. Enforcement Procedure for the Occupational Exposure to Blood Born Pathogens under 29 CFR 1910.1030, March 6, 1992.

Pillat A. Epidemic of keratoconjunctivitis epidemica 1938 in Vienna. *Wien Klin Woschenr.* 1953;65(3):41-3.

OCULAR TRAUMA

Alper BS. Using the pressure patch to treat corneal abrasions. *Am Fam Phys.* 1997;55(2):442.

Bains RA, Rubin PA. Blunt orbital trauma. *Int Ophthalmol Clin.* 1995;35(1): 37-46.

Barker NH, Hennis A. Interventions for recurrent corneal erosions (Protocol for a Cochrane Review). Cochrane Library 3; 2002.

Blais BR. Discrimination against contact lens wearers. *J Occup Environ Med.* 1998;40(10):876-80

Benson WH, Snyder IS, Granus V, et al. Tetanus prophylaxis following ocular injuries. *J Emerg Med.* 1993;11(6):677-83.

Burnstine MA. Clinical recommendations for repair of isolated orbital floor fractures: An evidence-based analysis. *Ophthalmology.* 2002;109(7):1207-10; discussion 1210-1; quiz 1212-3.

Chiapella AP, Rosenthal AR. One year in an eye casualty clinic. *Br J Ophthalmol.* 1985;69(11):865-70.

Classe JG, Semes LP. The initial assessment of ocular contusion injury. *Optometr Clin.* 1993;3(2):115-45.

Coe JE, Douglas RB. Objective measurement of ocular responses to chemical irritation. *J Physiol (Lond).* 1980;308:53.

Coe JE, Douglas RB. Ocular responses to chemical and physical injury. In: Zenz C, Dickerson OB, Horvath EP Jr, eds. *Occupational Medicine.* 3rd ed. St. Louis, Mo: Mosby; 1994:85-92.

Dannenberg AL, Parver LM, Brechner RJ, Khoo L. Penetration eye injuries in the workplace. The National Eye Trauma System Registry. *Arch Ophthalmol.* 1992;110(6):843-8.

DeBroff BM, Donahue SP, Caputo BJ, et al. Clinical characteristics of corneal foreign bodies and their associated culture results. *CLAO J.* 1994;20(2): 128-30.

Deutsch TS, Feller DB. *Paton and Goldberg's Management of Ocular Injuries.* 2nd ed. Philadelphia, Pa: Saunders; 1985.

Donnefeld ED, Selkin BA, Perry HD, et al. Controlled evaluation of a bandage contact lens and a topical nonsteroidal anti-inflammatory drug in treating traumatic corneal abrasions. *Ophthalmology.* 1995;102(6):979-84.

Dunya IM, Rubin PA, Shore JW. Penetrating orbital trauma. *Int Ophthalmol Clin.* 1995;35(1):25-36.

Dutton G. The GP and eye trauma. *Practitioner.* 1995;239(1549):265-6, 270-1.

Easty DL. Is an eye pad needed in cases of corneal abrasion? *BMJ.* 1993;307(6911):1022.

Endo EG, Mead MD. The management of traumatic hyphema. *Int Ophthalmol Clin.* 1994;34(3):1-7.

Fingeret M, Onofrey BE, Talley DK. Management of ocular emergencies. *Optometr Clin.* 1993;3(2):147-52.

Fong LP. Secondary hemorrhage in traumatic hyphema: predictive factors for selective prophylaxis. *Ophthalmology.* 1994;101(9):1583-8.

Grossman MD, Roberts DM, Barr CC. Ophthalmic aspects of orbital injury: a comprehensive diagnostic and management approach. *Clin Plast Surg.* 1992;19(1):71-85.

Guy PR, Taggart I, Adeniran A, et al. Corneal burns with eyelid sparing and their treatment. *Burns.* 1994;20(6):561-3.

Ham WT Jr. Ocular hazards of light sources: review of current knowledge. *J Occup Med.* 1983;25:101.

Hammerton ME. Burns to the eye: an overview. *Aust Fam Phys.* 1995;24(6): 998-1001, 1003.

Hammerton ME. Management of ocular burns. *Aust Fam Phys.* 1995;24(6): 1006-10.

Hartstein ME, Roper-Hall G. Update on orbital floor fractures: indications and timing for repair. *Facial Plast Surg.* 2000;16(2):95-106

Health C, Becker LA. Are eye patches necessary for corneal abrasions? *J Fam Pract.* 1996;42(5):454.

Hoflin-Lima AL, Roizenblatt R. Therapeutic contact lens-related bilateral fungal keratitis. *CLAO J.* 2002;28(3):149-50.

Holds JB, Patrinely JR, Zimmerman PL, et al. Hydraulic orbital injection injuries. *Ophthalmology.* 1993;100(10):1475-82.

Hulbert MF. Efficacy of eyepad in corneal healing after corneal foreign body removal. *Lancet.* 1991;16:337(8742):643.

Jampel HD. Patching for corneal abrasions. *JAMA.* 1995;274(19):1504. Comment in: *JAMA.* 1996;275(11):837; *JAMA.* 1996;275(11):837.

Kaiser PK. A comparison of pressure patching versus no patching for corneal abrasions due to trauma or foreign body removal. Corneal Abrasion Patching Study Group. *Ophthalmology.* 1995;102(12):1936-42.

Kaiser PK, Pineda R II. A study of topical nonsteroidal anti-inflammatory drops and no pressure patching in the treatment of corneal abrasions. Corneal Abrasion Patching Study Group. *Ophthalmology.* 1997;104(8): 1353-9.

Kenyon KR, Kenyon BM, Starck T, et al. Penetrating keratoplasty and anterior segment reconstruction for severe ocular trauma. *Geriatr J Ophthalmol.* 1994;3(2):90-9.

Khani SC, Mukai S. Posterior segment intraocular foreign bodies. *Int Ophthalmol Clin.* 1995;35(1):151-61.

Kirkpatrick JN, Hoh HB, Cook SD. No eye pad for corneal abrasion. *Eye.* 1993;7(3):468-71; comment in *Eye.* 1994;8(3):371-2.

Koch PS. Managing the torn posterior capsule and vitreous loss. *Int Ophthalmol Clin.* 1994;34(2):113-30.

Koster HR, Kenyon KR. Complications of surgery associated with ocular trauma. *Int Ophthalmol Clin.* 1992;32(4):157-78.

Kuhn F, Morris R, Witherspoon CD, Heimann J, Jeffers JB, Treister G. A standardized classification of ocular trauma. *Graefes Arch Clin Exp Ophthalmol.* 1966;234(6):399-403.

Kylstra JA, Lamkin JC, Runyan DK. Clinical predictors of scleral rupture after blunt ocular trauma. *Am J Ophthalmol.* 1993;115(4):530-5.

Lam SR, Devenyi RG, Berger AR, Dunn W. Visual outcome following penetrating globe injuries with retained intraocular foreign bodies. *Can J Ophthalmol.* 1999;34(7):389-93.

Leone CR Jr. Periorbital trauma. *Int Ophthalmol Clin.* 1995;35(1):1-24.

Liggett PE, Pince KI, Barlow W. Ocular trauma in an urban population. *Ophthalmology.* 1990;97:581.

Linden JA, Renner GS. Trauma to the globe. *Emerg Med Clin North Am.* 1995;13(3):581-605.

McCulley JP, Whiting DW, Petitt MG, et al. Hydrofluoric acid burns of the eye. *J Occup Med.* 1983;25:447.

Meyer DR, Kersten RC, Kulwin DR, et al. Management of canalicular injury associated with eyelid burns. *Arch Ophthalmol.* 1995;113(7):900-3.

Mindlin AM. Treatment of corneal abrasions. *JAMA.* 1996;275(11):837.

Morgan SJ. Chemical burns of the eye: causes and management. *J Ophthalmol [Br].* 1987;71:854-7.

Nanda SK, Mieler WF, Murphy ML. Penetrating ocular injuries secondary to motor vehicle accidents (see comments). *Ophthalmology.* 1993;100(2): 201-71.

Navon SE. Management of the ruptured globe. *Int Ophthalmol Clin.* 1995; 35(1):71.

Ng CS, Strong NP, Sparrow JM, et al. Factors related to the incidence of secondary haemorrhage in 462 patients with traumatic hyphema. *Eye.* 1992;6(Pt 3):308-12.

Onofrey BE. Injury to the cornea. *Optometr Clin.* 1993;3(2):1-19.

Onofrey BE. Management of corneal burns. *Optometr Clin.* 1995;4(3):31-40.

OSHA. 29 CFR 1910.132. Personal Protective Equipment. OSHA 3077.1994, revised. Washington, DC: Occupational Safety and Health Administration, 1994.

Owens JK, Scibilia J, Hezoucky N. Corneal foreign bodies: First aid, treatment, and outcomes. Skills review for an occupational health setting. *AAOHN J.* 2001;49(5):226-30.

Pastor JC, Calonge M. Epidermal growth factor and corneal wound healing: a multicenter study. *Cornea.* 1992;11(4):311-4.

Patterson J, Fetzer D, Krall J, Wright E, Heller M. Eye patch treatment for the pain of corneal abrasion. *South Med J.* 1996;89(2):227-9.

Pfister RP. Chemical corneal burns. *Common Corneal Problems.* 1984;157-69.

Rao GP, Scott JA, King A, et al. No eye pad for corneal abrasion. *Eye.* 1994;8(3):371-2.

Recchia FM, Saluja RK, Hammel K, Jeffers JB. Outpatient management of traumatic microhyphema. *Ophthalmology.* 2002;109(8):1465-70; discussion 1470-1.

Roll D, Duffie K. Eyewash standards and guidelines for the workplace. *Occup Health Saf.* 2000;4. Available at *www.stevenspublishing.com/Stevens/OHS-Pub.nsf/frame?open&redirect=http://www.stevenspublishing.com/stevens/OHSpub.nsf/PubArchive?openview.*

Scardovi C, DeFelice GP, Gazzaniga A. Epidermal growth factor in the topical treatment of traumatic corneal ulcers. *Ophthalmologica.* 1993;206(3):119-24.

Seal DV, Kirkness CM. Criteria for intravitreal antibiotics during surgical removal of intraocular foreign bodies. *Eye.* 1992;6(5):465-8.

Schein OD. Contact lens abrasions and the nonophthalmologist. *Am J Emerg Med.* 1993;11(6):606-8.

Schein OD, Hibbard PL, Shingleton BJ. The spectrum and burden of ocular injury. *Ophthalmology.* 1988;95:300-5.

Shingleton BJ, Hersh VS, Kenyon KR, ed. *Eye Trauma.* St. Louis, Mo: Mosby-Year Book; 1991.

Smolin G, Thoft RA. Corneal trauma. In: *The Cornea Scientific Foundations and Clinical Practice.* 3rd ed. Boston, Mass: Little, Brown and Company; 1994: Chapter 12.

Taher AA. Diplopia caused by orbital floor blowout fracture. *Oral Surg Oral Med Oral Pathol.* 1993;75(4):433-5.

Tervo T, van Setten GB, Paallysaho T, et al. Wound healing of the ocular surface. *Ann Med.* 1992;24(1):19-27.

Thompson JT, Parver LM, Enger CL, et al. Infectious endophthalmitis after penetrating injuries with retained intraocular foreign bodies: National Eye Trauma System. *Ophthalmology.* 1993;100(10):1468-74.

Tredici TR. Lecture Notes. Management of Eye Injuries; 2001.

Trevino MA, Herrmann GH, Sprout WL. Treatment of severe hydrofluoric acid exposures. *J Occup Med.* 1983;25:861.

Vinger PF, Sliney D. Eye disorders. In: Levy BS, Wegman DH, eds. *Occupational Health: Recognizing and Preventing Work-Related Disease.* 2nd ed. Boston, Mass: Little, Brown and Company; 1988:387-97.

Walton W, Von Hagen S, Grigorian R, Zarbin M. Management of traumatic hyphema. *Surv Ophthalmol.* 2002;47(4):297.

Werner MS, Dana MR, Viana MA, et al. Predictors of occult scleral rupture. *Ophthalmology.* 1994;101(12):1941-4.

Williams C, Laidlaw A, Diamond J, et al. Outpatient management of small traumatic hyphaemas: is it safe? *Eye.* 1993;7(1):155-7.

Williams J Sr. Lecture Notes. American Occupational Health Conference (AOHC), San Francisco; 2001.

Williams-Steiger Occupational Safety and Health Act of 1970 (OSHA). 84 Stat 1593.

Wolf MA. The management of corneal abrasions and corneal foreign bodies. *Occup Health Nurs.* 1981;29(6):32-3.

Wright P. The chemically injured eye. *Trans Ophthalmol Soc UK.* 1982;102:85.

INITIALIZING AN EYE AND FACE SAFETY PROGRAM

Ben-zvi S. Laser safety: guidelines for use and maintenance. *Biomed Instr Technol.* 1989;23:360-8.

Henderson D. Ocular trauma: One in the eye for safety glasses. *Arch Emerg Med.* 1991;8(3):401-4.

Keeney A. The eye and the workplace: special considerations. In: Tassman W, Jaeger E, eds. *Duane's Clinical Ophthalmology.* Vol. 5. Philadelphia, Pa: Lippincott; 1991:(5)Chapter 47, 1-14.

Keller JJ. *Head, Body and Foot Protection: Government and Industry Standard Cross References.* Neenah, Wis: OSHA; 1998.

Keller JJ. *Personal Protective Equipment: OSHA Compliance Manual Application of Key OSHA Topics.* Neenah, Wis: OSHA; 1998.

OSHA. 29 CFR 1910.133. Eye and Face Protection, Parts 1900-1910, 1994 revised. Washington, DC: OSHA; 1994.

Sliney D. Biohazards of ultraviolet, visible and infrared radiation. *J Occup Med.* 1983;25:203.

Sliney D, Wolbarsht M. *Safety with Lasers and Other Optical Sources.* New York, NY: Plenum Press; 1990.

NONTRAUMATIC OCULAR DISEASE

Miserocchi E, Waheed NK, Dios E, et al. Visual outcome in herpes simplex virus and varicella zoster virus uveitis: a clinical evaluation and comparison. *Ophthalmology.* 2002;109(8):1532-7.

ASSESSING RED FLAGS AND INDICATORS FOR IMMEDIATE REFERRAL

Flitcroft DI, Westcott M, Wormald R, et al. Who should see eye casualties? a comparison of eye care in an accident and emergency department with a dedicated eye casualty. *J Accid Emerg Med.* 1995;12(1):23-7.

INITIAL AND DEFINITIVE CARE

Folwer PD. Aspirin, paracetamol and nonsteroidal anti-inflammatory drugs: A comparative review of side effects. *Med Toxicol.* 1987;2:338-66.

King JW, Brison RJ. Do topical antibiotics help corneal epithelial trauma? *Can Fam Phys.* 1993;39:2349-52.

Muncie HL Jr, King DE, DeForge B. Treatment of mild to moderate pain of acute soft tissue injury: diflunisal vs. acetaminophen with codeine. *J Fam Pract.* 1986;23:125-7.

Physicians Desk Reference for Ophthalmology. Oradell, NJ: Medical Economics Company; 2002.

Sheikh A, Hurwitz B. Topical antibiotics for acute bacterial conjunctivitis: a systematic review. *Br J Gen Pract.* 2001;51(467):473-7.

Titcomb LC. Eye disorders: over-the-counter ophthalmic preparations. *Pharmaceutical J.* 2000;264(7082):212-8.

Weaver CS, Terrell KM. Evidence-based emergency medicine. Update: do ophthalmic nonsteroidal anti-inflammatory drugs reduce the pain associated with simple corneal abrasion without delaying healing? *Ann Emerg Med.* 2003;41(1):134-40.

BLURRED VISION

Dickersin K, Manheimer E. Surgery for nonarteritic anterior ischemic optic neuropathy. *Cochrane Database Syst Rev.* 2000;(2):CD001538.

FDA. Ophthalmic drug products for over-the-counter human use; proposed amendment of final monograph—FDA proposed rule. *Fed Reg.* 1998; 63(35):8888-90.

Fraser S, Siriwardena D. Interventions for acute nonarteritic central retinal artery occlusion. *Cochrane Database Syst Rev.* 2002;(1):CD001989.

VISUAL FATIGUE

Blais BR. Visual ergonomics of the office workplace. *Health Saf.* 1999;July-Aug:31-8.

Coe JV, Cuttle K, McClellan WC, Worden MJ. *Visual Display Units: A Review of Potential Health Problems Associated with Their Use.* Wellington, NZ: Department of Health Regional Unit; 1980.

Shen C, Chiu S, Wang A, et al. Accommodation and visual fatigue in visual display terminal (VDT) work. *Acta Ophthalmol Suppl (Copenh).* 1988;185: 175-6.

Rhee DJ, Pyfer MF, Rhee DM, eds. *Wills' Eye Manual: Office and Emergency Room Diagnosis and Treatment of Eye Disease.* 3rd ed. Baltimore, Md: Lippincott Williams & Wilkins; 1999.

WORK-RELATEDNESS

Lipscomb HJ. Effectiveness of interventions to prevent work-related eye injuries. *Am J Prevent Med.* 2000;18(4 Suppl):27-32.

Additional Resources

Fundamental Clinical Signs of Ocular Inflammation

Inflammation of the conjunctiva and cornea produces only a few clinical signs. Some of these, such as hyperemia of conjunctival vessels, edema, and conjunctival papillae, are nonspecific and may not be helpful in determining the etiology of inflammation. Others, such as conjunctival follicles, giant papillae, membranes, phlyctenules, and marginal infiltrates, are more specific and can be helpful in determining etiology.

CONJUNCTIVA

Morphologically, the conjunctiva consists of two layers, the epithelium and the underlying stroma (substantia propria). In a few areas, the overlying conjunctival epithelium is attached to an underlying structure, such as the tarsus or bulbar limbus, by fine fibrous strands or anchoring septa.

Papillary Response of the Conjunctiva. A conjunctival papillary response is a nonspecific clinical sign that can result from any type of inflammation. Papillae in the palpebral conjunctiva or at the limbus are the equivalent of simple hyperemia elsewhere in the conjunctiva. Only where fine fibrous strands are present and are attached to subjacent tissues can conjunctiva fully develop. A papillary response presents with a fine, mosaic-like pattern of elevated, polygonal, hyperemic areas separated by pale channels. A central fibrovascular core is present within each papilla. This gives rise to a central vessel that, on reaching the surface of the structure, erupts into a spokelike pattern that is readily evident on biomicroscopic examination. The papillae result from leakage of fluid and acute inflammatory cells (polymorphonuclear leukocytes, etc.) from the vascular core, resulting in swelling of the tissue. The connective tissue septa that anchor the overlying epithelium to the deeper collagenous tissue are responsible for forming the papillae. The connective tissue septa restrict the size of papillae to less that 1 millimeter.

Various types of papillae can develop in essentially three conjunctival areas: (1) upper palpebral conjunctiva; (2) lower palpebral conjunctiva; and (3) bulbar limbus. Each area will have a somewhat different clinical appearance of papillae owing to variations in anatomy.

Giant papillae are a unique form. They are greater than 1 millimeter in size and have several different clinical appearances and etiologies.

There is a different clinical spectrum of giant papillae from various etiologies, including palpebral vernal conjunctivitis, limbal vernal conjunctivitis, atopic keratoconjunctivitis, giant papillary conjunctivitis (GPC) of contact lenses, and giant papillae from prostheses and ends of nylon sutures.

The giant papillae seen with the atopic diseases of palpebral vernal and atopic keratoconjunctivitis are polygonal in shape with a flat surface. These are usually much larger than follicles and vary in size and shape. The giant papillae produced by contact lenses have a wide spectrum of clinical appearance. The common, mild form of GPC has giant papillae larger than 1 millimeter, but the papillae do not have the polygonal shapes or flat surfaces that are typical of giant papillae of vernal conjunctivitis.

In other areas, inflammation causes simple hyperemia rather than papillae. Normally, small blood vessels exist that extend into the conjunctival stroma among the fibrous strands. Conjunctival lymphoid follicles also are present within the stroma and can be commonly seen in the inferior conjunctival sac in young individuals and occasionally in older people.

Follicular Response of the Conjunctiva. A follicular response of the conjunctiva is a much more specific clinical sign and narrows the differential diagnosis as to the etiology of the inflammation. The conjunctival follicle is a smooth elevation of the conjunctiva that represents a lymphocytic response with an active germinal center. Vessels may encroach on the surface of the follicles but are not seen within the follicle. A papillary response is nonspecific and can occur along with any follicular response. These pathologic etiologies produce a more severe follicular response in the inferior conjunctival cul-de-sac than in the upper tarsal conjunctiva, with the exception of trachoma. Unfortunately, the clinical sign of pathologic follicles can be obscured by an overlying papillary response or an overlying inflammatory membrane or pseudomembrane.

Conjunctival Pseudomembrane or Membrane. The conjunctival pseudomembrane or membrane is another condition that has some specificity. A transudation of fluid, rich in protein and fibrin, is extruded through the walls of the altered conjunctival blood vessels, coagulating on the surface of the conjunctiva and producing a pseudomembrane or membrane. The difference in the two is one of severity; because pseudomembranes are less firmly adherent, they do not produce bleeding when stripped from the conjunctival surface.

CORNEA

Edema. There are two types of corneal epithelial edema:

- *Intracellular epithelial edema*, a swelling within the epithelial cells as a result of local epithelial inflammation or nutritional compromise of the corneal epithelium, can be localized or generalized. Examples of intracellular epithelial edema are Sandler's veil, seen with scleral-corneal contact lenses and rarely with soft contact lenses, and circumscribed epithelial edema seen with polymethylmethacrylate (PMMA) contact lenses. This intracellular epithelial edema is due to hypoxia.

- *Intercellular epithelial edema* manifests as fluid between the epithelial cells, maintained within the epithelial layer by the zonula occludens and macular adherens, the cellular adhesions among the corneal epithelial cells. Intercellular epithelial edema results from fluid that passes from the corneal stroma into the epithelial layer whenever the IOP exceeds the corneal stromal swelling pressure. Intercellular epithelial edema is seen clinically as microcystic epithelial edema or in the more severe form as epithelial bullae.

Epithelial Filaments. Epithelial filaments of the cornea may occur in various types of keratitis. Epithelial filaments are coils of epithelial cells attached to the cornea at their base. Mucus and other debris adhere to these epithelial filaments. The corneal epithelial filament is a clinical sign that can occur from a variety of etiologies.

Active Corneal Stromal Inflammation. Active corneal stromal inflammation is most readily identified clinically by infiltrates of leukocytes and edema within the corneal stroma. The infiltrates appear as focal opacities on biomicroscopic examination and can lie at any level of the stroma. In an avascular cornea, a stromal infiltrate is usually composed predominantly of polymorphonuclear leukocytes. These cellular elements can originate from the limbal vascular arcades and migrate to the site of corneal injury. Alternatively, they can enter the stroma from the tear film or the aqueous humor when defects occur in the layers of the cornea that act as barriers. In a vascularized cornea, inflammatory cells make their way into stroma by way of the new vascular channels, and the infiltrates are comprised of mixed cellular components.

Stromal Edema. Stromal edema from an inflammatory etiology almost invariably coexists with inflammatory infiltrates. This is evident clinically by increased thickness of the corneal stroma, which is roughly proportional to its water content. Stromal edema may be localized or generalized.

Corneal Scarring. Corneal scarring results wherever the inflammatory process is severe enough to cause tissue destruction. This process interrupts the regular lamellar arrangement of corneal collagen, resulting in loss of transparency. The scarring process involves manufacture of new collagen from active stromal keratocytes. Pigment, particularly melanin, is sometimes included in the structure of the scar. A number of deposits—calcium, lipid, proteinaceous material, or iron are encountered most often—in the corneal stroma can appear in cases of long-standing inflammation.

Neovascularization. Neovascularization is an additional indicator of active corneal inflammation. The new vessels can lie in the superficial or deep cornea depending on the nature of the inflammatory stimulus. It is important to recognize that there is a normal superficial vascular arcade at the corneal limbus. The distance that the vascular arcade extends onto the corneal limbus varies from person to person, but once the vessels leave the normal arcade and extend onto the cornea:

- A superficial micropannus can develop, extending 1 to 2 millimeters beyond the normal vascular arcade or as a gross pannus that extends more than 2 millimeters beyond the normal vascular arcade. It is important to distinguish between micropannus and gross pannus because the differential diagnosis of each varies.
- Deep stromal (interstitial) vascularization, which has a less specific etiology, can be caused by any chronic inflammation associated with stromal edema.

Chronic Inflammation. This can result from several etiologies and can produce various superficial opacities in a horizontal band across the interpalpebral area of the cornea; this is known clinically as band-shaped keratopathy.

Epithelial Keratitis. Epithelial keratitis is a common clinical sign with several possible etiologies. The term superficial punctate keratitis (SPK) should be reserved for the specific clinical entity described by Braley and Thygeson. Other etiologies of epithelial keratitis are not specific entities but are secondary to a number of other causes. Morphologic and distribution differences may help to differentiate the many causes of epithelial keratitis.

Corneal Endothelium. The corneal endothelium can be involved secondarily by inflammatory processes in the corneal stroma (keratitis) or in the anterior uveal tract (anterior uveitis). In the latter instance, inflammatory cells are present in the anterior chamber and appear on the biomicroscope as white or gray specks circulating in the aqueous humor. Aggregates of these cells can accumulate on the endothelial surface of the cornea, where they are referred to as keratic precipitates (KPs). Several clinical forms of KPs are recognized. In the punctate or granular form, the cells are primarily polymorphonuclear leukocytes and lymphocytes. Larger cellular aggregates are known as "mutton fat" KPs; macrophages predominate in this type of deposit. Finally, the fibrinous KP, in which the endothelial deposits are composed largely of fibrin with few inflammatory cells, also is recognized. KPs usually resolve completely, but residual hyalinized deposits can remain on the posterior cornea.

Retrocorneal Membranes. Retrocorneal membranes (thin, filmy membranes of connective tissue that cover the posterior corneal surface) can develop following inflammation and occur especially following hyphema, penetrating keratoplasty, or corneal perforation due to trauma or infection. These membranes can, at times, be vascularized or pigmented. It is thought that endothelial cell damage or death precedes proliferation of a retrocorneal membrane, and in the vast majority of cases, its occurrence is accompanied by edema of the corneal stroma.

ANTERIOR CHAMBER

Examining the depth and contents of the anterior chamber is extremely important and correlates well with the symptoms and signs previously obtained.

- *Depth.* In the case of narrow-angle glaucoma, the edema of the cornea is associated with a narrow-angle *iris bombé* where the anterior surface of the iris almost touches the peripheral cornea and where the anterior chamber is extremely shallow. An ancillary finding in these cases is an increase in IOP averaging 40 to 60 mmHg.
- *Content.* The content of the anterior chamber is significant because it correlates with the other findings of the conjunctiva and cornea.
    - In cases of a uveitis (purulent cyclitis), the presence of protein and cells in the anterior chamber is classic.
    - When the number of cells develop sufficiently that they precipitate, a hypopyon will be present. A hypopyon is associated with layering of cells in up to 50% of the inferior anterior chamber.
    - A hyphema is an accumulation of red blood cells secondary to trauma in the anterior chamber generally in the inferior half, but it can occupy the entire anterior chamber. When there is an associated IOP increase, the blood will be forced into the cornea, causing blood staining of the cornea.

Examination for Disorders Associated with Red Eye

Any patient who complains of a red or painful eye (see Tables 16-1 and 16-2) should be examined to detect any of the conditions described below:

CONJUNCTIVA/SCLERA

- *Conjunctivitis* is manifested by hyperemia of the conjunctival blood vessels; the cause may be bacterial, viral, allergic, or irritative; the condition is common and often not serious.
- *Episcleritis* is an inflammation (often sectorial) of the episclera, the vascular layer between the conjunctiva and the sclera. It is neither common nor serious, nor does it produce a discharge. It may be allergic and is occasionally painful.
- *Scleritis* is an inflammation (localized or diffuse) of the sclera. Although it is potentially serious to the eye, it is uncommon, often protracted, usually accompanied by pain, and may indicate serious systemic disease such as a collagen-vascular disorder.
- *Subconjunctival hemorrhage* is an accumulation of blood in the potential space between the conjunctiva and the sclera. It is rarely serious except as related to orbital trauma.
- *Pterygium* is an abnormal growth consisting of a triangular fold of tissue that advances progressively over the cornea, usually from the

nasal side. It is usually not serious. Localized conjunctival inflammation may be associated with pterygiae. Most cases occur in tropical climates. Surgical excision is indicated if the pterygium encroaches on the visual axis.

CORNEA

- *Herpes simplex keratitis* is an inflammation of the cornea caused by the herpes simplex virus. It is common, potentially serious, and can lead to corneal ulceration.
- *Abrasions* and *foreign bodies* may be associated with hyperemia ciliary flush (circumcorneal hyperemia).

ANTERIOR CHAMBER

- *Acute angle-closure glaucoma* is an uncommon form of glaucoma due to sudden and complete occlusion of the anterior chamber angle by its tissue. It is serious. The more common chronic open-angle glaucoma causes no redness of the eye.
- *Iritis or iridocyclitis* is a serious inflammation of the iris, alone or with the ciliary body; it often is manifested by ciliary flush (circumcorneal hyperemia).

ADNEXA

- *Adnexal disease* affects the eyelids, lacrimal apparatus, and orbit. It includes dacryocystitis, styes, and blepharitis. Red eye also can occur secondary to lid lesions (such as basal cell carcinoma or squamous cell carcinoma), thyroid disease, and vascular lesions in the orbit.
- *Abnormal lid function* can result in a red eye. Potentially serious lesions such as Bell's palsy, thyroid ophthalmopathy, and others allow ocular exposure.

Laboratory Diagnosis

Most mild cases of conjunctivitis are managed without laboratory assistance. While representing a compromise with ideal management, it is justified by the economic waste of obtaining routine smears and cultures in such a common and benign disease. Most clinicians prescribe broad-spectrum topical ophthalmic antibiotic treatment. Cases of presumed bacterial conjunctivitis that do not improve after 2 days of antibiotic treatment should be referred to an ophthalmologist to confirm the diagnosis and to conduct appropriate laboratory studies. In cases of hyperpurulent conjunctivitis, when copious purulent discharge is produced, conjunctival cultures and ophthalmologic consultation are necessary because of a possible gonococcal cause. Gonococcal hyperpurulent conjunctivitis is a serious, potentially blinding disease.

In doubtful cases, smears of exudate or conjunctival scrapings can confirm clinical impressions regarding the type of conjunctivitis. Generally, the amount of exudate in an ocular infection is very small, especially in corneal ulcers, and this task should be left to the ophthalmologist with his or her microsurgical techniques. Typical findings include polymorphonuclear cells and bacteria in bacterial conjunctivitis. Cultures for bacteria and determinations of antibiotic sensitivity also are useful in cases that are resistant to therapy.

Current Testing Methods Visual (Ocular) Screening

Most required visual tests may be provided by using visual screeners. Currently, in the United States the following instruments provide:

- Titmus Model 2a Screener (Titmus Optical, Inc., Petersburg, Va)
    1. VA. D, INT. (20-40 inches) near: monocular and binocular
    2. Binocularity, monocularity, or diplopia
    3. Color vision red or green
    4. Muscle balance—heterophoria or heterotropia, horizontal and vertical
    5. Stereopsis
    6. Peripheral vision—horizontal plane
- The Titmus Model 2c Vision Screening System (Titmus Optical, Inc., Petersburg, Va). The Titmus Model 2c Vision Screening System is for the occupational models only. Its computerized vision screening system consists of a Titmus 2a Vision Screener, an encoder (interface device between a computer and vision screener), and Optimum for Windows, software that features:
    1. Control of vision screener from computer
    2. Elimination of manual scoring using record forms
    3. Recording of test results on the computer screen
    4. Comparison and interpretation of test results to preset job standards
    5. Printing of test results—interpretation report
    6. Export of test results in ASCII format
- Stereo Optical Model Optec 2000c Vision Tests (Stereo Optical C., Inc., Chicago, Ill)
    1. VA. D, INT. (20-36 inches) near: monocular and binocular
    2. Binocularity, monocularity, or diplopia
    3. Color vision red or green
    4. Muscle balance—heterophoria or heterotropia, horizontal and vertical
    5. Stereopsis
    6. Peripheral vision—horizontal plane
    7. Contrast sensitivity available
- In addition to the capabilities of Models 2000c and 2500, the new model Optec 3500 Vision Testing System features

1. Target illumination for day and night testing
2. Glare illuminance at distance
3. Contrast sensitivity
4. Potential acuity (assessment macular functions in cataract patients)

The Department of Defense (DOD) uses an Armed Forces Visual Screener, the Bausch & Lomb Ortho-Rater, manufactured to specifications by Stereo Optical Company (Chicago), the Armed Forces Tester Model 3500 Vision Tester. Other instruments currently in use but not being manufactured include the Bausch & Lomb and American Optical instruments described previously. The tests may be conducted using separate, individual instruments.

In specific types of occupational testing (e.g., DOT, FAA, and the Federal Railroad Administration), the Farnsworth Lantern (now Stereo Optical Co. Model 900) must be passed when the patient fails the Ishihara color screening plates in many of these regulations.

Appendix Evidence-based Medicine:

What Does It Mean? Why Do We Care?

Evidence-based medicine focuses on the need for health care providers to rely on a critical appraisal of available scientific evidence rather than clinical opinion or anecdotal reports in reaching decisions regarding diagnosis, treatment, causation, and other aspects of health care decision making. This mandates that information regarding health outcomes in study populations or experimental groups be extracted from the medical literature, after which it can be analyzed, synthesized, and applied to individual patients.

To the extent that the literature has adequate high-quality studies of a given topic, it is possible to develop guidelines or conclusions regarding treatment and causation that are truly based on scientific evidence. Unfortunately many, if not most, of the treatments and tests we provide, and many of the hypotheses on which we base concerns regarding risk and exposure, have not been rigorously evaluated. Budget constraints and the absence of sponsors who would benefit from study results are only two of the reasons that there is a lack of funding for research in this area. Interventions that as yet have not been satisfactorily proved (or disproved) to be of value or relevance are continuously being introduced, and often integrated into clinical practice.

The scientific literature that serves as the foundation for the development of clinical guidelines is of mixed quality. While most clinical practice guidelines cite the literature on which they are based, the final decision regarding the implications of the studies involved is the consensus opinion of those who develop the guidelines. It is critical that those opinions reflect a commitment to the use of the high-quality scientific evidence. When high-quality scientific data are used, high quality recommendations can be made regarding matters as important as clinical practice patterns, exposure assessments, and the like.

Guidelines can be evidence based only to the extent that there is appropriate scientific literature on which they can be based. That a particular intervention or hypothesis has not been "proved" to be valid does not necessarily mean that it is invalid or not useful—only that we have not yet devised a study that conclusively supports or refutes it. Unfortunately, guideline development most often requires reaching a consensus regarding "best practice" in areas in which there is no definitive literature. Guideline developers must then base their recommendations on something other than science. Frequently, recommendations are premised on the apparent reasonableness of the intervention in question, the degree to which it puts a patient at a risk for harm, and the apparent cost-effectiveness of the intervention.

Despite the lack of high-quality studies on a number of topics, it remains desirable for clinical practice guidelines to be as evidence based as is currently possible. This requires a comprehensive review and critical evaluation of the available literature. The goal of such a review is to ascertain whether the design, results/outcomes, and statistical power of individual studies warrant their use as a basis for treatment or other health care decisions.

Study Design

Assessment of study design is the initial task that must be performed by those who develop guidelines, as this dictates the degree to which one can comfortably extrapolate results from a given piece of literature to patients with similar clinical presentations.

Types of Studies

EXPERIMENTAL STUDIES

Studies can be experimental or observational. Experimental randomized controlled studies are the best foundation ("gold standard") for evaluating a particular treatment, or assessing whether an exposure leads to a given outcome. With regard to treatment, one can randomize the choice of subjects, controlling for those variables that might affect treatment response. One also can randomize the use of a given treatment in the study population and then attempt to blind patients with regard to whether they are receiving a treatment or a placebo. Those who analyze the data also can be kept unaware as to whether a given subject received treatment (double-blind studies). In those circumstances where experimental studies are successfully randomized, double-blinded, and analyze outcomes in a large population, one can generally feel reasonably comfortable in placing some reliance on the conclusions.

Unfortunately in many experimental studies, despite attempts to blind subjects, this cannot be performed reliably. For example, in studies of procedures, especially invasive ones, it is difficult, and often impossible, to design a true "placebo." If symptomatic response (subjective benefit) is the primary treatment outcome under analysis (as is often the case) and the study is not adequately blinded, even with the use of the experimental model, it becomes difficult to know if those who received the "real" treatment are exhibiting a true or a placebo response. Conversely, when studies are successfully blinded, a placebo response in the nontreatment group (if the placebo is convincing enough) will mandate a larger experimental population to manifest a statistically significant result than would otherwise be necessary. Consequently, while experimental studies have a greater ability than observational studies to yield reproducible results, they are by no means infallible and should never be considered as such.

Regardless of their shortcomings, variables can be better controlled in experimental rather than in observational studies, leading to their widespread use in evaluating the merit of new or established treatments. It is, however, difficult to ethically justify further evaluation of treatments that already are held to be of potential benefit with experimental studies, especially when the treatment can slow down or prevent a process with considerable morbidity. This is the case even when the initial basis for classifying the treatment as of potential benefit was weak. It is even more difficult to ethically justify experimental studies of exposure using human populations. Even when experimental studies of a given exposure are designed in a manner that meets all ethical considerations, they are difficult to blind.

Animals can be substituted for humans in exposure studies, and this is one way in which problems inherent in the studies that use human subjects can be avoided. However, the degree to which one can extrapolate the results of animal studies to human populations (referred to as "analogy") is never clear. Given difficulties in the design and interpretation of experimental studies, there is considerable ambiguity regarding the merits and demerits of various testing and treatment options that is matched by controvery regarding the causal roles that workplace activities and exposures play in the genesis of occupational disease.

OBSERVATIONAL STUDIES

Epidemiology is the study of disease in populations. Epidemiologic studies are, by definition, observational rather than experimental, and draw conclusions with regard to the degree to which two events are associated by analyzing the response of populations (groups of people) to a given exposure or treatment. In observational studies, researchers do not control the exposure or treatment and do not select subjects randomly. They instead must work with existing data. The degree to which one can rely on the results of observational studies is based both upon their design and the methodology applied to the analysis of data. Even when studies are impeccable in design, it is important to remember that observational studies can never be described as "proving" cause and effect, though they may certainly provide information regarding the strength of a postulated association.

Observational studies can be analytical or descriptive. Case reports and case series are examples of descriptive studies. In these, the author simply describes the characteristics of a given disease process or treatment response among a group of individuals, attempting to ascertain what factor the individuals had in common that could explain the outcome. This type of study does not, by definition, include individuals without the treatment or condition. Consequently, while one can look at the affected population and generate hypotheses regarding the relationship(s) between the exposure or treatment and the observed outcome (which then can be tested in future studies), case reports cannot be used as grounds to assert the existence of a causal relationship between the two.

Analytic studies are designed to evaluate hypotheses. There are three types of studies that do so—prevalence, case-control, and cohort studies. Data can be collected either at a single point in time as in prevalence and case control studies, or longitudinally as is done in both cohort studies and case-control studies that use incident cases (i.e., wait for cases to occur before analyzing them). In these studies, direct evaluation of hypotheses is possible as those who have been exposed to a putatively harmful factor, or received a potentially beneficial treatment, are compared with those who have not. Careful matching of cases with controls in terms of all potentially relevant variables is mandatory for conclusions to be valid. To the extent that this does not occur (the main flaw of observational studies), the degree to which one can confidently assert the existence of a causal relationship between an exposure or treatment and a given outcome is diminished.

Prevalence (cross-sectional) studies are the weakest form of analytic studies, and entail evaluation of the prevalence of a "condition" in a population at a point in time. One then assesses the impact of risk factors or prior treatment on those with and without the condition of interest. Since cases included are prevalent and not incident, the relationship of cause and effect cannot be readily evaluated for the exposure and outcomes being assessed. In other words, it may well be that patients self-selected themselves to be exposed (or not exposed) to a given factor or receive a particular treatment before the study began. For example, one could survey a population and find that those with sedentary jobs were more likely to have back pain than those who were in more demanding positions. While this might represent a causal relationship between sedentary work and back pain, it is equally possible that workers with prior back pain, or in worse physical condition, were more likely to choose sedentary jobs over more physically demanding employment (selection bias). Alternatively one might find that those who did well with a given treatment had chosen to receive it due to a prior positive response in family members, thus biasing the study toward indicating a benefit from the treatment when indeed no clinical benefit was present. Prevalence studies cannot differentiate between these scenarios.

Experimental Versus Observational Studies

Study Characteristics	Experimental	Observational
Single-blind	Generally*	Rarely
Double-blind	Sometimes	Never
Investigator controls treatment or exposure	Yes	No
Subjects randomly selected	Yes	No
Possible selection bias	No	Yes
Possible recall bias	No	Yes
Possible nonresponse bias	Sometimes	Depends
Possible confounders (noncausal)	Sometimes	Sometimes
Suggests "cause and effect" if positive	Yes	Rarely
Only suggests "association" if positive	No	Yes

*Though degree to which blinding is "real" is often controversial.

In case-control studies, individuals who have received a given treatment or have a particular disease are matched to control persons who share those characteristics that might otherwise be sources of bias, after which the two groups are comparatively analyzed. There usually are predetermined, and equal, numbers of cases and controls. In order for the study to be valid, cases and controls must be matched for all factors except the one under evaluation. To the extent that this does not occur, or cases and controls differ in the degree to which they accurately remember past exposures and history (recall bias), the analysis of the data may be flawed. This is less likely when the study is prospective and uses incident cases, though prospective studies are more difficult to perform and hence require greater amounts of time and money to reach completion.

The optimal type of observational study is a cohort study, a longitudinal prospective (or retrospective, though prospective is best) study of a group of healthy people in a well-defined source population. Baseline information about the persons under evaluation and their risk factors for disease and/or general responses to treatment are collected before a disease or treatment intervention occurs. One then observes the population (cohort) over time (with the period of follow-up dependent on the treatment or exposure under investigation) to evaluate their status both in terms of medical conditions and response to treatment or other health interventions.

Compared to other observational studies, cohort studies offer the best evidence regarding etiology, as they most closely approximate the randomized controlled trial. Before performing them it is best to have data (from prior descriptive or prevalence studies) that lead one to suspect that a particular treatment or exposure is associated with the health outcome of interest in a given population, as simply following large populations to see what happens is otherwise prohibitively expensive. It also is possible to "nest" case-control studies inside large cohort studies once one has identified a treatment response or condition of interest, as this reduces costs by limiting the analysis to a well-defined and, presumably, clinically relevant subset of the study population.

Sources of Error in Study Design

As demonstrated in the discussion of prevalence studies, the existence of an association between two events does not automatically imply that they are causally related. Associations can be causal, but can also be noncausal, artifactual, or reflective of multiple causation. If one wants to review experimental or observational studies in the literature, or analyze one's own data to assess the relationship between a given treatment or exposure and clinical outcomes, it is mandatory to understand the multiple potential sources of error and the shortcomings of statistical analysis, even when done properly.

MULTIPLE CAUSATION

Multiple causation is common in medicine, and happens when the occurrence of a given disease or when a response to treatment is, or can be, due to one or more of several processes/interventions. This obviously makes it impossible to state with certainty that a given intervention or exposure was the sole cause of a given outcome. One is then obliged to estimate the degree to which each of the multiple potential factors led to the outcome being evaluated. Then the concepts of apportionment, aggravation, and exacerbation (see Chapter 4) become important in causation analysis and why it is best, in experimental studies of treatment, to be as specific as possible in defining an intervention. (For example, in chiropractic care is a positive outcome due to the manipulation *per se* or the attention that the patient is receiving while the manipulation is being performed (i.e., the laying on of hands).

NONCAUSAL RELATIONSHIPS

Noncausal relationships are imputed as indicative of causality when there is a third, or "confounding," factor that is associated with both the exposure and the disease (and may be what we are actually measuring—e.g., a link between coffee drinking and heart disease was ultimately found to reflect an increased rate of cigarette smoking in the group that drank coffee—once this was controlled for the association disappeared).

ARTIFACTUAL ASSOCIATIONS / BIAS

Artifactual associations occur when the studies or analyses on which the assumption of causality is based fail to appropriately consider sources of bias or are flawed in the statistical analysis of the data. Bias is a systematic or measurement error in the design or analysis of a study, which leads to an overestimation or underestimation of the strength and significance of a given association. There are different types of bias, one or several of which may be present in a given study.

1. *Selection bias* occurs when two groups are compared that initially were not comparable in terms of a relevant factor (though this may not have been necessarily obvious). An example would be when one finds a decreased rate of a disease process in workers as compared with their nonworking peers, only to find that this is because the workers are actually healthier (the "healthy worker effect," which is why they are working and their peers are not).
2. A similar effect can be seen as a consequence of *prevalence bias* in which those with the greatest degree of disease as a result of an exposure have already died (if fatal) or left the workforce by the time the study is performed, thus, again, leading to an artifactually low rate of illness.
3. *Procedure selection bias* can be found in both observational and experimental studies, occurring when the characteristics of patients assigned to different treatment groups differ in a fashion that affects their response (such as whether an injury was sustained at work versus recreationally, etc.). Procedure bias differs in that subject characteristics are matched across groups, but the groups of subjects themselves do not receive identical treatment.
4. *Compliance bias* is another form of bias that is seen only in experimental

studies, where it is of major importance in the characterization of treatment effects. Noncompliance with the treatment arm of a study due to side effects or because one treatment is clearly easier to perform or follow than another may be justifiable, but clearly lessens the degree to which results can be extrapolated, especially if subjects who fail to comply with the treatment due to adverse effects are also lost to follow-up.

5. When members in one group are more likely to recall certain events or exposures than those in another, *recall bias* is said to occur. This type of bias is frequently found in prevalence, case-control, and retrospective studies in general as those who have a condition, or have undergone a particular treatment (such as breast implants) are generally more likely to recall an exposure or focus on potential side effects of the procedure than do those who did not have the condition or receive the treatment.

6. *Detection bias* also can lead to an increased rate of association between an exposure or treatment and a health outcome, but rather than reflecting patient recall it occurs when diagnostic testing is differentially applied to one group more than to another group. This type of bias occurs most frequently when a new treatment is accompanied by potential health risks, leading to an increased rate of screening in the treatment group and, in turn, detection of the condition of interest at an earlier stage than it otherwise would have been found (or when it is still asymptomatic).

7. *Measurement bias* occurs when the instruments used to measure the results of an exposure or treatment are not of sufficient validity to produce reliable results. This is often seen when results are "measured" by using

Comparison of Observational Studies

Study Characteristics	Cross-sectional	Case Control	Historical Cohort	Nested Case Control	Prospective Cohort
Data collected at single point in time	Yes	Yes	Yes	Y/N: cases are incident	No
Data collected longitudinally	No	Y/N incident	Yes	Yes	Yes
Work "backward" to identify exposures	Yes	Yes	Yes	No	No
Used to calculate disease incidence	Yes	No	Yes	Yes	Yes
Prone to recall bias	Yes	Yes	No (?)	No	No
Prone to artifactual associations	Yes	Yes	Y/N	No	No
Suitable for rare disease processes	Yes	Yes	Yes	Yes	No
Appropriateness for diseases with long latency	Yes	Yes	Yes	Yes	No
Expense	Low	Low	Low	Medium	High
Strength of evidence	Low	Low	Medium	Medium	Good

diagnostic tests that are of low positive or negative predictive value in the population under evaluation. When this lack of reliability preferentially occurs (by chance if nothing else) in one group rather than another, outcome analysis will be based on flawed data and will then be flawed as well. A variant of measurement bias occurs when study analysts are not blinded to participant group assignments, as this is likely to subtly bias the analysis of results, especially when the analysis is at least in part based on the significance one ascribes to "soft" findings.

8. *Nonresponse bias* either can falsely elevate or falsely reduce the association between a given treatment or exposure and a health outcome. In the case of exposure analysis, if those who do not respond fail to do so because they have not developed the condition of interest (despite exposure) or recovered from a disease, analysis solely of those who respond will lead to a falsely elevated estimate of the risk of the adverse outcome based on its prevalence in the remaining population studied. When response to a treatment intervention is being studied, failure of those who have done well to respond will lead to underestimation of benefit. On the other hand, if nonresponse reflects the development of health outcomes or side effects so severe as to preclude those who did poorly from responding, the converse will obviously be the case—i.e., adverse effects will be underestimated. In order to adjust for the characteristics and outcomes of those who left, the study must be analyzed (in the case of experimental studies described as "intention to treat analysis"). If those who withdrew were not comparable to those who remained, or if withdrawals were preferentially from one group (experimental or control) rather than another, analysis of the study must compensate for this.

It is clear that study design can have a major impact upon the accuracy of conclusions. The type of statistical analysis used in reaching conclusions is also of significance as goals are to maximize "significance" and minimize "error."

Statistical Analysis

MEASUREMENTS OF DISPERSION

Standard deviation is a measure of dispersion, or spread, of a sample or a population around the mean (average) value. This dispersion is graphically characterized as a bell curve, with the greatest concentration of values around the mean and lesser concentrations as one moves away from the mean (to the "tails"). The calculation for standard deviation (SD or σ) is the square root of the summation of the absolute value of the squares of each test value minus the mean value, divided by the total number measurements minus 1. Stated as a formula, standard deviation is:

$$\text{SD} = \sqrt{\frac{\sum(x - \bar{x})^2}{n - 1}}$$

The coefficient of variation is the standard deviation divided by the mean and multiplied by 100%. The smaller the coefficient of variation, the greater the reproducibility of the measurement, as the standard deviation is then small relative to the mean. The expected values for normal distributions are based on use of calculations derived from a baseline bell-shaped dispersion of values that has been adjusted via commonly accepted statistical calculations to reflect the actual mean, the standard deviation, and the number of subjects in the study.

STATISTICAL SIGNIFICANCE

The analysis of statistical significance is based upon the premise that 95% of a given sample of "normal" values will fall within 2 standard deviations of the mean (average) and 99% will be within 3 standard deviations. In a "two-tailed test," i.e., a test in which the researcher has no expectation that values will necessarily be either lower or higher than expected, it is generally held that values that fall within the 2.5% of values that fall to either side of the mean are 95% likely to represent a real difference from what would be "normal" as they are over 2 standard deviations from the mean, with a study leading to results of this nature described as having a "*P* value" of .05. Those that yield results that fall only within the top .5% of values on either side of the normal curve are considered to be 99% likely to be representative of true differences (and the *P* value is .01.)

In creating a study one generally begins with the hypothesis that a given intervention or exposure will *not* make a difference—i.e., will lead to results that fall at least within the 95% of values considered "normal" or "expected." A test statistic is calculated based on the observed data (details are beyond the scope of this appendix) and, depending on what level of significance is desired, is indicative of the cut-off values at 2 SD from the mean in either direction. If values fall above or below this "statistic," there is a 5% probability that they are still reflective of a normal distribution (and simply represent outliers) and a 95% probability that they are "statistically significant." When values are larger or smaller than the 99% of values found within 3 SD of the mean, the level of significance—i.e., the degree to which one can feel confident that they are statistically relevant and represent a true difference as opposed to a normal outlier value—increases to 99%. Hence, in analyzing a study, one compares the mean of the distribution of study values with that of the values one expected. Those study means that fall outside 2 or 3 SD of the "true" or "expected" mean are held to be statistically significant, with the degree of significance dependent upon how far from the expected mean they fall.

Another way to use the same data is by calculating confidence intervals, ranges of values that represent 2 ($P < .05$) or 3 ($P < .01$) standard deviations from where one would have expected the mean to have fallen. Results are statistically significant in demonstrating a difference (rejecting the null hypothesis of no difference) if the observed results after exposure or treatment do not fall into this confidence limit. The new hypothesis is then that the external event or situation was a causal factor in shifting the confidence interval away from the "original" mean. Again, this is reflective of an association between the exposure or treatment and the outcome rather than absolute proof of causality.

Alternatively one can calculate likelihood or odds ratios indicating the chances of observing the value seen in a given study in the normal population. If the likelihood ratio is, for example, 1.0, then the outcome was no more likely to occur (or not occur) as a result of the exposure or intervention than it was in its absence. Likelihood or odds ratio values are always listed in conjunction with a range representing, as a rule, the 95% confidence level for significance. Clearly, if the value 1.0 is included within the confidence limits of the calculated ratio the observed value most likely is *not* of statistical relevance.

ERROR AND POWER ANALYSIS

A causal relationship is generally postulated to exist between an exposure or treatment and a given health outcome in a given study if the use of the treatment, or occurrence of the exposure leads to a mean result that is greater than 2 to 3 (depending upon the *P* value one is using) standard deviations from the mean of the values that was either expected or found in a control, or baseline, group. Type I error occurs when one concludes there is a causal relationship between an exposure and a disease, or a treatment and clinical improvement, when there really is not. Type I error is equal to *P* value—and indeed, when one selects the *P* value one will use (i.e., how many standard deviations from the mean to accept as "normal") one is in essence determining the amount of Type I error (also referred to as alpha) one is willing to accept.

Type II error, the converse, occurs when a difference or causal relationship is *not* found, but exists. Type II error is defined as 1 minus the power, hence if one knows the power of a study one can determine the chance of Type II error.

		Reality	
		Difference exists (H_1)	No difference (H_0)
Conclusions from test	Difference exists (reject H_0)	Power or $1 - B$	Type I error, or a
	No difference (Do not reject H_0)	Type II error, or B	

Power is the ability of a test to appropriately reject the null hypothesis when it is false. In other words, power describes the ability of a study to detect a given difference of a given size between two outcomes if the difference really exists. The power of a statistical test is analogous to the sensitivity of a diagnostic test (Dawson-S), i.e., the ability to find a difference that is present. Power analysis consists of determining how large a sample is required to detect an actual difference of some specified magnitude. The larger the sample, or the size of the difference one is expecting, the greater the power. Conversely, if the power is large—i.e. if there is a high chance of finding a difference, the greater the likelihood of erroneously rejecting the null hypothesis.

In other words, small studies that are looking for small differences in response to a treatment or exposure are most likely to be negative—i.e., have a Type I error. Large studies that are looking for large differences (such as mortality rates) are likely to have a high degree of Power, but at an increased risk of rejecting the null hypothesis—i.e., of finding a difference when one really does not exist.

There are formulae used to make these calculations but a more in-depth discussion of statistical analysis is beyond the scope of this text. Suffice it to state that before ascribing significance to the results of a study it is important to know the results of the power analysis, as well as the *P* value, and then determine their significance based on the parameters that are being evaluated.

Analyzing and Applying Study Results

When using medical literature to make recommendations regarding clinical practice, it is necessary to determine the degree of confidence one has in the conclusions that have been reached. This is especially the case when a previously accepted treatment, test, or hypothesis has been formally evaluated and found to be lacking. A number of formats are used to describe the overall conclusions research panels or groups have reached regarding the efficacy of a given intervention (or effect of a given exposure). They rate the sum total of health care interventions or assumptions in support of a given premise, by placing them into categories, each of which represents the minimum level of scientific evidence required for inclusion. The system adopted by the Agency for Healthcare Research and Quality (AHRQ) and the Cochrane Review uses four categories, though there is no reason why further categorization could not occur.

Level A. Strong research-based evidence provided by generally consistent findings in multiple (more than one) high-quality randomized control trials (RCTs).

Level B. Moderate research-based evidence provided by generally consistent findings in one high-quality RCT and one or more low-quality RCTs, or generally consistent findings in multiple low quality RCTs.

Level C. Limited research based evidence provided by one RCT (either high- or low-quality) or inconsistent or contradictory evidence findings in multiple RCTs.

Level D. No research-based evidence, no RCTs.

The Clinical Evidence series uses a different set of categorizations that perhaps are more relevant clinically, classifying treatments and tests as one of the following:

Beneficial. Interventions for which effectiveness has been demonstrated by clear evidence from RCTs, and for which expectation of harms is small compared with the benefits.

Likely to be beneficial. Interventions for which effectiveness is less well established than for those listed under "beneficial."

Trade off between benefit and harms. Interventions for which clinicians and patients should weigh the beneficial and harmful effects according to individual circumstances and priorities.

Unknown effectiveness. Interventions for which there are currently insufficient data or data of inadequate quality.

Unlikely to be beneficial. Interventions for which lack of effectiveness is less well established than for those listed under "likely to be ineffective or harmful."

Likely to be ineffective or harmful. Interventions for which ineffectiveness or harmfulness has been demonstrated by clear evidence.

There is no particular reason why one could not choose other forms of categorization as well, but regardless of the categorization one chooses, one clearly must be able to assess the quality of the studies reviewed in order to determine which level most appropriately conveys the strength of the available evidence.

In analyzing studies that purport to provide "evidence" supporting or refuting a given health care intervention or causal association, one should then ask the following questions:

1. What was the aim (hypothesis) of the study?
   - Was it an exploratory study, surveying a population for interesting cases of a disease in order to generate hypotheses (case-report or case series) or to assess whether a potential association exists between two concurrent events (cross-sectional)?
   - Was it an anecdotal report of a change in the status of a patient, or a group of patients, in association with a particular treatment?
   - Was a specific hypothesis being examined, and, if so, how?

2. How were study subjects selected?
   - Were the main features of the study population well described?
   - If an exposure study, were cases and controls drawn from populations matched for potentially relevant variables? Were prevalent or incident cases used?
   - In studies of treatment (or testing) were both treatment and control groups comparable at entry?
   - Were all relevant variables controlled for?

3. How were treatments or exposures defined and quantified?
   - Was there a placebo group? If so, were placebos indistinguishable from treatment or exposures both initially and subsequently, so as to allow for blinding?

- If not, or if the treatment or exposure was one that could not be adequately concealed, how was this adjusted for or considered in the analysis of data—and did this adjustment or consideration have merit?
- Were treatment providers blinded to treatment status? If not, could this have affected the results?

4. If a study of exposure, were there any factors that would bias the study?
   - Were the instruments used to measure exposure valid and reliable?
   - Was exposure measured in an identical fashion in cases and controls?
   - Were exposures measured retrospectively or prospectively?
   - Were all potentially relevant exposures considered?
   - Was data collected soon after initial manifestations of the disease occurred?

5. Were there any obvious potential sources of error in initial outcome analysis?
   - Were outcome measures clearly defined?
   - Were those who analyzed the study results blinded to subject treatment or exposure status both at the initiation of the study and subsequently?
   - Over what period of time were outcomes measured? Was this reasonable given the treatment or exposure under analysis?
   - Were the outcomes of participants who withdrew (intentionally or unintentionally) or were lost to follow-up described and included in the analysis? Did the analysis discuss whether these individuals differed in any substantive fashion from those who continued in the study (intention to treat analysis)?

6. How were potential sources of bias or error accounted for in the study analysis?
   - Did the investigators describe sources of bias (especially selection and recall bias), and state whether they felt that these may have led to artifactual associations?
   - Did the study account for possible confounding or co-existing factors (by considering all potentially relevant prior or current exposures or treatments that subjects may have experienced)?
   - Were all other possible sources of error described, with focus upon their potential impact upon study results?

7. What type of statistical analysis was used, and how were the results conveyed?
   - Specifically, were *P* values, confidence limits, likelihood estimates, or odds ratios consistent with the existence of a statistically significant relationship between the exposure and the disease?
   - If so, how significant were they (the greater the significance the less the likelihood that there was a Type I error)?
   - Was the sample size large enough to make meaningful conclusions?

8. Does the association make sense and correspond with what is already known or with what one might suspect to be true?
   - If the study was evaluating the relationship between an exposure and a health effect, did the cause precede the effect in time? Does increased exposure increase the risk—i.e., is there a dose-response relationship? Does decreased exposure, or the elimination of exposure, reduce or eliminate the risk of disease?
   - If the study was evaluating a treatment option, is there a scientifically sound rationale linking the treatment to the observed outcome? Would one expect similar outcomes if a physiologically equivalent treatment were offered? Have there been other studies of this treatment leading to similar outcomes?

Even when studies are well designed, with conclusions that are statistically sound, there other questions that still must be answered before one uses their conclusions to shape clinical practice. Specifically, one should ask:

1. Regardless of the strength of the study, were the outcomes concrete enough to suggest a change in, or maintenance of, clinical practice?
   - Were they subjective or objective? If the former, what tools, if any, were used to measure subjective responses and of what reliability are they? What allowances were made for potential bias (as this is of major import when outcomes are defined subjectively)?
   - If outcomes were measured objectively, how was this performed? If diagnostic tests were used to assess outcome, were the tests valid—i.e., were they of sufficient positive (or negative) predictive value in the population analyzed to accurately reflect the presence or absence of pathology? Do the tests, or do interpretations of the tests, exhibit high degrees of inter-rater and intra-rater reliability?
   - Was the study comparative in nature, or without controls and/or placebo? If so, was the treatment, test, or exposure in the comparison group one that already has been investigated via high-quality studies? If not, how can one be certain that any difference, or lack of difference, between study groups means anything, or is any way clinically applicable?
2. Of what clinical relevance were the outcomes?
   - Did the outcomes represent a significant change in what was experienced, or held to be true, previously?
   - If so, was the change of such magnitude as to mandate an immediate reconsideration of current practice patterns?
   - If the documented change in outcome was small, is the health condition under treatment or evaluation sufficiently serious as to make even a small change in outcome based on an intervention or exposure worthy of serious consideration?
3. Who were the authors?
   - Were they invested financially in the outcome of the study?

- If not, could their results be reflective predominantly of practice skills and other factors that are unique to them or their situation?

4. What are the costs (both direct and indirect) that would be associated with adoption of a new test, procedure, or means of reducing or mitigating exposure?
   - Is the intervention more difficult to perform, or does it require more staff, than those currently used?
   - Will the intervention lead to additional testing or treatment that would not have been required otherwise? If so, what is the cost (both financial and emotional)?
   - Overall, is the incremental cost of adopting the intervention justified by the clinical benefit gained? In other words, what are the results of an analysis of "cost versus benefit?" Proponents of new tests and treatments are apt to lose sight of this very pragmatic concept, especially when they are invested financially or emotionally.

Conclusions

Despite an overall trend toward the use of "evidence-based" practice parameters, it is difficult to achieve this goal when evaluating treatments, tests, and causes of musculoskeletal and other disorders that are defined, at least in part, subjectively. While there are clear guidelines for the identification of high-quality studies, there is a dearth of such studies available for review.

Of equal importance in reaching decisions regarding practice parameters is comparison of a new test or treatment (with regard to both efficacy and cost) to those that are already available. Regardless of whether or data support a given intervention, a guideline generally should not be adopted if it does not provide clinical benefit above and beyond that provided from those currently in existence. This is particularly so when the new intervention increases direct or indirect costs.

Hence, though we may endeavor to make "evidence-based medicine" the source of our conclusions, the available evidence often is not of the highest quality and the applicability of the evidence is not necessarily clear. Under such circumstances the use of lower quality scientific evidence is necessary. Guideline recommendations then are based on the analysis of less than ideal data, an inventory of current practices, and a discussion of both that will hopefully produce a consensus conclusion regarding the "best clinical practices."

References

Annas GJ. Burden of proof: judging science and protecting public health in (and out of) the courtroom. *Am J Pub Health.* 1999;89(4):490-3.

Bombardier C, Kerr MS, Shannon HS, Frank JW. A guide to interpreting epidemiologic studies on the etiology of back pain. *Spine.* 1994;19(18S): 2047S-56S.

Bouter LM, van Tulder MW, Koes BW. Methodologic issues in low back pain research in primary care. *Spine.* 1998;23(18):2014-20.

Dawson-Saunders B, Trapp RG. *Basic and Clinical Biostatistics.* 2nd ed. Norwalk, Conn: Appleton and Lange; 1994.

Harber P, Shusterman D. Medical causation analysis heuristics. *J Occ Environ Med.* 1996;38(6): 577-86.

Macklin R. Ethics, epidemiology and law: the case of silicone breast implants. *Am J Pub Health.* 1999;89(4):487-9.

Morton RF, Hebel JR, McCarter RJ. *A Study Guide to Epidemiology and Biostatistics*; Gaithersburg, Md; Aspen; 1990.

Van Tulder MW, Assendelft WJ, Koes BW, Bouter LM. Method guidelines for systematic reviews in the Cochrane Collaboration Back Review Groups for Spinal Disorders. *Spine.* 1997;22(20):2323-30.

Index